EXTREMITIES	HEART	GUT, ABDOMEN	LUNG	UROGENITAL	OTHER
					Early blastocyst with inner cell mass and cavitation (58 cells) lying free within the uterine cavity
		Yolk sac			Early amnion sac Extraembryonic mesoblast, angioblast Chorionic gonadotropin
	Merging mesoblast anterior to prechordal plate	Stomatodeum Cloaca		Allantois	Primitive streak Hensen's node Notochord Prechordal plate Blood cells in yolk sac
	Single heart tube Propulsion	Foregut		Mesonephric ridge	Yolk sac larger than amnion sac
Arm bud	Ventric. outpouching Gelatinous reticulum	Rupture stomatodeum Evaination of thyroid, liver, and dorsal pancreas	Lung bud	Mesonephric duct enters cloaca	Rathke's pouch Migration of myotomes from somites
Leg bud	Auric. outpouching Septum primum	Pharyngeal pouches yield parathyroids, lat. thyroid, thymus Stomach broadens	Bronchi	Ureteral evag. Urorect. sept. Germ cells Gonadal ridge Coelom, Epithelium	
Hand plate, Mesench. condens. Innervation	Fusion mid. A-V canal Muscular vent. sept.	Intestinal loop into yolk stalk Cecum Gallbladder Hepatic ducts Spleen	Main lobes	Paramesonephric duct Gonad ingrowth of coelomic epith.	Adrenal cortex (from coelomic epithelium) invaded by sympathetic cells = medulla Jugular lymph sacs
Finger rays, Elbow	Aorta Pulmonary artery Valves Membrane ventricular septum	Duodenal lumen obliterated Cecum rotates right Appendix	Tracheal cartil.	Fusion urorect. sept. Open urogen. memb., anus Epith. cords in testicle	Early muscle
Clearing, central cartil.	Septum secundum			S-shaped vesicles in nephron blastema connect with collecting tubules from calyces	Superficial vascular plexus low on cranium
Shell, Tubular bone				A few large glomeruli Short secretory tubules Tunica albuginea Testicle, interstitial cells	Superficial vascular plexus at vertex

EX LIBRIS

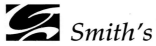 *Smith's*

Recognizable Patterns of Human Malformation

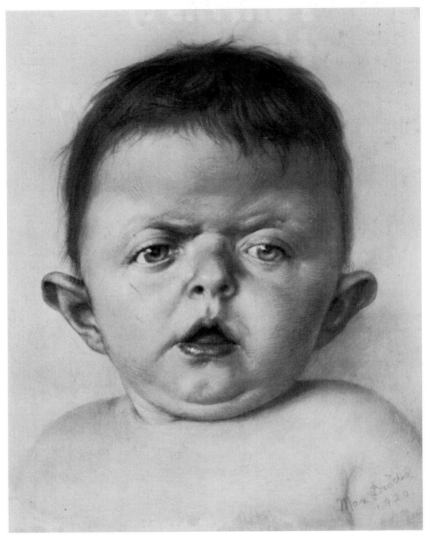

A Girl with Apert Syndrome
Original Max Brödel drawing No. 506. Property of The Johns Hopkins University School of Medicine, Department of Art as Applied to Medicine.

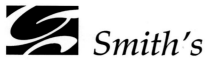 Smith's
Recognizable
Patterns of
Human
Malformation

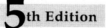**5**th Edition

Kenneth Lyons Jones, M.D

Professor of Pediatrics
Chief, Division of Dysmorphology and Teratology
University of California, San Diego
School of Medicine
La Jolla, California

W.B. SAUNDERS COMPANY

A Division of Harcourt Brace & Company
Philadelphia   London   Toronto   Montreal   Sydney   Tokyo

W.B. SAUNDERS COMPANY
A Division of Harcourt Brace & Company

The Curtis Center
Independence Square West
Philadelphia, Pennsylvania 19106

Library of Congress Cataloging-in-Publication Data

Jones, Kenneth Lyons.
    Smith's recognizable patterns of human malformation /
Kenneth Lyons Jones.—5th ed.
        p.   cm.
    Includes bibliographical references and index.
    ISBN 0–7216–6115–7
    1. Abnormalities. Human.   I. Smith, David W., 1926–1981
Recognizable patterns of human malformation.   II. Title.
    [DNLM: 1. Abnormalities.   QS 675 J77s 1997]
RG627.5.S57   1997
616'.043—dc20
DNLM/DLC   96–16722

SMITH'S RECOGNIZABLE PATTERNS OF HUMAN MALFORMATION   ISBN 0–7216–6115–7

Last digit is the print number: 9   8   7   6   5   4   3   2   1

Dedication of the First Edition

To my wife, Ann, beloved inspirational companion

To my father, William H. Smith,
accomplished engineer and would-be physician

To my teachers Dr. Lawson Wilkins,
molder of clinicians and humanist, and
Professor Dr. Gian Töndury,
complete anatomist, who brings embryology
into living perspective

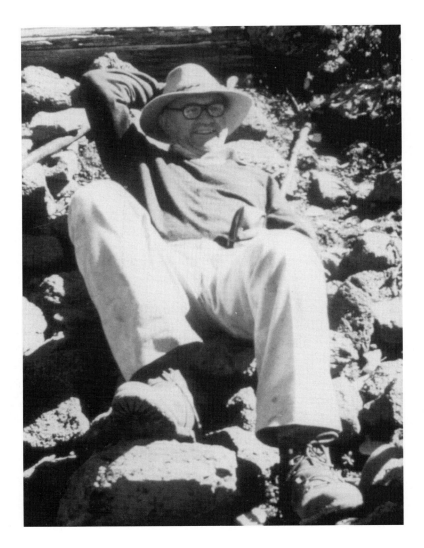

Dedicated to the Memory of

David W. Smith, M.D.
1926–1981

"Far better it is to dare mighty things, to win glorious triumphs, even though checkered by failure, than to take rank with those poor spirits who neither enjoy much nor suffer much, because they live in the great twilight that knows neither victory nor defeat."

Theodore Roosevelt, in a speech before the
Hamilton Club, Chicago, April 10, 1899

ACKNOWLEDGMENTS

The information set forth in this book represents an amalgamation of the knowledge, commitment and hard work of many individuals. I would like to acknowledge a number of those who have made significant contributions to the development of this 5th edition.

Dr. Kurt Benirschke, University of California School of Medicine, San Diego whose breadth of knowledge, intellectual curiosity, creativity and enthusiasm is a continuing stimulus to me.

Dr. Marilyn C. Jones, who has tirelessly contributed her knowledge, advice, patience, writing skills and love. She has made it possible for life to go on during the preparation of this edition.

Kathleen A. Johnson, who has labored long hours editing and transcribing the text of this edition while at the same time providing leadership and direction for the Division of Dysmorphology and Teratology. She continues to be a great support to me.

Fellows in Dysmorphology at UCSD: Dr. Marilyn C. Jones, University of California, San Diego; Dr. H. Eugene Hoyme, University of Arizona; Dr. Luther K. Robinson, State University of New York, Buffalo; Dr. Ronald Lacro, Boston Children's Hospital; Dr. Christopher Cunniff, University of Arizona; Dr. Rick Martin, University of California Irvine; Dr. Leah W. Burke, Allegheny-Singer Research Institute, Pittsburgh; Dr. Stephen R. Braddock, University of Missouri, Columbia; Dr. Lynne M. Bird, University of California, San Diego, and Dr. Kenjiro Kosaki, University of California, San Diego. All have made their own significant contribution to the development of this edition and have been a great inspiration to me.

Colleagues: Many individuals have contributed photos, information and expertise. Especially helpful have been the following: Dr. John Carey, University of Utah School of Medicine; Dr. John Opitz, Helena, Montana; Dr. Robert Gorlin, University of Minnesota Medical and Dental School; Dr. Michael Cohen, Jr., Dalhousie University; Dr. Judith Hall, University of British Columbia; Dr. David Rimoin, Cedars Sinai Medical Center, Los Angeles; Dr. Jaime Frias, University of South Florida, Tampa; Dr. Jon Aase, University of New Mexico; Dr. Bryan Hall, University of Kentucky Medical School, Dr. James Hanson, Washington, D.C.; Dr. Sterling Clarren, University of Washington Medical School; Dr. John Graham, Cedars Sinai Medical Center; Dr. Cynthia Curry, Valley Children's Hospital, Fresno, CA; Dr. Roger Stevenson, Greenwood Genetics Center, Greenwood, S.C., and Dr. Buzz Chernoff, Sacramento, CA.

Tina Chambers, Lyn M. Dick, Robert J. Felix, and Kelly Kim have provided invaluable assistance which is greatly appreciated.

CONTENTS

Introduction
including dysmorphology approach and classification

We ought not to set them aside with idle thoughts or idle words about "curiosities" or "chances." Not one of them is without meaning; not one that might not become the beginning of excellent knowledge, if only we could answer the question—why is it rare? or being rare, why did it in this instance happen?—JAMES PAGET, *Lancet*, 2:1017, 1882.

The questions set forth by Paget are still applicable today. Every structural defect represents an inborn error in morphogenesis. Just as the study of inborn metabolic errors has extended our understanding of normal biochemistry, so the accumulation of knowledge concerning defects in morphogenesis may assist us in further unraveling the story of structural development. The major portion of this text is devoted to patterns of malformation, as contrasted with patterns of deformation due to mechanical factors, which is the subject of a separate text, *Smith's Recognizable Patterns of Human Deformation*. You will also find relevant chapters on normal and abnormal morphogenesis, genetics and genetic counseling, minor anomalies and their relevance, a clinical approach toward a specific diagnosis for certain categorical problems, and normal standards of measurement for a variety of features. It is hoped that the design of the book will lend itself to practical clinical application, as well as provide a basic text for the education of those interested in a better understanding of altera-

tions in morphogenesis. Furthermore, many of the charts have been developed for direct use in the counseling of patients and parents.

Accurate diagnosis of a specific syndrome among the 0.7 per cent of babies born with multiple malformations is a necessary prerequisite of providing a prognosis and plan of management for the affected infant, as well as genetic counseling for the parents.

DYSMORPHOLOGY APPROACH

The following is the author's approach toward the evaluation of an individual with multiple defects:

I. Gather information. The family history is an essential aspect of such an evaluation. A question such as "Are there any individuals in the family with a similar type of problem?" may be helpful. The early history should usually include information about the onset and vigor of fetal activity, gestational timing, indications of uterine constraint, mode of delivery, size at birth, neonatal adaptation, and problems in postnatal growth and development. The physical examination should be complete, with the physician searching for minor as well as ma-

1

SINGLE LOCALIZED ANOMALY
in early morphogenesis

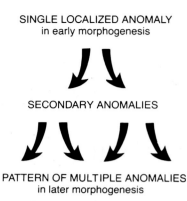

SECONDARY ANOMALIES

PATTERN OF MULTIPLE ANOMALIES
in later morphogenesis

FIGURE 1. Sequence designates a single localized anomaly plus its subsequently derived structural consequences, as depicted above.

jor anomalies. When possible, measurements should be taken to determine whether a given feature, such as apparent ocular hypertelorism or a small-appearing ear, is truly abnormal. The charts of normal measurements in Chapter 6 are provided for this purpose. An unusual feature ideally should be interpreted in relation to the findings in other family members before its relevance is determined.

II. Interpret the patient's anomalies from the viewpoint of developmental anatomy and strive to answer the following questions:

   A. Which anomaly in the individual represents the earliest defect in morphogenesis? A table for this purpose is found in Chapter 3 (Table 3–1). From such information one can determine that the problem in development must have existed *prior* to a particular prenatal age and any factor *after* that time could not be the cause of that structural defect.

   B. Can all the anomalies in the patient be explained on the basis of a single problem in morphogenesis that leads to a cascade of subsequent defects, as shown in Figure 1? These types of patterns of structural defects, referred to as *sequences*, may be divided into four categories from the developmental pathology viewpoint, as summarized in Figure 2. The first category is the *malformation sequence*, in which there has been a single localized poor formation of tissue that initiates a chain of subsequent defects. Malformation sequences occur in all gradation, the manifestations ranging from nearly normal to more severe, and have a recurrence risk that is most commonly in the 1 to 5 per cent range.

   Deformation sequence is the second category, in which there is no problem in the embryo or fetus (collectively referred to as fetus in this text), but mechanical forces such as uterine constraint result in altered morphogenesis, usually of

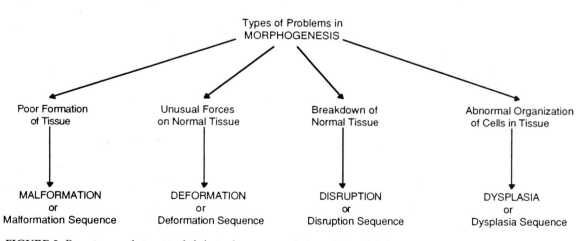

FIGURE 2. Four types of structural defects that can result in a chain of defects (sequence) by the time of birth.

the molding type. One example is the oligohydramnios deformation sequence, due to chronic leakage of amniotic fluid; another is the breech deformation sequence, the manifold effects of prolonged breech position late in fetal life. The deformations and deformation sequences are the subject of a separate text entitled *Smith's Recognizable Patterns of Human Deformation*. Most deformations have a very good to excellent prognosis in contrast with many malformations. The recurrence risk for deformation is usually of very low magnitude, unless the cause of the deformation problem is a persisting one, such as a bicornuate uterus.

The third category is the *disruption sequence*, in which the normal fetus is subjected to a destructive problem and its consequences. Such disruptions may be of vascular, infectious, or even mechanical origin. One example of the latter is disruption of normally developing tissues by amniotic bands. The spectra of consequences are set forth under *Amnion Rupture Sequence* in Chapter 1. In the final category, the *dysplasia sequence*, the primary defect is a lack of normal organization of cells into tissues. One example is the lack of migration of melanoblastic precursors from the neural crest. The spectra of consequences is referred to as the *neurocutaneous melanosis sequence* (see Chapter 1), in which melanocytic hamartosis of the skin occurs in conjunction with similar changes in the pia and arachnoid.

C. Does the patient have multiple structural defects that cannot be explained on the basis of a single initiating defect and its consequences, but rather appear to be the consequence of multiple defects in one or more tissues? These are referred to as *malformation syndromes* and are most commonly thought to be due to a single

cause. The known modes of etiology for malformation syndromes include chromosomal abnormalities, mutant gene disorders, and environmental teratogens. However, there are still many for which the mode of etiology has not been resolved.

III. Attempt to arrive at a specific overall diagnosis within the six categories shown in Figure 3, confirm when possible, and counsel accordingly. When possible, counseling should include the following: an understanding of how the altered structures came to be as they are; the natural history of the condition and what measures can be utilized to assist the child; and the mode of etiology and genetic counseling (recurrence risks).

IMPORTANT GENERAL PRINCIPLES

The following are some of the important principles and information that should be appreciated in the evaluation of a patient with multiple defects.

1. Nonspecificity of Individual Defects

With rare exceptions, a clinical diagnosis of a pattern of malformation cannot be made on the basis of a single defect, as is evident in the differential diagnosis in the appendix. Even a rare defect may be a feature in several syndromes of variant etiology. A specific diagnosis is usually dependent on recognition of the overall *pattern of anomalies*, and the detection of minor defects may be as helpful as that of major anomalies in this regard.

2. Variance in Expression

Variance in extent of abnormality (expression) among individuals with the same etiologic syndrome is a usual phenomenon. Except for such nonspecific general features as mental deficiency and small stature, it is unusual to find a given anomaly in 100 per

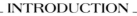

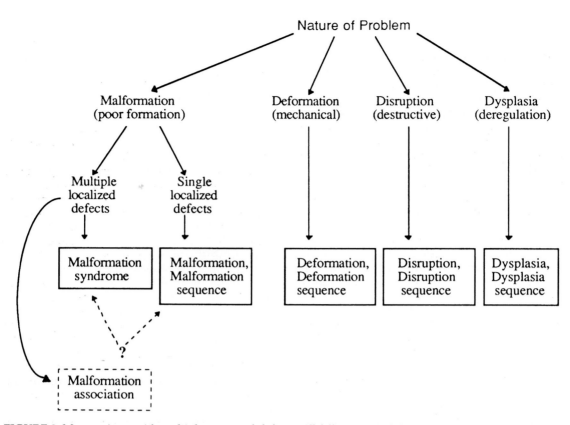

FIGURE 3. Most patients with multiple structural defects will fall into one of these six categories. The prognosis, management, and recurrence risk counseling may vary considerably among these categories.

cent of patients with the same etiologic syndrome. For example, in full 21 trisomy Down syndrome, only mental deficiency is ubiquitous; hypotonia is a frequent feature, but most of the other individual clinical features are found in less than 80 per cent of such patients. However, a specific diagnosis of Down syndrome can generally be rendered, based on the *total pattern of anomalies*. It is especially important to appreciate that the environmentally determined disorders occur in all gradations of severity. Thus, as one example, prenatal exposure to alcohol leads to a spectrum of defects including spontaneous abortion, the pattern of structural defects referred to as the fetal alcohol syndrome, growth deficiency, and mental retardation.

Intraindividual variability in expression is also frequent, with variance in the degree of abnormality on the left versus the right side of the individual.

3. Heterogeneity

Similar phenotypes (overall physical similarity) may result from different etiologies. Only by finer discrimination of the phenotype or mode of etiology can such similar entities be distinguished. For example, the Marfan syndrome and homocystinuria were initially discriminated on the basis of homocystinuria, next by a difference in mode of etiology (autosomal dominant for the Marfan syndrome and autosomal recessive in homocystinuria), and finally by closer scrutiny of the phenotype. As another example, achondroplasia is frequently misdiagnosed among individuals who have chondrodystrophies that only superficially resemble true achondroplasia. A diagnosis should be rendered only when there is close resemblance in the overall pattern of malformation between the patient and the disorder under consideration.

4. Etiology

Most of the disorders herein set forth have a genetic basis. Chapter 4 provides the background information relative to genetic counseling for these conditions.

Besides the following established disorders, roughly one half of the individuals with multiple defects have conditions that have not yet been recognized as specific disorders. A small percentage of such patients have a structural chromosomal abnormality. In such cases, genetic counseling should be withheld until it has been determined whether either parent is a balanced translocation carrier of the chromosomal abnormality. In the absence of an evident chromosomal abnormality or familial data suggesting a particular mode of etiology, it is generally impossible to state any accurate risk of recurrence for unknown patterns of multiple malformation. It is presumptuous to inform the parents that "this is a rare condition and therefore unlikely to recur in your future children." Under these circumstances, the author's present approach is to inform the parents that the lowest recurrence risk is zero and the highest risk with each pregnancy would be 25 per cent. The latter figure is predicated on the possibility of recessive inheritance or a nondetectable chromosomal abnormality from a balanced translocation carrier parent.

5. Nomenclature

Some of the recommendations of an international committee on "Classification and Nomenclature of Morphologic Defects," published in *Lancet*, 1:513, 1975, are utilized in this text. The recommendations of a more recent international group, which met in Mainz, Germany, under the direction of Professor Jurgen Spranger in November 1979 and again in Seattle in February 1980, have also been utilized.

Most of the nomenclature has already been alluded to; the following recommendations relate to the naming of single defects and patterns of malformation.

Naming of Single Malformations

Utilize an adjective or descriptive term and the name of the structure or the classic equivalent in common use (e.g., small mandible or micrognathia).

Naming of Patterns of Malformations

1. When the etiology is known and easily remembered, utilize the appropriate term to designate the disorder.
2. Continue time-honored designations unless there is good reason for change.
3. In the absence of a reasonably descriptive designation, eponyms, some of them multiple, may be used until the basic defect for the disorder is recognized. However, usage of an eponym should, in the future, be limited to one proper name.
4. The possessive use of an eponym should be discontinued, since the author neither had nor owned the disorder.
5. Designation of a disorder by one or more of its manifestations does not necessarily imply that they are either specific or consistent components of that disorder.
6. Avoid names that may have an unpleasant connotation for the family or affected individual.
7. The syndrome should not be designated by the initials of the originally described patients.
8. Names that are too general for a specific syndrome should be avoided.
9. Avoid acronyms unless they are extremely pertinent or appropriate.

Nomenclature Used to Describe Chromosomal Syndromes

Many of the disorders set forth in this book are the result of chromosomal abnormalities. This section is intended to familiarize those readers who are not versed in cytogenetics with some of the basic nomenclature used in describing chromosomal syndromes. Several shorthand systems have been devised. The examples shown employ the "short system," which is the most commonly used in the recent literature. By comparing the karyotype examples with those in the text, the reader should be able to decipher the cytogenetic shorthand. No attempt has been made to include every possible abnormality. For a comprehensive discussion of nomenclature, the reader is referred to the following source: *ISCN(1995): An International System for Human Cytogenetic Nomenclature.* F. Mitelman (Ed.); S. Carger, Basel, 1995.

METHOD AND UTILITY OF PRESENTATION OF PATTERNS OF MALFORMATION

The arrangement of the disorders in this book is predominantly based on the similarity in overall features or in one major feature among the patterns of malformation, as set forth in the table of contents. Thus, the order of presentation is designed to be of assistance in the diagnosis of the patient for whom a firm diagnosis has not been established. With the exception of the chromosomal abnormality syndromes, which share many features, and the disorders determined by an environmental agent, the conditions are not arranged in accordance with the mode of etiology. Each disorder has a listing of anomalies. The features that together tend to distinguish the syndrome from other known disorders are set forth in italic print. The main list consists of defects that occur in at least 25 per cent and usually more than 50 per cent of patients. Sometimes the actual percentage or number is stated for each anomaly. Below these are listed the occasional defects that occur with a frequency of 1 to 25 per cent, most commonly 5 to 10 per cent. The occurrence of these "occasional abnormalities" is of interest and has been loosely ascribed to "developmental noise." In other words, an adverse influence that usually causes a particular pattern of malformation may occasionally cause other anomalies as well. Possibly it is differences of genetic background, environment, or both that allow some individuals to express these "occasional" anomalies. The important feature is that they are not random for a particular syndrome. For example, clinicians who have seen a large number of children with the Down syndrome are not surprised to see "another" Down syndrome baby with duodenal atresia, webbed neck, or tetralogy of Fallot.

The references listed for each disorder have been selected as those that give the best account of that disorder, provide recent additional knowledge, or represent the initial description. They are arranged in chronological order.

A word of caution is indicated. This book does not contain a number of vary rare syndromes. Furthermore, information that appeared after December 1995, regarding the identification of specific genes responsible for disorders set forth in this book, is not always included.

Other Sources of Information

In addition to this text, there are many others that may be of value in the recognition, management, and counseling of particular problems and patterns of malformation.

References

General

Bergsma, D. S.: Birth Defects Atlas and Compendium, 2nd ed. Baltimore, Williams & Wilkins Co., 1979.

Emery, A. E. H., and Rimoin, D. L.: Principles and Practice of Medical Genetics, 2nd ed. New York, Churchill Livingstone, 1990.

Gorlin, R. J., Cohen, M. M., Jr., and Levin, L. S.: Syndromes of the Head and Neck, 3rd ed. New York, Oxford University Press, 1990.

Graham, J. M.: Smith's Recognizable Patterns of Human Deformation, 2nd ed. Philadelphia, W. B. Saunders Co., 1988.

McKusick, V. A.: Mendelian Inheritance in Man: Catalogs of Autosomal Dominant, Autosomal Recessive, and X-Linked Phenotypes, 11th ed. Baltimore, The Johns Hopkins University Press, 1995.

Stevenson, R. E., Hall, J. G., and Goodman, R. M.: Human Malformations and Related Anomalies. New York, Oxford University Press, 1993.

Warkany, J.: Congenital Malformations. Chicago, Year Book Medical Publishers, 1971.

Chromosomal Abnormalities

Borgaonkar, D. S.: Chromosomal Variations in Man: A Catalog of Chromosomal Variants and Anomalies. New York, Wiley-Liss, 1994.

de Grouchy, J., and Turleau, C.: Clinical Atlas of Human Chromosomes. New York, John Wiley & Sons, 1984.

Schinzel, A.: Catalogue of Unbalanced Chromosome Aberrations in Man. New York, Walter de Gruyter, 1984.

Connective Tissue, and Skeletal Dysplasias

Beighton, P.: McKusick's Heritable Disorders of Connective Tissue, 5th ed. St. Louis, Mosby, 1993.

Ornoy, A., Borochowitz, A., Lachman, R., and Rimoin, D. L.: Atlas of Fetal Skeletal Radiology. Chicago, Year Book, 1988.

Spranger, J. W., Langer, L. O., and Wiedemann, H. R.: Bone Dysplasias, An Atlas of Constitutional Disorders of Skeletal Development. Philadelphia, W. B. Saunders Co., 1974.

Wynne-Davies, R., Hall, C. M., and Apley, A. G.: Atlas of Skeletal Dysplasias. New York, Churchill Livingstone, 1985.

Hereditary Deafness with Associated Anomalies

Gorlin, R. J., Toriello, H. V., and Cohen, M. M.: Hereditary Hearing Loss and its Syndromes. New York, Oxford University Press, 1995.

Ocular Abnormalities

Waardenburg, P. J.: Genetics and Ophthalmology, Vols. I and II. Oxford, Blackwell Scientific Publications, 1963.

Teratology

Briggs, G. G., Freeman, R. K., and Yaffe, S. J.: Drugs in Pregnancy and Lactation, 4th ed. Baltimore, Williams & Wilkins Co., 1994.

Shepard, T. H.: Catalog of Teratogenic Agents, 7th ed. Baltimore, The Johns Hopkins University Press, 1992.

1
Recognizable Patterns of Malformation

A

A. CHROMOSOMAL ABNORMALITY SYNDROMES

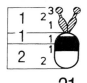

DOWN SYNDROME

(Trisomy 21 Syndrome)

Hypotonia, Flat Facies, Slanted Palpebral Fissures, Small Ears

Down's report of 1866 on the ethnic classification of idiots stated that a "large number of congenital idiots are typical Mongols," and he set forth the clinical description of the Down syndrome. The textbook by Penrose and Smith provides an overall appraisal of this disorder that has an incidence of 1 in 660 newborns, making it the most common pattern of malformation in man.

ABNORMALITIES

General. Hypotonia with tendency to keep mouth open and protrude the tongue; diastasis recti. Hyperflexibility of joints. Relatively small stature with awkward gait. Increased weight in adolescence.

Central Nervous System. Mental deficiency.

Craniofacial. Brachycephaly with relatively flat occiput and tendency toward midline parietal hair whorl. Mild microcephaly with upslanting palpebral fissures. Thin cranium with late closure of fontanels. Hypoplasia to aplasia of frontal sinuses, short hard palate.

Small nose with low nasal bridge and tendency to have inner epicanthal folds.

Eyes. Speckling of iris (Brushfield spots) with peripheral hypoplasia of iris. Fine lens opacities by slit lamp examination (59 per cent). Refractive error, mostly myopia (70 per cent); nystagmus (35 per cent); strabismus (45 per cent); blocked tear duct (20 per cent). Acquired cataracts in adults (30 to 60 per cent).

Ears. Small; overfolding of angulated upper helix; sometimes prominent; small or absent earlobes. Hearing loss (66 per cent) of conductive, mixed, or sensorineural type. Fluid accumulation in middle ear (60 to 80 per cent).

Dentition. Hypoplasia, irregular placement, fewer caries than usual. Periodontal disease.

Neck. Appears short.

Hands. Relatively short metacarpals and phalanges. Fifth finger: hypoplasia of midphalanx of fifth finger (60 per cent) with clinodactyly (50 per cent), a single crease (40 per cent),

8

or both. Simian crease (45 per cent). Distal position of palmar axial triradius (84 per cent). Ulnar loop dermal ridge pattern on all digits (35 per cent).

Feet. Wide gap between first and second toes. Plantar crease between first and second toes. Open field dermal ridge patterning in hallucal area of sole (50 per cent).

Pelvis. Hypoplasia with outward lateral flare of iliac wings and shallow acetabular angle.

Cardiac. Anomaly in about 40 per cent; endocardial cushion defect, ventricular septal defect, patent ductus arteriosus, auricular septal defect, and aberrant subclavian artery, in decreasing order of frequency. Mitral valve prolapse with or without tricuspid valve prolapse and aortic regurgitation by 20 years of age. Risk for regurgitation occurs after 18 years of age.

Skin. Loose folds in posterior neck (infancy). Cutis marmorata, especially in extremities (43 per cent). Dry, hyperkeratotic skin with time (75 per cent). Infections in the perigenital area, buttocks, and thighs that begin as follicular pustules in 50 to 60 per cent of adolescents.

Hair. Fine, soft, and often sparse; straight pubic hair at adolescence.

Genitalia. Relatively small penis and decreased testicular volume. Primary gonadal deficiency is common, is progressive from birth to adolescence, and is definitely present in adults. Although fertility has rarely been reported in females, no male has reproduced.

OCCASIONAL ABNORMALITIES. Seizures (less than 9 per cent); keratoconus (6 per cent); congenital cataract (3 per cent); low placement of ears; webbed neck; two ossification centers in manubrium sterni; funnel or pigeon breast; tracheal stenosis with hourglass trachea and midtracheal absence of tracheal pars membranacea; gastrointestinal tract anomalies (12 per cent) including tracheoesophageal fistula; duodenal atresia; omphalocele, pyloric stenosis, annular pancreas, Hirschprung disease, and imperforate anus. Incomplete fusion of vertebral arches of lower spine (37 per cent); only 11 ribs; atlantoaxial instability (12 per cent); posterior occipitoatlantal hypermobility (8.5 per cent); abnormal odontoid process (6 per cent); hypoplastic posterior arch C1 (26 per cent). Hip abnormality (8 per cent) including dysplasia, dislocation, avascular necrosis, and/or slipped capital femoral epiphyses; syndactyly of second and third toes; prune belly anomaly. The incidence of leukemia is about 1 in 95, or close to 1 per cent. Thyroid disorders are more common, including athyreosis, simple goiter, and hyperthyroidism. Fatal perinatal liver disease has been reported.

PRINCIPAL FEATURES IN NEONATE. The diagnosis can generally be made shortly after birth, and therefore, the following ten features of Down syndrome in the neonate are presented as set forth by Hall, who found at least four of these abnormalities in all of 48 neonates with Down syndrome and six or more in 89 per cent of them.

Hypotonia	80%
Poor Moro reflex	85%
Hyperflexibility of joints	80%
Excess skin on back of neck	80%
Flat facial profile	90%
Slanted palpebral fissures	80%
Anomalous auricles	60%
Dysplasia of pelvis	70%
Dysplasia of midphalanx of fifth finger	60%
Simian crease	45%

NATURAL HISTORY. Muscle tone tends to improve with age, whereas the rate of developmental progress slows with age. For example, 23 per cent of a group of Down syndrome children under 3 years had a developmental quotient above 50, whereas none of those in the 3- to 9-year group had intelligence quotients above 50. Though the I.Q. range is generally said to be 25 to 50 with an occasional individual above 50, the mean I.Q. for older patients is 24. Fortunately, social performance is usually beyond that expected for mental age, averaging $3^{4}/_{12}$ years above mental age for the older individuals. Generally "good babies" and happy children, individuals with Down syndrome tend toward mimicry, are friendly, have a good sense of rhythm, and enjoy music. Mischievousness and obstinacy may also be characteristics, and 13 per cent have serious emotional problems. Coordination is often poor, and the voice tends to be harsh. Early developmental enrichment programs for Down syndrome children have resulted in improved rate of progress during the first 4 to 5 years of life. Whether such training programs will appreciably alter the ultimate level of performance remains to be determined.

Sleep-related upper airway obstruction occurs in approximately one third of cases.

Growth is relatively slow, and during the first 8 years, secondary centers of ossification are often late in development. However, during later childhood, the osseous maturation is more "normal," and final height is usually attained around 15 years of age. Adolescent sexual development is usually somewhat less complete than normal. Because thyroid dysfunction is common and can be easily missed, periodic thyroid function studies should be performed.

The major cause for early mortality is congenital heart defects. For patients with Down syndrome with congenital heart defects, survival to age 1 year is 76.3 per cent; to age 5, 61.8 per cent; to age 10, 57.1 per cent; to age 20, 53.1 per cent; and to age 30, 49.9 per cent, respectively. For patients with Down syndrome who do not have congenital heart defects, survival to the same ages is 90.7 per cent, 87.2 per cent, 81.9 per cent, and 79.2 per cent, respectively. Mortality from respiratory disease, mainly pneumonia, as well as other infectious diseases is much higher than in the general population. Low-grade problems that occur frequently are chronic rhinitis, conjunctivitis, and periodontal disease, none of which are easy to "cure." Immunologic dysfunction including both T-cell and B-cell derangement, has been demonstrated, as has the frequent occurrence of hepatitis B surface antigen carrier state. Therefore, HBV vaccination is advised.

Although asymptomatic atlantoaxial dislocation occurs in 12 to 20 per cent of individuals with Down syndrome, symptoms referable to compression of the spinal cord are rare. Unfortunately, the literature regarding radiographic screening for this finding is controversial. No study to date has documented that radiographic findings can predict which children will develop neurologic problems. Any child with Down syndrome who develops changes in bowel or bladder function, neck posturing, or loss of ambulatory skills should be evaluated carefully with plain roentgenograms of the cervical spine. The majority of patients develop symptoms before 10 years of age, when the ligamentous laxity is most severe.

ETIOLOGY. Trisomy for all or a large part of chromosome 21. The combined results of 11 unselected surveys totaling 784 cases showed the following relative frequencies of particular types of chromosomal alteration for Down syndrome:

Full 21 trisomy	94%
21 Trisomy/normal mosaicism	2.4%
Translocation cases (with about equal occurrence of D/G and G/G translocations)	3.3%

Faulty chromosome distribution leading to Down syndrome is more likely to occur at older maternal age, as shown in the following figures of incidence for Down syndrome at term delivery for particular maternal ages: 15 to 29 years, 1 in 1500; 30 to 34 years, 1 in 800; 35 to 39 years, 1 in 270; 40 to 44 years, 1 in 100; and over 45 years, 1 in 50.

Though the general likelihood for recurrence of Down syndrome is 1 per cent, the principal task in giving recurrence risk figures to parents is to determine whether the Down syndrome child is a translocation case with a parent who is a translocation carrier and thereby has a relatively high risk for recurrence. The likelihood of finding a translocation in the Down syndrome child of a mother under 30 years of age is 6 per cent, and of such cases only one out of three will be found to have a translocation carrier parent. Therefore, the estimated probability that either parent of a Down syndrome patient born of a mother under 30 years is a G/D or G/G translocation carrier is 2 per cent versus 0.3 per cent when the Down syndrome patient is born of a mother over 30 years of age. Having excluded a translocation carrier parent, the risk for recurrence may be stated as about 1 per cent. Though a low figure, it is enough to justify prenatal diagnosis for any future pregnancy. The recurrence risk for the rare translocation carrier parent will depend on the type of translocation and the sex of the parent. Mosaicism usually leads to a less severe phenotype. Any degree of intellectual ability from normal or nearly normal to severe retardation is found, and this does not always correlate with the clinical phenotype. Patients with the features of Down syndrome and relatively good performance are likely to have mosaicism (which is not always easy to demonstrate).

References

Down, J. L. H.: Observations on an ethnic classification of idiots. Clinical Lecture Reports, London Hospital, 3:259, 1866.

Richards, B. W., et al.: Cytogenetic survey of 225 patients diagnosed clinically as mongols. J. Ment. Defic. Res., 9:245, 1965.

Hall, B.: Mongolism in newborn infants. Clin. Pediatr. (Phila.), 5:4, 1966.

Penrose, L. S., and Smith, G. F.: Down's Anomaly. Boston, Little, Brown & Co., 1966.

Smith, D. W., and Wilson, A. C.: The Child with Down's syndrome. Philadelphia, W. B. Saunders Co., 1973.

Baird, P. A., and Sadovnick, A. D.: Life expectancy in Down syndrome. J Pediatr., 110:849, 1987.

Davidson, R. G.: Atlantoaxial instability in individuals with Down syndrome: A fresh look at the evidence. Pediatrics, 81:857, 1988.

Pueschel, S. M.: Atlantoxial instability and Down syndrome. Pediatrics, 81:879, 1988.

Pueschel, S. M.: Clinical aspects of Down syndrome from infancy to adulthood. Am. J. Med. Genet. Suppl. 7:52, 1990.

Ugazio, A. G., et al.: Immunology of Down syndrome: A review. Am. J. Med. Genet. Suppl., 7:204, 1990.

Pueschel, S. M., et al.: A longitudinal study of atlanto-dens relationships in asymptomatic individuals with Down syndrome. Pediatrics, 89:1194, 1992.

Cremers, M. J. G., et al.: Risks of sports activities in children with Down's syndrome and atlantoaxial instability. Lancet, 342:511, 1993.

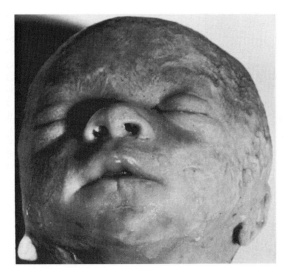

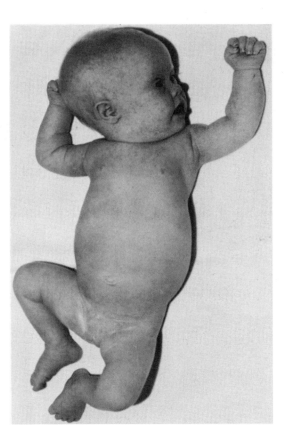

FIGURE 1. *Left*, At least 20 per cent of trisomy 21 fetuses are stillborn. This 20-week fetus showed few signs of Down syndrome, the diagnosis having been made by chromosome study. *Right*, The surviving term infant shows many signs, including hypotonia. (Left photo courtesy of Dr. Renée Bernstein, University of Johannesburg, S. Africa.)

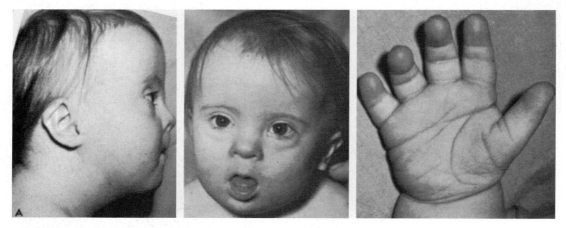

FIGURE 2. Down syndrome. *A,* Young infant. Flat facies, straight hair; protrusion of tongue; single crease on inturned fifth finger.

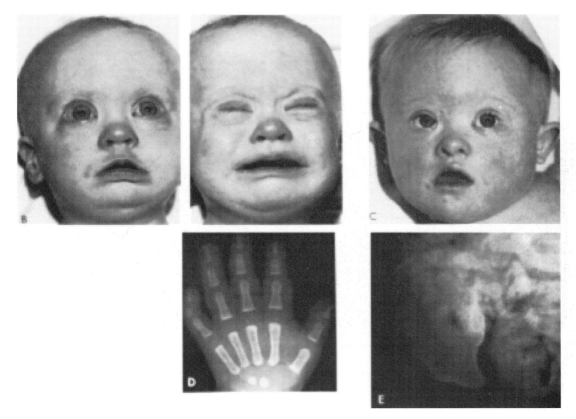

FIGURE 2. *Continued. B* and *C*, Inner canthal folds. Speckling of iris with lack of peripheral patterning. Small auricles, prominent at right. "Pouting" expression when crying. (*B* and *C*, from Smith, D. W.: J. Pediatr., *70*:474, 1967, with permission).) *D*, Hypoplasia, midphalanx of fifth finger. *E*, shallow acetabular angle with small iliac wings having the shape of elephant ears.

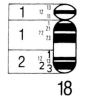

18

TRISOMY 18 SYNDROME

*Clenched Hand, Short Sternum, Low
Arch Dermal Ridge Patterning on Fingertips*

This condition was first recognized as a specific entity in 1960 by discovery of the extra 18 chromosome in babies with a particular pattern of malformation (Edward et al., Patau et al., and Smith et al.). It is the second most common multiple malformation syndrome, with an incidence of about 0.3 per 100 newborn babies. There has been a 3:1 preponderance of females to males. Several good reviews set forth a full appraisal of this syndrome. More than 130 different abnormalities have been noted in the literature on patients with the 18 trisomy syndrome, and therefore the listing of abnormalities has been divided into those that occur in 50 per cent or more of patients, in 10 to 50 per cent of patients, and in less than 10 per cent of patients.

ABNORMALITIES FOUND IN 50 PER CENT OR MORE OF PATIENTS

General. Feeble fetal activity, weak cry, altered gestational timing; one third premature, one third postmature. Polyhydramnios, small placenta, single umbilical artery, Growth deficiency; mean birth weight, 2340 g. Hypoplasia of skeletal muscle, subcutaneous and adipose tissue. Mental deficiency, hypertonicity (after neonatal period). Diminished response to sound.

Craniofacial. Prominent occiput, narrow bifrontal diameter. Low-set, malformed auricles. Short palpebral fissures. Small oral opening, narrow palatal arch. Micrognathia.

Hands and Feet. Clenched hand, tendency for overlapping of index finger over third, fifth finger over fourth. Absence of distal crease on fifth finger with or without distal creases on third and fourth fingers. Low arch dermal ridge pattern on six or more fingertips. Hypoplasia of nails, especially on fifth finger and toes. Short hallux, frequently dorsiflexed.

Thorax. Short sternum, with reduced number of ossification centers. Small nipples.

Abdominal Wall. Inguinal or umbilical hernia and/or diastasis recti.

Pelvis and Hips. Small pelvis, limited hip abduction.

Genitalia. Male: cryptorchidism.

Skin. Redundancy, mild hirsutism of forehead and back, prominent cutis marmorata.

Cardiac. Ventricular septal defect, auricular septal defect, patent ductus arteriosus.

ABNORMALITIES FOUND IN 10 TO 50 PER CENT OF CASES

Craniofacial. Wide fontanels, microcephaly, hypoplasia of orbital ridges. Inner epicanthal folds, ptosis of eyelid, corneal opacity. Cleft lip, cleft palate, or both.

Hands and Feet. Ulnar or radial deviation of hand, hypoplastic to absent thumb, simian crease. Equinovarus, rocker-bottom feet, syndactyly of second and third toes.

Thorax. Relatively broad, with or without widely spaced nipples.

Genitalia. Female: hypoplasia of labia majora with prominent clitoris.

Anus. Malposed or funnel-shaped anus.

Cardiac. Bicuspid aortic and/or pulmonic valves, nodularity of valve leaflets, pulmonic stenosis, coarctation of aorta.

Lung. Malsegmentation to absence of right lung.

Diaphragm. Muscle hypoplasia with or without eventration.

Abdomen. Meckels diverticulum, heterotopic pancreatic and/or splenic tissue, omphalocele. Incomplete rotation of colon.

Renal. Horseshoe defect, ectopic kidney, double ureter, hydronephrosis, polycystic kidney.

ABNORMALITIES FOUND IN LESS THAN 10 PER CENT OF CASES

Central Nervous System. Facial palsy, paucity of myelination, microgyria, cerebellar hypoplasia, defect of corpus callosum, hydrocephalus, meningomyelocele.

Craniofacial. Wormian cranial bones, shallow elongated sella turcica. Slanted palpebral fissures, hypertelorism, colobomata of iris, cataract, microphthalmos, choanal atresia.

Hands. Syndactyly of third and fourth fingers, polydactyly, short fifth metacarpals, ectrodactyly.

Other Skeletal. Radial aplasia. Incomplete ossification of clavicle. Hemivertebrae, fused vertebrae, short neck, scoliosis, rib anomaly, pectus excavatum, dislocated hip.

Genitalia. Male: hypospadias, bifid scrotum. Female: bifid uterus, ovarian hypoplasia.

Cardiovascular. Anomalous coronary artery, transposition, tetralogy of Fallot, coarctation of aorta, dextrocardia, aberrant subclavian artery, intimal proliferation in arteries with arteriosclerotic change and medial calcification.

Abdominal. Pyloric stenosis, extrahepatic biliary atresia, hypoplastic gallbladder, gallstones, imperforate anus.

Renal. Hydronephrosis, polycystic kidney (small cysts). Wilms tumor.

Endocrine. Thyroid or adrenal hypoplasia.

Other. Hemangiomata, thymic hypoplasia, tracheoesophageal fistula, thrombocytopenia.

NATURAL HISTORY. Babies with the trisomy 18 syndrome are usually feeble and have a limited capacity for survival. Resuscitation is often performed at birth, and they may have apneic episodes in the neonatal period. Poor sucking capability may necessitate nasogastric tube feeding, but even with optimal management, they fail to thrive. Fifty per cent die within the first week and many of the remaining die in the next 12 months. Only 5 to 10 per cent survive the first year as severely mentally defective individuals. Although most children who survive the first year are unable to walk in an unsupported fashion and verbal communication is usually limited to a few single words, it is important to realize that some older children with trisomy 18 smile, laugh, and interact with and relate to their families. All achieve some psychomotor maturation and continue to learn. There are at least ten reports of affected children older than 10 years of age. Once the diagnosis has been established, limitation of extraordinary medical means for prolongation of life should be seriously considered. However, the personal feelings of the parents and the individual circumstances of each infant must be taken into consideration. Baty et al. have documented the natural history of this disorder. For children who survive, the average number of days in the neonatal intensive care unit was 16.3, average days on a ventilator was 10.1, and 13 per cent had surgery in the neonatal period. There was no evidence for an increase in adverse reactions to immunizations. Growth curves for length, weight, and head circumference are provided in that study.

ETIOLOGY. Trisomy for all or a large part of the number 18 chromosome. The great majority of cases have full 18 trisomy, the result of faulty chromosomal distribution, which is most likely to occur at older maternal age; the mean maternal age at birth of babies with this syndrome is 32 years. Translocation cases, the result of chromosomal breakage, can only be excluded by chromosomal studies. When such a case is found, the parents should also have chromosomal studies to determine whether one of them is a balanced translocation carrier with high risk for recurrence in future offspring. Though no adequate studies of recurrence risk exist for full 18 trisomy cases, it seems safe to presume that the recurrence risk would be even lower than the 1 per cent for full 21 trisomy syndrome cases. This latter statement is predicated on the indication that most 18 trisomic individuals die in embryonic or fetal life, as suggested by the chromosomal findings in spontaneous abortuses.

Mosaicism for an additional chromosome 18 leads to a partial clinical expression of the pattern of trisomy 18, with longer survival and any degree of variation between nearly normal and the full pattern.

Partial trisomy 18: Trisomy of the short arm causes a very nonspecific clinical picture and mild or no mental deficiency. Cases with familial trisomy of the short arm, centromere, and proximal one third of the long arm show features of trisomy 18, although not the full pattern. Trisomy for the entire long arm is clinically indistinguishable from full trisomy 18. Trisomy for the distal one third to one half of the long arm leads to a partial picture of trisomy 18 with longer survival and less profound mental deficiency. In early childhood, the patients resemble trisomy 18 cases, whereas adolescents and adults display a more nonspecific pattern of malformation, including prominent orbital ridges, broad and prominent nasal bridge, everted upper lip, receding mandible, poorly modeled ears, short neck, and long, hyperextendible fingers. Muscular tone tends to be decreased, mental deficiency is severe, and about one third of the patients suffer from seizures.

References

Edwards, J. H., et al.: A new trisomic syndrome. Lancet, 1:787, 1960.

Patau, K., et al.: Multiple congenital anomaly caused by an extra autosome. Lancet, 1:790, 1960.

Smith, D. W., et al.: A new autosomal trisomy syndrome. J Pediatr., 57:338, 1960.

Smith, D. W., Autosomal abnormalities. Am. J. Obstet. Gynecol., 90:1055, 1964.

Taylor, A., and Polani, P. E.: Autosomal trisomy syndromes, excluding Down's. Guy's Hosp. Rep., 13:231, 1964.

Warkany, J., Passarge, E., and Smith, L. B.: Congenital malformations in autosomal trisomy syndromes. Am. J. Dis. Child., 112:502, 1966.

Weber, W. W.: Survival and the sex ratio in trisomy 17–18. Am. J. Hum. Genet., 19:369, 1967.

Turleau, C., and de Grouchy, J.: Trisomy 18 qter and trisomy mapping of chromosome 18. Clin. Genet., 12:361, 1977.

Carey, J. C.: Health supervision and anticipatory guidance for children with genetic disorders (including specific recommendations for trisomy 21, trisomy 18 and neurofibromatosis I). Pediatr. Clin. North Am., 39:25, 1992.

Baty, B. J., et al.: Natural history of trisomy 18 and trisomy 13: I. Growth, physical assessment, medical histories, survival, and recurrence risk. Am. J. Med. Genet., 49:175, 1994.

Baty, B. J., et al.: Natural history of trisomy 18 and trisomy 13: II. Psychomotor development. Am. J. Med. Genet., 49:189, 1994.

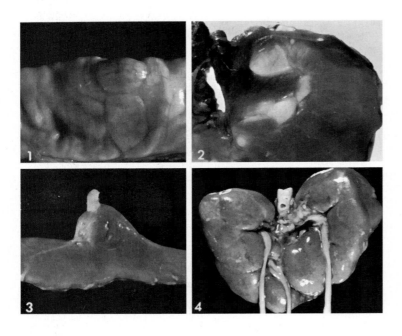

FIGURE 1. Some pathologic features of trisomy 18 syndrome. *1,* Ectopic pancreatic tissue in duodenum. *2,* Meckel's diverticulum. *3,* Defects of muscle development in diaphragm. *4,* Horseshoe fused kidneys with extra ureter.

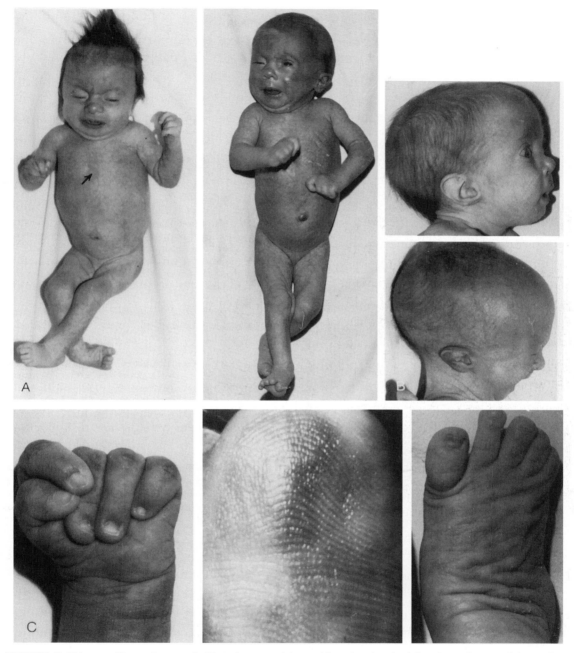

FIGURE 2. Trisomy 18 syndrome. *A,* Note hypertonicity evident in clenched hands and crossed legs; short sternum (*arrow* marks lower end); narrow pelvis. *B,* Prominent occiput; low-set slanted auricle. *C,* Clenched hand with index finger overlying third; hypoplasia of fifth fingernail; low arch dermal ridge configuration on fingertip; dorsiflexed short hallux (From Smith, D. W.: Am. J. Obstet. Gynecol., *90*:1055, 1964, with permission.)

TRISOMY 13 SYNDROME

(D₁ Trisomy Syndrome)

*Defects of Eye, Nose, Lip, and Forebrain of
Holoprosencephaly Type; Polydactyly; Narrow
Hyperconvex Fingernails; Skin Defects of Posterior Scalp*

Apparently described by Bartholin in 1657, this syndrome was not generally recognized until its trisomic etiology was discovered by Patau et al. in 1960. The incidence is about 1 in 5000 births.

ABNORMALITIES FOUND IN 50 PER CENT OR MORE OF PATIENTS

Central Nervous System. Holoprosencephaly type defect with varying degrees of incomplete development of forebrain and olfactory and optic nerves. Minor motor seizures, often with hypsarrhythmic EEG pattern. Apneic spells in early infancy. Severe mental defect.

Hearing. Apparent deafness (defects of organ of Corti in the two cases studied).

Cranium. Moderate microcephaly with sloping forehead. Wide sagittal suture and fontanels.

Eyes. Microphthalmia, colobamata of iris, or both. Retinal dysplasia, often including islands of cartilage.

Mouth. Cleft lip (60 to 80 per cent), cleft palate, or both.

Auricles. Abnormal helices with or without low-set ears.

Skin. Capillary hemangiomata, especially forehead. Localized scalp defects in parieto-occipital area. Loose skin, posterior neck.

Hands and Feet. Distal palmar axial triradii. Simian crease. Hyperconvex narrow fingernails. Flexion of fingers with or without overlapping and camptodactyly. Polydactyly of hands and sometimes feet. Posterior prominence of heel.

Other Skeletal. Thin posterior ribs with or without missing rib. Hypoplasia of pelvis with shallow acetabular angle.

Cardiac. Abnormality in 80 per cent with ventricular septal defect, patent ductus arteriosus, auricular septal defect, and dextroposition, in decreasing order of frequency.

Genitalia. Male: cryptorchidism, abnormal scrotum. Female: bicornuate uterus.

Hematologic. Increased frequency of nuclear projections in neutrophils. Unusual persistence of embryonic and/or fetal type hemoglobin.

Other. Single umbilical artery. Inguinal or umbilical hernia.

ABNORMALITIES FOUND IN LESS THAN 50 PER CENT OF PATIENTS

Growth. Congenital hypoplasia; mean birth weight, 2480 g.

Central Nervous System. Hypertonia, hypotonia, agenesis of corpus callosum, hydrocephalus, fusion of basal ganglia, cerebellar hypoplasia, meningomyelocele.

Eyes. Shallow supraorbital ridges, slanting palpebral fissures, absent eyebrows, hypotelorism, hypertelorism, anophthalmos, cyclopia.

Nose, Mouth, and Mandible. Absent philtrum, narrow palate, cleft tongue, micrognathia.

Hands and Feet. Retroflexible thumb, ulnar deviation at wrist, low arch digital dermal ridge pattern, fibular S-shaped hallucal dermal ridge pattern, syndactyly, cleft between first and second toes, hypoplastic toenails, equinovarus, radial aplasia.

Cardiac. Anomalous venous return, overriding aorta, pulmonary stenosis, hypoplastic aorta, atretic mitral and/or aortic valves, bicuspid aortic valve.

Abdominal. Omphalocele, heterotopic pancreatic or splenic tissue, incomplete rotation of colon, Meckel's diverticulum.

Renal. Polycystic kidney (31 per cent), hydronephrosis, horseshoe kidney, duplicated ureters.

Genitalia. Male: hypospadias. Female: duplication and/or anomalous insertion of fallopian tubes, uterine cysts, hypoplastic ovaries.

Other. Thrombocytopenia, situs inversus of lungs, cysts of thymus, calcified pulmonary arterioles, large gallbladder, radial aplasia, flexion deformity of large joints, diaphragmatic defect.

NATURAL HISTORY. The median survival for children with this disorder is 2.5 days. Eighty-two per cent of these babies die within the first month. Only 5 per cent survive the first 6 months. Survivors have severe mental defects, often seizures, and fail to thrive. Only one adult, 33 years of age, has been detected. Because of the high infant mortality, surgical or orthopedic corrective procedures should be withheld in early infancy to await the outcome of the first few months. Furthermore, because of the severe brain defect, limitation of extraordinary medical means to prolong the life of individuals with this syndrome should be seriously considered. However, it is important to emphasize that each case must be taken on an individual basis. The individual circumstances of each child as well as the personal feelings of the parents must be acknowledged. Baty et al. have documented the natural history of this disorder. For children who survive, the average number of days in the neonatal intensive care unit was 10.8, average days on a ventilator was 13.3, and 23 per cent had surgery in the neonatal period. There was no evidence for an increase in adverse reactions to immunizations. Growth curves, in that study are provided.

ETIOLOGY. Trisomy for all or a large part of chromosome 13. Older maternal age has been a factor in the occurrence of this aneuploidy syndrome. Although no accurate empiric recurrence risk data are presently available, it is presumed that the likelihood for recurrence is of very low magnitude for the full 13 trisomy cases. As with Down syndrome, chromosomal studies are indicated on 13 trisomy syndrome babies in order to detect the rare translocation patient having a balanced translocation parent for whom the risk of recurrence would be of major concern.

Cases with *trisomy 13 mosaicism* most often show a less severe clinical phenotype with every degree of variation, from the full pattern of malformation seen in trisomy 13 to a near-normal phenotype. Survival is usually longer. The degree of mental deficiency is variable.

Partial trisomy for the proximal segment (13pter→q14) is characterized by a nonspecific pattern, including a large nose, short upper lip, receding mandible, fifth finger clinodactyly, and usually severe mental deficiency. The overall picture shows little similarity to that of full trisomy 13, and survival is not significantly reduced.

Partial trisomy for the distal segment (13q14→qter) has a characteristic phenotype associated with severe mental deficiency. The facies is marked by frontal capillary hemangiomata, a short nose with upturned tip, and elongated philtrum, synophrys, bushy eyebrows and long, incurved lashes, and a prominent antihelix. Trigonocephaly and arhinencephaly have occasionally been seen. About one fourth of the patients die during early postnatal life.

COMMENT. The defects of midface, eye, and forebrain, which occur in variable degree as a feature of this syndrome, appear to be the consequence of a single defect in the early (3 weeks) development of the prechordal mesoderm, which is not only necessary for morphogenesis of the midface but also exerts an inductive role on the subsequent development of the prosencephalon, the forepart of the brain. This type of defect has been referred to as holoprosencephaly or arhinencephaly and varies in severity from cyclopia to cebocephaly to less severe forms.

References

Patau, K., et al.: Multiple congenital anomaly caused by an extra chromosome. Lancet, 1:790, 1960.

Warburg, M., and Mikkelsen, M.: A case of 13–15 trisomy or Bartholin-Patau's syndrome. Acta Ophthalmol. (Kbh.), 41:321, 1963.

Smith, D. W.: Autosomal abnormalities. Am. J. Obstet. Gynecol., 90:1055, 1964.

Warkany, J., Passarge, E., and Smith, L.B.: Congenital malformations in autosomal trisomy syndromes. Am. J. Dis. Child., 112:502, 1966.

Schinzel, A.: Autosomale Chromosomenaberationen. Arch. Genet., 52:1, 1979.

Goldstein, H., and Nielsen, K. G.: Rates and survival of individuals with trisomy 13 and 18: Data from a 10-year period in Denmark. Clin. Genet., 34:366, 1988.

Baty, B. J., et al.: Natural history of trisomy 18 and trisomy 13: I. Growth, physical assessment, medical histories, survival and recurrence risk. Am. J. Med. Genet., 49:175, 1994.

Baty, B. J., et al.: Natural history of trisomy 18 and trisomy 13: II. Psychomotor development. Am. J. Med. Genet., 49:189, 1994.

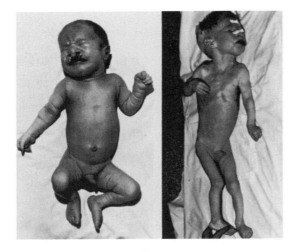

FIGURE 1. Trisomy 13 patient at 6 weeks (22 inches, 9 pounds) and again at 2 years (30 inches, 15 pounds).

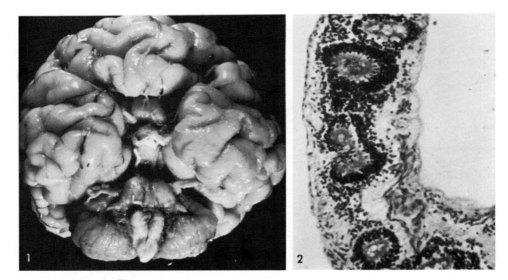

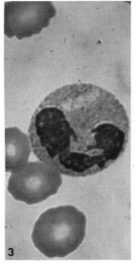

FIGURE 2. Some pathologic features of trisomy 13 syndrome. *1*, Lack of septation of forebrain (holoprosencephaly). *2*, Dysplastic retina with rosette formation. *3*, Excess nuclear projections in polymorphonuclear leukocyte.

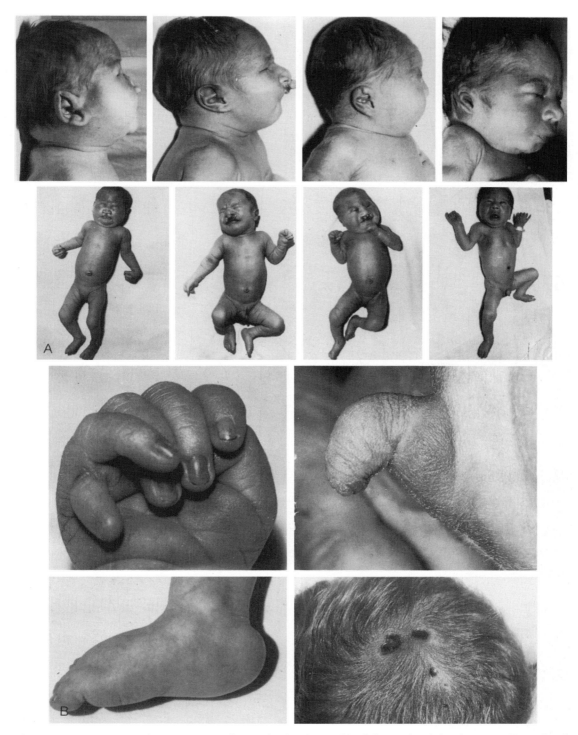

FIGURE 3. Trisomy 13 syndrome. *A*, Note sloping forehead, variable defect in facial development. (From Smith, D. W., et al.: J. Pediatr., *62*:326, 1963, with permission.) *B*, Narrow hyperconvex fingernails, anomalous scrotum, prominent heel, and posterior scalp lesions. (From Smith, D. W.: Am. J. Obstet. Gynecol., *90*:1055, 1964, with permission.)

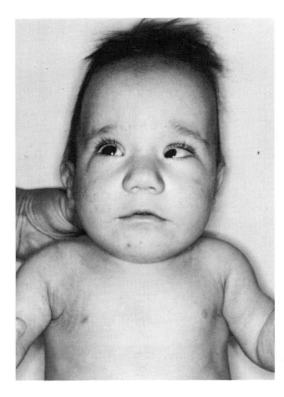

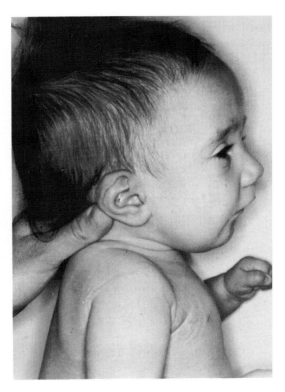

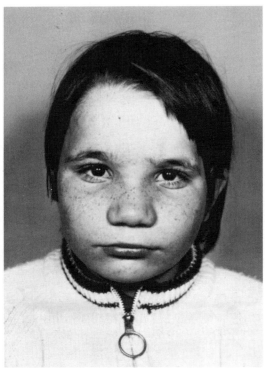

FIGURE 4. Partial 13 trisomy, proximal segment Q. *Above*, A 6-month-old patient. High forehead; left esotropia; large, broad-based nose; receding mandible. (From Schinzel, A., et al.: Humangenetik, 22:287, 1974, with permission.) *Below*, Same patient at 11 years of age. Hypertelorism; prominent and broad-based nose; no strabismus; normal size of the mandible. (From Schinzel, A.: Arch. Genet., 52:180, 1979, with permission.)

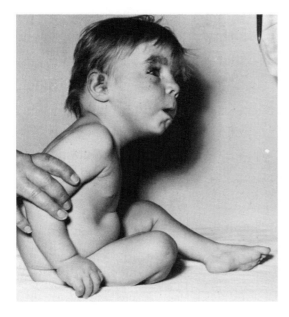

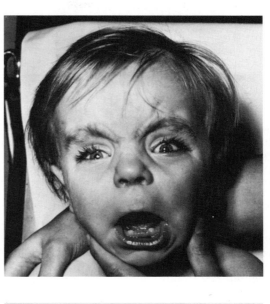

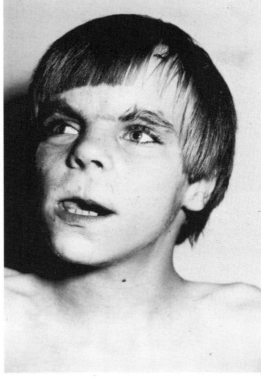

FIGURE 5. Partial 13 trisomy, distal segment Q. *Above*, Patient at 1⁶/₁₂ years of age. Note bushy eyebrows, long and curled lashes, small nose, increased distance between nose and upper lip, and prominent antihelix. (From Schinzel, A.: Arch. Genet., *52*:178, 1979, with permission.) *Below*, Same patient at 12 years of age (From Schinzel, A., et al.: Humangenetik, 22:287, 1974, with permission.)

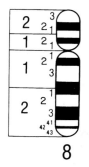

8

TRISOMY 8 SYNDROME
(Usually Trisomy 8/Normal Mosaicism)

Thick Lips, Deep-Set Eyes, Prominent Ears, Camptodactyly

Patients with trisomy for a C-group autosome have been recognized since 1963. Most of them have been mosaics of trisomy C/normal. The phenotype tends to be similar, and, more recently, chromosomal banding techniques have identified the extra chromosome as number 8. More than 100 cases have been reported.

ABNORMALITIES
Growth. Variable, from small to tall.

Performance. Mild to severe mental deficiency with tendency to poor coordination.

Craniofacial. Tendency toward prominent forehead, deep-set eyes, strabismus, hypertelorism with broad nasal root and prominent nares, full lips, everted lower lip, micrognathia, high arched palate, cleft palate, and prominent cupped ears with thick helices.

Limbs. Camptodactyly of second through fifth fingers and toes; limited elbow supination; deep creases, palms and soles; single transverse palmar crease; major joint contracture; abnormal nails.

Other. Long, slender trunk; abnormal scapula, abnormal sternum, short or webbed neck; narrow pelvis; hip dysplasia; widely spaced nipples; ureteral-renal anomalies; cardiac defects.

OCCASIONAL OR UNCERTAIN INCIDENCE.
Absent patellae, conductive deafness, seizures, vertebral anomaly (bifid vertebrae, extra lumbar vertebra, spina bifida occulta), scoliosis, cryptorchidism, jejunal duplication, agenesis of corpus callosum. Hypoplastic anemia, leukopenia, coagulation factor VII deficiency, mediastinal germ cell tumor, gastric leiomyosarcoma.

NATURAL HISTORY. The natural history is largely dependent on the severity of mental deficiency. There appears to be a lack of correlation between the phenotype and the percentage of trisomic cells.

ETIOLOGY. Trisomy 8, the majority of patients being mosaics. Apparently, full trisomy 8 is usually an early lethal disorder.

References

Stalder, G. R., Buhler, E. M., and Weber, J. R.: Possible trisomy in chromosome group 6–12. Lancet, *1*:1379, 1963.

Schinzel, A., et al.: Trisomy 8 mosaicism syndrome. Helv. Pediatr. Acta., *29*:531, 1974.

Riccardi, V. M.: Trisomy 8: An international study of 70 patients. Birth Defects, *XIII*(3C):171, 1977.

Kurtyka, Z. E., et al.: Trisomy 8 mosaicism syndrome. Clin. Pediatr. 27:557, 1988.

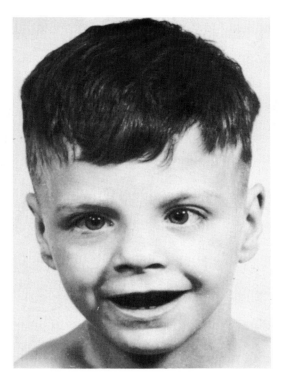

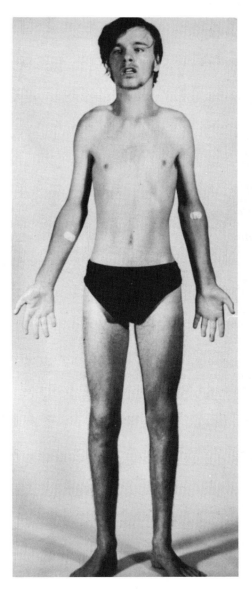

FIGURE 1. Amiable, tall individual at 4 years and at 16 years who has trisomy 8/normal mosaicism, with a normal karyotype from cultured leukocytes but trisomy 8 in skin fibroblast cells. He has a moderate hearing deficit and an I.Q. estimated in the 70s. He is quite active and skates, swims, and bowls. Note the facies, the small, widely spaced nipples, and the general body stance. There is some limitation of full extension of the fingers, which are partially webbed, and limited extension of the right elbow. There is hypoplasia of the supraspinatus, trapezius, and upper pectoral musculature. (Courtesy of Dr. G. Howard Valentine, War Memorial Children's Hospital, London, Ontario.)

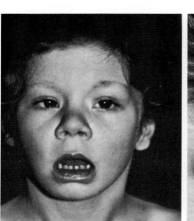
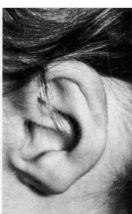
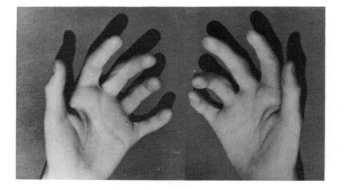

FIGURE 2. Boy with trisomy 8/normal mosaicism. (From Riccardi, V. M., et al.: J. Pediatr., 77:664, 1970, with permission.)

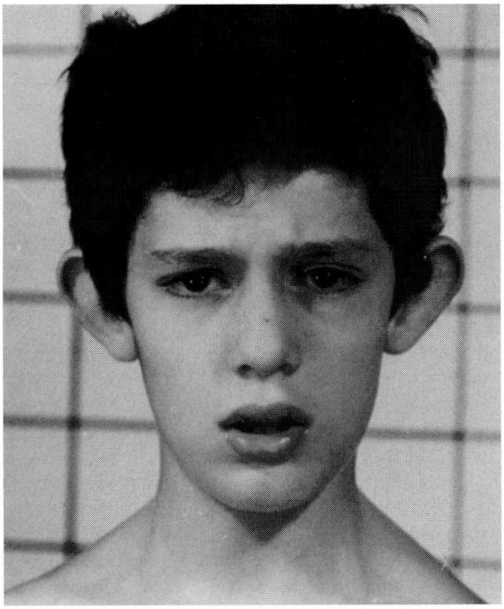

FIGURE 3. Mentally deficient 10-year-old with trisomy 8/ normal mosaicism. Note the prominent ears. (From De Grouchy, J., et al.: Ann. Genet., *14*:69, 1971, with permission.)

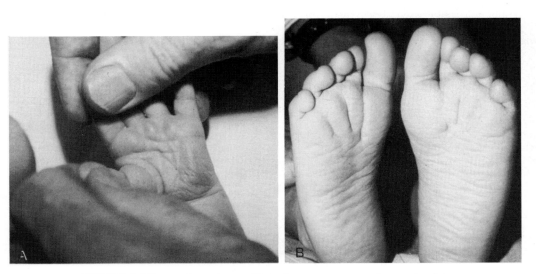

FIGURE 4. Trisomy 8 syndrome. Note deep creases on palms and soles.

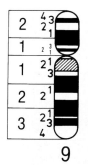

9

TRISOMY 9 MOSAIC SYNDROME

*Joint Contractures, Congenital
Heart Defects, Low-Set Malformed Ears*

In 1973, Haslam et al. reported the first case of trisomy 9 mosaicism. In the same year, Feingold et al. reported the first example of a child with full trisomy 9 utilizing blood lymphocytes.

ABNORMALITIES
Growth. Prenatal onset growth deficiency.
Performance. Severe mental deficiency.
Craniofacial. Sloping forehead with narrow bifrontal diameter; up-slanting, short palpebral fissures, deeply set eyes; prominent nasal bridge with short root, small fleshy tip, and slit-like nostrils; prominent lip covering receding lower lip; micrognathia, low-set, posteriorly rotated, and misshapen ears.
Skeletal. Joint anomalies including abnormal position and/or function of hips, knees, feet, elbows, and digits; kyphoscoliosis; narrow chest; hypoplasia of sacrum, iliac wings, and pubic arch; hypoplastic phalanges of toes.
Other. Congenital heart defects in about two thirds of cases.

OCCASIONAL ABNORMALITIES.
Subarachnoid cyst, choroid plexus cyst, cystic dilatation of fourth ventricle with lack of midline fusion of cerebellum, hydrocephalus, lack of gyration of cerebral hemispheres, meningocele, microphthalmia, corneal opacities, Peters anomaly, absence of optic tracts, preauricular tags, short neck, cleft lip and/or palate, velopharyngeal insufficiency, bile duct proliferation in absence of a demonstrable stenosis or atresia, gastroesophageal reflux, punctate mineralization in developing cartilage, 13 ribs and 13 thoracic vertebrae. Diaphragmatic hernia. Nonpitting edema of legs, simian crease, nail hypoplasia, genitourinary anomalies including hypoplastic external genitalia, cryptorchidism, cystic dilatation of renal tubules, diverticulae of bladder, hydronephrosis, and hydroureter.

NATURAL HISTORY. The majority of patients die during the early postnatal period. In those that survive, failure to thrive and severe motor and mental deficiency are the rule. Some patients remain bedridden throughout their lives, whereas others achieve the ability to walk and minimal speech.

ETIOLOGY. Trisomy for chromosome 9. The incidence and severity of malformations and mental deficiency correlate with the percentage of trisomic cells in the different tissues.

References

Haslam, R. H. A., et al.: Trisomy 9 mosaicism with multiple congenital anomalies. J. Med. Genet., *10*: 180, 1973.
Feingold, M., et al.: A case of trisomy 9. J. Med. Genet., *10*:184, 1973.
Bowen, P., et al.: Trisomy 9 mosaicism in a newborn infant with multiple malformations. J. Pediatr., *85*: 95, 1974.
Akatsuka, A., et al.: Trisomy 9 mosaicism with punctate mineralization in developing cartilages. Eur. J. Pediatr., *131*:271, 1979.
Frohlich, G. S.: Delineation of trisomy 9, J. Med. Genet., *19*:316, 1982.
Kamiker, C. P., et al.: Mosaic trisomy 9 syndrome with unusual phenotype. Am. J. Med. Genet., 22:237, 1985.
Levy, I., et al.: Gastrointestinal abnormalities in the syndrome of mosaic trisomy 9. J. Med. Genet., *26*: 280, 1989.

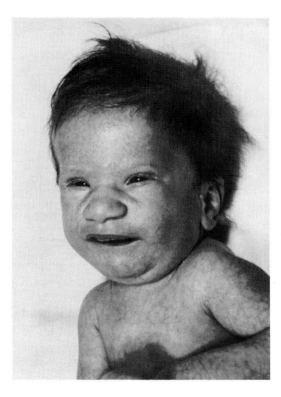
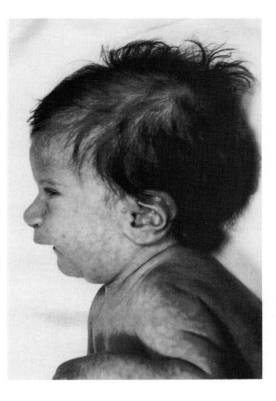
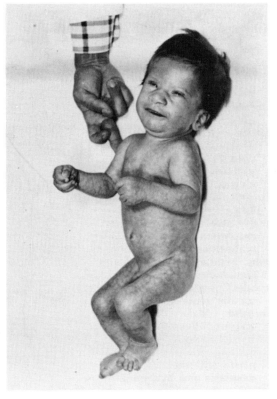

FIGURE 1. Trisomy 9 mosaic syndrome. A 2-month-old boy. Long and narrow face with narrow eyelids in mongoloid position, broad and bulbous nose with a broad and prominent bridge, short upper lip covering the receding lower lip, small mandible, left preauricular pit, cutis marmorata, inability to lie on the back because of congenital thoracic kyphosis, and flexion position of hands and fingers. (From Schinzel, A., et al.: Humangenetik, 25:171, 1974, with permission.)

TRIPLOIDY SYNDROME AND DIPLOID/ TRIPLOID MIXOPLOIDY SYNDROME

Large Placenta With Hydatidiform Changes, Growth Deficiency, Syndactyly of Third and Fourth Fingers

Triploidy, a complete extra set of chromosomes, is estimated to occur in about 2 per cent of conceptuses. Most are lost as miscarriages, accounting for about 20 per cent of all chromosomally abnormal spontaneous abortuses. Triploid pregnancies may be accompanied by varying degrees of toxemia. Fetal wastage may be due to hydatidiform placental changes or to specific cytogenetic characteristics, with only 3 per cent of 69,XYY conceptuses surviving to be recognized. Partial hydatidiform moles are usually associated with a triploid fetus and very rarely undergo malignant changes. Classic moles show more pronounced trophoblastic hyperplasia in the absence of a fetus. These moles show a diploid karyotype and are totally androgenic in origin.

Infrequently, triploid infants survive to be born after 28 weeks' gestation with severe intrauterine growth retardation. Instances of diploid/triploid mixoploidy have been less frequently recognized. Asymmetric growth deficiency with mild syndactyly and occasional genital ambiguity in 46,XX/69,XXY individuals are the key diagnostic features in mixoploid individuals.

ABNORMALITIES FOUND IN 50 PER CENT OR MORE OF CASES

Placenta. Large, with tendency toward hydatidiform changes.
Growth. Disproportionate prenatal growth deficiency that affects the skeleton more than the cephalic region. In mixoploid individuals skeletal growth may be asymmetric.
Craniofacial. Dysplastic calvaria with large posterior fontanel, ocular hyperterlorism with eye defects ranging from colobomata to microphthalmia, low nasal bridge, low-set, malformed ears, micrognathia.
Limbs. Syndactyly of third and fourth fingers, simian crease, talipes equinovarus.
Cardiac. Congenital heart defect (atrial and ventricular septal defects).
Genitalia. Male: hypospadias, micropenis, cryptorchidism, Leydig cell hyperplasia.
Other. Brain anomalies, including hydrocephalus and holoprosencephaly; adrenal hypoplasia; and renal anomalies, including cystic dysplasia and hydronephrosis.

ABNORMALITIES FOUND IN LESS THAN 50 PER CENT OF CASES

Aberrant skull shape; choanal atresia; cleft lip and/or palate; iris heterochromia; patchy cutaneous hyperpigmentation, hypopigmentation or a mixture of both referred to as pigmentary dysplasia; meningomyelocele; macroglossia; omphalocele or umbilical hernia; biliary tract anomalies, including aplasia of the gallbladder; incomplete rotation of colon; proximally placed thumb; clinodactyly of fifth finger; splayed toes.

NATURAL HISTORY. Partial hydatidiform molar pregnancies associated with a triploid fetus should not raise concern regarding the development of choriocarcinoma. All cases of full triploidy have either been stillborn or have died in the early neonatal period, with 5 months being the longest recorded survival. Individuals with diploid/triploid mixoploidy usually survive and manifest some degree of psychomotor retardation. As a result of body asymmetry, patients with mixoploidy may require a heel lift for the shorter leg to prevent compensatory scoliosis, and some of these people may resemble those having Russell-Silver syndrome. Diagnosis of mixoploidy usually requires skin fibroblast cultures, since the triploid cell line may have disappeared from among peripheral blood leukocytes. The degree of skeletal asymmetry does not appear to correspond to the proportions of triploid cells present, and triploid cells in culture grow with the same variability as diploid cells, except for those with the XYY complement, which grow much more slowly.

ETIOLOGY. In most instances, the extra set of chromosomes is paternally derived, with 66 per cent attributed to double fertilization, 24 per cent due to fertilization with a diploid sperm, and 10 per cent a result of fertilization of a diploid egg (failure to shed a polar body). About 60 per cent of the cases have been XXY, with most of the remainder being XXX. It is not unusual for more than one X chromosome to remain active in triploidy. Older maternal age has not been a factor, and there are no data to indicate an increased recurrence risk, such as that seen for chromosomal disorders due to nondisjunction. In several instances, a triploid pregnancy has been followed or preceded by a molar pregnancy.

References

Book, J. A., and Santesson, B.: Malformation syndrome in man associated with triploidy (69 chromosomes). Lancet, 1:858, 1960.

Ferrier, P., et al.: Congenital asymmetry associated with diploid-triploid mosaicism and large satellites. Lancet, 1:80, 1964.

Niebular, E.: Triploidy in man: Cytogenetical and clinical aspects. Humangenetik, 21:103, 1974.

Wertelecki, W., Graham, J. M., and Sergovich, F. R.: The clinical syndrome of triploidy. Obstet. Gynecol., 47:69, 1976.

Jacobs, P. A., et al.: The origin of human triploids. Ann. Hum. Genet., 42:49, 1978.

Poland, B. J., and Bailie, D. L.: Cell ploidy in molar placental disease. Teratology, 18:353, 1978.

Jacobs, P. A., et al.: Late replicating X chromosomes in human triploidy. Am. J. Hum. Genet., 31:446, 1979.

Graham, J. M., et al.: Diploid-triploid mixoploidy: Clinical and cytogenetic aspects. Pediatrics, 68:23, 1981.

Wulfsberg, E. A., et al.: Monozygotic twin girls with diploid/triploid chromosome mosaicism and cutaneous pigmentary dysplasia. Clin. Genet., 39:370, 1991.

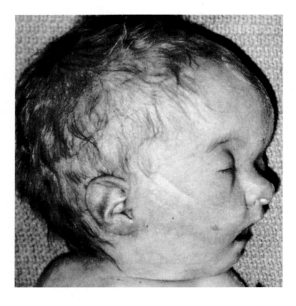

FIGURE 1. Stillborn infant with triploidy showing relatively large-appearing upper head in relation to very small face.

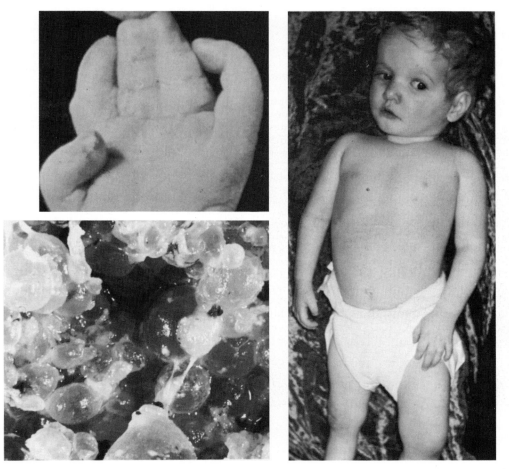

FIGURE 2. Hand (*upper left*) and placenta (*lower left*) of stillborn infant showing syndactyly and hydatidiform cystic changes, respectively. Infant (*right*) with asymmetric growth deficiency (*right side smaller*), syndactyly of third and fourth fingers, and mild developmental delay who has triploid/diploid mixoploidy syndrome that is evident only in cultured fibroblasts. (Courtesy of Dr. John M. Graham, Cedars Sinai Medical Center, Los Angeles, CA.)

DELETION 3p SYNDROME

Mental and Growth Deficiency, Ptosis, Postaxial Polydactyly

Partial deletion of the distal part of the short arm of chromosome 3 was first reported by Verjaal and De Nef in 1978. Subsequently, 15 patients have been reported. In all cases the deleted segment has been 3p25→pter.

ABNORMALITIES

Growth. Prenatal onset growth deficiency, most striking postnatally.

Performance. Severe to profound mental retardation. Hypotonia.

Craniofacial. Microcephaly with flat occiput. Synophrys. Epicanthal folds. Ptosis. Prominent nasal bridge. Small nose with anteverted nares. Long philtrum. Malformed ears. Micrognathia. Downturned corners of mouth.

Other: Postaxial polydactyly of hands and less frequently the feet.

OCCASIONAL ABNORMALITIES. Trigonocephaly with prominent metopic sutures, upslanting palpebral fissures, preauricular pits and/or fistula, cleft palate, cardiac defects including ventricular septal defect (two patients) and one patient with double mitral valve, atrioventricular canal and tricuspid atresia; inguinal hernia, hiatal hernia, common mesentery, anteriorly placed anus, renal anomalies including pelvic and cystic kidney; cryptorchidism.

NATURAL HISTORY. Two children have died, one at 3 days of age with a complex cardiac defect and the other at 3 months of age of aspiration pneumonia. The survivors, the oldest of which is 24 years old, all have severe mental retardation. Many are blind and deaf and interact only minimally with their environment.

ETIOLOGY. Partial deletion of the short arm of chromosome 3, del(3p25→pter). In all but one case the deletion has occurred de novo.

References

Verjaal, M., and DeNef, J.: A patient with a partial deletion of the short arm of chromosome 3. Am. J. Dis. Child., *132*:43, 1978.

Higginbottom, M. C., et al.: A second patient with partial deletion of the short arm of chromosome 3: Karyotype 46XY,del(3) (p25). J. Med. Genet., *19*:71, 1982.

Tolmie, J. L., et al.: Partial deletion of the short arm of chromosome 3. Clin. Genet., *29*:538, 1986.

Schwyzer, U., et al.: Terminal deletion of the short arm of chromosome 3, del(3pter-p25): A recognizable syndrome. Helv. Paediatr. Acta, *42*:309, 1987.

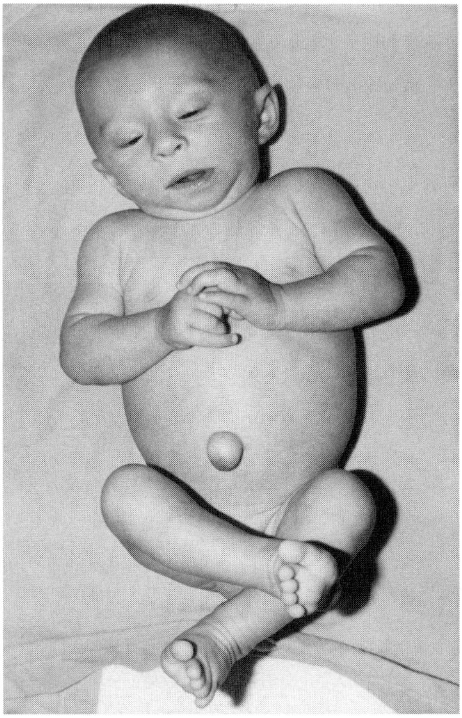

FIGURE 1. A 5-month-old male. Note the bilateral ptosis, long philtrum, micrognathia, and umbilical hernia. (From Higginbottom, M. C., et al.: J. Med. Genet., *19*:71, 1982, with permission.)

DUPLICATION 3q SYNDROME

Mental and Growth Deficiency,
Broad Nasal Root, Hypertrichosis

First described by Falek et al. in 1966, this disorder initially was confused with the Brachmann–de Lange syndrome. Hirschhorn et al. performed chromosome banding studies in 1973 that associated duplication of the 3q21→qter region with a distinct phenotype that Francke and Opitz subsequently emphasized can be clinically distinguished from Brachmann–de Lange. Greater than 40 cases of the duplication 3q syndrome now have been reported.

ABNORMALITIES

Growth. Severe postnatal growth deficiency (100 per cent).

Performance. Severe mental deficiency (100 per cent) with brain anomalies/seizures (83 per cent).

Craniofacies. Abnormal head shape frequently due to craniosynostosis (92 per cent). Hypertrichosis and synophrys (86 per cent). Up-slanting palpebral fissures (56 per cent). Broad nasal root (100 per cent). Anteverted nares (91 per cent). Prominent maxilla (86 per cent). Long philtrum (85 per cent). Downturned corners of mouth (82 per cent). High arched palate (100 per cent). Cleft palate (79 per cent). Micrognathia (100 per cent). Malformed ears (79 per cent). Short webbed neck (93 per cent).

Limbs. Fifth finger clinodactyly (90 per cent). Hypoplastic nails (64 per cent). Simian crease (74 per cent). Talipes equinovarus (64 per cent). Arch dermal ridge pattern or digital pattern with low ridge counts (86 per cent).

Other. Cardiac defects (75 per cent). Chest deformities (89 per cent). Renal or urinary tract anomalies (48 per cent). Genital anomalies in 61 per cent (primarily cryptorchidism). Umbilical hernia (50 per cent).

OCCASIONAL ABNORMALITIES. Microphthalmia, glaucoma, cataract, coloboma, strabismus, syndactyly, polydactyly, camptodactyly, short limbs, cubitus valgus, dislocated radial head, ulnar or fibular deviation of hands or feet, omphalocele, hemivertebrae.

NATURAL HISTORY. Death prior to 12 months has occurred in 36 per cent of cases. For survivors, prognosis is grim with severe mental deficiency, growth retardation, and pulmonary infections the rule.

ETIOLOGY. Duplication for 3q21→qter. In the majority of cases duplication of 3q occurs concurrently with monosomy of another chromosomal region, frequently 3p. However, the clinical phenotype of duplication 3q is the same irrespective of the accompanying monosomy. Seventy-five per cent of cases have arisen from segregation of parental rearrangements. Trisomy of genes in the distal part of 3q26 and the proximal part of 3q27 are most likely essential for the characteristic phenotype.

COMMENT. Although superficial resemblance exists between the duplication 3q syndrome and the Brachmann–de Lange syndrome, they are clearly distinct disorders that can be differentiated clinically.

References

Falek, A., et al.: Familial de Lange syndrome with chromosome abnormalities. Pediatrics, *37*:92, 1966.

Hirschhorn, K., et al.: Precise identification of various chromosomal abnormalities. Ann. Hum. Genet., *36*: 3875, 1973.

Francke, U., and Opitz, J.: Chromosome 3q duplication and the Brachmann–de Lange syndrome (BDLS). J. Pediatr., *95*:161, 1979.

Steinbach, P., et al.: The dup (3q) syndrome: Report of eight cases and review of the literature. Am. J. Med. Genet., *10*:159, 1981.

Wilson, G. N., et al.: Further delineation of the dup (3q) syndrome. Am. J. Med. Genet., *22*:117, 1985.

Van Essen, A. J., et al.: Partial 3q duplication syndrome and assignment of D355 to 3q25→3q28. Hum. Genet., *87*:151, 1991.

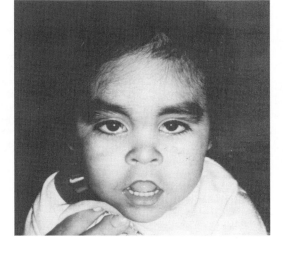

FIGURE 1. A 3-month-old male. Note the hypertrichosis, long philtrum, and downturned corners of the mouth.

DELETION 4p SYNDROME

(Chromosome Number 4 Short-Arm Deletion Syndrome, 4p− Syndrome)

Ocular Hypertelorism With Broad or Beaked Nose; Microcephaly and/or Cranial Asymmetry; and Low-Set, Simple Ear With Preauricular Dimple

After delineation of the cri du chat syndrome, occasional patients with deletions of the short arm of a B-group chromosome were found who lacked the typical cry and some other features of that condition. Autoradiographic labeling studies revealed that the deficit chromosome was a number 4 rather than a number 5, and the detection of further cases with consistent clinical findings has allowed the definition of the syndrome.

ABNORMALITIES

Growth. Marked growth deficiency, prenatal onset. Microcephaly.

Performance. Feeble fetal activity. Hypotonia. Severe mental deficiency; seizures.

Craniofacial. Stabismus, iris deformity, ocular hypertelorism, epicanthal folds; prominent glabella, cleft lip and/or palate, downturned "fishlike" mouth, short upper lip and philtrum, and micrognathia. Posterior midline scalp defects. Cranial asymmetry. preauricular tag or pit.

Extremities. Hypoplastic dermal ridges, low dermal ridge count. Simian creases. Talipes equinovarus. Hyperconvex fingernails.

Other. Hypospadias, cryptorchidism, sacral dimple or sinus. Cardiac anomaly, primarily atrial septal defect. Scoliosis.

OCCASIONAL ABNORMALITIES.

Exophthalmos, ptosis, Rieger anomaly, nystagmus, fused teeth, defect of the medial half of the eyebrows, hearing loss, hypodontia of permanent teeth, low hairline with webbed neck, metatarsus adductus, polydactyly, hip dislocation, accessory ossification centers in proximal metacarpals, absence of pubic rami, delayed bone age, abnormalities in sternal ossification centers, "bottle opener" deformity of clavicles, precocious puberty, renal anomaly, malrotation of small bowel, cavum septum pellucidum, absent septum pellucidum, interventricular cysts.

NATURAL HISTORY.

These children are profoundly mentally defective and tend to have severe grand mal and minor motor seizures. Those who survive beyond early childhood have shown continued slow growth, with a propensity for respiratory tract infections.

ETIOLOGY.

Partial deletion of the short arm of chromosome 4. About 87 per cent of cases represent de novo deletions, while in 13 per cent of cases one of the parents is a balanced translocation carrier. In the cases in which there is a familial translocation, there is a 2 to 1 excess of maternally derived 4p deletions, while in the de novo deletions, the origin of the deleted chromosome is paternal in approximately 80 per cent of cases. The phenotype does not differ based on the size of the deletion, which can vary from almost one half of the short arm to so small as to be cytogenitically undetectable. In those latter cases in which the disorder is suspected clinically but standard chromosome studies are normal, a molecular deletion on the short arm of chromosome 4 at 4p16.3, the critical region for determination of the phynotype, often can be detected using flurorescent in situ hybridization (FISH) analysis.

References

Leao, J. C., et al.: New syndrome associated with partial deletion of short arms of chromosome no. 4. J. A. M. A., 202:434, 1967.

Wolf, U., and Reinwein, H.: Klinische und cytogenetische Differentialdiagnose der Defizienzen an den kurzen Armen der B-Chromosomen. Z. Kinderheilkd, 98:235, 1967.

Guthrie, R. D., et al.: The 4p− syndrome. Am. J. Dis. Child., 122:421, 1971.

Lurie, I. W., et al.: The Wolf-Hirschorn syndrome. Clin. Genet., 17:375, 1980.

Quarrell, O. W. J., et al.: Paternal origin of the chromosomal deletion resulting in Wolf-Hirschorn syndrome. J. Med. Genet., 28:256, 1991.

Katz, D. S., and Smith, T. H.: Wolf syndrome. Pediatr. Radiol., 21:369, 1991.

Estabrooks, L. L., et al.: Molecular characterisation of chromosome 4p deletions resulting in Wolf-Hirschhorn syndrome. J. Med. Genet., 31:103, 1994.

Fagan-Bagric, K., et al.: A practical application of fluorescent in situ hybridication to the Wolfe-Hirshhorn syndrome. Pediatrics, 93:826, 1994.

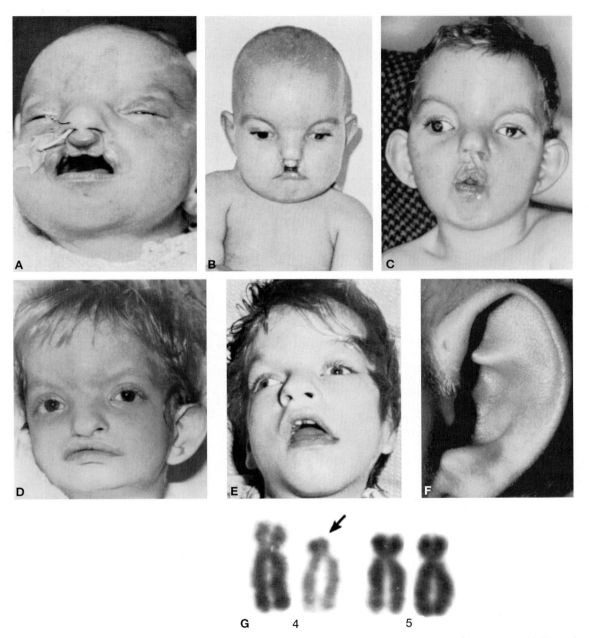

FIGURE 1. Deletion 4p syndrome. *A to C*, A 2-week-old, 11-month-old, and 33-month-old. (From Wolf, U., and Reinwein, H.: Z Kinderheilkd., *98*:235, 1967, with permission.) *D*, Child, $5^9/_{12}$ years old, with height age of 10 months and I.Q. of less than 20. *E*, A 7-year-old with height age of $3^6/_{12}$ years and performance age of less than 6 months. *F*, Relatively simple form of ear with cutaneous pit. *G*, B-group chromosomes from patient shown in *E*.

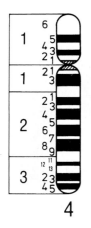

4

DUPLICATION 4p SYNDROME

(Trisomy for the Short Arm of Chromosome 4, Trisomy 4p Syndrome)

Characteristic Facies, Severe Mental Deficiency With or Without Seizures, Growth Deficiency

First described by Wilson et al. in 1970, the overall pattern of malformation was more completely delineated by Gonzalez et al. in 1977. At least 85 cases have now been described.

ABNORMALITIES

Growth. Prenatal onset growth deficiency. A tendency toward obesity. Adult height ranges from 145 to 150 cm.

Performance. Severe mental deficiency present in 100 per cent of cases. Language is more severely delayed than social and fine motor skills.

Neurologic. Hypertonia during infancy followed by hypotonia. Seizures. Abnormal EEGs.

Craniofacies. Microcephaly; small, flat forehead; prominent supraorbital ridges fused across the glabella. Depressed or flat nasal bridge with bulbous nasal tip; synophrys, macroglossia, irregular teeth; small pointed mandible; frequently enlarged ears with abnormal helix and antihelix; short neck. In childhood the face is round with chubby cheeks. Later the face becomes triangular with poor dentition and elongated chin.

Limbs. Clinodactyly of fifth fingers, camptodactyly, hypoplastic fingernails and toenails.

Genitalia. Micropenis, hypospadias, cryptorchidism.

Other. Kyphoscoliosis; hypoplastic, widely spaced nipples; absent or additional ribs.

OCCASIONAL ABNORMALITIES.

Serious ocular defects including microphthalmos and colobomata of uveal tract (15 per cent), cleft lip, preauricular tags, cardiac defects, renal malformations and atresia, absence of corpus callosum, congenital hip dislocations, talipes equinovarus, foot position anomalies, two-three syndactyly of toes, preaxial polydactyly, vertebral anomalies.

NATURAL HISTORY. Approximately one third of reported cases died during early infancy. Without visceral anomalies, life span does not seem to be impaired. Feeding problems are frequent in the neonatal period, and respiratory difficulties are a common complication. Of the survivors, the majority are severely mentally retarded with very poor if any speech. Fine motor development is severely compromised. Epilepsy, joint contractures, significant neurologic complications, and behavioral problems are consistent features with advancing age.

ETIOLOGY. Trisomy for part or most of the short arm of chromosome 4. The clinical phenotype is most likely due to the duplicated 4p15.2→16.1 segment.

References

Wilson, M. G., et al.: Inherited pericentric inversion of chromosome No. 4. Am. J. Hum. Genet., 22:679, 1970.

Dallapiccola, B., et al.: Trisomy 4p: Five new observations and overview. Clin. Genet., 12:344, 1977.

Gonzalez, C. H., et al.: The trisomy 4p syndrome: Case report and review. Am. J. Med. Genet., 1:137, 1977.

Crane, J., Sujanski, W., and Smith, A.: 4p Trisomy syndrome: Report of 4 additional cases and segregation analysis of 21 families with different translocations. Am. J. Med. Genet., 4:219, 1979.

Kleczkowska, A., et al.: Trisomy of the short arm of chromosome 4: The changing phenotype with age. Ann. Genet., 35:217, 1992.

Lurie, I. W., and Samochvalov, V. A.: Trisomy 4p and ocular defects. Br. J. Ophthalmol., 78:415, 1994.

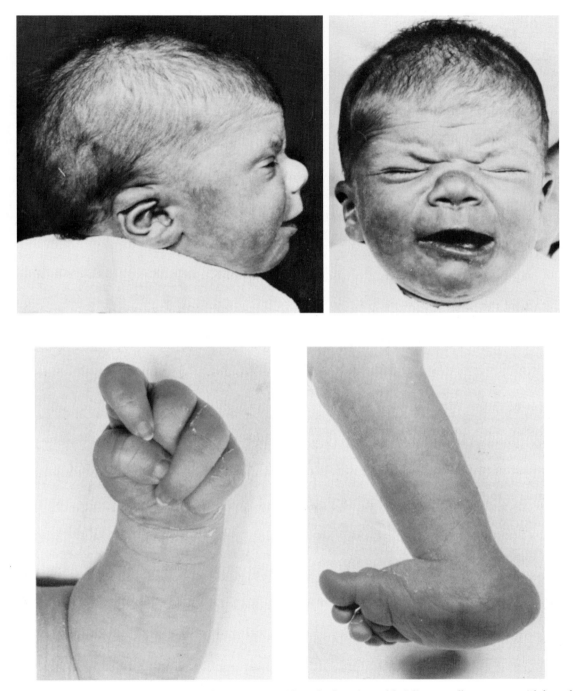

FIGURE 1. Duplication 4p syndrome. *Above,* Neonate. Note the low frontal hairline, small pug nose with broad and depressed bridge, asymmetric crying mouth, small, misshapen ears with overfolding of the upper helix, and prominent antihelix. *Below,* Same patient. Flexion position of the fingers of the left hand and rocker-bottom foot with prominent heel. (From Schinzel, A., and Schmid, W.: Humangenetik, *15*:163, 1972, with permission.)

DELETION 4q SYNDROME

Mental and Growth Deficiency, Cleft Palate, Limb Anomalies

Partial deletion of the long arm of chromosome 4 was initially reported by Ockey et al. in 1967. Townes et al. proposed the existence of a 4q− syndrome in 1981. The phenotype was further delineated by Mitchell et al. in 1981 and by Lin et al. in 1988. The deleted segment associated with this disorder is 4q31→qter.

ABNORMALITIES
Growth. Postnatal onset growth deficiency (83 per cent).
Performance. Moderate to severe mental deficiency (92 per cent). Hypotonia (28 per cent). Seizures (17 per cent).
Craniofacies. Ocular hypertelorism (56 per cent). Short nose (67 per cent). Broad nasal bridge (94 per cent). Cleft palate (94 per cent). Micrognathia (94 per cent). Low-set, posteriorly rotated ears (56 per cent). Abnormal pinnae (67 per cent).
Limbs. Fifth finger clinodactyly (44 per cent). Tapering fifth finger (50 per cent). Pointed/duplicated fifth fingernail (33 per cent). Absent to hypoplastic flexion creases on fifth fingers (56 per cent). Abnormal thumb/hallux implantation (44 per cent). Simian crease (61 per cent). Overlapping toes (22 per cent).
Other. Cardiac defects (61 per cent) including ventricular septal defect, patent ductus arteriosus, peripheral pulmonic stenosis, aortic stenosis, tricuspid atresia, atrial septal defect, aortic coarctation, tetralogy of Fallot. Genitourinary defects (50 per cent). Gastrointestinal defects (22 per cent).

OCCASIONAL ABNORMALITIES.
Asymmetric face (17 per cent), small, up-slanting palpebral fissures (22 per cent), epicanthal folds (39 per cent), anteverted nares (33 per cent), cleft lip (39 per cent), Robin sequence (28 per cent), camptodactyly (17 per cent), missing digits (11 per cent).

NATURAL HISTORY. Fifty per cent of patients with a terminal deletion (q31→qter) have died prior to 15 months of age of cardiopulmonary difficulties including asphyxia, apnea, and congestive heart failure. Of those who survived, moderate to severe mental deficiency occurred in the vast majority. One child who is at least 15 years has profound mental deficiency, behavioral disorder, and seizures.

ETIOLOGY. Deletion of 4q31→qter. Virtually all cases represent de novo defects.

COMMENT. Deletions of 4q32 seem to be similar to 4q31. More distal deletions at 4q33 and 4q34 are associated with a less severe clinical phenotype. Patients with interstitial deletion of 4q differ completely from those with terminal deletions.

References

Ockey, C. H., et al.: A large deletion of the long arm of chromosome no. 4 in a child with limb abnormalities. Arch. Dis. Child., 42:428, 1967.

Townes, P. L., et al.: 4q− syndrome. Am. J. Dis Child., 133:383, 1979.

Mitchell, J. A., et al.: Deletions of different segments of the long arm of chromosome 4. Am. J. Med. Genet., 8:73, 1981.

Davis, J. M., et al.: Brief clinical report: The del (4) (q31) syndrome—a recognizable disorder with atypical Robin malformation sequence. Am. J. Med. Genet., 9:113, 1981.

Lin, A. E., et al.: Interstitial and terminal deletions of the long arm of chromosome 4: Further delineation of phenotypes. Am. J. Med. Genet., 31:533, 1988.

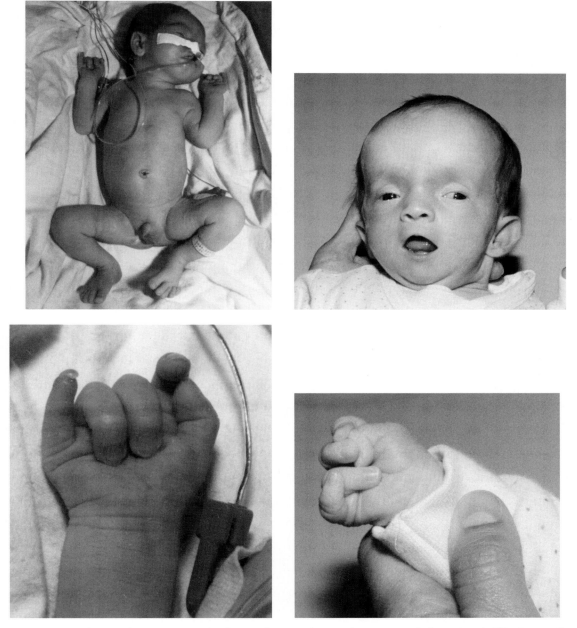

FIGURE 1. Newborn infants. Note ocular hypertelorism, abnormal pinnae, and the pointed fifth fingernail. (Courtesy of Dr. Marilyn C. Jones, Children's Hospital of San Diego, San Diego, Calif.)

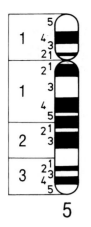

5

DELETION 5p SYNDROME

(Cri du Chat Syndrome, Partial Deletion of the Short Arm of
Chromosome Number 5 Syndrome, 5p− Syndrome)

*Cat-Like Cry in Infancy, Microcephaly,
Downward Slant of the Palpebral Fissures*

Lejeune et al. first described this condition in 1963. Further reports have raised to over 100 the number of cases described.

ABNORMALITIES
General

Low birth weight (less than 2.5 kg)	72%
Slow growth	100%
Cat-like cry	100%

Performance

Mental deficiency	100%
Hypotonia	78%

Craniofacial

Microcephaly	100%
Round face	68%
Hypertelorism	94%
Epicanthal folds	85%
Downward slanting of the palpebral fissures	81%
Strabismus, often divergent	61%
Low-set and/or poorly formed ears	58%
Facial asymmetry	—

Cardiac

Congenital heart disease (variable in type)	30%

Hands

Simian crease	81%
Distal axial triradius	40%
Slightly short metacarpals	—

OCCASIONAL ABNORMALITIES. Cleft lip and cleft palate, myopia, optic atrophy, preauricular skin tag, bifid uvula, dental malocclusion, short neck, clinodactyly, inguinal hernia, cryptorchidism, absent kidney and spleen, hemivertebra, scoliosis, flat feet, premature graying of hair.

NATURAL HISTORY. As babies, the patients tend to be unusually squirmy in their activity. The mewing cry, ascribed to abnormal laryngeal development, becomes less pronounced with the increasing age of the patient, thus making the diagnosis more difficult in older patients. A study by Wilkins et al. of 65 children with cri du chat syndrome reared in the home suggests that a much higher level of intellectual performance can be achieved than was previously suggested from studies performed on institutionalized patients. With early special schooling and a supportive home environment, some affected children attained the social and psychomotor level of a normal 5- to 6-year-old. One half of the children older than 10 years had a vocabulary and sentence structure adequate for communication. Scoliosis is a frequent occurrence.

ETIOLOGY. The underlying chromosomal aberration is partial deletion of the short arm of chromosome number 5. Approximately 85 per cent of cases result from sporadic de novo deletions, while 15 per cent arise secondary to unequal segregation of a parental translocation. Although the size of the deletion is variable, a critical region for the high-pitched cry maps to 5p15.3, while the chromosomal region involved in the remaining features maps to 5p15.2. The deleted chromosome is of paternal origin in 80 per cent of cases in which the syndrome is the result of a de novo deletion.

References

Lejeune, J., et al.: Trois cas de délétion partielle du bras court du chromosome 5. C. R. Acad. Sci. [D] (Paris), 257:3098, 1963.

Berg, J. M., et al.: Partial deletion of short arm of a chromosome of the 4 and 5 group (Denver) in an adult male. J. Ment. Defic. Res., 9:219, 1965.

Breg, W. R., et al.: The cri-du-chat syndrome in adolescents and adults. J. Pediatr., 77:782, 1970.

Wilkins, L. E., Brown, J. A., and Wolf, B.: Psychomotor development in 65 home-reared children with cri-du-chat syndrome. J. Pediatr., 97:401, 1980.

Overhauser, J., et al.: Parental origin of chromosome 5 deletions in the cri-du-chat syndrome. Am. J. Med. Genet., 37:83, 1990.

Overhauser, J., et al.: Molecular and phenotypic mapping of the short arm of chromosome 5: Sublocalization of the critical region of the cri-du-chat syndrome. Hum. Mol. Genet., 3:247, 1994.

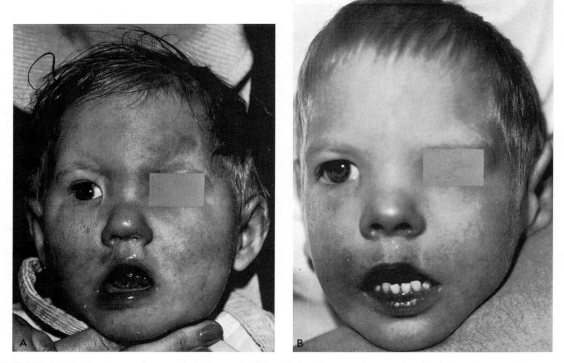

FIGURE 1. Deletion 5p syndrome. *A,* A 9-month-old with height age of 5 months; birth length, 18 inches. Note the delay in dentition. *B,* Child, $3^{10}/_{12}$ years old with height age of $1^6/_{12}$ years. Note the inner epicanthal fold and relatively small cranium with narrow forehead. (From Smith, D. W.: J. Pediatr., *70:*475, 1967, with permission.)

DELETION 9p SYNDROME

(9p Monosomy, 9p− Syndrome)

Craniostenosis With Trigonocephaly, Up-slanting Palpebral Fissures, Hypoplastic Supraorbital Ridges

Since the initial delineation of this disorder in 1973 by Alfi et al., at least 40 similarly affected patients with 9p− as the sole chromosomal anomaly have been reported.

ABNORMALITIES

Growth. Usually normal.

Performance. Mean I.Q. is 49 with a range from 33 to 73. Social adaptation is often good.

Craniofacies. Craniostenosis involving the metopic suture leading to trigonocephaly; flat occiput; up-slanting palpebral fissures; epicanthal folds, prominent eyes secondary to hypoplastic supraorbital ridges; highly arched eyebrows; midfacial hypoplasia with a short nose, depressed nasal bridge, anteverted nares, and long philtrum; small mouth, micrognathia; posteriorly rotated, poorly formed ears with hypoplastic, adherent ear lobes; short broad neck with low hairline.

Limbs. Long middle phalanges of the fingers with extra flexion creases; short distal phalanges with short nails; excess in whorl patterns on fingertips; foot positioning defects; simian crease.

Cardiovascular. Ventricular septal defects, patent ductus arteriosus, and/or pulmonic stenosis in one third to one half of patients.

Other. Scoliosis, widely spaced nipples, diastasis recti, inguinal and/or umbilical hernia, micropenis and/or cryptorchidism in males; hypoplastic labia majora in females.

OCCASIONAL ABNORMALITIES. Cleft palate; choanal atresia; postaxial polydactyly; diaphragmatic hernia; hydronephrosis; radiographic anomalies of ribs, clavicles, and vertebrae.

ETIOLOGY. Deletion of the distal portion of the short arm of chromosome 9. In most cases, the breakpoint is located at band 9p22 and the deletion is de novo.

COMMENT. In cases in which the 9p deletion is associated with another unbalanced chromosome segment, the break point usually occurs at 9p24. Most of them are inherited from a balanced translocation carrier parent. Mean I.Q. in those cases is 46 with a range from 33 to 57. Trigonocephaly, long philtrum, digital anomalies, and hernias are all usually present despite the variability of the associated unbalanced chromosome segment.

References

Alfi, O. S., et al.: Deletion of the short arm of chromosome 9(46,9p−): A new deletion syndrome. Ann. Genet., *16*:17, 1973.

Alfi, O. S., et al.: The 9p− syndrome. Ann. Genet., *19*: 11, 1976.

Mattei, J. F., et al.: Pericentric inversion, inv(9)(p22q32), in the father of a child with a duplication-deletion of chromosome 9 and gene dosage effect for adenylate kinase-I. Clin. Genet., *17*, 129, 1980.

Huret, J. L., et al.: Eleven new cases of del (9p) and features from 80 cases. J. Med. Genet., *25*:741, 1988.

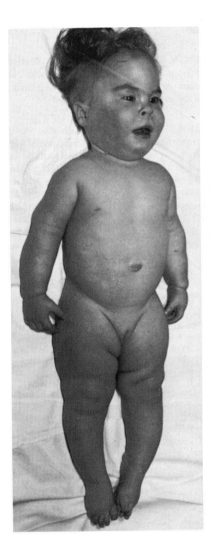

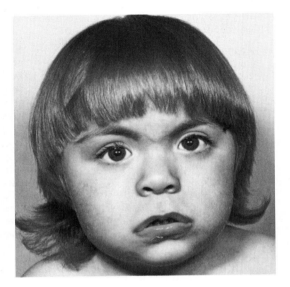

FIGURE 1. Deletion 9p syndrome. *Left*, A 10-month-old patient. Note trigonocephalic configuration of the skull with metopic prominence, up-slanting palpebral fissures, short nose with anteverted nostrils, and short and broad neck. *Right*, An 18-month-old patient. Full, round face with low, narrow forehead, synophrys, and short nose with anteverted nostrils. (Courtesy of Dr. Albert Schinzel, University of Zürich.)

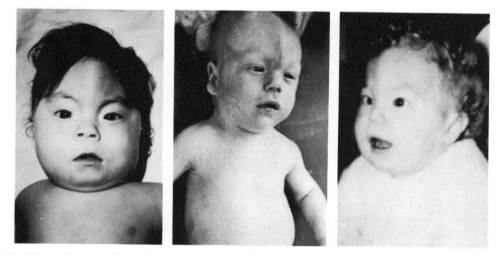

FIGURE 2. Three affected individuals with deletion 9p syndrome. (From Alfi, O., et al.: Ann. Genet., *19*:11, 1976, with permission.)

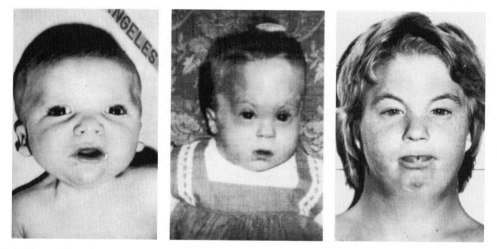

FIGURE 3. Three affected individuals with deletion 9p syndrome (From Alfi, O., et al.: Ann. Genet., *19*:11, 1976, with permission.)

DUPLICATION 9p SYNDROME

(Trisomy 9p Syndrome)

*Distal Phalangeal Hypoplasia, Delayed
Closure of Anterior Fontanel, Ocular Hypertelorism*

First reported in 1970 by Rethoré et al., the pattern of malformation was set forth by Centerwall and Beatty-DeSana in 1975. Approximately 100 patients have now been described.

ABNORMALITIES

Growth. Growth deficiency, primarily of postnatal onset. Delayed puberty such that some patients continue to grow up to the middle of their third decade.

Performance. Severe mental deficiency. Language tends to be most significantly delayed.

Craniofacies. Microcephaly, hypertelorism, down-slanting palpebral fissures, deep-set eyes, prominent nose, downturned corners of the mouth, cup-shaped ears.

Limbs. Short fingers and toes with small nails and short terminal phalanges; fifth finger clinodactyly with single flexion crease. Single palmar crease.

Other Skeletal. Kyphoscoliosis, usually developing during the second decade; hypoplasia of periscapular muscles with deep acromial dimples; defective ossification of the pubic bone, broad ischial tuberosity; pseudoepiphysis of metacarpals, metatarsals, and middle phalanges of fifth fingers; delayed closure of cranial sutures and fontanels.

OCCASIONAL ABNORMALITIES.
Micrognathia; epicanthal folds, short or webbed neck; partial two-three syndactyly of toes and three-four syndactyly of fingers, congenital heart defects in 5 to 10 per cent of cases and cleft lip and/or palate in 5 per cent; hydrocephalus, renal malformations, micropenis, cryptorchidism, hypospadias, talipes equinovarus, and congenital hip dislocation.

NATURAL HISTORY. Approximately 5 to 10 per cent of reported patients have died in early childhood.

ETIOLOGY. The degree of clinical severity correlates with the extent of triplicated material. However, mental retardation occurs in virtually all patients. Partial trisomy 9pter→p21 is associated with mild craniofacial features and rare skeletal or visceral defects. Partial trisomy 9pter→p11 is associated with the typical craniofacial features, while partial trisomy 9pter→q11-13 is associated not only with the typical craniofacial features but also skeletal and cardiac defects. Partial trisomy 9pter→q22-32 is associated with the typical craniofacial features, intrauterine growth deficiency, cleft lip/palate, micrognathia, cardiac anomalies, and congenital hip dislocation. If the trisomic segment is larger than that (9pter→9q31 or 32), the clinical findings no longer fit into the trisomy 9p syndrome but rather resemble trisomy 9 mosaic syndrome.

References

Rethoré, M. O., et al.: Sur quatre cas de trisomie pour le bras court du chromosome 9. Individualisation d'une nouvelle entité morbide. Ann. Genet., *13*:217, 1970.

Centerwall, W. R., and Beatty-Desana, J. W.: The trisomy 9p syndrome. Pediatrics, *56*:748, 1975.

Centerwall, W. R., et al.: Familial "partial 9p" trisomy: Six cases and four carriers in three generations. J. Med. Genet., *13*:57, 1976.

Schinzel, A.: Trisomy 9p, a chromosome aberration with distinct radiologic findings. Radiology, *130*: 125, 1979.

Wilson, G. N., et al.: The phenotypic and cytogenetic spectrum of partial trisomy 9. Am. J. Med. Genet., *20*:277, 1985.

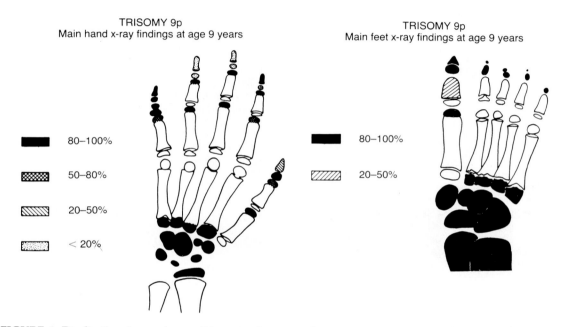

FIGURE 1. Duplication 9p syndrome. Diagram of major radiologic findings in hand and foot of a 9-year-old patient. Pseudoepiphyses on metacarpals and metatarsals 2 to 5; notches on metacarpal 1, metatarsal 1, and proximal and middle phalanges of fingers; hypoplasia of the middle phalanx of fifth finger, terminal phalanges of fingers, and middle and terminal phalanges of toes; thick epiphyses, especially of terminal phalanges of big toe, thumb, and little finger; and clinodactyly of fifth finger. (From Schinzel, A.: Radiology, *130*:125, 1979, with permission.)

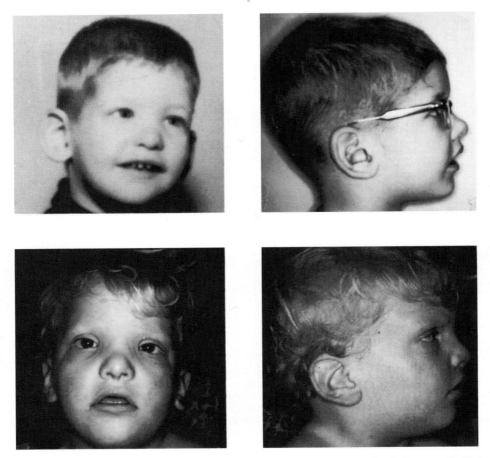

FIGURE 2. Two children with duplication 9p syndrome. (Courtesy of Dr. Willard Centerwall, University of California, Davis, Calif.)

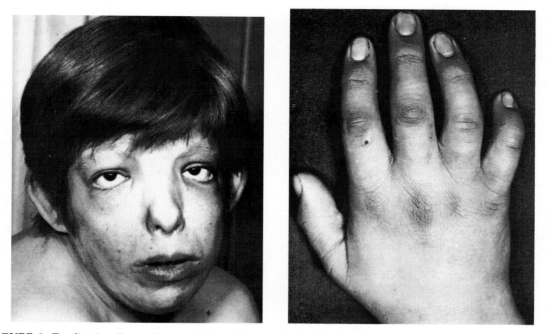

FIGURE 3. Duplication 9p syndrome. *Left,* A 21-year-old female patient. Note low forehead, hypertelorism, down-slanting palpebral fissures, bulbous nose, short distance between nose and upper lip, thick lips, protruding ears, and short neck. *Right,* Hand from a 17-year-old patient. Short hand and fingers, clinodactyly of little finger, and hypoplastic terminal phalanges of thumbs and nails of thumb and little finger. (Right photo from Schinzel, A., et al.: Hum. Genet., *30*:307, 1975, with permission.)

DUPLICATION 10q SYNDROME

Ptosis, Short Palpebral Fissures, Camptodactyly

First set forth as a specific phenotype by Yunis and Sanchez in 1974, this disorder has been further delineated by Klep-de Pater et al. in 1979.

ABNORMALITIES
Growth. Prenatal onset growth deficiency; mean birth weight of 2.7 kg.
Performance. Severe mental deficiency.
Craniofacies. Microcephaly; flat face with high forehead and high, arched eyebrows; ptosis; short palpebral fissures; microphthalmia; broad and depressed nasal bridge, anteverted nares, bow-shaped mouth with prominent upper lip; cleft palate; malformed posteriorly rotated ears.
Limbs. Camptodactyly, proximally placed thumbs, syndactyly between second and third toes, foot position anomalies, hypoplastic dermal ridge patterns.
Other. Heart and renal malformations—each occurs in approximately one half of affected patients; kyphoscoliosis; pectus excavatum; 11 pairs of ribs; cryptorchidism.

OCCASIONAL ABNORMALITIES. Brain malformations, ocular anomalies, malrotation of the gut, hypospadias, vertebral malformations, postaxial hexadactyly of hands, streak gonads.

NATURAL HISTORY. Approximately one half of reported patients died within the first year of life, usually from congenital heart defects and other malformations. Surviving children showed marked mental deficiency and usually are bedridden without the ability to communicate.

ETIOLOGY. Trisomy 10q24→qter, the distal segment of the long arm of chromosome 10.

References

Yunis, J. J., et al.: A new syndrome resulting from partial trisomy for the distal third of the long arm of chromosome 10. J. Pediatr., *84*:567, 1974.
Klep-de Pater, J. M., et al.: Partial trisomy 10q. A recognizable syndrome. Hum. Genet. *46*:29, 1979.

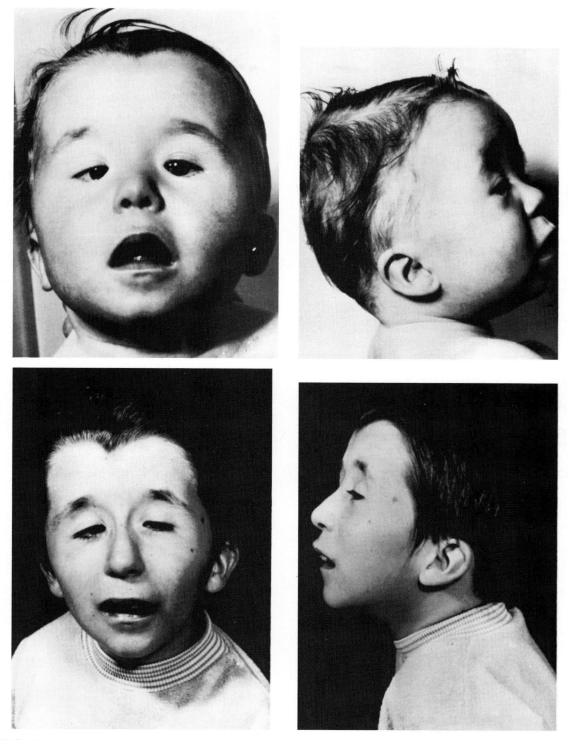

FIGURE 1. Duplication 10q syndrome. *Above*, A 2-year-old patient. Note high forehead, down-slanting palpebral fissures, narrow lids, small nose, and low-set ears. *Below*, Same patient at 10 years of age. (From Bühler, E., et al.: Helv. Pediatr. Acta, 22:41, 1967, with permission.)

ANIRIDIA–WILMS TUMOR ASSOCIATION

(WAGR Syndrome)

11

Numerous cases of the association of Wilms tumor and aniridia have been reported, and it is estimated that 1 in 70 patients with aniridia also has Wilms tumor. In 1978, Riccardi et al. identified an interstitial deletion of 11p in a group of patients with aniridia and Wilms tumor, who also had genitourinary anomalies and mental retardation, a pattern of malformation referred to as WAGR syndrome. The features of that disorder are set forth below.

ABNORMALITIES

Performance. Moderate to severe mental deficiency in most patients.

Growth. Growth deficiency and microcephaly in at least one half of the patients.

Craniofacial. Prominent lips, micrognathia, poorly formed ears.

Eyes. Aniridia in most patients; congenital cataracts, nystagmus, ptosis, blindness.

Genitalia. Cryptorchidism, hypospadias.

Wilms Tumor. In one half of the patients.

OCCASIONAL ABNORMALITIES.
Glaucoma, kyphoscoliosis, inguinal hernias, ambiguous external genitalia, cystic lesions of the kidney, streak gonads, gonadoblastoma, fifth finger clinodactyly, ventricular septal defects.

ETIOLOGY.
Most cases represent a de novo 11p13 deletion. Differences in the size of the deleted segment (especially distal to 11p13) in individual cases may account for the observed variability in concomitant features and in the degree of growth and mental deficiency. Deletions of segments in 11p, not including 11p13, do not cause the aniridia–Wilms tumor association. Familial occurrence resulting from unbalanced transmission of a balanced insertional translocation has been recorded. An interstitial deletion in 11p should be particularly sought in the cytogenetic investigation of mentally retarded patients with Wilms tumor and/or aniridia.

COMMENT.
It has been estimated that one third of patients with sporadic aniridia develop Wilms tumor, while 50 per cent of patients with aniridia, genitourinary anomalies, and mental retardation develop Wilms tumor. The risk of Wilms tumor in patients with aniridia who have a cytogenetically detectable deletion of 11p13 increases to 60 per cent. Patients with sporadic cases of aniridia should be monitored for Wilms tumor even if the chromosomes and phenotype are otherwise normal.

References

Anderson, S. R., et al.: Aniridia, cataract and gonadoblastoma in a mentally retarded girl with deletion of chromosome 11. Ophthalmologica, 176:171, 1978.

Riccardi, V. M., et al.: Chromosomal imbalance in the aniridia–Wilms' tumor association: 11p interstitial deletion. Pediatrics, 61:604, 1978.

Francke, U., et al.: Aniridia–Wilms' tumor association: Evidence for specific deletion of 11p13. Cytogenet. Cell Genet., 24:;185, 1979.

Hittner, H. M., Riccardi, V. M., and Francke, U.: Aniridia caused by a heritable chromosome 11 deletion. Ophthalmology, 86:1173, 1979.

Yunis, J. J., and Ramsay, N. K. C.: Familial occurrence of the aniridia–Wilms tumor syndrome with deletion 11p13-14.1. J. Pediatr., 96:1027, 1980.

Clericuzio, C. L.: Clinical phenotypes and Wilms' tumor. Med. Pediatr. Oncol., 21:182, 1993.

Pavilack, M. A., and Walton, D. S.: Genetics of aniridia: The aniridia–Wilms' tumor association. Int. Ophthalmol. Clin., 33:77, 1993.

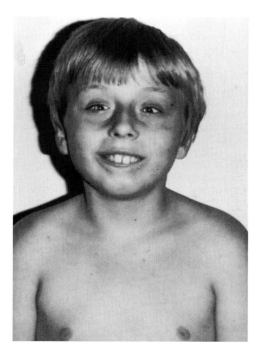
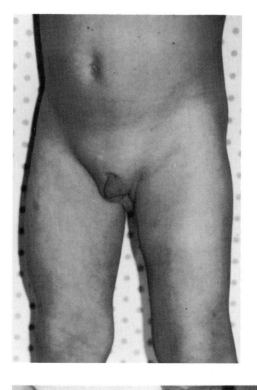
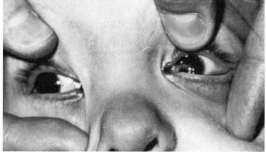
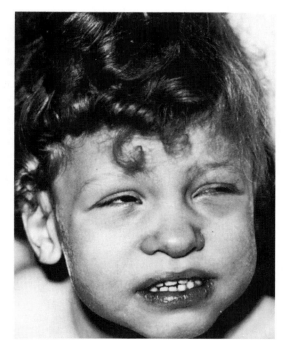

FIGURE 1. *Above*, Facies and micropenis in a boy with aniridia–Wilms tumor association. (Courtesy of Dr. Vincent M. Riccardi.) *Below*, A 2-year-old boy with microcephaly, bilateral aniridia, ptosis, and cataract. The patient also has Wilms tumor on the right side. (Courtesy of Dr. B. Zabel, Mainz, Germany.)

DELETION 11q SYNDROME

Trigonencephaly; Large, Carp-Shaped Mouth; Cardiac Defects

Described initially by Jacobsen et al. in 1973, greater than 30 cases of this disorder have now been reported. In the majority of cases the deletion involves band 11q23→qter. However, it appears than the clinical phenotype is due to deletion of subband 11q24.1.

ABNORMALITIES.
Growth. Intrauterine growth retardation (76 per cent). Failure to thrive (35 per cent).
Performance. Mental deficiency (96 per cent). Approximately one half are in the moderate range, the remainder are more severely effected. Hypotonia in infancy frequently progressing toward spasticity.
Craniofacies. Trigonencephaly (90 per cent). Microcephaly (40 per cent). Epicanthal folds (60 per cent). Ocular hypertelorism (70 per cent). Ptosis (67 per cent). Strabismus (75 per cent). Depressed nasal bridge (93 per cent). Short nose with upturned nasal tip (91 per cent). Large, carp-shaped mouth (78 per cent). Micrognathia (77.7 per cent). Low-set and/or malformed ears (85 per cent).
Other. Joint contractures (65 per cent). Cardiac defect (60 per cent). Hypospadius and/or cryptorchidism (50 per cent).

OCCASIONAL ABNORMALITIES. Macrocephaly, hydrocephalus, holoprosencephaly, ocular coloboma, optic atrophy, retinal reduplication, retinal dysplasia, abnormality of supratentorial white matter on CT scan, short neck, digital anomalies including hammer position of great toes, fifth finger clinodactyly, brachydactyly, pyloric stenosis, inguinal hernia, renal malformations, vesico-vaginal fistula, hypoplasia of labia and clitoris.

NATURAL HISTORY. Death related to their cardiac defect has occurred in approximately 25 per cent of cases. The remainder except for recurrent respiratory infections are healthy. Mental deficiency, which occurs in 100 per cent of patients, ranges from moderate to severe.

ETIOLOGY. Partial deletion of the long arm of chromosome 11 involving 11q23→qter; most commonly a simple deletion and occasionally as part of a ring-11 chromosome. The critical subband responsible for this disorder is most likely 11q24.1. Seventy-five per cent of affected individuals are female.

References

Jacobsen, P. H., et al.: An (11;21) translocation in four generations with chromosome 11 abnormalities in the offspring. Hum. Hered., 23:568, 1973.

Schinzel, A., et al.: Partial deletion of long arm of chromosome 11[del(11)(q23)]: Jacobsen syndrome. J. Med. Genet., 14:438, 1977.

O'Hare, A. E., et al.: Deletion of the long arm of chromosome 11 [46,XX,del(11)(q24.1→qtr)]. Clin. Genet., 25:373, 1984.

Fryns, J. P., et al.: Distal 11q monosomy. The typical 11q monosomy syndrome is due to deletion of subband 11q24.1. Clin Genet., 30:255, 1986.

Wardinsky, T. D., et al.: Partial deletion of the long arm of chromosome 11[del(11)(q23.3→qtr)] with abnormal white matter. Am. J. Med. Genet., 35:60, 1990.

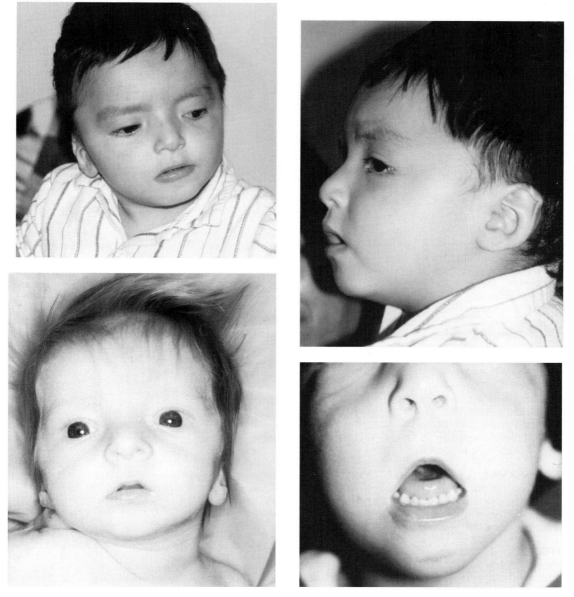

FIGURE 1. Three affected children. Note the ocular hypertelorism, malformed ears, and carp-shaped mouth.

DELETION 13q SYNDROME

(13q– Syndrome)

Microcephaly With High Nasal Bridge, Eye Defect, Thumb Hypoplasia

Partial deletion of the long arm of one of the D-group chromosomes was initially reported in 1963 by Lele et al. in a mentally deficient and growth deficient patient with retinoblastoma. Subsequently, well over 100 cases have been recorded, and the deleted chromosome has been considered to be number 13. The phenotype has been variable, but a pattern of malformation is emerging that should allow for suspicion of this disorder. A similar phenotype has been noted in 13 ring chromosome patients who are missing part of the short arm as well as part of the long arm of chromosome 13. The features listed below are those found in del(13q) patients.

ABNORMALITIES

Growth. Growth deficiency, usually of prenatal onset.

Central Nervous System. Mental deficiency. Microcephaly with tendency toward trigonocephaly and holoprosencephaly-type of brain defects.

Facial. Prominent nasal bridge, hypertelorism. Ptosis, epicanthal folds, microphthalmia, colobomata. Retinoblastoma, usually bilateral. Prominent maxilla, micrognathia. Prominent ears, slanting, low placement.

Neck. Short, webbing.

Limbs. Small to absent thumbs, clinodactyly of fifth finger, fused metacarpal bones 4 and 5. Talipes equinovarus, short big toe.

Cardiac. Cardiac defect.

Genitalia. Hypospadias, cryptorchidism.

Other. Focal lumbar agenesis.

OCCASIONAL ABNORMALITIES.
Optic nerve and retinal dysplasia, colobomata, facial asymmetry, posterior auricular pits, narrow palate, imperforate anus, Hirschsprung disease, bifid scrotum, pelvic anomaly, renal anomaly.

ETIOLOGY.
Deletion of part of the long arm of a 13 chromosome. Ring 13 chromosome individuals may have a similar pattern of malformation.

COMMENT.
The natural history is dependent on the deleted segment. Patients with proximal deletions not extending into q32 have mild to moderate mental retardation, variable minor anomalies, and growth retardation. If the q14 region is involved, a significant risk exists for retinoblastoma. Patients with more distal deletions including at least part of q32 usually have severe mental retardation; growth deficiency; and major malformations including microcephaly and CNS defects, distal limb anomalies, eye defects, and gastrointestinal malformations. Patients with the most distal deletions, involving q33-q34, have severe mental retardation but usually lack growth deficiency or gross structural malformations.

Although the majority of patients with deletions of chromosome 13 involving the q14 region develop retinoblastoma, it has been estimated that 13 to 20 per cent remain unaffected. Chromosome studies would seem merited in all patients with retinoblastoma.

References

Lele, K. P., Penrose, L. S., and Stallarf, H. B.: Chromosome deletion in a case of retinoblastoma. Ann. Hum. Genet., 27:171, 1963.

Allerdice, P. W., et al.: The 13q-deletion syndrome. Am. J. Hum. Genet., 21:499, 1969.

Taylor, A. I.: Dq–, Dr and retinoblastoma. Humangenetik, 10:209, 1970.

Yunis, J. J., and Ramsay, N.: Retinoblastoma and sub band deletion of chromosome 13. Am. J. Dis. Child., 132:161, 1978.

Riccardi, V. M., et al.: Partial triplication and deletion of 13q: Study of a family presenting with bilateral retinoblastoma. Clin. Genet., 18:332, 1979.

Wilson, W. G., et al.: Deletion (13) (q14.1q14.3) in two generations: Variability of ocular manifestations and definition of the phenotype. Am. J. Med. Genet., 28:675, 1987.

Tranebjaerg, L., et al.: Interstitial deletion 13q: Further delineation of the syndrome by clinical and high-resolution chromosome analysis of five patients. Am. J. Med. Genet., 29:739, 1988.

Brown, S., et al.: Preliminary definition of a "critical region" of chromosome 13 in q32: Report of 14 cases with 13q deletions and review of the literature. Am. J. Med. Genet., 45:52, 1993.

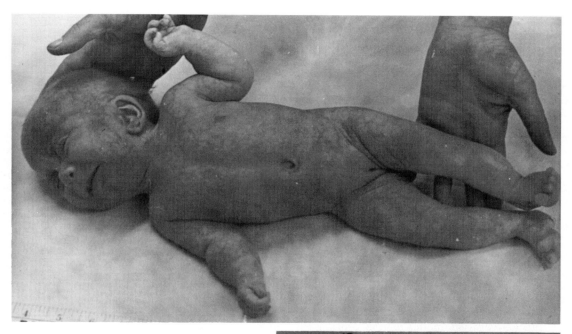

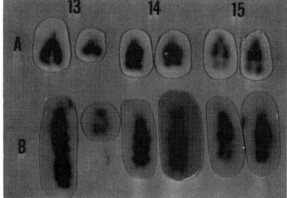

FIGURE 1. *Above*, Patient who died at 3 months, with microcephaly, cleft palate, low-set ears, short neck with slight webbing, relatively short limbs with clenched hands, short sternum, and marked cutis marmorata. *Right*, D-group chromosomes showing del(13q) in the patient (*A*) and her mother (*B*), who is a 13/13 balanced translocation carrier. (Courtesy of Dr. M. Jansch.)

DUPLICATION 15q SYNDROME

Prominent Nose With Broad Nasal Bridge, Camptodactyly, Cardiac Defects

Initially described by Fujimoto et al., duplication of distal 15q has been described now in at least 28 additional cases. The breakpoints have all been between bands 15q21 and 15q23 except for two families with breakpoints at 15q25 and two families with breakpoints at 15q15. The clinical phenotype is consistent and recognizable.

ABNORMALITIES

Growth. Prenatal growth deficiency (15 per cent). Postnatal growth deficiency (60 per cent). Tall stature (11 per cent).

Performance. Severe to profound mental deficiency (92 per cent). Two patients with duplication of 15q25→qter were only mildly retarded.

Craniofacies. Microcephaly (37 per cent). Sloping forehead (71 per cent). Short palpebral fissures (78 per cent). Down-slanting palpebral fissures (71 per cent). Ptosis (56 per cent). Prominent nose with broad nasal bridge (96 per cent). Long, well-defined philtrum (77 per cent). Midline crease in lower lip (86 per cent). Micrognathia (88 per cent). Puffy cheeks (70 per cent).

Skeletal. Pectus excavatum (46 per cent). Scoliosis (60 per cent). Short neck with or without vertebral anomalies (68 per cent).

Hands. Arachnodactyly (75 per cent). Camptodactyly (100 per cent).

Other. Cardiac defects (69 per cent).

OCCASIONAL ABNORMALITIES. Genital abnormalities including cryptochidism and hypoplastic labia majora, preauricular pit.

NATURAL HISTORY. Death primarily related to congenital heart defects, recurrent respiratory infections, and aspiration pneumonia has occurred in one third of patients. A 27-year-old mentally retarded male is the oldest known survivor.

ETIOLOGY. Duplication of distal 15q. The majority of cases have resulted from unbalanced translocations, all but one of which were the offspring of a balanced carrier parent. Despite the fact that the second chromosome involved in the reciprocal translocation has varied, the clinical phenotype is consistent.

References

Fujimoto, A., et al.: Inherited partial duplication of chromosome No. 15. J. Med. Genet., *11*:287, 1974.

Lacro, R. V., et al.: Duplication of distal 15q: Report of five new cases from two different translocation kindreds. Am. J. Med. Genet., *26*:19, 1987.

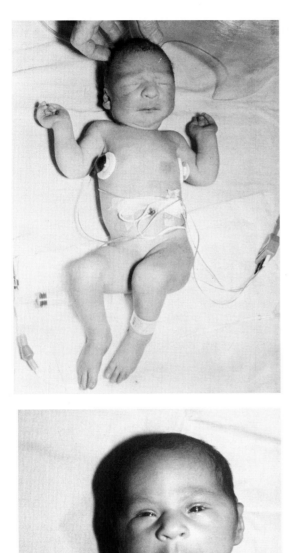

FIGURE 1. *Above*, Newborn female infant. Note the sloping forehead, down-slanting palpebral fissures, and prominent nose with broad nasal bridge. *Below*, Affected female at birth and 41 months. (From Lacro, R. V., et al.: Am. J. Med. Genet., 26:719, 1987, with permission of Wiley-Liss, a division of John Wiley & Sons.)

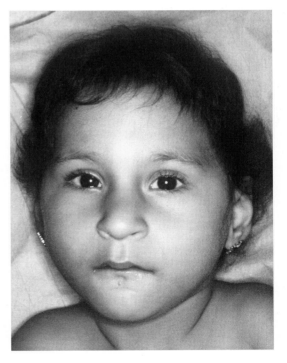

DELETION 18p SYNDROME

(18p– Syndrome)

Mental and Growth Deficiencies,
Ptosis or Epicanthal Folds, Prominent Auricles

Deletion of the short arm of chromosome 18 was first noted by de Grouchy et al. in 1963. Subsequently, more than 100 cases have been reported. There is rather broad variability in the phenotype.

ABNORMALITIES. The most consistent features are listed below.
Growth. Mild to moderate growth deficiency.
Central Nervous System. Mental deficiency, tendency toward hypotonia. Microcephaly (mild) (29 per cent).
Facial. Ptosis (38 per cent), epicanthal folds (40 per cent), low nasal bridge, hypertelorism (41 per cent) rounded facies, micrognathia (25 per cent), wide mouth, downturning corners of mouth, large protruding ears.
Dental. High frequency of caries (29 per cent).
Limbs. Relatively small hands and feet.
Other. Pectus excavatum.

OCCASIONAL OR UNCERTAIN INCIDENCE

Immunologic. IgA absence or deficiency, usually asymptomatic.
Central Nervous System and Facial. Holoprosencephaly arhinencephaly-type defect (12 per cent).
Skin and Hair. Alopecia (three cases), hypopigmentation.
Other. Cataract, strabismus (15 per cent), webbed neck, broad chest, cleft palate, kyphoscoliosis, clinodactyly of fifth fingers (21 per cent), syndactyly (11 per cent), simian crease, cubitus valgus, pectus excavatum (17 per cent), inguinal hernia, dislocation of hip (9 per cent), talipes equinovarus (13 per cent), genital anomalies (18 per cent). Development of rheumatoid arthritis–like signs and symptoms. Polymyositis. Cardiac defects (10 per cent). Ulerythema ophryogenes (i.e., reticular erythema, small horny papules, atrophy, and permanent loss of hairs in outer halves of eyebrows sometimes extending to adjacent skin, scalp, and cheeks).

NATURAL HISTORY. Mild to severe mental deficiency. I.Q.s range from 25 to 75, with an average of about 45 to 50. There is a dissociation between language ability and practical performance; many do not speak even simple sentences before 7 to 9 years of age. Restlessness, emotional lability, fear of strangers, and lack of ability to concentrate. They can best be helped in small groups intended especially for the mentally deficient. The prognosis is poor for those patients with holoprosencephaly-type defect. Otherwise, life expectancy does not seem to be impaired. Alopecia, when a problem, develops during infancy. Adequate adaptation has occurred in some patients, and they can be capable of reproduction.

ETIOLOGY. Short arm 18 deletion, sometimes as part of the deficiency in a ring 18 chromosome. Parents should be studied to determine whether either is a balanced translocation carrier or has the unbalanced 18p– deletion. Offspring from a parent with the same deletion have been affected, who presumably would have a 50 per cent risk.

Sex ratio (female:male) is 3:2. The mean parental ages of 32 years for the mothers and 38 for the fathers are older then average.

References

De Grouchy, J., et al.: Dysmorphie complexe avec oligophrénie: Délétion des bras courts d'un chromosome 17–18. D. R. Acad. Sci. [D] (Paris), 256:1028, 1963.

Uchida, I. A., et al.: Familial short arm deficiency of chromosome 18 concomitant with arhinencephaly and alopecia congenita. Am. J. Hum. Genet., 17:410, 1965.

Reinwein, H., et al.: Defizienz am kurzen Arm eines Chromosoms Nr. 18 (46,XX,18p–). Ein einheitliches Missbildungs syndrom. Monatsschr. Kinderheilkd., 116:511, 1968.

Schinzel, A., et al.: The 18p– syndrome. Arch. Genetik, 47:1, 1974.

Movahhedian, H. R., et al.: Heart disease associated with deletion of the short arm of chromosome 18. Del. Med. J., 63:285, 1991.

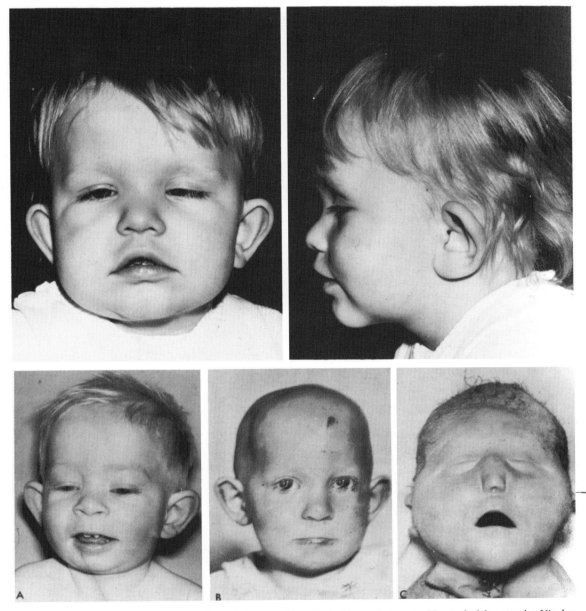

FIGURE 1. Deletion 18p syndrome. *Above,* A 3-year-old patient. (From Reinwein, H., et al.: Monatsschr. Kinderheilkd., *116*:511, 1968, with permission.) *Below,* Mother (mosaic 18p−/normal) shown as a child (*B*) and two of her affected offspring (*A* and *C*), showing variability in expression for the same inherited del(18p), including alopecia (*B*) and cebocephaly (*C*). (From Uchida, I. A., et al.: Am. J. Hum. Genet., *17*:410, 1965, with permission.)

DELETION 18q SYNDROME

(Long Arm 18 Deletion Syndrome, 18q– Syndrome

Midfacial Hypoplasia, Prominent Antihelix, Whorl Digital Pattern

Discovered by de Grouchy et al. in 1964, this genetic imbalance syndrome has been documented in more than 29 cases.

ABNORMALITIES. The most consistent features are listed below.
Growth. Small stature.
Performance. Mental deficiency with hypotonia, poor coordination, nystagmus, conductive deafness, seizures.
Craniofacial. Microcephaly. Midfacial hypoplasia with deep-set eyes. Carp-shaped mouth, narrow palate.
Ears. Prominent antihelix, antiragus, or both. Narrow or atretic external canal.
Limbs. Long hands, tapering fingers, and short first metacarpal with proximal thumb. High-frequency whorl digital pattern, distal axial triradius, simian crease. Distal hypoplastic tapering of lower legs. Abnormal toe placement. Vertical talus with or without talipes equinovarus.
Genitalia. Female: hypoplastic labia minora. Male: cryptorchidism with or without small scrotum and penis.
Other. Skin dimples over acromion and knuckles. Cardiac defect.

OCCASIONAL ABNORMALITIES
Eyes. Inner epicanthal folds, slanted palpebral fissures, ocular hypertelorism, microphthalmia, corneal abnormality, iris hypoplasia, cataract, retinal defect, abnormal optic disk, myopia.
Ears. Atretic middle ear, low-set ears.
Other. Cleft palate (30 per cent), cleft lip, widely spaces nipples, extra rib, horseshoe kidney, lipomata at lateral border of feet. Choreoathetotic movements. Eczema. Absence of IgA. Atrophy of olfactory and optic nerves. Poor myelination of central white matter tracts with relatively normal myelination of corpus callosum. Hydrocephalus, porencephaly, cerebellar hypoplasia.

NATURAL HISTORY. Mental deficiency, with I.Q.s from 40 to 85, and growth deficiency, coupled with various visual and hearing problems, may leave these individuals seriously handicapped. Behavioral problems, including obnoxious or autistic behavior, may be features. However, some patients with this deletion have not been severely affected. For example, a 10-year-old child studied by Wertelecki and Gerald was not obviously debilitated.

ETIOLOGY. Variable deletions of part of the long arm of chromosome 18 from 18q21.3 or 18q22.2 to qter. In general the size of the deletion correlates with the severity of the phenotype.

References

De Grouchy, J., et al.: Délétion partielle du bras long du chromosome 18. Path. Biol. (Paris), *12*:579, 1964.
Wertelecki, W., and Gerald, P. S.: Clinical and chromosomal studies of the 18q– syndrome. J. Pediatr., *78*:44, 1971.
Miller, G., et al.: Neurologic manifestations in 18q– syndrome. Am. J. Med. Genet., *37*:128, 1990.
Kline, A. D., et al.: Molecular analysis of the 18q– syndrome and correlation with phenotype. Am. J. Hum. Genet., *52*:895, 1993.

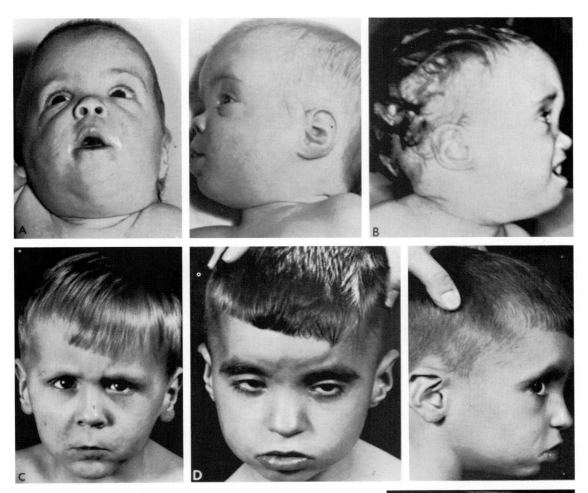

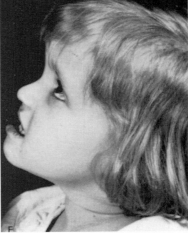

FIGURE 1. Deletion 18q syndrome. *A*, Young infant. Note shape of mouth, midfacial hypoplasia, and prominent antihelix. (Courtesy of E. Engel, Vanderbilt University.) *B*, Infant. Note prominent antihelix and absence of external auditory canal openings. *C*, Note mild slant to palpebral fissures, strabismus, and facial asymmetry. *D*, Note mouth and micrognathia. *E*, Note prominent forehead in relation to hypoplasia of midface. (*B* to *E* courtesy of W. Wertelecki, National Cancer Institute— NIH, P. S. Gerald, Boston Children's Hospital.)

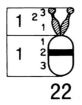

CAT-EYE SYNDROME

(Coloboma of Iris–Anal Atresia Syndrome)

*Coloboma of Iris, Down-Slanting
Palpebral Fissures, Anal Atresia*

Anal atresia and colobomata of the iris, initially considered the hallmarks of this disorder, are present in combination in only a minority of the 40 patients reported.

ABNORMALITIES

Performance. Usually mild mental deficiency. Some patients have been of normal intelligence but emotionally retarded.

Growth. Normal in the majority of cases.

Craniofacial. Mild hypertelorism; down-slanting palpebral fissures; inferior coloboma of iris, choroid, and/or retina; micrognathia, preauricular pits, and/or tags.

Cardiac. Cardiac defects in more than one third of cases, including total anomalous pulmonary venous return and persistence of the left superior vena cava.

Anus. Anal atresia with rectovestibular fistula.

Renal. Renal agenesis.

OCCASIONAL ABNORMALITIES. Microphthalmos; low-set, malformed ears with stenotic external canals; biliary atresia; dislocation of hip; radial aplasia; cleft palate; malrotation of gut; agenesis of uterus and fallopian tubes.

ETIOLOGY. Usually the result of an extra chromosome derived from two identical segments of chromosome 22, consisting of the satellites, the entire short arm, the centromere, and a tiny piece of the long arm (22pter→q11). That segment is thus present in quadruplicate.

The phenotype can also result from an interstitial duplication of the 22q11 region. In this latter situation the segment is present in triplicate, which may explain the few reported cases of cat-eye syndrome in which an extra chromosome is not present. Fluorescent in situ hybridization studies have been used successfully to document typical as well as atypical cases in which only a few of the features are present.

References

Schachenmann, G., et al.: Chromosomes in coloboma and anal atresia. Lancet, 2:290, 1965.

Darby, C. W., and Hughes, D. T.: Dermatoglyphics and chromosomes in cat-eye syndrome. Br. Med. J., 3:47, 1971.

Balci, S., et al.: The cat-eye syndrome with unusual skeletal malformations. Acta Paediatr. Scand., 63: 623, 1974.

Schinzel, A., et al.: The "cat eye syndrome": Dicentric small marker chromosome probably derived from a No. 22 (tetrasomy 22pter q11) associated with a characteristic phenotype. Report of 11 patients and delineation of the clinical picture. Hum. Genet., 57: 148, 1981.

McDermid, H. E., et al.: Characterization of the supernumerary chromosome in cat eye syndrome. Science, 232:646, 1986.

Liehr, T., et al.: Typical and partial cat eye syndrome: Identification of the marker chromosome by FISH. Clin. Genet., 42:91, 1992.

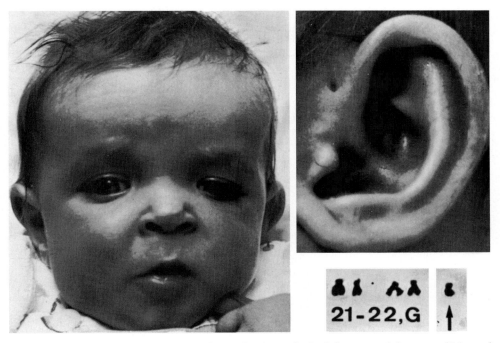

FIGURE 1. Cat-eye syndrome. Infant showing down-slanting palpebral fissures, colobomata of iris, and preauricular pits. *Arrow* denotes extra chromosome. (From Schmid, W.: J. Hum. Genet., *16*:89, 1967, with permission.)

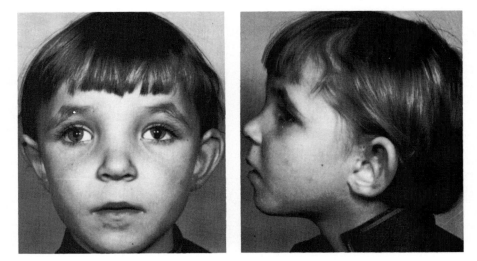

FIGURE 2. Cat-eye syndrome. A 4-year-old girl with hypertelorism, down-slanting palpebral fissures, total coloboma on left and peripheral coloboma on right iris, exotropia, and preauricular pit. (Courtesy of Dr. Albert Schinzel, University of Zürich Medical School.)

XYY SYNDROME

Tall Stature, Aberrant Behavior

Despite an incidence of 1 in 840 newborn males, the XYY individual is seldom detected during childhood or even in the adult. Based on studies of unselected newborns with sex chromosome anomalies who have been followed longitudinally, it is now recognized that the majority of XYY males are phenotypically normal. However, a pattern of variable abnormalities has come to be appreciated, which may allow for clinical suspicion of the XYY syndrome in childhood.

ABNORMALITIES. Variable features from among the following:

Growth. Acceleration in midchildhood.

Performance. Dull mentality. Full-scale I.Q. is within normal limits although usually lower than siblings (range, 80 to 140). Relative weakness, with poor fine motor coordination and sometimes a fine intentional tremor. Speech delay common. Learning disabilities (50 per cent).

Dentition. Large teeth.

Facies. Prominent glabella, asymmetry, long ears.

Skeletal. Increased length versus breadth; evident in cranial vault, hands, and feet. Mild pectus excavatum.

Skin. Severe nodulocystic acne at adolescence.

OCCASIONAL ABNORMALITIES

Skeletal. Radioulnar synostosis.

Genital. Cryptorchidism, small penis, hypospadias.

Other. EEG abnormality, EKG showing prolonged PR interval.

NATURAL HISTORY. Though affected patients are occasionally long at birth, the tendency toward tall stature is usually not evident until they reach 5 to 6 years of age. Despite the large size, these boys are usually not strong or well coordinated and tend to have poor development of the pectoral and shoulder girdle musculature. Behavioral problems, especially distractability, hyperactivity, and temper tantrums are present in childhood and early adolescence. Aggressive behavior is not usually a problem and they learn to control anger as they get older. Onset of puberty is approximately 6 months delayed. Heterosexual activity is normal. The majority of 47XYY males are fertile and have chromosomally normal offspring. However, an increased risk for offspring with chromosomal abnormalities as well as miscarriage and perinatal death has been suggested.

Although early reports suggested that there existed an overrepresentation of 47XYY individuals among institutionalized male juvenile delinquents, prospective longitudinal studies of unselected 47XYY males suggest that behavior disorders are not a significant problem for these individuals in childhood and adolescence.

COMMENT. Based on normal testicular biopsies on seven men with 47XYY to look for carcinoma in situ, it is concluded that men with a 47XYY karyotype are not at increased risk of developing gonadal tumors.

ETIOLOGY. The diagnosis is confirmed by chromosomal analysis revealing a 47XYY karyotype.

References

Sandberg, A. A., et al.: XYY human male. Lancet, 2: 488, 1961.

Daly, R. F.: Neurological abnormalities in XYY males. Nature, 221:472, 1969.

Sundequist, U., and Hellstrome, E.: Transmission of 47,XYY karyotype. Lancet, 2:1367, 1969.

Nielsen, J., Friedrich, U., and Zeuthen, E.: Stature and weight in boys with the XYY syndrome. Humangenetik, 14:66, 1971.

Voorhees, J. J., et al.: Nodulocystic acne as a phenotypic feature of the XYY genotype. Report of five cases, review of all known XYY subjects with severe acne, and discussion of XYY cytodiagnosis. Arch. Dermatol., 105:913, 1972.

Grass, F., et al.: Reproduction in XYY males: Two new cases and implications for genetic counseling. Am. J. Med. Genet., 19:533, 1984.

Muller, J., and Skakkeback, N. D.: Gonadal malignancy in individuals with sex chromosome anomalies. Birth Defects, 26(4):247, 1991.

Robinson, A., et al.: Sex chromosome aneuploids: The Denver prospective study. Birth Defects, 26(4):59, 1991.

Robinson, A., et al.: Summary of clinical findings in children and young adults with sex chromosome anomalies. Birth Defects, 26(4):225, 1991.

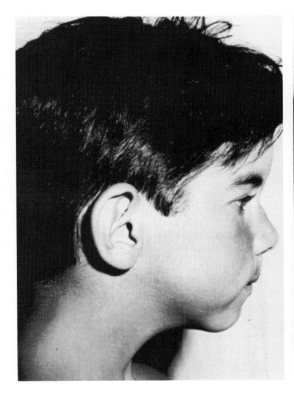
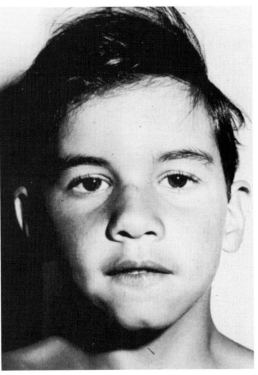
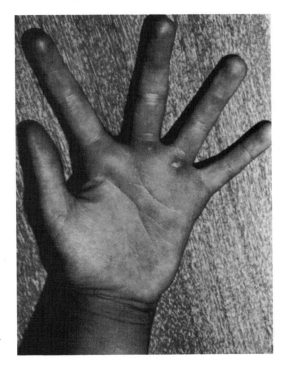

FIGURE 1. XYY syndrome. An 8-year-old boy, evaluated because of behavioral problems and poor school performance. Note the prominent glabella, relatively long face, and long fingers.

XXY SYNDROME, KLINEFELTER SYNDROME

Hypogenitalism and Hypogonadism, With or Without Long Legs, Dull Mentality, and/or Behavioral Problems

This disorder, initially described by Klinefelter et al. in 1942, is now appreciated as being the most common single cause of hypogonadism and infertility, affecting about 1 in 500 males.

ABNORMALITIES Variable features from among the following:

Performance. Although a wide range of I.Q.s has been noted from well below to well above average, mean full-scale I.Q. is between 85 and 90. Verbal I.Q. is usually higher than performance, with significant problems in expressive language, auditory processing abilities, and auditory memory leading to decreased ability to read and spell. Between 20 and 50 per cent have a fine to moderate intention tremor. Tendency toward behavior problems, especially immaturity, insecurity, shyness, poor judgment, and unrealistic boastful and assertive activity. The formation of peer relationships is difficult. Problems with psychosocial adjustment are increased, although significant psychiatric difficulties are not often encountered.

Growth. Tendency from childhood toward long limbs, with low upper to lower segment ratio and relatively tall and slim stature. Height ranges from the 25th to 99th percentile with a mean at the 75th percentile. Weight and head circumference at the 50th percentile.

Hypogonadism with Hypogenitalism. Childhood: Relatively small penis and testes. Adolescence and adulthood: Testes remain small, usually less than 2.5 cm in length. With rare exception, testosterone production is inadequate, with the average serum testosterone values in the adult being less than one half the normal value. Infertility is the rule, with hyalinization and fibrosis of the seminiferous tubules because of excess gonadotropin. Virilization is partial and inadequate, with gynecomastia occurring in one third of adolescents.

Other. Mild elbow dysplasia, fifth finger clinodactyly.

OCCASIONAL ABNORMALITIES. Genital: Cryptorchidism, hypospadias. Scoliosis during adolescent years. As adults, diabetes mellitus (8 per cent) and chronic bronchitis are more common. Mild to moderate ataxia occasionally occurs, and ulcerative breakdown of the skin over the anterior lower legs may develop. Germ cell tumors of the mediastinum.

NATURAL HISTORY. Most 47XXY boys enter puberty normally. Testosterone levels decrease in late adolescence and early adulthood. The majority of affected individuals require some help in school, particularly in reading and spelling. Some have been placed in full-time special education programs. A significant number of affected individuals can be expected to complete a college degree.

ETIOLOGY AND DIAGNOSIS. The diagnosis is confirmed by chromosomal analysis revealing a 47XXY karyotype. Paternal meiosis I errors account for about one half of 47XXY males while the remainder are due to maternal meiosis I errors, maternal meiosis II errors, and in a very small number of cases to a postzygotic mitotic error. There was no increase in paternal age associated with the paternally derived 47XXY males, but a marked increase in maternal age associated with maternally derived 47XXY males, the increase associated with maternal meiosis I but not meiosis II errors. Individuals with XXY/XY mosaicism have a better potential prognosis for testicular function. Other variants include XXYY, in which the patient is more likely to be mentally deficient and have behavioral problems, and XXXY, an abnormality that is characterized by mental deficiency, possible growth deficiency, and multiple minor anomalies, including radioulnar synostosis at the elbow.

MANAGEMENT. Diagnosis during childhood of XXY (or XXYY or XXXY) syndrome is helpful in allowing for prospective testosterone replacement therapy beginning at the age of 11 to 12 years, if and when studies show deficient testosterone and elevated gonadotropin values for maturational age. This will bring about a more usual adolescent development and prevent many of the features of adult Klinefelter syndrome that are due to testosterone insufficiency. Unfortunately, none of the commercially available androgen preparations is completely satisfactory. Injections of testosterone enanthate or cypionate at intervals no more frequently than every 2 weeks is most suitable.

References

Klinefelter, H. F., Jr., Reifenstein, E. C., Jr., and Albright, F.: Syndrome characterized by gynecomastia, aspermatogenesis without aleydigism and increased secretion of follicle-stimulating hormone (gynecomastia). J. Clin. Endocrinol. Metab., 2:615, 1942.

Caldwell, P. D., and Smith, D. W.: The XXY syndrome in childhood: Detection and treatment. J. Pediatr., 80:250, 1972.

Baughman, F. H., Higgin, J. V., and Mann, J.: Sex chromosome anomalies and essential tremor. Neurology, 23:623, 1973.

Jacobs, P. A., et al.: Klinefelter's syndrome: An analysis of the origin of the additional sex chromosome using molecular probes. Ann. Hum. Genet., 52:93, 1988.

Graham, J. M., et al.: Oral and written language abilities of XXY boys: Implications for anticipatory guidance. Pediatrics, 81:795, 1988.

Robinson, A., et al.: Summary of clinical findings in children and young adults with sex chromosome anomalies. Birth Defects 26(4):225, 1991.

Mandocki, M. W., and Summer, G. S.: Klinefelter syndrome: The need for early identification and treatment. Clin. Pediatr., 30:161, 1991.

Muller, J., and Skakkeback, N. E.: Gonadal malignancy in individuals with sex chromosome anomalies. Birth Defects, 26(4):247, 1991.

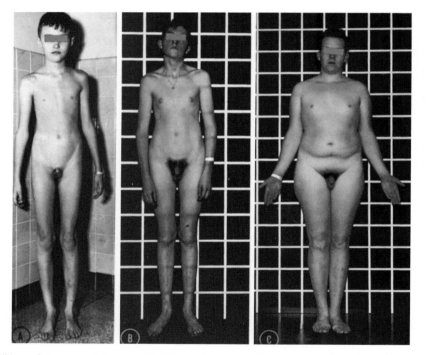

FIGURE 1. XXY syndrome. *A*, A 9-year-old child; note the small penis, long legs. *B*, A 16-year-old untreated XXY adolescent; note the gynecomastia and scoliosis. *C*, A 21-year-old untreated XXY adult; note the obesity, hypovirilization.

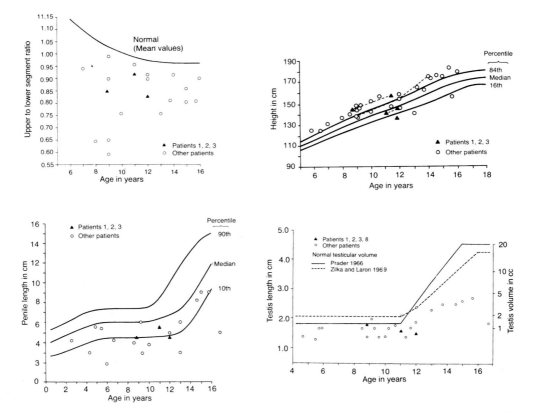

FIGURE 2. *D*, Measurements in XXY syndrome during childhood versus normals. (*D*, From Caldwell, P. D., and Smith, D, W.: J. Pediatr., *80*:250, 1972, with permission.)

XXXY AND XXXXY SYNDROMES

Hypogenitalism, Limited Elbow Pronation, Low Dermal Ridge Count on Fingertips

The greater the aneuploidy, from XXY to XXXXY, the more severe the growth deficiency, mental deficiency, hypogenitalism, and other features. The abnormalities listed below are for XXXXY syndrome, and the findings for XXXY syndrome extend from the milder XXY features toward this more severe end of the spectrum.

ABNORMALITIES

Performance. Mental deficiency, intelligence quotient of 20 to 70, mean I.Q. of 35. Hypotonia, joint laxity, or both, in about one third.

Growth. Tendency to low birth weight, shortness of stature, retarded osseous maturation — 53%

Craniofacial.
Sclerotic cranial sutures	57%
Wide-set eyes	80%
Upward slant to palpebral fissures	79%
Inner epicanthal folds	82%
Strabismus	59%
Low nasal bridge; wide, upturned nasal tip	95%
Mandibular prognathism	50%
Auricular anomaly (large, low-set, malformed)	70%

Neck
Short	72%

Thorax
Thick undersegmented sternum	75%

Limbs
Limited pronation at elbow	95%
Radioulnar synostosis	42%
Clinodactyly of fifth finger	90%
Coxa valga	25%
Genu valgum	50%
Pes planus	73%
Epiphyseal dysplasia, usually mild	—

Dermal ridge patterns. High frequency of low arch pattern on fingertips, with mean total ridge count of only 50, versus the average male total ridge count of 144.

Genitalia
Small penis	80%
Small testes, hypoplastic tubules, diminished Leydig cells	94%
Cryptorchidism	28%
Hypoplastic scrotum	80%

OCCASIONAL ABNORMALITIES. Obesity, flat occiput, microcephaly, arhinencephaly, hypoplasia of corpus callosum, seizures, antimongoloid slant to palpebral fissures, Brushfield speckled iris, myopia, cleft palate, cleft lip, small peg-shaped teeth, delayed eruption of teeth, taurodontism and enamel defects leading to premature loss of deciduous anterior teeth, webbed neck (12 per cent), pectus excavatum, gynecomastia, congenital heart defect (especially patent ductus arteriosus), umbilical hernia, scoliosis, simian creases, talipes, abnormal toes, wide gap between first and second toes, hypospadias, bifid scrotum, growth hormone deficiency.

NATURAL HISTORY. Perinatal problems in adaptation have been frequent; linear growth is generally slow, with moderately short final height attainment. Infertility and inadequate virilization may be anticipated. Depending on the overall life situation, testosterone replacement therapy should be considered at 11 to 12 years of age. A decline in intellectual performance occurs with advancing age. Behavioral problems including irritability and agitation, hyperactivity and noncompliance, and inappropriate speech occur. Poor language development has been documented with a significant discrepancy between expressive ability and comprehension.

ETIOLOGY. The diagnosis is confirmed by chromosomal analysis revealing an XXXY or XXXXY karyotype. Molecular methods have indicated that the X chromosomes are maternally derived.

COMMENT. Although some of the features may initially suggest Down syndrome, the total pattern of anomalies is usually at variance with this diagnosis.

References

Fraccaro, M., Kaijser, K., and Lindsten, J.: A child with 49 chromosomes. Lancet, 2:899, 1960.

Zaleski, W. A., et al.: The XXXXY chromosome anomaly: Report of three new cases and review of 30 cases from the literature. Can. Med. Assoc. J., 94:1143, 1966.

Schmid, R., Pajewski, M., and Rosenblatt, M.: Epiphyseal dysplasia: A constant finding in XXXXY syndrome. J. Med. Genet., 15:282, 1978.

Borghgraef, M., et al.: The 49 XXXXY syndrome. Clinical and psychological follow-up data. Clin. Genet., 33:429, 1988.

Plaha, D. S., et al.: Origin of the X chromosomes in a patient with the 49 XXXXY syndrome. J. Med. Genet., 27:203, 1990.

Lomelino, C. A., and Reiss, A. L.: 49 XXXXY syndrome: Behavioral and developmental profiles. J. Med. Genet., 28:609, 1991.

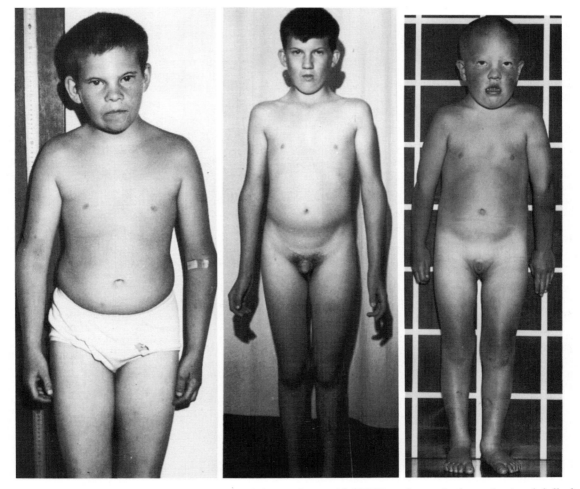

FIGURE 1. *Left* and *middle*, Preadolescent and adolescent boys with XXXY syndrome; both are short and dull of mentality. Note the facial dysmorphia, elbow aberrations, and hypogonadism (*middle*). *Right*, A 6-year-old with XXXXY syndrome. Note some resemblance to Down syndrome and the more severe hypogenitalism. (Right photo from Smith, D. W.: J. Pediatr., *70*:476, 1976, with permission.)

XXX AND XXXX SYNDROMES

Initially described by Jacobs et al. in 1959 in a woman of normal intelligence who had secondary amenorrhea, the XXX syndrome is recognized to occur in 1 in 1000 newborn females. There is no pattern of malformation associated with this karyotype. Based on studies of unselected newborns with sex chromosome anomalies who have been followed longitudinally, the following can be stated relative to females with a 47XXX karyotype: Affected individuals are usually tall with average height of 172 cm. Mean occipitofrontal circumference is about the 20th percentile. Pubertal development is normal with an average age of menarche of $12^8/_{12}$ years. Fertility is probably normal. Delay in achievement of motor milestones, poor coordination, and awkwardness are common. I.Q. scores cluster in the 85 to 90 range (generally lower than their sibs). Problems with verbal learning and expressive language are frequent. Special education classes in high school are required in 60 per cent. Behavior problems including mild depression, having a conduct disorder, or being undersocialized occur in 30 per cent. However, most cope well and adapt as young adults without major problems.

This is in contrast to the XXXX syndrome, initially described by Carr et al. in 1961, in which only 40 cases have been reported. Individuals with the XXXX syndrome have a variable phenotype with the facies suggestive of the Down syndrome in several cases.

ABNORMALITIES IN THE XXXX SYNDROME. For other than mental deficiency, all of the other features have been variable. The patients are usually of normal to tall stature.

Performance. I.Q. of 30 to 80, average of 55. Speech development is most prominently affected.

Facies. Midfacial hypoplasia, upward slanting palpebral fissures, mild hypertelorism, epicanthal folds, mild micrognathia.

Limbs. Occasional fifth finger clinodactyly, radioulnar synotosis, reduced total finger ridge count.

Other. Tall stature. Narrow shoulder girdle, taurondontism. Variable amenorrhea, irregular menses.

OCCASIONAL ABNORMALITIES. Seizures. Variable EEG abnormalities. Mild ventricular enlargement on CT scan. Webbed neck.

NATURAL HISTORY. Besides mental deficiency, speech and behavioral problems are frequent in the XXXX syndrome. The patient initially reported by Carr et al., now 56 years old, is in good physical health with no evidence of intellectual deterioration. Her full-scale I.Q. is 56. Although menstrual disorders are common and fertility is reduced, offspring of these individuals tend to be normal.

ETIOLOGY. The diagnosis is confirmed by chromosomal analysis revealing a XXX or XXXX karyotype. Nondisjunction at maternal meiosis I is the most common cause of 47XXX. Although not as striking an effect as is seen with trisomy 21, an increased maternal age effect has been seen for 47XXX females.

References

Jacobs, P. A., et al.: Evidence for the existence of the human "super female." Lancet, 2:423, 1959.

Carr, D. H., Barr, M. L., and Plunkett, E. R.: An XXXX sex chromosome complex in two mentally defective females. Can. Med. Assoc. J., 84:131, 1961.

Telfer, M. A., et al.: Divergent phenotypes among 48,XXXX and 47,XXXX females. Am. J. Hum. Genet., 22:326, 1970.

Gardner, R. J. M., Veale, A. M. O., and Sands, V. E.: XXXX syndrome: Case report, and a note on genetic counselling and fertility. Humangenetik, 17:323, 1973.

Berg, J. M., et al.: Twenty-six years later: A woman with tetra-X chromosomes. J. Mental Defic. Res., 32:67, 1988.

Robinson, A., et al.: Sex chromosome aneuploidy: The Denver prospective study. Birth Defects, 26(4):59, 1991.

Robinson, A., et al.: Summary of clinical findings in children and young adults with sex chromosome anomalies. Birth Defects, 26(4):225, 1991.

FIGURE 1. A 6⁶/₁₂-year-old girl with XXXX syndrome.

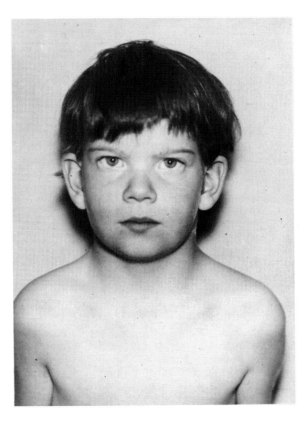

XXXXX SYNDROME

(Penta X Syndrome)

Upward Slant to Palpebral Fissures, Patent Ductus Arteriosus, Small Hands With Clinodactyly of Fifth Fingers

The first description of an individual with XXXXX was by Kesaree and Wooley in 1963.

ABNORMALITIES. Mental deficiency, moderate to severe. Prenatal onset growth deficiency, failure to thrive, short stature. Microcephaly. Mild upward slant (mongoloid) to palpebral fissures. Low nasal bridge, short neck. Hypertelorism. Epicanthal folds. Low hairline. Dental malocclusion. Taurodontism and enamel defects leading to premature loss of deciduous anterior teeth. Small hands with mild clinodactyly of fifth fingers. Congenital heart defect (patent ductus arteriosus or ventricular septal defect).

OCCASIONAL ABNORMALITIES. Colobomata of iris, low-set ears. preauricular tags, macroglossia, cleft palate, micrognathia, high-frequency low arch dermal ridge patterns, simian creases, equinovarus, overlapping toes, multiple joint dislocations including shoulder, elbow, hips, wrists, and fingers. Renal dysplasia. Horseshoe kidney. Ovarian agenesis.

NATURAL HISTORY. I.Q. varies from 20 to 75. The oldest known affected individual, a 16-year-old, had small nipples, prepubertal external genitalia, and an atrophic vaginal smear. Information on fertility is lacking.

COMMENT AND ETIOLOGY. Of interest is the occurrence in these XXXXX individuals of many of the nonspecific anomalies found in Down syndrome, a diagnosis that was initially considered in some of the patients. The diagnosis is confirmed by chromosomal analysis revealing an XXXXX karyotype. Molecular methods have indicated that the X chromosomes are maternally derived.

References

Kesaree, N., and Wooley, P. V.: A phenotypic female with 49 chromosomes, presumably XXXXX. A case report. J. Pediatr., 63:1099, 1963.

Sergovich, F., Vilenberg, C., and Pozaonyi, J.: The 49,XXXXX condition. J. Pediatr., 78:285, 1971.

Dryer, F. R., et al.: Pentasomy X with multiple dislocations. Am. J. Med. Genet., 4:313, 1979.

Funderburk, S. J., et al.: Pentasomy X: Report of a patient and studies of X-inactivation. Am. J. Med. Genet., 8:27, 1981.

Deng, H. X., et al.: Parental origin and mechanism of formation of polysomy X: An XXXXX case and four XXXXY cases determined with RFLPs. Hum. Genet., 86:541, 1991.

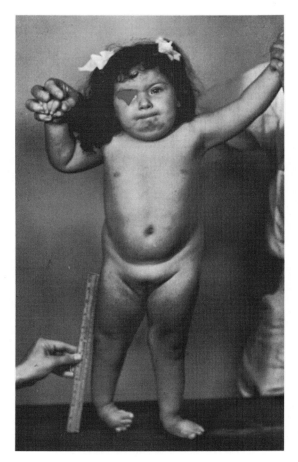

FIGURE 1. XXXXX syndrome. A 28-month-old girl with height age of 18 months and a performance level of about 1 year. A patent ductus arteriosus had been repaired. The hands were small, with incurved fifth fingers, and the ears were slightly low in placement. (From Brody, J., et al.: J. Pediatr., 70:105, 1967, with permission.)

XO SYNDROME

(Turner Syndrome)

Short Female, Broad Chest With Wide Spacing of Nipples, Congenital Lymphedema or Its Residua

An association between small stature and defective ovarian development had been noted as early as 1922 by Rossle, who classified the disorder under "sexagen dwarfism." A more expanded syndrome of small stature, sexual infantilism, webbed neck, and cubitus valgus in seven females was described by Turner in 1938. Most XO conceptuses are early lethals. It is estimated that approximately 1 in 2000 live-born phenotypic females are affected. Recommendations for diagnosis, treatment, and management of affected individuals have been established and published by Rosenfeld et al.

ABNORMALITIES. The following list of abnormalities, with the approximate percentage for each anomaly, includes those of the full monosomic XO syndrome. Patients with only a part of the cells XO (XX/XO mosaics, XY/XO mosaics with varying degrees of male-type genitalia) or in whom only a part of one X is missing (X-isochromosome X or X-deleted X) generally have a lesser degree of malformation. The most consistent features for the entire group are small stature and gonadal dysgenesis. Because the latter feature is not evident during childhood, a chromosomal study is indicated in any girl with short stature of unknown cause whose clinical phenotype is not incompatible with the XO syndrome. In addition, any adolescent with absent breast development by 13 years of age, pubertal arrest, or primary or secondary amenorrhea with elevated follicle-stimulating hormone should have a karyotype performed.

Growth. Small stature, often evident by birth. Tendency to become obese.

Performance. Mean I.Q. about 90 with performance usually below verbal scores. Although early development is usually normal, delays in motor skills are common, as is poor coordination. Specific neuropsychological deficits are as follows: Visual-spatial organization deficits such as difficulty driving; deficits in social cognition such as failure to appreciate subtle social cues, problems with nonverbal problem solving such as math, and psychomotor deficits such as clumsiness. A tendency for low self-esteem and depression in teenagers and young adults.

Gonads. Ovarian dysgenesis with hypoplasia to absence of germinal elements (90+ per cent).

Lymph Vessels. Congenital lymphedema with residual puffiness over the dorsum of the fingers and toes (80+ per cent). Can be seen at any age; often associated with initiation of growth hormone and/or estrogen therapy.

Thorax. Broad chest with widely spaced nipples that may be hypoplastic, inverted, or both (80+ per cent); often mild pectus excavatum.

Auricles. Anomalous auricles, most commonly prominent (80+ per cent).

Facies. Narrow maxilla (palate) (80+ per cent). Relatively small mandible (70+ per cent). Inner canthal folds (40+ per cent).

Neck. Low posterior hairline, appearance of short neck (80+ per cent). Webbed posterior neck (50 per cent).

Extremities. Cubitus valgus or other anomaly of elbow (70+ per cent). Knee anomalies such as medial tibial exostosis (60+ per cent). Short fourth metacarpal, metatarsal, or both (50+ per cent).

Other Skeletal. Bone dysplasia with coarse trabecular pattern, most evident at metaphyseal ends of long bones (50+ per cent). Dislocation of hip.

Nails. Narrow, hyperconvex, and/or deep-set nails (70+ per cent).

Skin. Excessive pigmented nevi (50+ per cent). Distal palmar axial triradii (40+ per cent). Loose skin, especially about the neck in infancy. Tendency toward keloid formation.

Renal. Most commonly horseshoe kidney, double or cleft renal pelvis, and minor alterations (60+ per cent).

Cardiac. Cardiac defects, the majority of which are bicuspid aortic valve (30 per cent), coarctation of aorta (10 per cent), valvular aortic stenosis, mitral valve prolapse, and aortic dissection later in life. Hypertension.

Central Nervous System. Perceptive hearing impairment (50+ per cent).

OCCASIONAL ABNORMALITIES

Skeletal. Abnormal angulation of radius to carpal bones, Madelung deformity, short midphalanx of fifth finger, short third to fifth metacarpals and/or metatarsals, scoliosis, kyphosis, spina bifida, vertebral fusion, cervical rib, abnormal sella turcica.

Eyes. Ptosis (16 per cent), strabismus, amblyopia, blue sclerae, cataract.

Central Nervous System. Mental retardation.

Other. Hemangiomata, rarely of the intestine. Long hair on arms. Idiopathic hypertension, diabetes mellitus, Crohn disease, primary hypothyroidism (10 to 30 per cent), agenesis of corpus callosum (two cases), partial anomalous pulmonary venous return, hypoplastic left heart, persistent left superior vena cava.

NATURAL HISTORY. The congenital lymphedema usually recedes in early infancy, leaving only puffiness of the dorsum of the fingers and toes, although there may be recrudescence of the lymphedema with growth hormone and/or estrogen replacement therapy. At birth, the skin tends to be loose, especially in the posterior neck where excess skin may persist as the pterygium colli. Small size is often evident at birth, the mean birth weight being 2900 g. From birth up to 3 years of age the growth rate is normal, although there is a delay in bone maturation. Between 3 and 12 years bone age progression is normal, but height velocity decreases. After 12 years of age there is a decreased growth rate, deceleration of bone age progression, and relative increase in weight. Final height of 50 to 60 inches with a mean of 55 inches is achieved at a usual age, despite the roentgenographic evidence of "retarded osseous maturation." Studies of XO abortuses have disclosed near-normal development of the ovaries in early fetal life. Apparently they usually do not make primary follicles, and the ovary degenerates rather rapidly. In the majority of affected individuals, by adolescence there is seldom any functional ovarian tissue remaining. Gonadotropin values may be helpful before 5 years in early childhood and again after 10 years. If they are elevated, the patient probably will not have functional ovarian tissue by adolescence. However, it is important to recognize that 10 to 20 per cent will have spontaneous pubertal development and 2 to 5 per cent will have spontaneous menses, although this is generally transient; at least several XO individuals have been fertile. Generally, estrogen replacement therapy is indicated, beginning at the appropriate psychologic time for each individual. Premarin, for example, may be started at a very low dosage and gradually increased to mimic normal adolescence, and the adult dosage is reached, with cycling of therapy to allow for menstruation, at 13 to 15 years of age. Although treatment with anabolic steroids is controversial, recent studies have shown a mean gain in final height of 3 to 4 cm following 2 years of oxandrolone in girls with Turner syndrome who begin treatment when bone age is less than 13 years while girls with a bone age greater than 13 years at the beginning of treatment do not improve final height. Regarding growth hormone therapy, the data suggest that human growth hormone, alone or in combination with anabolic steroids, stimulates short-term growth in girls with XO Turner syndrome. At some time between 8 years and adolescence, these patients should be told that the ovaries are probably incompletely developed and that they should plan on adopting children and taking "the same kind of medicine the ovary makes" at adolescence.

The actual incidence of early mortality due to congenital heart defects is unknown because there is no large series of cases diagnosed from birth. An increased risk for dissection of the aorta has been documented in adults—even in those without coarctation. In addition, hypertension is common even in those without cardiac or renal disease. The types of renal anomalies that occur generally pose no problem to health, which is generally good. Enhancement of physical appearance by plastic surgery for prominent inner canthal folds, protruding auricles, and especially for webbed neck should be given serious consideration prior to school age. However, there is a markedly increased incidence of keloid formation that must be taken into account.

At the present time, we do not have adequate information on the longevity and cause of death beyond the age of childhood for individuals with the XO syndrome. However, it is encouraging to note that Dr. Judith Hall (University of British Columbia) knows of one 90-year-old woman with XO syndrome.

If the chromosomal studies show XO/XY mosaicism, an exploratory laparotomy in childhood seems indicated to remove any gonadoblastoma, which such patients have an increased risk of developing.

If the child is mentally deficient, a careful search should be made for a chromosome abnormality in addition to that of the sex chromosome. For example, X-autosome translocation patients are more likely to be mentally deficient. Mental retardation has also been seen more frequently in individuals with a small ring X chromosome.

ETIOLOGY. Faulty chromosomal distribution leading to XO individual with 45 chromosomes. The paternal sex chromosome is the one more likely to be missing. There has been no significant older maternal age factor for this aneuploidy syndrome. It is generally a sporadic event in a family, although there are as yet no adequate data on risk for recurrence. Mosaicism does not ensure survival to term. However, the incidence of sex chromosome mosaicism is higher in liveborn than in aborted 45XO fetuses.

References

Rossle, R. I.: Wachstum und Altern. München, 1922.

Turner, H. H.: A syndrome of infantilism, congenital webbed neck, and cubitus valgus. Endocrinology, 23:566, 1938.

Weiss, L.: Additional evidence of gradual loss of germ cells in the pathogenesis of streak ovaries in Turner's syndrome. J. Med. Genet., 8:540, 1971.

Kastrup, K. W.: Oestrogen therapy in Turner's syndrome. Acta Paediatr. Scand. Suppl., 343:43, 1988.

Rosenfeld, R. G.: Update on growth hormone therapy for Turner's syndrome. Acta Paediatr. Scand. Suppl., 356:103, 1989.

Chang, H. J., et al.: The phenotype of 45X/46XY mosaicism: An analysis of 92 prenatally diagnosed cases. Am. J. Hum. Genet., 46:156, 1990.

Robinson, A., et al.: Sex chromosome aneuploidy: The Denver prospective study. Birth Defects, 26(4):59, 1991.

Hassold, T., et al.: Molecular studies of parental origin and mosaicism in 45X conceptuses. Hum. Genet., 89:647, 1992.

Rosenfeld, R. G., et al.: Recommendations for diagnosis, treatment and management of individuals with Turner syndrome. The Endocrinologist, 4:351, 1994.

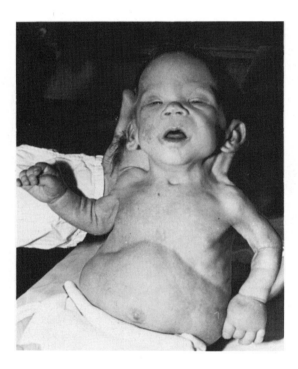

FIGURE 1. A 10-day-old XO patient who still has lymph-filled bilateral cysts in the posterior neck area, the cause for the webbed neck and for the prominent ears. This patient had abdominal muscle hypoplasia with bulging flanks, possibly secondary to earlier undue distention of the abdomen by fluid. Thus, this baby survived fetal life and was born with a more severe degree of lymphedema than usual.

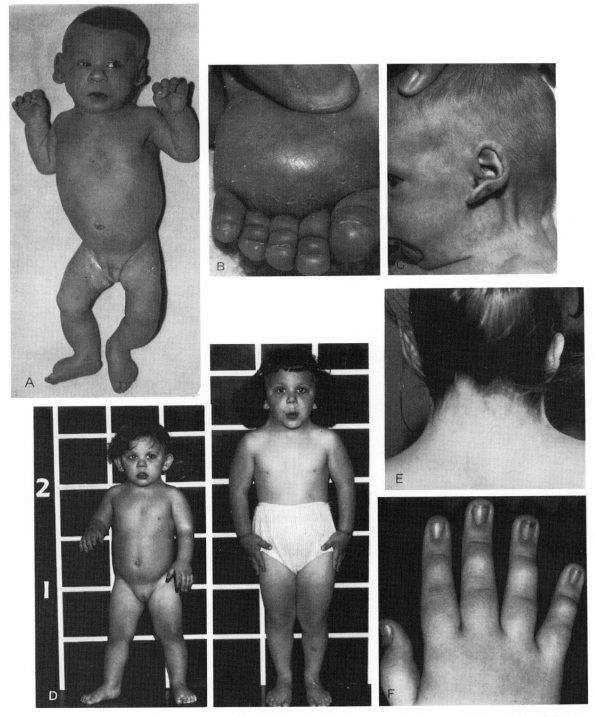

FIGURE 2. XO syndrome. *A* to *C*, A 1-month-old. Note lymphedema, prominent ears, and loose folds of skin in posterior neck with low hairline. *D*, Same girl at 2 years and at 4 years, with height ages of 17 months and 3 years, respectively. *E*, Low posterior hairline and residual lateral neck web. *F*, Narrow, hyperconvex, deep-set fingernails; residual puffiness. (*A* to *C*, *E*, and *F* from Lemli, L., and Smith, D. W.: J. Pediatr., *63*:577, 1963, with permission.)

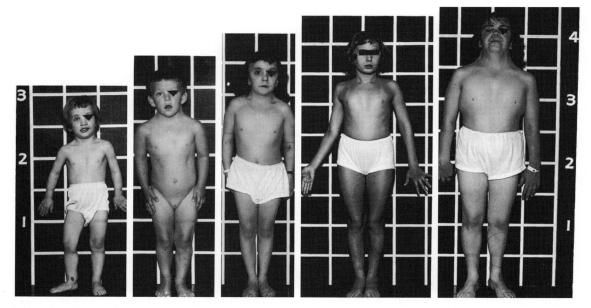

FIGURE 3. Five girls with the XO syndrome. Note the variability of such features as webbed neck and broad chest.

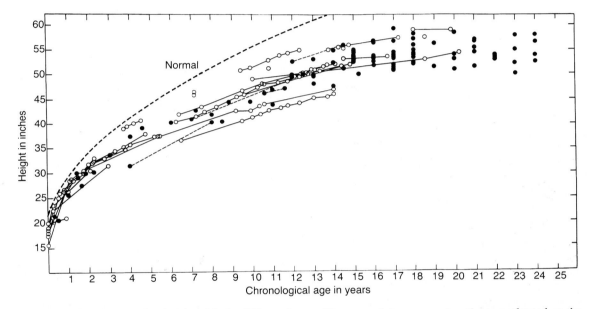

FIGURE 4. Linear growth of girls with the XO syndrome. The open dots represent patients evaluated at the University of Wisconsin; the others were taken from the literature. (From Lemli, L., and Smith, D. W.: J. Pediatr., 63:577, 1963, with permission.)

B

B. VERY SMALL STATURE, NOT SKELETAL DYSPLASIA

BRACHMANN–DE LANGE SYNDROME

(Cornelia de Lange Syndrome, de Lange Syndrome)

Synophrys, Thin Downturning Upper Lip, Micromelia

The syndrome was originally reported in 1933 by Cornelia de Lange. Brachmann had described a child with similar features at autopsy in 1916.

ABNORMALITIES

Growth. Prenatal onset growth deficiency with respect to length and weight.

Retarded osseous maturation	100%
Low-pitched, weak, growling cry in infancy	74%

Performance. Mental retardation and sluggish physical activity. Average I.Q. ranges from below 30 to 86 with an average of 53. Those with higher I.Q.'s tend to have better birth weight and head circumference.

Initial hypertonicity	100%
Low-pitched, weak, growling cry in infancy	74%

Cranium
Microbrachycephaly	93%

Eyes
Bushy eyebrows and synophrys	98%
Long, curly eyelashes	99%

Nose
Depressed nasal bridge	83%
Anteverted nares	85%

Mouth
Long philtrum, thin upper lip and downturned angles of mouth	94%
High arched palate	86%
Late eruption of widely spaced teeth	86%

Mandible
Micrognathia	84%
Spurs in the anterior angle of the mandible, prominent symphysi	66%

Skin
Hirsutism	78%
Cutis marmorata and perioral pale "cyanosis"	56%
Hypoplastic nipples and umbilicus	50%

Hands and Arms
Micromelia	93%
Phocomelia and oligodactyly	27%
Clinodactyly of fifth fingers	74%
Simian crease	51%
Proximal implantation of thumbs	72%
Flexion contracture of elbows	64%

Feet
Micromelia	93%
Syndactyly of second and third toes	86%

Male Genitalia
Hypoplasia	57%
Undescended testes	73%
Hypospadias	33%

Radiographic. Mandibular spur present up to 3 months of age. Dislocated/hypoplastic radial head. Hypoplastic first metacarpal and fifth middle phalanx. Short sternum with precocious fusion and 13 ribs.

Other. Ocular abnormalities including myopia, ptosis, and mystagmus in 57 per cent. Low posterior hairline (92 per cent). Short neck (66 per cent). Gastrointestinal problems including gastroesophagal reflux (30 per cent) and various forms of obstruction including duplication of gut, malrotation of colon with volvulus, and pyloric stenosis. Hearing loss (60 per cent).

OCCASIONAL ABNORMALITIES. Seizures (23 per cent), microcornea, astigmatism, optic atrophy, coloboma of the optic nerve, strabismus, proptosis, choanal atresia, low-set ears, cleft palate, congenital heart defect most commonly ventricular septal defect, hiatus hernia, diaphragmatic hernia, brachyesophagus, inguinal hernia, small labia majora, radial hypoplasia, absent second to third interdigital triradius, thrombocytopenia.

NATURAL HISTORY AND MANAGEMENT. These patients show a marked retardation of growth, evident by the time of birth, and as a rule, they fail to thrive. Feeding difficulties, including regurgitation, projectile vomiting, chewing, and swallowing difficulties, often continue beyond 6 months. Although a high percentage of affected children have severe mental retardation, a significant number have a much higher potential relative to performance than earlier studies have suggested. Hearing loss associated with speech delay occurs frequently. Their gait tends to be broad based. They sometimes show autistic behavior, including self-destructive tendencies. The patients may avoid and reject social interactions and physical contact. Though rapid movement may be pleasurable, they show infrequent facial emotion and tend to have stereotypic behavior. The majority of patients followed beyond 13 years had onset of puberty, with normal menses documented in several women. Episodes of aspiration in infancy, apnea, complications related to bowel obstruction, and cardiac defects appear to constitute the major hazards for survival in these patients.

ETIOLOGY AND RECURRENCE RISK. Unknown. Most cases are sporadic. Autosomal dominant inheritance has been suggested based on four instances in which a mildly affected parent and one or more of his/her children were affected. Recurrence risk is negligible if, after careful evaluation, both parents are determined to be normal, or 50 per cent if one parent is affected. The observed low recurrence risk most likely represents the inability of more severely affected individuals to reproduce. Clinically, there appears to be a gradation in severity, and it is very difficult to be secure about a diagnosis in the more mildly affected cases. Duplication of the q26-27 band region of chromosome 3 tends to yield a phenotype that is similar to that of the Brachmann–de Lange syndrome. Hence, cautious chromosome studies are indicated in some of the atypical Brachmann–de Lange syndrome patients.

References

Brachmann, W.: Ein Fall von symmetrischer Monodaktylie durch ulnadefekt mit symmetrischer Flughautbildung in den Ellenbeugen, sowie anderen Abnormitaten (Zwerghaftigheit, Halsrippen, Behaarung). Jahrb. Kinderkeilk, *84*:224, 1916.

de Lange, C.: Sur un type nouveau de génération (typus Amstelodamensis). Arch. Med. Engant., *36*:713, 1933.

Ptacek, L. J., et al.: The Cornelia de Lange syndrome. J. Pediatr., *63*:1000, 1963.

Vischer, D.: Typus degenerativus Amstelodamensis (Cornelia de Lange syndrome). Helv. Paediatr. Acta, *20*:415, 1965.

Barr, A. N., et al.: Neurologic and psychometric findings in Brachmann-de Lange syndrome. Neuropaediatrie, *3*:46, 1971.

Johnson, H. G., et al.: A behavioral phenotype in the de Lange syndrome. Pediatr. Res., *10*:843, 1976.

Wilson, G. N., Hieber, V. C., and Schmickel, R. D.: The association of chromosome 3 duplication and the Cornelia de Lange syndrome. J. Pediatr., *93*:783, 1978.

Robinson, L. K., Wolfsberg, E., and Jones, K. L.: Brachmann-de Lange syndrome: Evidence for autosomal dominant inheritance. Am. J. Med. Genet., *22*:109, 1985.

Jackson, L., et al.: de Lange syndrome: A clinical review of 310 individuals. Am. J. Med. Genet., *47*:940, 1993.

Braddock, S. R., et al.: Radiological features in Brachmann-de Lange syndrome. Am. J. Med. Genet., *47*: 1006, 1993.

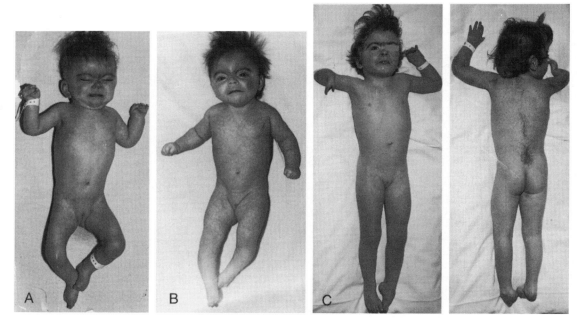

FIGURE 1. De Lange syndrome. *A,* Neonate with small hands and feet. *B,* A 3-month-old with newborn length. *C,* A 5⁶/₁₂-year-old with height age of 2 years and severe defect of right distal limb.

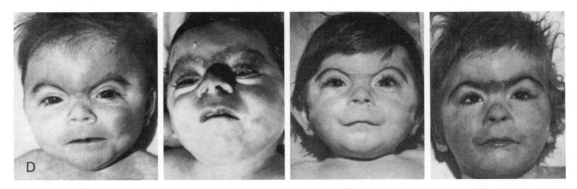

FIGURE 1. *Continued. D,* Similar facies of four affected individuals. (From Ptacek, L. J., et al.: J. Pediatr., *63*:1000, 1963, with permission.)

RUBINSTEIN-TAYBI SYNDROME

*Broad Thumbs and Toes, Slanted
Palpebral Fissures, Hypoplastic Maxilla*

Rubinstein and Taybi set forth this clinical entity in 1963. More than 550 cases have been reported.

ABNORMALITIES

Growth. Postnatal onset growth deficiency. In adults average height of 153 cm in males and 147 cm in females. Average weight of 48 kg in males and 55 kg in females.

Retarded osseous maturation	49%

Performance. I.Q. 30 to 79 with an average of 51; 52 per cent have an I.Q. less than 50.

Speech difficulties	90%
EEG abnormality	30%
Seizures	23%
Stiff, unsteady gait	85%
Hypotonia	67%
Hyperreflexia	40%

Cranium

Microcephaly	35%
Large anterior fontanel	41%
Delayed closure of fontanel	24%
Frontal bossing	33%

Facies

Palpebral fissures slant downward (50 per cent below age 5 years)	88%
Hypoplastic maxilla with narrow palate	100%
Small opening of mouth	56%
Prominent and/or beaked nose with or without nasal septum extending below alae nasi	90%
Deviated nasal septum	71%
Frontal hair up-sweep	20%
Auricles low-set and/or malformed	84%
Low anterior hairline	24%
Low posterior hairline	42%
Micrognathia	49%

Ocular

Heavy eyebrows	76%
Highly arched eyebrows	73%
Long eyelashes	87%
Stenosis nasolacrimal duct	43%
Ptosis	36%
Epicanthal folds	55%
Strabismus	69%
Enophthalmia	22%

Hands and Feet

Broad thumbs with radial angulation	87%
Broad great toes	100%
Other fingers broad	87%
Fifth finger clinodactyly	62%
Persistent fetal fingertip pads	31%
Deep plantar crease between first and second toes	33%
Flat feet	72%

Other Skeletal

Scoliosis	42%
Spina bifida occulta	47%
Cervical hyperkyphosis	37%
Small, flared iliac wings	26%

Genitalia

Cryptorchidism	78% of males

Skin

Hirsutism	75%
Capillary hemangioma	25%
Keloid formation	22%

Cardiac. Defects most frequent of which are patent ductus arteriosus, ventricular septal defect, and atrial septal defect occur in 25 per cent

OCCASIONAL ABNORMALITIES

Skeletal. Large foramen magnum, parietal foramina, micrognathia, sternal anomalies, syndactyly, polydactyly.

Other. Cataract, glaucoma, colobomata, ptosis of eyelid, nystagmus, myopia, exophthalmia, camptodactyly, polydactyly, simian crease, distal axial triradius, duplicated halluces, pectus excavatum, renal anomaly, angulated penis, hypospadias, shawl scrotum, absence of corpus callosum, café au lait spots, stereotypic movements, mirror movements.

NATURAL HISTORY. Respiratory infections, obstipation, and feeding difficulties are frequent problems in infancy. Average ages for childhood milestones are as follows: crawl, 15 months, sit up, 11 months; walk, 30 months; say first word, 25 months; and toilet trained, 62 months. In addition to speech therapy, the majority of affected children require physical therapy; 67 per cent of patients 6 years of age or older can read, although for the majority it does not progress beyond the first-grade level. Recurrent ear infections with mild hearing loss and dental problems primarily associated with overcrowding of the teeth occur frequently. Hand and/or foot surgery frequently improves grasp, oppositional function, and comfort. Unusual reactions to anesthesia (respiratory distress and cardiac arrhythmias) have been reported.

ETIOLOGY. The majority of cases of this disorder are sporadic. The locus for this disorder appears to be at 16p13.3, a region which encodes the human cAMP-regulated enhancer-binding protein (CBP). About one fourth of cases are due to submicroscopic deletions detectable by fluorescence in situ hybridization. Point mutations in the CBP gene, a transcriptional co-activator which mediates cAMP-regulated gene expression have been demonstrated.

COMMENT. The author has been impressed by the variability among affected individuals. Thus, presumed Rubinstein-Taybi syndrome patients have had broad thumbs but not broad toes, broad toes but not broad thumbs, and neither broad thumbs nor broad toes. The diagnosis in the latter category is, of course, a tentative one.

References

Rubinstein, J. H., and Taybi, H.: Broad thumbs and toes and facial abnormalities. A possible mental retardation syndrome. Am. J. Dis. Child., *105*:588, 1963.

Rubinstein, J. H.: The broad thumbs syndrome—progress report 1968. Birth Defects, 5:25, 1969.

Simpson, N. E., and Brissenden, J. E.: The Rubinstein-Taybi syndrome: Familial and dermatoglyphic data. Am. J. Hum. Genet., 25:225, 1973.

Hannekam, R. C. M., et al.: Rubinstein-Taybi syndrome in the Netherlands. Am. J. Med. Genet. Suppl., 6:17, 1990.

Stevens, C. A., et al.: Rubinstein-Taybi syndrome. A natural history study. Am. J. med. Genet. Suppl., 6: 30, 1990.

Stevens, C. A., et al.: Growth in Rubinstein-Taybi syndrome. Am. J. Med. Genet. Suppl., 6:51, 1990.

Breuning, M. J., et al.: Rubinstein-Taybi syndrome caused by submicroscopic deletions within 16p13.3 Am. J. Med. Genet., 52:249, 1993.

Petri, F., et al.: Rubinstein-Taybi syndrome caused by mutations in the transcriptional co-activator CBP. Nature *346*:348, 1995.

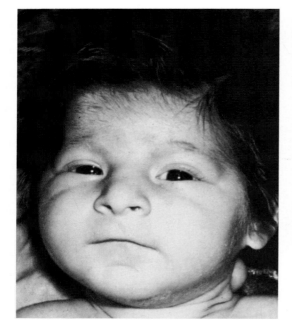

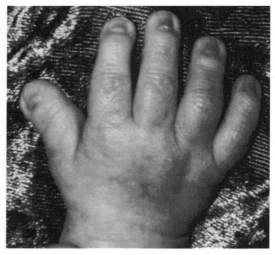

FIGURE 1. Young infant with Rubinstein-Taybi syndrome.

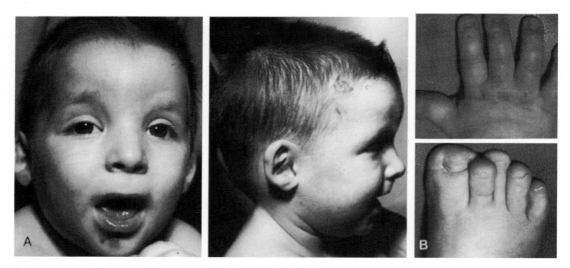

FIGURE 1. *Continued.* Rubinstein-Taybi syndrome. *A*, A 3⁶/₁₂-year-old. Height age of 2 years. I.Q. 45. Slight down-slant to palpebral fissures. *B*, Hand and foot of patient shown in *A*.

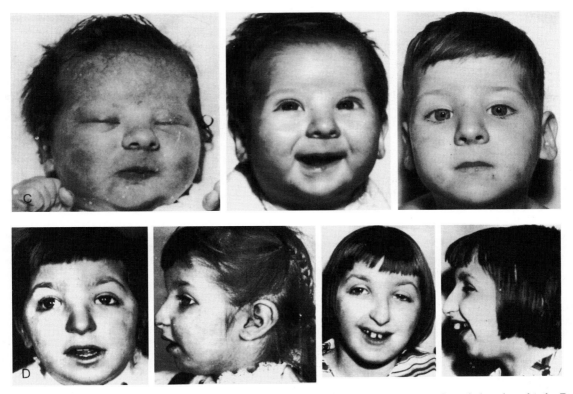

FIGURE 1. *Continued. C,* Changes in facies from birth to several years of age. Note broad thumb at birth. *D,* Changes in facies from 3⁶/₁₂ to 14 years. (*C* and *D* are gratefully acknowledged to J. Rubinstein, Cincinnati, Ohio.)

RUSSELL-SILVER SYNDROME

(Silver Syndrome)

Short Stature of Prenatal Onset, Skeletal Asymmetry, Small Incurved Fifth Finger

This pattern of malformation was independently described by Silver et al. and by Russell in 1953 and 1954. Silver emphasized the skeletal asymmetry as a feature of the disorder. This was a variable finding in the patients described by Russell. Gareis et al. have summarized the data on this syndrome and also noted that asymmetry of the prenatal onset growth deficiency is a variable feature in this disorder.

ABNORMALITIES

Growth and Skeletal. Small stature, prenatal onset. Immature osseous development in infancy and early childhood, with late closure of anterior fontanel. Asymmetry, most commonly of limbs. Short and/or incurved fifth finger.

Facies. Small, triangular facies with frontal prominence and a normal head circumference. Downturning corners of mouth. The sclerae may be bluish in early infancy. Micrognathia.

Skin. Café au lait spots.

Other. Tendency toward excess sweating, especially on the head and upper trunk, during infancy. Liability to fasting hypoglycemia from about 10 months until 2 to 3 years of age.

OCCASIONAL ABNORMALITIES. Developmental delay. Syndactyly of second to third toes, Sprengel deformity, renal anomaly, posterior urethral valves, hypospadias, cardiac defects, malignancy including craniopharyngioma, testicular seminoma, hepatocellular carcinoma, and Wilms tumor.

NATURAL HISTORY. The patients are usually slim and underweight for length during early childhood. There tends to be a gradual improvement in growth in weight and appearance during childhood and especially during adolescence. As a result, the adult usually appears more normal than the infant with this disorder. Final height attainment can be up to 5 feet. During infancy, patients tend to be weak and may be slow in major motor progress. However, intelligence is usually normal. Because of the small facies, the upper head may *appear* large, though head circumference is well within the normal range. This appearance, plus the relatively large fontanels in early infancy, may give rise to a false impression of hydrocephalus—which they do not have. Somewhat frequent feedings and adequate glucose intake during illnesses should be ensured from 6 months of age until 3 years, the period of enhanced liability to fasting hypoglycemia. Documentation of growth hormone deficiency in at least six patients suggests that an endocrine evaluation should be considered if the linear growth rate reaches a plateau.

ETIOLOGY. Unknown. The majority of cases are sporadic. A study by Saal et al. indicates the marked heterogeneity of this disorder. Some of the rare chromosomal abnormalities may initially resemble Russell-Silver syndrome. Such has occurred for del(18p) syndrome, for 18 trisomy/normal mosaicism, and for triploidy/normal mosaicism. Recently, reports of a number of chromosomal rearrangements have been reported in patients with features of Russell-Silver syndrome including ring chromosome 15; an interstitial deletion of proximal 8q (q11-q13); and two patients with translocations involving chromosome 17 in which an identical break point occurred at q25 in both. Finally, maternal uniparental disomy (UPD) 7 has been found in at least seven cases although it has been excluded in a number of others.

COMMENT. Strict conformity to the diagnostic features is vital. The diagnosis frequently is made incorrectly in any infant who is small for gestational age with a normal head circumference.

References

Silver, H. K., et al.: Syndrome of congenital hemihypertrophy, shortness of stature and elevated urinary gonadotrophins. Pediatrics, 12:368, 1953.

Russell, A.: A syndrome of "intra-uterine" dwarfism recognizable at birth with craniofacial dysostosis, disproportionately short arms and other anomalies. Proc. R. Soc. Med., 47:1040, 1954.

Silver, H. K.: Asymmetry, short stature, and variations in sexual development. A syndrome of congenital malformations. Am. J. Dis. Child., 107:495, 1964.

Gareis, F. J., Smith, D. W., and Summitt, R. L.: The Russell-Silver syndrome without asymmetry. J. Pediatr., 79:775, 1971.

Haslam, R. H. A., Berman, W., and Heller, R. M.: Renal abnormalities in the Russell-Silver syndrome. Pediatrics, 51:216, 1973.

Escobar, V., Gleiser, S., and Weaver, D. D.: Phenotypic and genetic analysis of Silver-Russell syndrome. Clin. Genet., 13:278, 1978.

Nishi, Y., et al.: Silver-Russell syndrome and growth hormone deficiency. Acta Paediatr. Scand., 71:1035, 1982.

Saal, H. M., Pagon, R. A., and Pepin, M. G.: Reevaluation of Russell-Silver syndrome. J. Pediatr., 107:733, 1985.

Donnai, et al.: Severe Silver-Russell syndrome. J. Med. Genet., 26:447, 1989.

Kotzot, D., et al.: Uniparental disomy 7 in Silver-Russell syndrome and primordial growth retardation. Hum. Molec. Genet., 4:583, 1995.

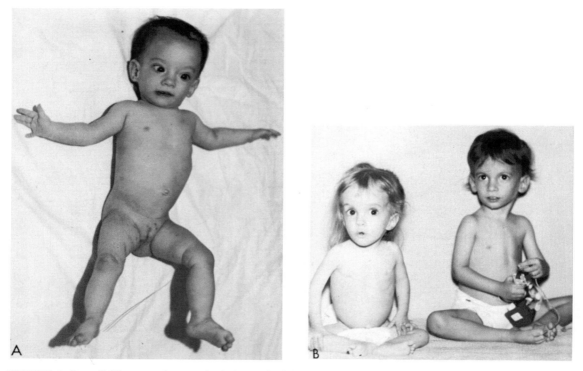

FIGURE 1. Russell-Silver syndrome. *A,* A 6-month-old; height age, 2 months. Asymmetric leg length. (From Smith, D. W.: J. Pediatr., *70*:483, 1967, with permission.) *B,* A 17-month-old girl with height age of 6 months and 2-year-old boy with height age of 15 months. Neither has asymmetry. Note the small facies, slimness, and "loose" sitting posture. (From Gareis, F. J., et al.: J. Pediatr., *79*:775, 1971, with permission.)

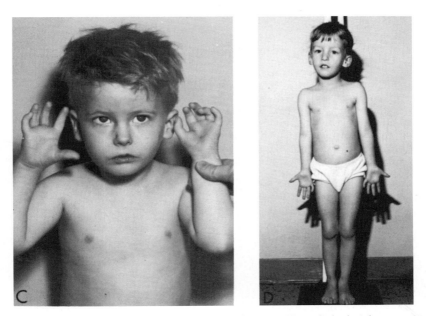

FIGURE 1. *Continued. C,* Child, $3^9/_{12}$ years old; height age, $1^6/_{12}$ years. Note slight facial asymmetry. *D,* A 6-year-old with height age of 2 years. Note clinodactyly of fifth fingers. (Courtesy of J. Aase, University of New Mexico, Albuquerque, N.M.)

MULIBREY NANISM SYNDROME

(Perheentupa Syndrome)

Small Stature, Pericardial Constriction, Yellow Dots in Fundus

Perheentupa et al. described the disorder in 1970, and more than 40 cases have been reported. The term "mulibrey" is an acronym used to denote the organs most frequently involved: *mu*scle, *li*ver, *br*ain, and *ey*es.

ABNORMALITIES

Growth. Prenatal onset growth deficiency. Mean birth weight and length at term is 2.4 kg and 45 cm, respectively. Adult height ranges from 136 to 161 cm for males and from 126 to 151 cm for females. Hands and feet appear relatively large in relation to body.

Craniofacies. Dolichocephaly with J-shaped sella turcica. Triangular facies with frontal bossing. Relatively small tongue. Decreased retinal pigmentation with dispersion and clusters of pigment and yellowish dots in the midperipheral region. Dental crowding. Missing or small frontal and/or sphenoidal sinuses.

Other. Development of thick adherent pericardium with hepatomegaly with prominent neck veins. Variable fibrous dysplasia, especially in tibia. Muscle hypotonia. High-pitched voice. Hypodontia of second bicuspid.

OCCASIONAL ABNORMALITIES. Growth hormone deficiency. Humoral immunodeficiency consisting of disturbed antibody response and impaired opsonization.

NATURAL HISTORY. Normal intelligence. Onset of pericardial constrictive problems from infancy to late childhood. Whether the hepatomegaly is secondary to pericardial constriction remains to be resolved.

ETIOLOGY. Autosomal recessive. Thirty-one of the cases have been reported from Finland.

References

Perheentupa, J., et al.: Mulibrey-nanism. Dwarfism with muscle, liver, brain and eye involvement. Acta Paediatr. Scand., *50*(Suppl. 206):74, 1970.

Voorhees, M. L., Husson, G. S., and Blackman, M. S.: Growth failure with pericardial constriction. Am. J. Dis. Child., *130*:1146, 1976.

Tarkkanen, A., Raitta, C., and Perheentupa, J.: Mulibrey nanism, an autosomal recessive syndrome with ocular involvement. Acta Ophthalmol., *60*:628, 1982.

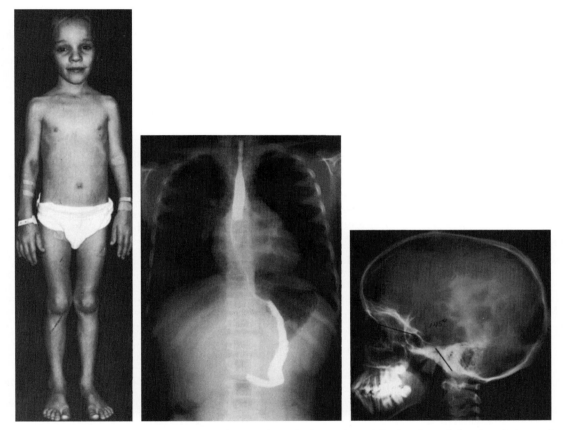

FIGURE 1. Girl with mulibrey nanism syndrome. Note the large size of the hands and feet in relation to her small stature, the aberrant cardiac silhouette and enlarged liver relating to constriction of the pericardium, and the dolichocephaly with J-shaped sella turcica. (From Voorhees, M. L., et al.: Am. J. Dis. Child., *130*:1146, 1976, with permission.)

DUBOWITZ SYNDROME

Peculiar Facies, Infantile Eczema,
Small Stature, Mild Microcephaly

This disorder was initially reported by Dubowitz in 1965, and Wilroy et al. summarized 21 cases, eight of their own, in 1978. More than 50 cases have now been described.

ABNORMALITIES

Growth. Prenatal growth deficiency with average birth weight of 2.3 kg, birth length of 44 cm, and head circumference of 30.6 cm. Retarded osseous maturation. Postnatal growth deficiency (80 per cent).

Performance. Mental retardation ranging from severe to mild (54 per cent). Hyperactivity (67 per cent). Short attention span, stubbornness, and shyness. High-pitched, hoarse cry. Muscular hypotonia (40 per cent).

Craniofacial. Microcephaly, small facies, shallow supraorbital ridge with nasal bridge at about same level as forehead, broad nasal tip, short palpebral fissures with lateral telecanthus and appearance of hypertelorism, variable ptosis and blepharophimosis, epicanthal folds, prominent or mildly dysplastic ears, and micrognathia.

Skin and Hair. Eczema-like skin disorder on face and flexural areas. Sparse scalp hair and of lateral eyebrows.

Dentition. Lag in eruption, caries, missing teeth.

Other. Brachyclinodactyly of fifth fingers. Syndactyly of second and third toes. Cryptorchidism. Ocular abnormalities including strabismus, microphthalmia, hyperopia, megalocornea, hypoplasia of iris, and coloboma. Abnormalities of the ocular fundus include abnormal veins, tapetoretinal degeneration, and ocular albinism.

Occasional. Submucous cleft palate, velopharyngeal insufficiency, pes planus, metatarsus adductus, hypospadias, pilonidal dimple, hypoparathyroidism. Bone marrow hypoplasia. Malignancies including a malignant lymphoma, a neuroblastoma, and an acute lymphatic leukemia. Fatal aplastic anemia. Cardiac defect.

NATURAL HISTORY. Eczema, noted in about one half of the patients, usually clears by 2 to 4 years. About one third have poor feeding. Respiratory and gastrointestinal infections occur frequently, raising the possibility of immunodeficiency. Teeth tend to become carious, and rhinorrhea and otitis media are frequent problems. Behavioral aberrations with lag in development of speech pose problems in function.

ETIOLOGY Autosomal recessive, based on affected male and female siblings from unaffected parents

COMMENT. The facies may appear similar to that of the fetal alcohol syndrome.

References

Dubowitz, V.: Familial low birth weight dwarfism with an unusual facies and a skin eruption. J. Med. Genet., 2:12, 1965.

Opitz, J. M., et al.: The Dubowitz syndrome. Further observations. Z. Kinderheilkd., *116*:1, 1973.

Winter, R. M.: Dubowitz syndrome. J. Med. Genet., 23: 11, 1986.

Kuster, W., and Majewski, F.: Dubowitz syndrome. Eur. J. Pediatr. 144:574, 1986.

Ilyina, H. G., and Lurie, I. W.: Dubowitz syndrome. Possible evidence for clinical subtype. Am. J. Med. Genet., *35*:561, 1990.

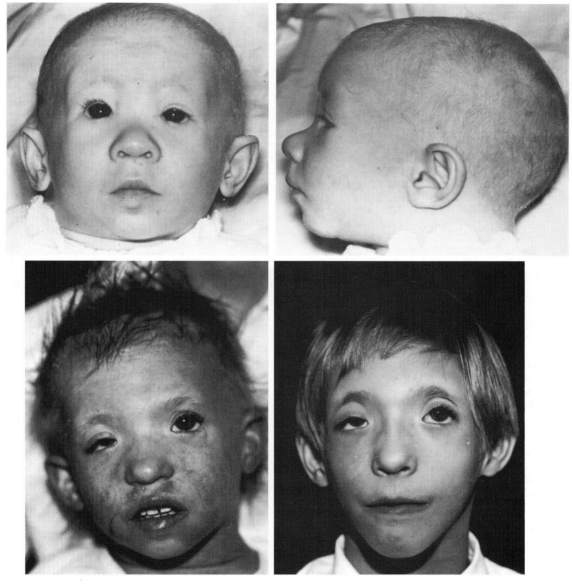

FIGURE 1. Dubowitz syndrome. *Above,* A 5-month-old showing short palpebral fissures, asymmetric ptosis, shallow supraorbital ridges, and mild micrognathia. *Below,* A 20-month-old showing eczema and above features; same patient at 6⁶/₁₂ years of age, at which time her I.Q. was 60. (From Grosse, R., et al.: Z. Kinderheilkd., *110:* 175, 1971, courtesy of J. M. Opitz, Helena, Mont.)

BLOOM SYNDROME

Short Stature, Malar Hypoplasia, Telangiectatic Erythema of the Face

Since Bloom's original description in 1954, more than 130 patients with this disorder have been reported.

ABNORMALITIES

Growth. Prenatal onset growth deficiency; average adult male height, 151 cm, and adult female height, 144 cm.

Craniofacial. Mild microcephaly with dolichocephaly. Malar hypoplasia, with or without small nose.

Skin. Facial telangiectatic erythema involves the butterfly midface region and is exacerbated by sunlight. It usually develops during the first year. Small and large areas of hyperpigmentation and hypopigmentation.

OCCASIONAL ABNORMALITIES.
Mild mental deficiency. Short attention span during childhood and learning, including reading, disabilities. Telangiectatic erythema of the dorsa of the hands and forearms. High-pitched voice, colloid-body–like spots in Bruch membrane of the eye. Absence of upper lateral incisors. Prominent ears. Ichthyotic skin, hypertrichosis, pilonidal cyst, sacral dimple. Syndactyly, polydactyly, clinodactyly of fifth finger, short lower extremity, talipes, café au lait spots. Immunoglobulin deficiency, with decreased serum levels of immunoglobulins and an impaired lymphocyte proliferation response to mitogens. Propensity to develop malignancy. Non–insulin-dependent diabetes mellitus.

NATURAL HISTORY.
These patients show a consistently slow pace of growth. Feeding problems are frequent during infancy. Susceptibility to infection decreases with age. However, chronic lung disease has been responsible for three deaths, at age 18, 19, and 24. The facial erythema is very seldom present at birth, usually appearing during infancy following exposure to sunlight; it may excoriate, but improves after childhood. Non–insulin-dependent diabetes mellitus occurs in about 8 per cent of patients in late adolescence or early adulthood. These are pleasant children, the majority being within the normal range in intelligence.

Malignancy has been the major known cause of death. About one in four patients has developed malignancy. Although leukemia occurs frequently, solid tumors with a variety of histologic types and sites of origin are the most common type of neoplasia. Of those with malignancy, the mean age at diagnosis was 24.8 years, with a range from 4 to 44 years. Gastrointestinal malignancy is common after the age of 30. Infertility due to lack of spermatogenesis is the rule in males. Subfertility in females may be common.

An increased rate of chromosomal breakage and sister chromatid exchange is found in cultured leukocytes and fibroblasts from all patients studied, but not reliably so in the heterozygotes.

ETIOLOGY.
Autosomal recessive, with the majority of individuals being of Ashkenazic Jewish ancestry. The gene has recently been assigned to chromosome 15q26.1. The frequency of the gene carrier in the Ashkenazic Jewish people is estimated at a minimum of 1:100. The excess of affected males to females is probably more apparent than real and relates to underdiagnosis of the disorder in females, in whom the skin lesion tends to be milder.

COMMENT.
The relation of the in vitro chromosomal breakage and the development of malignancies is not well understood at present.

References

Bloom, D.: Congenital telangiectatic erythema resembling lupus erythematosus in dwarfs. Am. J. Dis. Child., *88*:754, 1954.

Bloom, D.: The syndrome of congenital telangiectatic erythema and stunted growth. J. Pediatr., *68*:103, 1966.

Sawitsky, A., Bloom, D., and German, J.: Chromosomal breakage and acute leukemia in congenital telangiectatic erythema and stunted growth. Ann. Intern. Med., *65*:487, 1966.

German, J., Bloom, D., and Passarge, E.: Bloom's syndrome VII. Progress report for 1978. Clin. Genet., *15*:361, 1979.

German, J., Bloom, D., and Passarge, E.: Bloom's syndrome XI. Progress report for 1983. Clin. Genet., 25: 166, 1984.

German, J., and Passage, E.: Bloom's syndrome XII. Report from the Registry for 1987. Clin. Genet., *35*: 57, 1989.

German, J., et al.: Bloom syndrome. An analysis of consanguineous families assigns the locus mutated to chromosome band 15q26.1. Proc. Natl. Acad. Sci. U. S. A., *91*:6669, 1994.

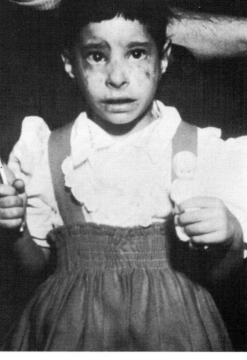

FIGURE 1. Bloom syndrome. A 4⁶/₁₂-year-old. Height age, 2⁶/₁₂ years. Died of leukemia at 13⁶/₁₂ years. (Courtesy of Dr. D. Bloom.)

JOHANSON-BLIZZARD SYNDROME

Hypoplastic Alae Nasi, Hypothyroidism, Deafness

In 1971 Johanson and Blizzard reported three cases of this disorder and found one from the past literature. At least 28 cases have now been reported. This syndrome incorporates elements of ectodermal dysplasia with endocrine and exocrine insufficiency plus growth and mental deficiency.

ABNORMALITIES

Growth. Prenatal onset growth deficiency (60 per cent).

Performance. Mental deficiency, sometimes severe (67 per cent). Sensorineural deafness (75 per cent). Hypotonia (80 per cent).

Craniofacial. Mild to moderate microcephaly (50 per cent). Midline scalp defect most typically posterior, but can be anterior or over vertex (87 per cent). Variable sparse hair with frontal up-sweep (96 per cent). Hypoplastic to aplastic alae nasi (100 per cent). Nasolacrimal duct cutaneous fistulae (66 per cent). Hypoplastic deciduous teeth, absent permanent teeth (90 per cent).

Anorectal. Imperforate and/or anteriorly placed anus (40 per cent). Recto-ureteral and/or rectovaginal fistula (18 per cent).

Genitourinary. Caliectasis to hydronephrosis. Defects occurring in 25 per cent include vagina septate or double, cryptorchidism, micropenis, hypospadias and/or single urogenital orifice.

Endocrine. Hypothyroidism of unknown etiology (30 per cent).

Exocrine. Pancreatic insufficiency with malabsorption (100 per cent).

OCCASIONAL ABNORMALITIES.
Strabismus, small nipples and absent areolae, radiolucent skull defects, abnormal EEG, cardiac defects, abdominal and thoracic situs inversus, diabetes mellitus, fifth finger clinodactyly, transverse palmar crease, café au lait spots.

NATURAL HISTORY. Although mental deficiency is frequent, normal intelligence has clearly been documented. Hypothyroidism only rarely noted in the neonatal period occurs in about one third of cases; it may progress in degree and is unusual in that the cholesterol level is not elevated. This unusual characteristic is possibly related to the concomitant malabsorption. Improvement in growth rate may occur with thyroid and pancreatin replacement therapy. However, the inadequate extent of catch-up growth implies a primary growth deficiency problem as well, as further implied by the prenatal onset of the growth deficiency.

ETIOLOGY. Autosomal recessive.

References

Grand, R. J., et al.: Unusual case of XXY Klinefelter's syndrome with pancreatic insufficiency, hypothyroidism, deafness, chronic lung disease, dwarfism and microcephaly. Am. J. Med., 41:478, 1966.

Johanson, A., and Blizzard, R.: A syndrome of congenital aplasia of the alae nasi, deafness, hypothyroidism, dwarfism, absent permanent teeth, and malabsorption. J. Pediatr., 79:982, 1971.

Daentl, D. L., et al.: The Johanson-Blizzard syndrome: Case report and autopsy findings. Am. J. Med. Genet., 3:129, 1979.

Moeschler, J. B., and Lubinsky, M. S.: Brief clinical report: Johanson-Blizzard syndrome with normal intelligence. Am. J. Med. Genet., 22:69, 1985.

Hurst, J. A. and Baraitser, M.: Johanson-Blizzard Syndrome. J. Med. Genet., 26:45, 1989.

Gershoni-Baruch, R., et al.: Johanson-Blizzard: Clinical spectrum and further delineation of the syndrome. Am. J. Med. Genet., 35:546, 1990.

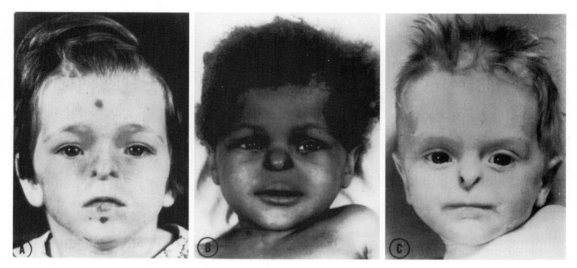

FIGURE 1. Johanson-Blizzard syndrome. Three affected children. (From Johanson, A., and Blizzard, R.: J. Pediatr., 79:982, 1971, with permission.)

SECKEL SYNDROME

Severe Short Stature, Microcephaly, Prominent Nose

Reported by Mann and Russell in 1959, this condition was extensively studied by Seckel in 1960. More precise criteria for diagnosis have recently been set forth.

ABNORMALITIES

Growth. Prenatal onset of marked growth deficiency. Average birth weight at term is 1543 g (1000 to 2005 g). Mean postnatal growth deficiency is −7.1 SD ± 2.08. One adult was 104 cm. Delayed bone age.

Central Nervous System. Mental deficiency, nearly one half with I.Q. less than 50.

Craniofacies. Microcephaly with secondary premature synostosis. In one half of cases, head circumference is more retarded than height, while for the remainder it is as retarded as height. Receding forehead. Prominent nose. Micrognathia. Low-set, malformed ears with lack of lobule. Relatively large eyes with down-slanting palpebral fissures.

Upper Extremities. Clinodactyly of fifth finger, simian crease, absence of some phalangeal epiphyses, hypoplasia of proximal radius with dislocation of radial head.

Lower Extremities. Dislocation of hip, hypoplasia of proximal fibula, gap between first and second toes. Inability to completely extend at knees.

Thorax. Only 11 pairs of ribs.

Genitalia. Male: cryptorchidism.

OCCASIONAL ABNORMALITIES. Facial asymmetry, strabismus, seizures, partial anodontia, enamel hypoplasia, sparse hair, scoliosis, talipes, pes planus, hypoplastic external genitalia, hypoplastic anemia, chromosome breakage, cleft palate.

NATURAL HISTORY. Gestational timing may be prolonged. Although moderate to severe mental deficiency occurs, early motor progress may be near normal. The cerebrum is small, with a simple primitive convolutional pattern resembling that of a chimpanzee. Though they tend to be friendly and pleasant, these patients are often hyperkinetic and easily distracted. Poor joint development and support may be evident by dislocations of the hip, elbow, or both, and by later development of scoliosis, kyphosis, or both. Survival to an age of 75 years has been recorded.

ETIOLOGY. Autosomal recessive.

References

Mann, T. P., and Russell, A.: Study of a microcephalic midget of extreme type. Proc. R. Soc. Med., *52*:1024, 1959.

Seckel, H. P. G.: Bird-Headed Dwarfs. Springfield, Ill., Charles C Thomas, 1960, p. 241.

Harper, R. G., Orti, E., and Baker, R. K.: Birdheaded dwarfs (Seckel's syndrome). A familial pattern of developmental, dental, skeletal, genital, and central nervous system anomalies. J. Pediatr., *70*:799, 1967.

McKusick, V. A., et al.: Seckel's birdheaded dwarfism. N. Engl. J. Med., *277*:279, 1967.

Majewski, F., and Goecke, T.: Studies of microcephalic primordial dwarfism I: Approach to a delineation of the Seckel syndrome. Am. J. Med. Genet., *12*:7, 1982.

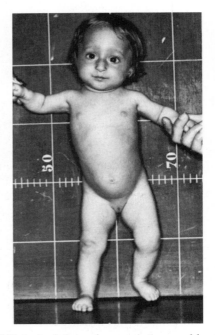

FIGURE 1. Seckel syndrome. A 1-year-old who at term birth was 1.2 kg with a length of 33.5 cm and at 1 year is 2.75 kg with a length of 48.5 cm and a head circumference of 34 cm. Note the disproportion of nose size to the size of the mandible and face, whereas general body proportions and adiposity are near normal for age (even though her size is still smaller than that of a neonate.) (Courtesy of Dr. D. Vischer, Kinderspital, Zúrich.)

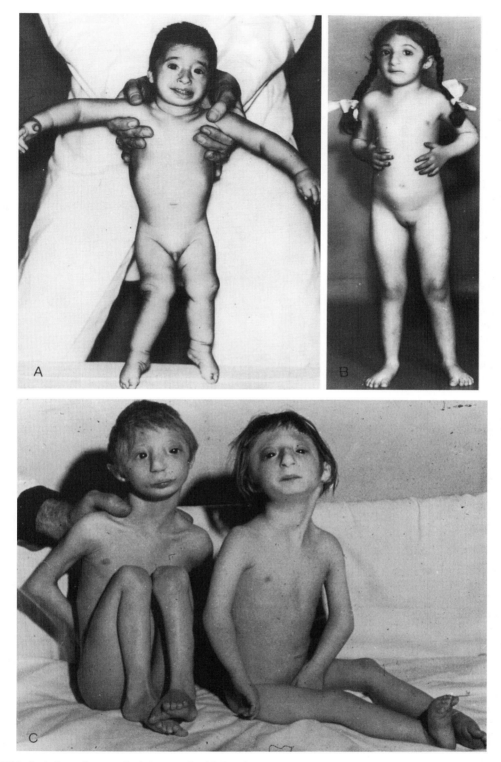

FIGURE 2. Seckel syndrome. *A*, A 14-month-old; height age, 2 months. *B*, A 5-year-old; height age, 19 months. (From Seckel, H. P. G.: Bird-Headed Dwarfs. Springfield, Ill., Charles C Thomas, 1960, with permission.) *C*, Mentally deficient brother (6-year-old) and sister (3-year-old) with height ages of 11 months and 4 months, respectively. (From Harper, R. G., et al.: J. Pediatr., *70*:799, 1967, with permission.)

HALLERMANN-STREIFF SYNDROME

(Oculomandibulodyscephaly With Hypotrichosis Syndrome)

Microphthalmia, Small Pinched Nose, Hypotrichosis

The first report of this disorder was by Audry, who described an incomplete case in 1893. Hallermann, in 1948, and Streiff, in 1950, independently described three cases, recognizing this syndrome as a separate entity. In 1958, Francois collected all the previously published cases and emphasized the cardinal features of the condition. Approximately 150 cases have been reported in the literature.

ABNORMALITIES

Growth. Prematurity and/or low birth weight in one third. Proportionate small stature. Postnatal growth deficiency in two thirds with mean final height of 152 cm in females and 155 to 157 cm in males.

Craniofacial. Brachycephaly with frontal and parietal bossing, thin calvarium, and delayed ossification of the sutures. Malar hypoplasia; micrognathia, with hypoplasia of the rami and anterior displacement of the temporomandibular joint. Nose is thin, small, and pointed, with hypoplasia of the cartilage, becoming parrot-like with age. Narrow and high arched palate. Dentition: hypoplasia of the teeth and/or malimplantation, neonatal teeth, and partial anodontia. Atrophy of the skin, most prominent over the nose and sutural areas of the scalp; thin and light hair with hypotrichosis, especially of the scalp, eyebrows, and eyelashes.

Ocular. Bilateral microphthalmia (80 per cent). Cataracts (94 per cent), total or incomplete, which may resorb spontaneously. Nystagmus. Strabismus.

Radiologic. Wormian bones. Obtuse or straight gonial angle. Thin, gracile long bones with widening at the metaphyseal ends. Thin ribs. Decreased number of sternal ossification centers. Thin, gracile metacarpals.

OCCASIONAL ABNORMALITIES. Scaphocephaly, microcephaly, platybasia, shallow sella turcica, absence of the mandibular condyles, tracheomalacia, double cutaneous chin. Microstomia. Blue sclerae, downward slant to palpebral fissures, optic disk colobomata, glaucoma, persistence of pupillary membrane, and various chorioretinal pigment alterations. Syndactyly, winging of the scapulae, lordosis, scoliosis, spina bifida, funnel chest. Mental retardation (15 per cent). Hyperactivity, choreoathetosis, and generalized tonic-clonic seizures. Hypogenitalism, cryptorchidism in the male.

NATURAL HISTORY. The narrow upper airway associated with the craniofacial configuration can lead to serious complications including severe early pulmonary infection, respiratory embarrassment, obstructive sleep apnea, and anesthetic complications. During early infancy, they may have feeding and respiratory problems, even necessitating tracheostomy. Respiratory infections may contribute to the cause of death. Laryngoscopy and endotrachial intubation at the time of anesthesia may be difficult because of the upper airway obstruction. The major handicap is the ocular defect, which usually culminates in blindness despite surgery. Though the majority of the reported patients have been of normal intelligence, motor and mental deficits, even to severe degree, have been reported.

ETIOLOGY. All cases have been sporadic occurrences.

References

Audry, C.: Variété d'alopécia congénitale; alopécie suturale. Ann. Dermatol. Syph. (Ser. 3), 4:899, 1893.

Hallermann, W.: Vogelgesicht und cataracta congenita. Klin. Monatsbl. Augenheilkd., 113:315, 1948.

Streiff, E. B.: Dysmorphie mandibulo-faciale (tête d'oiseau) et alterations oculaires. Ophthalmologica, 120:79, 1950.

Francois, J.: A new syndrome: Dyscephalis with bird face and dental anomalies, nanism, hypotrichosis, cutaneous atrophy, microphthalmia and congenital cataract. Arch. Ophthalmol., 60:842, 1958.

Hoefnagel, D., and Bernirschke, K.: Dyscephalia mandibulo-oculo-facialis. (Hallermann-Streiff syndrome). Arch. Dis. Child., 40:57, 1965.

Judge, C., and Chalcanovskis, J. F.: The Hallermann-Streiff syndrome. J. Ment. Defic. Res., 15:115, 1971.

Golomb, R. S., and Porter, P. S.: A distinct hair shaft abnormality in the Hallermann-Streiff syndrome. Cutis, 16:122, 1975.

Cohen, M. M.: Hallermann-Streiff syndrome. A review. Am. J. Med. Genet., 41:488, 1991.

Christian, C. L., et al.: Radiological findings in Hallermann-Streiff syndrome. Report of five cases and a review of the literature. Am. J. Med. Genet., 41:508, 1991.

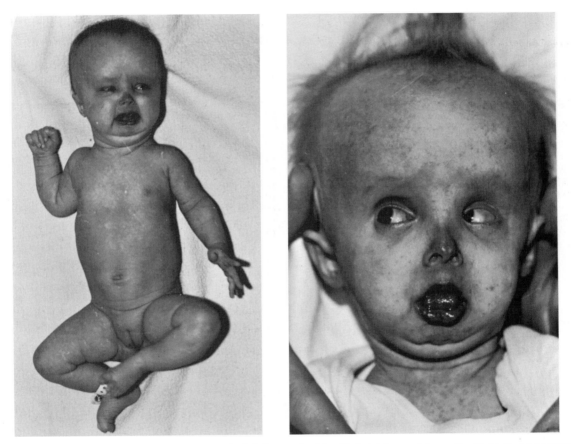

FIGURE 1. Hallermann-Streiff syndrome. *Left*, A 2^1/$_2$-month-old with height age of 1 month. *Right*, Same patient at 10 months, showing changes in facies. (From Smith, D. W.: J. Pediatr., 70:481, 1967, with permission.)

C

C. MODERATE SHORT STATURE, FACIAL, +/− GENITAL

SMITH-LEMLI-OPITZ SYNDROME

Anteverted Nostrils and/or Ptosis of Eyelids, Syndactyly of Second and Third Toes, Hypospadias and Cryptorchidism in Male

Four patients with this disorder were described by Smith et al. in 1964. Its birth prevalence has been estimated by Opitz to be 1 in 20,000, placing it third behind cystic fibrosis and phenylketonurina among North American Caucasian populations. Tint et al. in 1993 identified an abnormality in cholesterol biosynthesis in patients with this disorder that appears to explain much of the clinical phenotype.

ABNORMALITIES
Growth. Moderately small at birth, with subsequent failure to thrive.
Performance. Moderate to severe mental deficiency, with variable altered muscle tone.
Craniofacial. Microcephaly with narrow frontal area, auricles slanted or low-set, ptosis of eyelids, inner epicanthal folds, strabismus, broad nasal tip with anteverted nostrils, broad maxillary secondary alveolar ridges, micrognathia.
Limb. Simian crease, high frequency of digital whorl dermal ridge patterning, syndactyly of second and third toes.
Genitourinary. Genital abnormalities (70 per cent) including hypospadias, cryptorchidism, micropenis, hypoplastic scrotum, bifid scrotum, and microurethra. Upper tract anomalies (57 per cent) including ureteropelvic junction obstruction, hydronephrosis, renal cystic dysplasia, renal duplication, renal agenesis, reflux.

OCCASIONAL ABNORMALITIES
Central and Peripheral Nervous Systems. Seizures; abnormal EEG; demyelination found in cerebral hemispheres, cranial nerves, and peripheral nerves.
Optic. Cataract, demyelination of optic nerves, sclerosis of lateral geniculate bodies, lack of visual following, opsoclonus.
Limb. Flexed fingers, asymmetrically short finger(s), distal axial triradius, polydactyly, metatarsus adductus, vertical talus, dislocation of hip, dysplasia epiphysealis punctata.

Other. Cleft palate, cardiac anomaly, abnormal pulmonary lobation, hypoplasia of thymus, adrenal enlargement, inguinal hernia, hepatic dysfunction, giant cells in pancreatic islets, deep sacral dimple, rectal atresia, Hirschsprung disease, pit anterior to anus. Unusually blond hair.

NATURAL HISTORY. Many of these babies are born in a breech presentation. Stillbirth and early neonatal death are not uncommon. Feeding difficulty and vomiting have been frequent problems in early infancy, and of those who survive, 20 per cent have died during the first year. Death appeared to be related to pneumonia in most of them, one of whom had a hemorrhagic necrotizing pneumonia with varicella, suggesting an impaired immune response. Necropsy studies have shown serious defects in brain morphogenesis, including microencephaly, hypoplasia of the frontal lobes, hypoplasia of cerebellum and brain stem, dilated ventricles, irregular gyrus patterns, and irregular neuronal organization. Irritable behavior with shrill screaming may pose a problem during infancy. Muscle tone, which may be hypotonic in early infancy, tends to become hypertonic with time. The degree of mental deficiency is usually moderate to severe. Two adults described have had I.Q.s in the 20s.

ETIOLOGY. Autosomal recessive. A severe defect in cholesterol biosynthesis has been identified leading to abnormally low plasma cholesterol levels and elevated concentrations of the cholesterol precursor 7-dehydrocholesterol. Cholesterol is vitally important in normal development through its contribution to the cell membrane and outer mitochondrial membrane as well as its role in steroid, bile acid, and vitamin D metabolism, and myelination of the nervous system. Its relative deficiency explains many of the variable features of this disorder. Furthermore, it provides the potential for treatment. Although efficacy has not yet been determined, dietary trials are currently underway.

112

Conventional colorimetric techniques to measure cholesterol will not invariably detect the cholesterol abnormalities in this condition. At present only a chromatographic assay is suitable for measuring 7-dehydrocholesterol.

Prenatal diagnosis has been successfully accomplished at 16 weeks' gestation on an affected fetus on the basis of reduced amniotic fluid cholesterol, elevated 7-dehydrocholesterol with undetectable amniotic fluid unconjugated estriol.

COMMENT. A number of infants with female external genitalia and a 46 XY karyotype who have multiple structural anomalies, including postaxial polydactyly, cleft palate, small tongue, eye anomalies, and cardiac defects, have died in the neonatal period. Although some controversy exists as to whether this represents a distinct disorder referred to as Smith-Lemli-Opitz type II, the same defect of cholesterol biosynthesis exists in both type I and type II and both types have occurred in the same sibship, suggesting that they represent variable expression of the same disorder.

References

Smith, D. W., Lemli, L., and Opitz, J. M.: A newly recognized syndrome of multiple congenital anomalies. J. Pediatr., 64:210, 1964.

Gibson, R.: A case of the Smith-Lemli-Opitz syndrome of multiple congenital anomalies in association with dysplasia epiphysealis punctata. Can. Med. Assoc. J., 92:574, 1965.

Dallaire, L., and Fraser, F. C.: The syndrome of retardation with urogenital and skeletal anomalies in siblings. J. Pediatr., 69:459, 1966.

Fierro, M.: Smith-Lemli-Opitz syndrome: Neuropathological and ophthalmological observations. Dev. Med. Child. Neurol., 19:57, 1977.

Lowry, R. B.: Editorial comment: Variability in the Smith-Lemli-Opitz syndrome: Overlap with the Meckel syndrome. Am. J. Med. Genet., 14:429, 1983.

Curry, C. J. R., et al.: Smith-Lemli-Opitz syndrome. Type II: Multiple congenital anomalies with male pseudohermaphroditism and frequent early lethality. Am. J. Med. Genet., 26:45, 1987.

Joseph, D. B., et al.: Genitourinary abnormalities associated with the Smith-Lemli-Opitz syndrome. J. Urol., 137:179, 1987.

Tint, G. S., et al.: Defective cholesterol biosynthesis associated with the Smith-Lemli-Opitz syndrome. N. Engl. J. Med., 330:107, 1994.

Opitz, J. M., and de La Cruz, F.: Cholesterol metabolism in the RSH/Smith-Lemli-Opitz syndrome: Summary of an NICHD Conference. Am. J. Med. Genet., 50:326, 1994.

Opitz, J. M.: RSH/SLO ("Smith-Lemli-Opitz") syndrome. Historical, genetic and developmental considerations. Am. J. Med. Genet., 50:344, 1994.

Irons, M., et al.: Abnormal cholesterol metabolism in the Smith-Lemli-Opitz syndrome: Report of clinical and biochemical findings in four patients and treatment in one patient. Am. J. Med. Genet., 50:347, 1994.

Nwokoro, N. A., et al.: Smith-Lemli-Opitz syndrome: Biochemical before clinical diagnosis; early dietary management. Am. J. Med. Genet., 50:375, 1994.

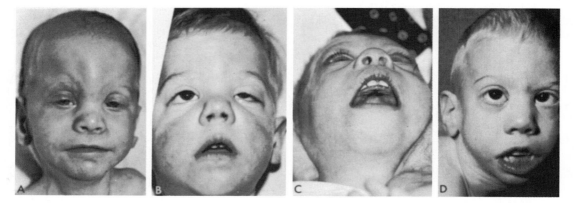

FIGURE 1. Smith-Lemli-Optiz syndrome. *First Row*: *A*, Young infant raised as female. *B*, A 10-month-old; height age, 6 months. *C*, Older infant. *D*, A 5-year-old; height age, 18 months. Note ptosis, nasal configuration, and prominent lateral palatine ridges.

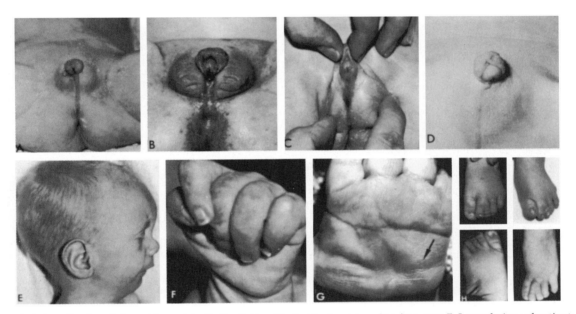

FIGURE 1. *Continued. Second Row*: *A* to *D*, Genitalia of individuals pictured in first row. *E*, Lateral view of patient *A*. Note prominent midforehead (gabella), micrognathia. *F*, Clenched hand (patient *A*), a variable feature. *G*, Simian crease and distal palmar axial triradius (*arrow*). *H*, Unusual appearance of syndactyly of the second and third toes in three of four patients. (*B, C, D, G,* and *H* from Smith, D. W., et al.: J. Pediatr., *64*:210, 1964, with permission.)

KABUKI SYNDROME

Initially reported in 1981 by Niikawa et al. and by Kuroki et al. in ten unrelated Japanese children, this disorder has now been reported in over 100 patients, many of them non-Japanese. Because of the facial resemblance of affected individuals to the make-up of actors in Kabuki, the traditional Japanese theater, this disorder has been referred to as the Kabuki syndrome.

ABNORMALITIES

Growth. Postnatal growth deficiency, with onset usually occurring in the first year, becomes more marked with increasing age. Mean height in children 12 months of age or over was −2.3 SD.

Performance. Mean developmental quotient in infants and children was 52, and in older patients, mean I.Q. was 62. Severe mental retardation is uncommon. Occasional individuals have had normal intelligence. Hypotonia.

Craniofacial. Long palpebral fissures with eversion of the lateral portion of the lower eyelid; ptosis; arching of eyebrows; strabismus; epicanthal folds; short nasal septum; large protuberant ears; preauricular pit; cleft palate; tooth abnormalities; open mouth with tented upper lip giving myopathic appearance.

Skeletal. Short, incurved fifth finger secondary to short fourth and fifth metacarpals; short middle phalanges; brachydactyly; rib anomalies; sagittal cleft of vertebral body; hip dislocation; scoliosis.

Cardiac. Defects occur in up to 50 per cent of patients and include malformations associated with altered hemodynamics such as coarctation of the aorta, bicuspid aortic valve, mitral valve prolapse, membranous ventricular septal defect, pulmonary, aortic, and mitral valve stenosis as well as tetralogy of Fallot, single ventricle with common atrium, double outlet right ventricle, and transportation of great vessels.

Other. Joint hyperextensibility; persistent fetal finger pad; excess digital ulnar loops.

OCCASIONAL ABNORMALITIES. Microcephaly; cleft lip; blue sclera; cutaneous syndactyly; nail hypoplasia; cryptorchidism; renal anomalies; imperforate anus; umbilical and inguinal hernias; malrotation of colon; premature thelarche; obesity; seizures; pectus excavatum; diaphragmatic eventration.

NATURAL HISTORY. The characteristic facial features become more obvious with age. The unusual length of the palpebral fissures and eversion of the lower lid is often difficult to appreciate in the neonatal period. Susceptibility to infection, particularly otitis media, is common.

ETIOLOGY. All cases have occurred sporadically in otherwise normal families.

COMMENT. Small marker ring chromosomes deriving most likely from the X chromosome have been described in at least three patients with the Kabuki syndrome. In addition, the phenotype of patients with Turner syndrome whose karyotype involves a very small marker X includes mental retardation and some features to suggest Kabuki syndrome. The relationship between these observations is at present unclear.

References

Niikawa, N., et al.: Kabuki make-up syndrome: A syndrome of mental retardation, unusual facies, large and protruding ears, and postnatal growth deficiency. J. Pediatr., *99*:565, 1981.

Kuroki, Y., et al.: A new malformation syndrome of long palpebral fissures, large ears, depressed nasal tip, and skeletal anomalies associates with postnatal dwarfism and mental retardation. J. Pediatr., *99*:570, 1981.

Niikawa, N., et al.: Kabuki make-up (Niikawa-Kuroki) syndrome: A study of 62 patients. Am. J. Med. Genet., *31*:565, 1988.

Philip, N., et al.: Kabuki make-up (Niikawa-Kuroki) syndrome: A study of 16 non-Japanese cases. Clin. Dysmorph., *1*:63, 1992.

Burke, L. W., and Jones, M. C.: Kabuki syndrome: Underdiagnosed recognizable pattern in cleft palate patients. Cleft Palate Craniofac. J., *32*:77, 1995.

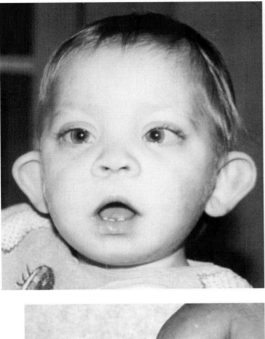

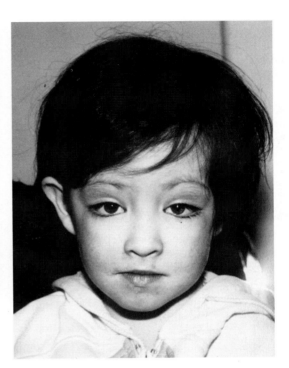

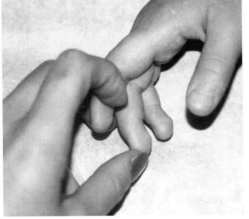

FIGURE 1. A 20-month-old boy and 4-year-old-girl. Note the long palpebral fissures, eversion of the lateral portion of the lower eyelid, and prominent fingertip pads.

WILLIAMS SYNDROME

Prominent Lips, Hoarse Voice, Cardiovascular Anomaly

In 1961, Williams et al. described this disorder in four unrelated children with mental deficiency, an unusual facies, and supravalvular aortic stenosis. Subsequently, well over 100 cases have been described. Hypercalcemia has been an infrequent finding; cardiovascular anomalies, including supravalvular aortic stenosis, have been variable; and features such as aberrations of growth and performance and the unusual facies are more consistent relative to diagnosis.

ABNORMALITIES. Varying features from among the following:

Growth. Mild prenatal growth deficiency. Postnatal growth rate about 75 per cent of normal. Mild microcephaly.

Performance. Average I.Q. of about 56, with a range from 41 to 80. Friendly, loquacious personality, hoarse voice, hypersensitivity to sound, mild neurologic dysfunction, primarily mild spasticity manifest by tight heel cords and hyperactive deep tendon reflexes and poor coordination. Perceptual and motor function more reduced (−3.0 to −3.9 SD) than verbal and memory performance (−2.0 SD). Level of general language ability is much greater than general cognitive ability.

Facies. Medial eyebrow flare, short palpebral fissures. Depressed nasal bridge. Epicanthal folds. Periorbital fullness of subcutaneous tissues. Blue eyes, stellate pattern in the iris. Anteverted nares, long philtrum, prominent lips with open mouth.

Limb. Hypoplastic nails, hallux valgus.

Cardiovascular. Supravalvular aortic stenosis, peripheral pulmonary artery stenosis, pulmonic valvular stenosis, ventricular and atrial septal defect. There may also be renal artery stenosis with hypertension, hypoplasia of the aorta, and other arterial anomalies.

Dentition. Partial anodontia, enamel hypoplasia.

Musculoskeletal. Joint limitations, lordosis, scoliosis, kyphosis, extra sacral crease.

Urinary. Renal anomalies including nephrocalcinosis, asymmetry in kidney size, small solitary and/or pelvic kidney. Bladder diverticula, urethral stenosis, vesicoureteral reflux.

OCCASIONAL ABNORMALITIES. Ocular hypotelorism, amblyopia, strabismus, refractive errors, tortuosity of retinal vessels, vocal cord paralysis, malar hypoplasia, fifth finger clinodactyly, radioulnar synostosis, small penis, pectus excavatum, inguinal and/or umbilical hernia, Chiari type I malformation, mucinous cystadenoma of ovary, hypercalcemia.

NATURAL HISTORY. In early infancy, these children tend to be fretful, have feeding problems, vomit frequently, are constipated, and are often colicky. During childhood they tend to be outgoing and loquacious, easily approach strangers, and have a strong interest in others. However, almost two thirds of children over 3 years display more difficult temperament characteristics than controls including higher activity, lower adaptability, greater intensity, more negative moods, less persistence, greater distractibility, and lower threshold arousal.

Over 20 adults have been carefully evaluated. Progressive medical problems were the rule, including hypertension; progressive joint limitations; recurrent urinary tract infections; and gastrointestinal problems including obesity, chronic constipation, diverticulosis and cholelithiasis, and hypercalcemia. The vast majority live with their parents, in group homes, or in supervised apartments.

Sudden death has been documented in a number of children. Some deaths were associated with the administration of anesthesia.

ETIOLOGY. Although most individuals with this disorder represent sporadic cases within otherwise normal families, parent-to-child transmission has been documented. Recent studies utilizing fluorescent in situ hybridization and quantitative Southern analysis indicate that both inherited and sporadic cases of Williams syndrome are caused by a deletion of one elastin allele located within chromosome subunit 7q11.23.

References

Joseph, M. C., and Parrott, D.: Severe infantile hypercalcemia with special reference to the facies. Arch. Dis. Child., 33:385, 1958.

Williams, J. C. P., Barratt-Boyes, B. G., and Lowe, J. B.: Supravalvular aortic stenosis. Circulation, 24:1311, 1961.

Jones, K. L., and Smith, D. W.: The Williams elfin facies syndrome. A new perspective. J. Pediatr., 86: 718, 1975.

Jensen, O. A., Marborg, M., and Dupont, A.: Ocular pathology in the elfin face syndrome. Ophthalmologica, 172:434, 1976.

Bennett, F. C., LaVeck, B., and Sells, C. J.: The Williams elfin facies syndrome: The psychological profile as an aid in syndrome identification. Pediatrics, *61*:303, 1978.

Culler, F. L., Jones, K. L., and Deftos, L. J.: Impaired calcitonin secretion in patients with Williams syndrome. J. Pediatr., *107*:720, 1985.

Morris, C. A., et al.: The natural history of the Williams syndrome. Physical characteristics. J. Pediatr., *113*:318, 1988.

Ewart, A. K., et al.: Hemizygosity at the elastin locus in a developmental disorder, Williams syndrome. Nat. Genet. *5*:11, 1993.

Pober, B. R., et al.: Renal findings in 40 individuals with Williams syndrome. Am. J. Med. Genet., *46*:271, 1993.

Bird, L. M., et al.: Sudden death in patients with supravalvular aortic stenosis and Williams syndrome. J. Pediatr. in press.

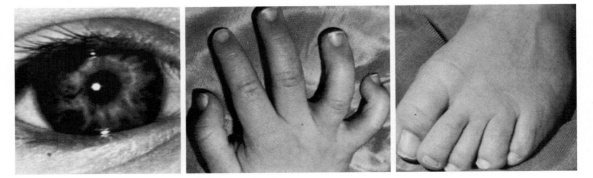

FIGURE 1. Stellate pattern to iris, relatively short nails, and valgus position of big toe—frequent features in Williams syndrome.

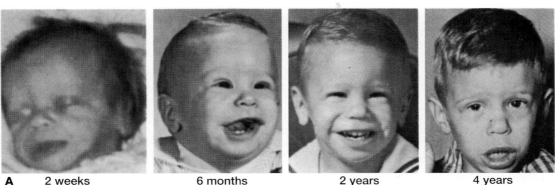

A   2 weeks   6 months   2 years   4 years
                                                         Height age 2¹⁰⁄₁₂
                                                         years

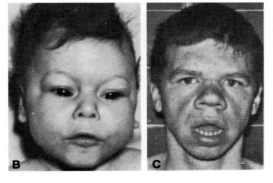

FIGURE 2. Williams syndrome. *A*, Facial appearance from the mother's photos of a boy with aortic stenosis, unusual facies, and relatively slow developmental progress. The serum calcium level is presently normal; serum calcium level during infancy is unknown. *B*, A 4 1/2-month-old with severe hypercalcemia, whose height age was 4 months at 7 months of age when the baby died. Necropsy showed nonspecific fibrous thickening in the intima of the aortic valve. (*B*, From Joseph, M. C., and Parrott, D.: Arch. Dis. Child., *33*:385, 1958, with permission.) *C*, A 17-year-old mentally deficient boy of short stature who has evidence of supravalvular aortic stenosis. (Courtesy of A. Reichert, Rainier State Training School, Buckley, Wash.)

NOONAN SYNDROME

(Turner-like Syndrome)

Webbing of the Neck, Pectus Excavatum, Cryptorchidism, Pulmonic Stenosis

Kobilinsky reported in 1883 a 20-year-old male with webbing of the neck, incomplete folding of the ears, and low posterior hairline, but no mention was made of other physical findings. The first complete description appears to be that of Weissenberg in 1928. In 1963, Noonan and Ehmke further delineated the clinical phenotype and documented its association with valvular pulmonic stenosis. Recently, Mendez and Opitz have set forth the entire phenotype based on a review of 63 publications since 1883.

ABNORMALITIES

Growth. Short stature of postnatal onset in 50 per cent.

Performance. Mental retardation (25 per cent).

Facies. Epicanthal folds, ptosis of eyelids, hypertelorism, low nasal bridge, down-slanting palpebral fissures, myopia, keratoconus, strabismus, nystagmus. Low-set and/or abnormal auricles. Anterior dental malocclusion. Increased width of mouth. Prominent, protruding upper lip; moderate retrognathia.

Neck. Low posterior hairline, short or webbed neck.

Thorax. Shield chest and pectus excavatum or pectus carinatum or both.

Other Skeletal. Cubitus valgus. Abnormalities of vertebral column.*

Heart. Pulmonary valve stenosis due to a dysplastic or thickened valve, left ventricular hypertrophy most frequently due to localized anterior septal hypertrophy and less often diffuse hypertrophy involving entire septum and free wall, septal defects, patent ductus arteriosus, branch stenosis of pulmonary arteries.

Genitalia. Small penis, cryptorchidism.

Bleeding Diathesis. A variety of defects in the coagulation and platelet systems including abnormalities in the intrinsic pathway (partial factor XI:C, XII:C, and VIII:C deficiencies), von Willebrand disease, and thrombocytopenia in approximately one third of cases.

OCCASIONAL ABNORMALITIES. High arched palate; large or asymmetric head; cerebral arteriovenous malformation, nerve deafness, hypoplastic nipples; kyphoscoliosis; winging of scapula, cervical ribs, edema of the dorsum of the hands and feet; lymphatic vessel dysplasia; chylothorax; simian creases; unusual wool-like consistency of the hair (curly); skin nevi, keloids, hyperelastic skin. Hypogonadism. Malignant hyperthermia.

NATURAL HISTORY. There is no apparent propensity to any special type of illness. The degree of mental retardation is seldom severe, and the social performance is usually better than anticipated from the intelligence quotient. Although impairment in fertility is present in some males, the major contributing factor is bilateral cryptorchidism. Fertility is normal in males with normally descended testes and in females.

Allanson et al. have documented changes in the clinical phenotype from birth through adulthood. In teenagers and in young adults, the face becomes more triangular and facial features are sharper. There is a tendency toward normalization.

ETIOLOGY. Usually a sporadic occurrence within families. Apparent autosomal dominant inheritance has been documented. A gene for this disorder has been mapped to 12q22-qter. However, nonlinkage has been documented in at least one family, indicating genetic heterogeneity for this disorder. Because of the wide variability in expression, careful evaluation of both parents must be undertaken prior to recurrence risk counseling.

COMMENT. The differential diagnosis for patients with the Noonan syndrome is extensive. XO/XY mosaicism, fetal hydantoin syndrome, fetal mysoline syndrome, and fetal alcohol syndrome have all been considered in patients with this phenotype. A number of patients have been described with features of both neurofibromatosis and Noonan syndrome. It is unclear if this is a distinct entity.

References

Kobilinsky, O.: Ueber eine flughautahnliche Ausbreitung am Halse. Arch. Anthropol., *14*:343, 1883.

Weissenberg, S.: Eine eigentumliche Hautflatengildung am Halse. Anthropol. Anz., *5*:141, 1928.

---

*Abnormal curvature of abnormal vertebrae (e.g., spina bifida occulta, hemivertebrae).

Noonan, J. A., and Ehmke, D. A.: Associated noncardiac malformations in children with congenital heart disease. J. Pediatr., *63*:469, 1963.

Opitz, J. M., and Weaver, D. D.: Editorial comment: The neurofibromatosis-Noonan syndrome. Am. J. Med. Genet., *21*:477, 1985.

Mendez, H. M. M., and Opitz, J. M.: Noonan syndrome: A review. Am J. Med. Genet., *21*:493, 1985.

Allanson, J. E., et al.: Noonan syndrome: The changing phenotype. Am. J. Med. Genet., *21*:507, 1985.

Witt, D. R., et al.: Bleeding diathesis in Noonan syndrome. A common association. Am. J. Med. Genet., *31*:305, 1988.

Sharland, M., et al.: Coagulation-factor deficiencies and abnormal bleeding in Noonan's syndrome. Lancet, *339*:19, 1992.

Sharland, M., et al.: Photoanthropometric study of facial growth in Noonan syndrome. Am. J. Med. Genet., *45*:430, 1993.

Bunch, M., et al.: Cardiologic abnormalities in Noonan syndrome: Phenotypic diagnosis and echocardiographic assessment of 118 patients. J. Am. Coll. Cardiol., *22*:1189, 1993.

Jamieson, C. R., et al.: Mapping a gene for Noonan syndrome to the long arm of chromosome 12. Nat. Genet., *8*:357, 1994.

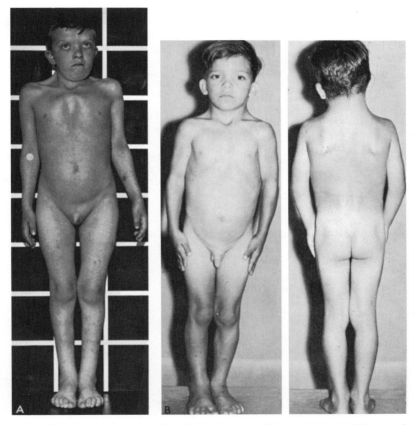

FIGURE 1. Noonan syndrome. *A,* A 12-year-old with height age of 7 years. Mental deficiency but a very affable personality. Cardiac defect. Cryptorchidism. (From Smith, D. W.: J. Pediatr., *70*:473, 1967, with permission.) *B,* A 9-year-old; height age at 10⁶/₁₂ years was 5⁸/₁₂ years. (From Ferrier, P. E.: Pediatrics, *40*:575, 1967, with permission.)

COSTELLO SYNDROME

This disorder initially was described by Costello in 1977. Subsequently, more than 20 cases have been reported.

ABNORMALITIES
Growth. Postnatal onset growth deficiency.
Performance. Mental deficiency with I.Q. ranging from 47 to 68; poor suck; sociable, warm personality.
Craniofacial. Macrocephaly; coarse face; low-set ears with thick lobes; epicanthal folds; strabismus; thick lips; depressed nasal bridge.
Skin/Hair/Nails. Thin, deep-set nails; cutis laxa (particularly hands and feet); dark skin pigmentation; curly hair; deep plantar, palmar, creases; hyperkeratotic palms and soles.
Musculoskeletal. Short neck; tight Achilles tendon; hyperextensible fingers; foot positional defects; increased anteroposterior diameter of chest; defective range of elbow motion.
Other. Papillomas in the perioral, nasal, and anal regions, with variable age of onset ranging from 2 to 15 years; hypertrophic cardiomyopathy; cerebral atrophy.

OCCASIONAL ABNORMALITIES.
Enamel dysplasia; acanthosis nigricans; palmar nevi; pulmonic stenosis; mitral valve prolapse; ventricular septal defect; epithelioma; ganglioneuroblastoma.

NATURAL HISTORY. Swallowing difficulties leading to failure to thrive frequently necessitates gavage feedings in the neonatal period. A disproportionate weight gain relative to linear growth has its onset in midchildhood when the facial changes become coarser. The cardiomyopathy can be associated with dysrhythmias and sudden death. The papillomas may undergo malignant change.

ETIOLOGY. Autosomal dominant inheritance. The fact that the majority of cases have occurred sporadically and that older mean paternal age has been documented suggests that fresh gene mutation is the most likely cause of this disorder. The occurrence of the disorder in siblings in two families is most likely related to gonadal mosaicism.

References

Costello, J. M.: A new syndrome: Mental subnormality and nasal papillomata. Aust. Pediatr. J., *13*:114, 1977.
Martin, R. A., and Jones, K. L.: Delineation of the Costello syndrome. Am. J. Med. Genet., *41*:345, 1991.
Zampino, G., et al.: Costello syndrome: Further delineation, natural history, genetic definition, and nosology. Am. J. Med. Genet., *47*:176, 1993.
Lurie, I. W.: Genetics of the Costello syndrome. Am. J. Med. Genet., *52*:358, 1994.

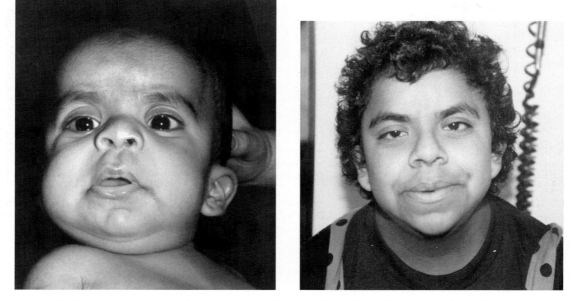

FIGURE 1. Affected female at 3 months and 15 years of age. *Illustration continued on following page*

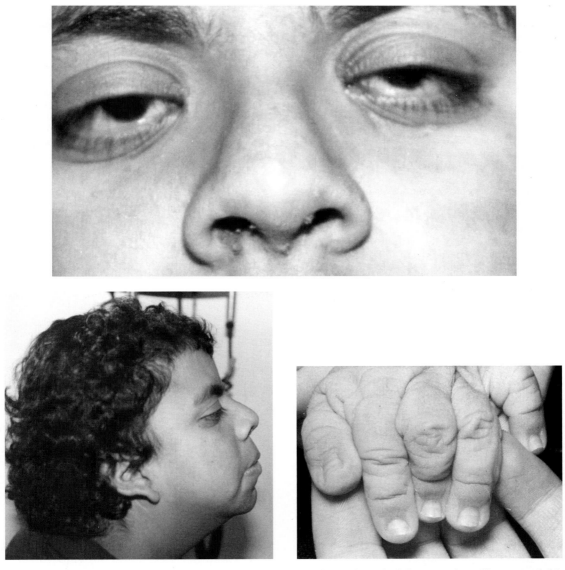

FIGURE 1. *Continued.* Note the coarse face, low-set ears with thick lobes, thick lips, nasal papillomas, and thin, deep-set nails with loose skin on hands. (From Martin, R. A., and Jones, K. L.: Am. J. Med. Genet., *41*:346, 1991, with permission.)

CARDIO-FACIO-CUTANEOUS (CFC) SYNDROME

Congenital Heart Defects, Ectodermal Anomalies, Frontal Bossing

Reynolds et al. reported eight patients with this disorder in 1986. More than 35 affected individuals have been described.

ABNORMALITIES

Neurologic. Mild to moderate mental retardation (80 per cent). Hypotonia. Nystagmus. Strabismus. Brain anomalies on CT scan including mild hydrocephalus, cortical atrophy, hypoplasia of frontal lobes, and/or brain stem atrophy.

Growth. Postnatal growth deficiency (68 per cent).

Craniofacies. Relative macrocephaly (88 per cent) with large prominent forehead (100 per cent), bitemporal narrowing (100 per cent), and shallow orbital ridges (100 per cent). Down-slanting palpebral fissures (71 per cent). Hypertelorism (84 per cent). Ptosis (53 per cent). Exophthalmos (55 per cent). Short upturned nose (92 per cent). Prominent philtrum (82 per cent). Posteriorly rotated ears (95 per cent).

Cardiac. Abnormalities in 77 per cent of cases, atrial septal defects and pulmonic stenosis being most common.

Skin and Hair. Sparse, curly, and/or slow-growing hair (100 per cent). Lack of eyebrows and eyelashes. Abnormalities of skin in 95 per cent varying from severe atopic dermatitis to hyperkeratosis/ichthyosis-like lesions.

OCCASIONAL ABNORMALITIES. Microcephaly. Seizures. Abnormal EEG. Hypertonia. Hearing loss. Submucous cleft palate. Hernia. Splenomegaly. Cavernous hemangiomas. Nail dysplasia.

NATURAL HISTORY. The extensive neurologic problems often associated with defects of the cortex, brain stem, and/or ventricular system represent the major problems for affected individuals. Language dysfunction is common and has not been well characterized. No information is available regarding the long-term follow-up of affected individuals.

ETIOLOGY. Unknown. All cases have been sporadic. An observed increase in paternal age has been noted, suggesting that all cases of this disorder have been due to an autosomal dominant mutation. However, no affected offspring of an affected parent has been documented.

References

Reynolds, J. F., et al.: New multiple congenital anomalies/mental retardation syndrome with cardio-facio-cutaneous involvement. The CFC syndrome. Am. J. Med. Genet., 25:413, 1986.

Bottani, A., et al.: The cardio-facio-cutaneous syndrome: Report of a patient and review of the literature. Eur. J. Pediatr., 150:486, 1991.

Raymond, G., and Holmes, L. B.: Cardio-facio-cutaneous (CFC) syndrome: Neurologic features in two children. Dev. Med. Child. Neurol., 35:727, 1993.

Borradori, L., et al.: Skin manifestations of cardio-facio-cutaneous syndrome. J. Am. Acad. Dermatol., 28:815, 1993.

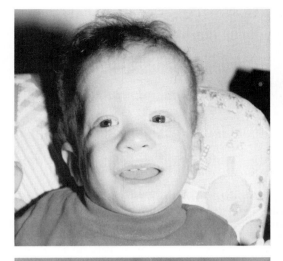

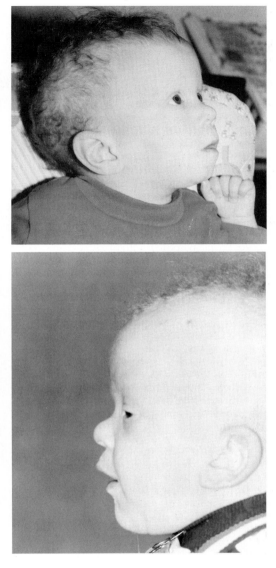

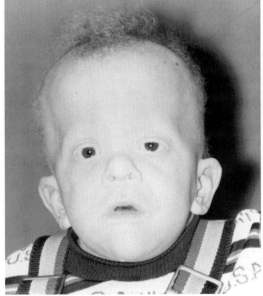

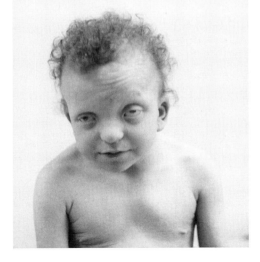

FIGURE 1. A 15-month-old boy, a $2^{6/12}$-year-old boy, and a $7^{10/12}$-year-old girl. Note bitemporal narrowing, prominent forehead, sparse curly hair, posteriorly rotated auricles, and ptosis. (From Reynolds, J. F., et al.: Am. J. Med. Genet., 25:413, 1991, with permission.)

AARSKOG SYNDROME

Hypertelorism, Brachydactyly, Shawl Scrotum

Set forth by Aarskog in 1970, there has been increasing recognition of this disorder. It can easily be misdiagnosed as the Noonan syndrome.

ABNORMALITIES

Growth. Slight to moderate short stature. Final adult height between 160 and 170 cm.

Performance. Mild to moderate mental deficiency (32 per cent). In the mentally normal males, dull normal intelligence is common. Hyperactivity and attention deficit disorders are common, particularly in the mentally subnormal.

Facies. Rounded. Facial edema in children less than 4 years of age. Hypertelorism with variable ptosis of eyelids and slight downward slant to palpebral fissures. Widow's peak. Small nose with anteverted nares, broad philtrum, maxillary hypoplasia, slight crease below the lower lip. Upper helices of ears incompletely outfolded. Hypodontia, retarded dental eruption, broad central upper incisors (permanent dentition), orthodontic problems.

Limbs. Brachydactyly with clinodactyly of fifth fingers, unusual position of extended fingers, simian crease, mild interdigital webbing. Broad thumbs and great toes.

Thorax. Mild pectus excavatum.

Abdomen. Prominent umbilicus, inguinal hernias.

Genitalia. "Shawl" scrotum in 90 per cent (see Fig., part E), cryptorchidism.

Other. Short neck with or without webbing. Cervical vertebral anomalies including hypoplasia and synostosis of one or more cervical vertebrae and spina bifida occulta.

OCCASIONAL ABNORMALITIES

Ocular. Strabismus, ambylopia, hyperopia, astigmatism, latent nystagmus, inferior oblique overaction, blue sclerae, anisometropia, posterior embryotoxon, corneal enlargement.

Skeletal. Scoliosis, cubitus valgus, splayed toes with bulbous tips, metatarsus adductus.

Genitalia. Cleft scrotum, phimosis.

Other. Scalp defects, anomalous cerebral venous drainage, Hirschsprung disease, midgut malrotation, hypoplastic kidney, dental enamel hypoplasia, delayed eruption of teeth, cleft lip and/or cleft palate, cardiac defects.

NATURAL HISTORY. Growth deficiency may be of prenatal onset. Marked failure to thrive in the first year with feeding difficulties and recurrent respiratory infections in 35 per cent. More commonly, mild growth deficiency is first evident at 1 to 3 years of age and may be associated with slow maturation and a late advent of adolescence. Fertility is normal. Orthodontic correction is often necessary. In the affected individuals with normal intelligence hyperactivity, when present, usually regresses between 12 and 14 years of age. For these patients social performance is usually good, and they tend to have a pleasant personality.

ETIOLOGY. X-linked recessive inheritance, with carrier females often showing some minor manifestations of the disorder, especially in the facies and hands. The gene for this disorder, designated FGDY1, has been mapped to Xp11.21. FDDY1 appears to code for a Rho/Rac guanine nucleotide exchange factor, a class of proteins involved in growth regulation and signal transduction suggesting a mechanism through which the growth anomalies seen in the Aarskog syndrome are produced. Genetic heterogeneity in this condition has not been excluded.

References

Aarskog, D.: A familial syndrome of short stature associated with facial dysplasia and genital anomalies. J. Pediatr., 77:856, 1970.

Furukawa, C. T., Hall, B. D., and Smith, D. W.: The Aarskog syndrome. J. Pediatr., 81:1117, 1972.

Halse, A., Bjorvatn, K., and Aarskog, D.: Dental findings in patients with the Aarskog syndrome. Scand. J. Dent. Res., 87:253, 1979.

Brodsky, M. C., et al.: Ocular and systemic findings in the Aarskog (facial-digital-genital) syndrome. Am. J. Ophthalmol., 109:450, 1990.

Fryns, J. P.: Aarskog syndrome: The changing phenotype with age. Am. J. Med. Genet., 43:420, 1992.

Glover, T. W., et al.: Translocation breakpoint in Aarskog syndrome maps to Xp11.21 between ALAS2 and DXS323. Hum. Mol. Genet., 2:1717, 1993.

Teebi, A. S., et al.: Aarskog syndrome: Report of a family with review and discussion of nosology. Am. J. Med. Genet., 46:501, 1993.

Pasteris, N. G., et al.: Isolation and characterization of the faciogenital dysplasia (Aarskog-Scott syndrome) gene: A putative Rho/Rac guanine nucleotide exchange factor. Cell, 79:669, 1994.

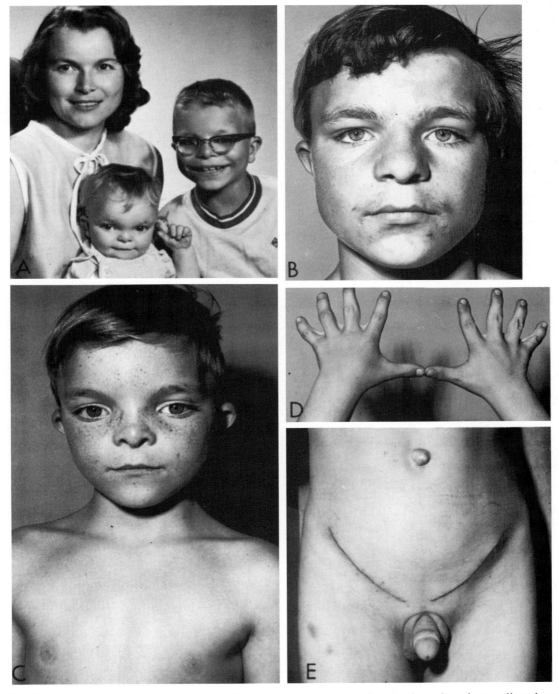

FIGURE 1. Aarskog syndrome. *A,* Mother with mild hypertelorism and widow's peak and two affected sons showing more striking hypertelorism. *B,* A 16-year-old, shown as a boy in *A.* Note the mild flare of the medial eyebrow and the less pronounced appearance of hypertelorism with age. *C,* A 7-year-old, shown as an infant in *A.* Note the mild overfolding of the ear helixes and the mild pectus excavatum. *D,* Mild brachyclinodactyly with mild syndactyly in patient shown in *C. E* "Pouting" umbilicus, scars of inguinal hernia repairs, and "shawl" scrotum in an 8-year-old boy. (From Furukawa, C. T., et al.: J. Pediatr., *81*:1117, 1972, with permission.)

ROBINOW SYNDROME

(Fetal Face Syndrome)

Flat Facial Profile, Short Forearms, Hypoplastic Genitalia

Initially reported by Robinow et al. in 1969, many additional cases of this disorder have been recognized. Butler and Wadlington have summarized the clinical phenotype and documented the natural history.

ABNORMALITIES

Growth. Slight to moderate shortness of stature of postnatal onset (93 per cent).

Craniofacial. Macrocephaly (44 per cent); large anterior fontanel, frontal bossing (94 per cent), hypertelorism (100 per cent), prominent eyes (86 per cent), down-slanting palpebral fissures (80 per cent), small upturned nose (100 per cent), long philtrum (88 per cent), triangular mouth with downturned angles (94 per cent) and micrognathia (87 per cent), hyperplastic alveolar ridges (66 per cent), crowded teeth (96 per cent), and posteriorly rotated ears (53 per cent).

Limbs. Short forearms (100 per cent). Small hands with clinodactyly (88 per cent). Nail dysplasia (48 per cent).

Other Skeletal. Hemivertebrae of thoracic vertebrae (70 per cent). Rib anomalies, primarily fusion of or absent ribs (40 per cent). Scoliosis (50 per cent).

Genitalia. Small penis, clitoris, labia majora (94 per cent); cryptorchidism (65 per cent).

OCCASIONAL ABNORMALITIES

Oral-Facial. Nevus flammeus (23 per cent), epicanthal folds, macroglossia, high arched palate, absent or bifid uvula (18 per cent), cleft lip and/or cleft palate (9 per cent), short frenulum of tongue with cleft tongue tip.

Limbs. Broad thumbs and toes, bifid terminal phalanges, clinodactyly of fifth finger, hyperextensible fingers, short metacarpals. Madelung-like anomaly of forearm, dislocation of hip, hypoplastic interphalangeal creases, single flexion creases on third and fourth fingers, hypoplastic middle and terminal phalanges of fingers and toes, transverse palmar crease, ectrodactyly.

Other. Seizures; developmental delay and mental retardation (18 per cent); language deficiency; pectus excavatum (19 per cent); superiorly positioned, broad, and poorly epithelialized umbilicus and inguinal hernia (20 per cent); pilonidal dimple; renal anomalies (29 per cent); cardiac defects especially right ventricular outlet obstruction (13 per cent).

NATURAL HISTORY. Early death secondary to pulmonary or cardiac complications occurs in 10 per cent of patients. The penile hypoplasia may be sufficient to initially raise the question of sex of rearing. Although partial primary hypogonadism evidenced by elevated serum follicle-stimulating hormone levels was documented in four affected males, normal pubertal virilization occurred in all three patients older than 16 years. Two adult females are 4 feet 10 inches and 5 feet respectively, and three adult males are 5 feet 3 inches, 5 feet 7 inches, and 5 feet 10 inches in height. The facial features become less pronounced with age owing to accelerated growth of the nose at adolescence. Performance has been normal in most individuals.

ETIOLOGY. Autosomal dominant inheritance was implied in the family reported by Robinow et al. However, Wadlington et al. reported affected siblings of normal parents, and other cases have been sporadic in the family. Therefore, as high as a 25 per cent recurrence risk must be discussed with unaffected parents who have one affected child. The possibility of etiologic heterogeneity for this disorder remains open. It has been suggested that vertebral and multiple rib anomalies, as well as more severe mesomelic brachymelia and more triangular shaped mouth are more indicative of autosomal recessive inheritance.

References

Robinow, M., Silverman, F. N., and Smith. H. D.: A newly recognized dwarfing syndrome. Am. J. Dis. Child., *117*:645, 1969.

Wadlington, W. B., Tucker, V. L., and Schimke, R. N.: Mesomelic dwarfism with hemivertebrae and small genitalia (the Robinow syndrome). Am. J. Dis. Child., *126*:202, 1973.

Bain, M. D., Winter, R. M., and Burn, J.: Robinow syndrome without mesomelic brachymelia: A report of five cases. J. Med. Genet., *23*:350, 1986.

Butler, M. G., and Wadlington, W. B.: Robinow syndrome: Report of two patients and review of the literature. Clin. Genet., *31*:77, 1987.

Webber, S. A., et al.: Congenital heart disease and Robinow syndrome: Coincidence or an additional component of the syndrome? Am. J. Med. Genet., *37*:519, 1990.

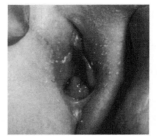

FIGURE 1. Robinow syndrome. Genitalia in an affected female, showing minute clitoris.

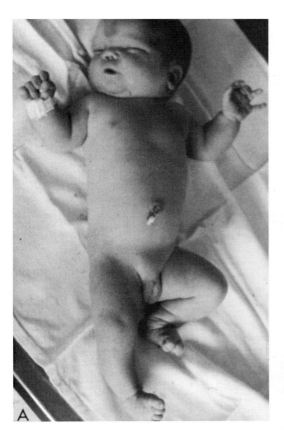

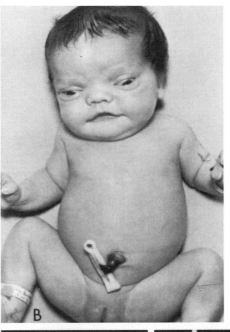

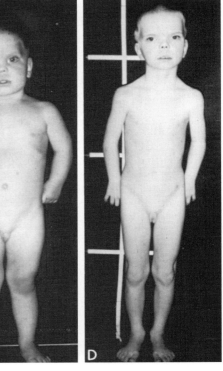

FIGURE 2. Robinow syndrome. *A,* A 3-day-old male with micropenis, hypertelorism, and capillary hemangioma on central forehead. *B,* A 2-day-old female with flat facies, hypertelorism, and minute clitoris *C* and *D,* Note small nose, hypertelorism, micropenis, and variable shortness of hands. (*A, C,* and *D* from Robinow, M., et al.: Am. J. Dis. Child., *117*:645, 1969. Copyright 1969, American Medical Association.)

OPITZ SYNDROME

(Hypertelorism-Hypospadias Syndrome, Opitz-Frias
Syndrome, Opitz Oculo-Genito-Laryngeal Syndrome)

Hypertelorism, Hypospadias, Swallowing Difficulties

In 1965 and again in 1969, Opitz, Smith, and Summitt reported this condition, previously referred to as the BBB syndrome, in three families in which affected males usually have apparent ocular hypertelorism and hypospadias and affected females have only hypertelorism. As the spectrum of defects in this disorder has evolved, it has become clear that the disorder described by Opitz et al. in 1969, previously referred to as the G syndrome or Opitz-Frias syndrome, is the same condition.

ABNORMALITIES
Performance. Mild to moderate mental deficiency in about two thirds of patients. Hypotonia.
Facial. Ocular hypertelorism. Upward or downward slanting of palpebral fissures and epicanthal folds. Broad flat nasal bridge with anteverted nostrils. Cleft lip with or without cleft palate. Short frenulum of tongue. Posterior rotation of auricles. Micrognathia.
Genital. Hypospadias, cryptorchidism. Bifid scrotum.
Other. Hernias.

OCCASIONAL ABNORMALITIES.
Cranial asymmetry, widow's peak, strabismus, grooving of nasal tip, flattened elongated philtrum, thin upper lip, bifid uvula, cleft tongue, dental anomalies. Brain magnetic resonance imaging findings including agenesis or hypoplasia of corpus callosum, cerebellar vermal hypoplasia, cortical atrophy and ventriculomegaly, macro cisterna magna, and a wide cavum septum pellucidum. Laryngotracheal cleft, malformation of larynx, tracheoesophageal fistula, hypoplastic epiglottis, high carina, and pulmonary hypoplasia. Renal defect. Cardiac defects, most commonly conotruncal lesions. Agenesis of gallbladder. Duodenal stricture. Imperforate anus. Hiatal hernia. Diastasis recti. Increased monozygotic twinning.

NATURAL HISTORY.
Swallowing problems with recurrent aspiration, stridulous respirations, intermittent pulmonary difficulty, wheezing, and a weak, hoarse cry should raise concern about a potentially lethal laryngoesophageal defect. In those individuals mortality is high unless vigorous efforts are made to repair the defect and protect the lungs with gastrostomy or jejunostomy. Although males tend to have more severe and more frequent laryngoesophageal defects, it is important to recognize that this disorder can express itself in both males and females with equal severity. Initial failure to thrive is followed by normal growth in survivors.

ETIOLOGY. Heterogeneity has been demonstrated with an X-linked locus linked to Xp22 and an autosomal dominant locus linked to 22q11.2. The two different forms appear indistinguishable clinically.

References

Opitz, J. M., Smith, D. W., and Summitt, R. L.: Hypertelorism and hypospadias (abst.) J. Pediatr., 67: 968, 1965.

Opitz, J. M., et al.: The G syndrome of multiple congenital anomalies. Birth Defects, 5:95, 1969.

Opitz, J. M., Summitt, R. L., and Smith, D. W.: The BBB syndrome. Familial telecanthus with associated anomalies. *In* Bergsma, D. (ed.): First Conference on Clinical Delineation of Birth Defects, Vol. 5. The National Foundation, 1969, pp. 86–94.

Gonzales, C. H., Hermann, J., and Opitz, J. M.: The hypertelorism-hypospadias (BBB) syndrome. Eur. J. Pediatr., 12:51, 1977.

Cordero, J. F., and Holmes, L. B.: Phenotypic overlap of the BBB and G syndromes. Am. J. Med. Genet., 2:145, 1978.

Stoll, C., et al.: Male-to-male transmission of the hypertelorism-hypospadias (BBB) syndrome. Am. J. Med. Genet., 20:221, 1985.

Brooks, J. K., et al.: Opitz (BBB/G) syndrome: Oral manifestations. Am. J. Med. Genet., 43:595, 1992.

MacDonald, M. R., et al.: Brain magnetic resonance imaging findings in the Opitz/G/BBB syndrome: Extension of the spectrum of midline brain anomalies. Am. J. Med. Genet., 46:706, 1993.

Robin, N. H., et al.: Opitz syndrome is genetically heterogeneous with one locus on Xp22 and a second locus on 22q11.2. Nat. Genet., 11:459, 1995.

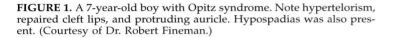

FIGURE 1. A 7-year-old boy with Opitz syndrome. Note hypertelorism, repaired cleft lips, and protruding auricle. Hypospadias was also present. (Courtesy of Dr. Robert Fineman.)

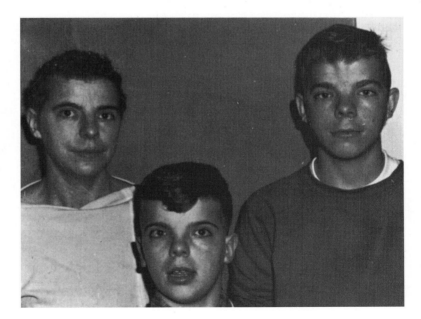

FIGURE 2. Opitz syndrome. An affected mother (mild hypertelorism) and two of her affected boys who show hypertelorism and also have hypospadias. (From the B. O. family pedigree of Opitz, J. M., et al.: Birth Defects, 5:86, 1969, with permission.)

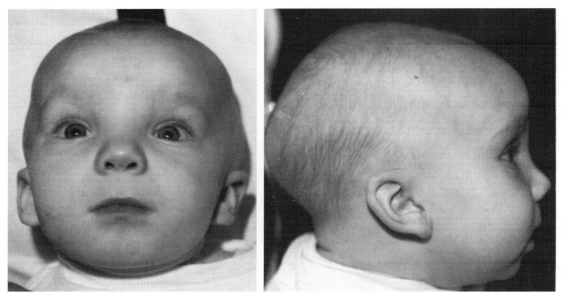

FIGURE 3. Opitz syndrome. A 1-month-old.

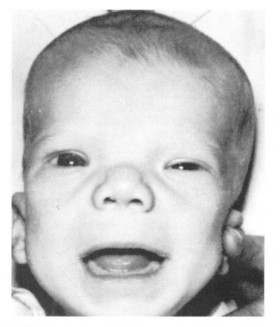

FIGURE 3. *Continued.* A 7$\frac{1}{2}$-month-old. (From Opitz, J. M., et al.: Birth Defects, *5*(2):95, 1969, with permission.)

FLOATING-HARBOR SYNDROME

Postnatal Growth Deficiency, Bulbous Nose, Speech Delay

Pelletier and Feingold described the initial patient with this disorder in 1973. One year later, Leisti et al. reported a child with almost identical features and suggested the term "Floating-Harbor syndrome," an amalgam of the names of the hospitals where the initial two patients were evaluated (Boston Floating and Harbor General, Torrance, Calif.). Approximately 15 patients have been reported with this condition.

ABNORMALITIES

Growth. Birth weight and length at third percentile. Striking postnatal growth deficiency. Delayed bone age.

Performance. Significant speech delay. Normal motor development. Mild mental retardation.

Craniofacies. Broad, bulbous nose with prominent nasal bridge and wide columella. Short, smooth philtrum. Wide mouth with thin lips. Prominent eyes in infancy which in older children give the appearance of being deep-set. Posteriorly rotated ears.

Other. Low posterior hairline. Short neck. Fifth finger clinodactyly. Brachydactyly. Broad thumbs. Joint laxity.

OCCASIONAL ABNORMALITIES. Abnormal EEG. Pulmonary stenosis. Triangular face. Rib anomalies. Accessory thumb. Cone-shaped epiphyses. Perthes disease. Clavicular pseudoarthrosis. Finger clubbing. Celiac disease. Abdominal distention. Constipation. Hirsutism. Long eye lashes.

NATURAL HISTORY. The facial features are most recognizable in midchildhood. During childhood, height and weight tend to parallel the third percentile, but 4 to 6 SD below the mean. The speech problem is related to deficient expressive language skills.

ETIOLOGY. Unknown. All cases have been sporadic events in otherwise normal families.

References

Pelletier, G., and Feingold, M.: Case report 1. Syndrome Identification, *1*:8, 1973.

Leisti, J., et al.: Case report 12. Syndrome Identification, *2*:3, 1973.

Robinson, P. L., et al.: A unique association of short stature, dysmorhpic features and speech impairment. (Floating-Harbor syndrome). J. Pediatr., *113*: 703, 1988.

Patton, M. R., et al.: Floating-Harbor syndrome. J. Med. Genet., *28*:201, 1991.

Houlston, R. S., et al.: Further observations on the Floating-Harbor syndrome. Clin. Dysmorph., *3*:143, 1994.

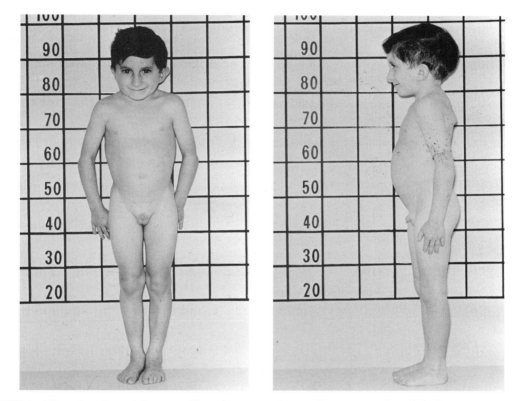

FIGURE 1. Affected male at 6⁸/₁₂ years. Note the proportionate short stature, broad, bulbous nose and short philtrum. (Courtesy of David L. Rimoin, Cedars-Sinai Medical Center, Los Angeles, Calif.)

D

D. SENILE-LIKE APPEARANCE

PROGERIA SYNDROME

(Hutchinson-Gilford Syndrome)

Alopecia, Atrophy of Subcutaneous Fat, Skeletal Hypoplasia and Dysplasia

The following entry was recorded in the *St. James Gazette* in 1752: "March 19, 1754 died in Glamorganshire of mere old age and a gradual decay of nature at seventeen years and two months, Hopkins Hopkins, the little Welshman, lately shown in London. He never weighed more than 17 pounds but for three years past no more than twelve."

In 1886, Hutchinson described a similar patient. Later, Gilford studied this boy and another patient and termed the condition progeria, meaning premature aging. DeBusk summarized the findings in 60 cases.

ABNORMALITIES

Alopecia. Onset at birth to 18 months, with degeneration of hair follicles.

Skin. Thin with onset in early to midinfancy. Prominent scalp veins. Localized scleroderma-like areas over lower abdomen, upper legs, and buttocks appearing at birth or early infancy. Irregular pigmentary changes over sun-exposed areas that become more prominent with age.

Nails. Hypoplastic with onset in infancy; nails may be brittle, curved, yellowish.

Subcutaneous Fat. Diminished with onset in infancy, last areas of adipose atrophy are cheeks and pubic areas.

Periarticular Fibrosis. Onset at 1 to 2 years; stiff or partially flexed prominent joints or both; leads to "horse-riding" stance.

Skeletal Hypoplasia, Dysplasia, and Degeneration. Deficient growth, which becomes evident between 6 and 18 months; subsequent growth rate one third to one half normal. Facial hypoplasia and micrognathia, slim tubular bones and ribs with small thoracic cage, and thin calvarium with marked delay in ossification of fontanels. Generalized osteoporosis. Skeletal dysplasia evident in coxa valga; tendency toward ovoid vertebral bodies. In the long bones, sclerotic changes with thinned shafts, reduced corticomedullary ratio, and pathological fractures, particularly of the humerus. Skeletal degenertion evident in loss of bone in clavicle and distal phalanges.

Dentition. Delayed eruption of deciduous and permanent dentition; crowding of teeth; anodontia and hypodontia, especially of permanent teeth; discoloration; high incidence of cavities.

Atherosclerosis. As early as 5 years, onset of generalized atherosclerosis, especially evident in coronary arteries, aorta, and mesenteric arteries; at later age, may have cardiac murmur, left ventricular hypertrophy.

OCCASIONAL ABNORMALITIES. Perceptive hearing deficit, congenital or acquired cataract, microphthalmia, absent breast and nipple, upper radial metaphyseal changes consisting of a waist-like defect in the region of the proximal radial metaphysis, relatively large thymus, lymphoid and reticular hyperplasia.

NATURAL HISTORY. Though the onset of disease manifestations is usually stated as 1 to 2 years, there may be subtle indicators of disease within the first year. The average birth weight for 17 patients was 2.7 kg. One patient whose scalp was shaved at 6 weeks had no regrowth of hair. The deficit of growth becomes severe after 1 year of age and there is absent sexual maturation. The tendency to fatigue easily is a factor that might limit full participation in childhood activities. The life span is shortened by the early advent of relentless arterial atheromatosis, and the usual cause of death is coronary occlusion. One instance of cerebral infarction has been reported. The life expectancy for 13 patients was 7 to 27 years, with an average of 14.2 years. Since intelligence and brain development do not appear to be impaired, children with progeria should be allowed as normal a social life as possible.

At the present time, there is no effective therapy. One affected child who suffered from severe angina pectoris underwent coronary angiography, saphenous and internal mammary artery–to–coronary artery bypass surgery, and percutaneous transluminal angioplasty at 14 years of age. At follow-up, 1 year after surgery, the child was having only infrequent episodes of chest pain. The use of a wig is recommended for cosmetic purposes.

ETIOLOGY. Unknown. Most cases are sporadic. Older mean paternal age suggests the possibility of a fresh mutant gene of an autosomal dominant disorder. However, there are at least three instances of affected siblings from normal parentage, suggesting autosomal recessive inheritance. Possibly, there is etiologic heterogeneity for this phenotype.

References

Hutchinson, J.: Congenital absence of hair and mammary glands with atrophic condition of the skin and its appendages in a boy whose mother had been almost wholly bald from alopecia areata from the age of six. Trans. Med. Chir. Soc. Edinb., *69*:473, 1886.

Gilford, H.: Progeria: A form of senilism. The Practitioner, *73*:188, 1904.

DeBusk, F. L.: The Hutchinson-Gilford progeria syndrome. J. Pediatr., *80*:697, 1972.

Dyck, J. D., et al.: Management of coronary artery disease in Hutchinson-Gilford syndrome. J. Pediatr., *711*:407, 1987.

Gillar, P. J., et al.: Progressive early dermatologic changes in Hutchinson-Gilford progeria syndrome. Pediatr. Dermatol. *8*:199, 1991.

Wagle, W. A., et al.: Cerebral infarction in progeria. Pediatr. Neurol., *8*:476, 1992.

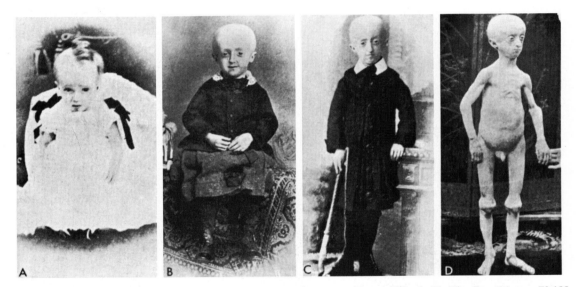

FIGURE 1. Progeria syndrome. *A* to *D*, Gilford's original patient. (From Gilford, H.: The Practitioner, 73:188, 1904, with permission)

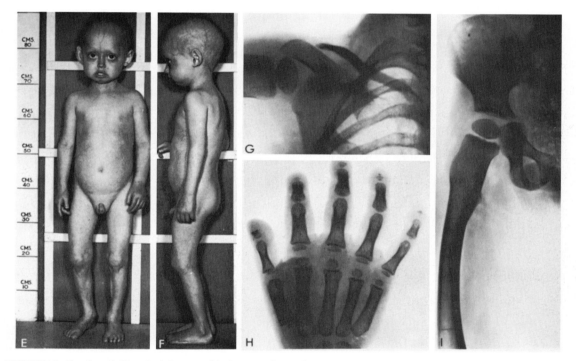

FIGURE 1. *Continued. E* to *I,* A 3-year-old showing loss of outer clavicle, distal phalanges, and straight femur. (From Macleod, W.: Br. J. Radiol., *39:*224, 1966, with permission.)

WERNER SYNDROME

*Early Adult—Cataract, Thin Skin With
Thick Fibrous Subcutaneous Tissue, Gray Sparse Hair*

The subject of Werner's doctoral thesis in 1904, this disease is usually not diagnosed until young adult life. More than 400 cases have been recorded.

ABNORMALITIES

Growth. Short stature; mean stature of affected males, 61 inches; females, 57.5 inches.

Deterioration. Loss of subcutaneous fat; slim, spindly extremities with small hands and feet; pinched facies with beak nose. Irregular dental development. Patches of stiffened skin, particularly on face and lower legs; skin ulcerations; atrophy of distal extremities. Thick, fibrous subcutaneous tissue with thin dermis. Osteoporosis, atherosclerosis with calcification. Muscle hypoplasia with patchy areas of fibrosis. Gray, sparse hair, premature balding. Cataract, retinal degeneration. Premature loss of teeth. Hypogonadism, reduced fertility. High-pitched, hoarse voice secondary to vocal chord atrophy. Liver atrophy. Adult-type diabetes (44 per cent). Mönckeberg sclerosis with organic brain syndrome. Metastatic calcifications. Excess urinary excretion of hyaluronic acid.

OCCASIONAL ABNORMALITIES. Propensity toward malignancy (10 per cent), especially sarcoma and meningioma. Mild hyperthyroidism. Adrenal atrophy. Valvular sclerosis. Hyperkeratosis of palms and soles.

NATURAL HISTORY. Often noted to be slim with a slow rate of growth in later childhood, these individuals have no adolescent growth spurt and reach their final height at 10 to 18 years, usually at approximately 13 years. Gray hair develops at around 20 years. Thereafter follows skin changes, primarily atrophy involving the face and distal extremities, hair loss, development of a high-pitched or hoarse voice, visual symptoms, detection of cataracts, skin ulcers, and lastly, diabetes at an average age of 34 years. Old age appearance is evident by 30 to 40 years, with the mean age of survival being 47 years with a range of 31 to 63 years. Calcification occurs not only in the atheromatous vessels but in the thick subcutaneous tissues as well. Hypertension occurs in about 50 per rcent of patients.

ETIOLOGY. Autosomal recessive. The gene responsible for this disorder (WRN) has been mapped to 8p12. Its product shows significant similarity to DNA helicases. As such, mutations of this gene could lead to abnormalities of DNA replication, recombination, chromosome segregation, DNA repair, transcription or other functions requiring DNA unwinding.

References

Werner, O.: Uber Katarakt in Verbindung mit Sklerodermie. (Doctoral dissertation, Kiel University.) Kiel, Schmidt and Klaunig, 1904.

Epstein, C. J., et al.: Werner's syndrome. Medicine. *45*: 177, 1966.

Fleischmajer, R., and Nedwich, A.: Werner's syndrome. Am. J. Med., *54*:111, 1973.

Murata, K., and Nakashima, H.: Werner's syndrome: 24 cases with a review of the Japanese literature. J. Am. Geriatr. Soc., *30*:303, 1982.

Salk, D.: Werner's syndrome: A review of recent research with an analysis of connective tissue metabolism, growth control of cultured cells, and chromosome aberrations. Hum. Genet., *62*:1, 1982.

Goto, M., et al.: Genetic linkage of Werner's syndrome to five markers on chromosome 8. Nature, *355*:733, 1992.

Chang-En, Y., et al.: Positional cloning of the Werner's syndrome gene. Science 272:258, 1996.

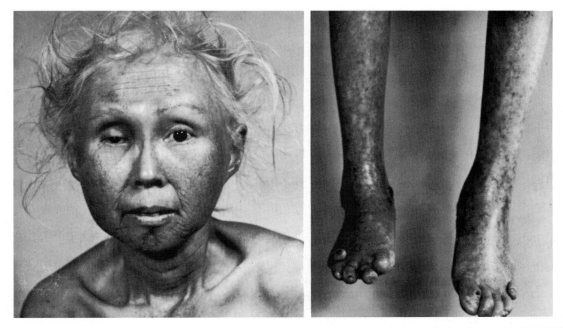

FIGURE 1. A 48-year-old woman with Werner syndrome. (From Epstein, C. J., et al.: Medicine, *45*:177, 1966, with permission.)

COCKAYNE SYNDROME

*Senile-like Changes Beginning
in Infancy, Retinal Degeneration and Impaired
Hearing, Photosensitivity of Thin Skin*

Cockayne reported this disorder in siblings in 1946. Subsequently, more than 150 other cases have been documented.

ABNORMALITIES

Growth. Profound postnatal growth deficiency with loss of adipose tissue beginning in the first year of life. Weight more affected than length. Final height and weight are rarely greater than 115 cm and 20 kg, respectively.

Central and Peripheral Nervous Systems. Microcephaly by 2 years of age in almost 100 per cent. Mental deficiency (borderline in 14 per cent; mild in 29 per cent; moderate in 38 per cent; severe in 19 per cent). Unsteady gait; ataxia, tremor, incoordination, dysarthric speech. Weakness with peripheral neuropathy. Sensorineural hearing loss (50 per cent). Seizures (5 to 10 per cent). Decreased lacrimation or sweating, miotic pupils. Increased ventricular size and/or cerebral atrophy. Calcifications in basal ganglia. Demyelination of subcortical white matter.

Ocular. Salt and pepper retinal pigmentation, optic atrophy, strabismus, hyperopia, corneal opacity, cataract, decreased lacrimation, nystagmus.

Facial. Relatively small cranium with radiographic evidence of a thickened calvarium. Loss of facial adipose tissue with slender nose, moderately sunken eyes, and thin skin that is photosensitive. Dental abnormalities including caries, delayed eruption of deciduous teeth, malocclusion, and absent/hypoplastic teeth.

Skin. Photosensitive dermatitis (75 per cent). Dry and sometimes scaly skin.

Extremities. Cool hands and feet, sometimes cyanotic. Mild to moderate joint limitation.

Trunk. Relatively short, with biconvex flattening of vertebrae and tendency toward dorsal kyphosis.

Other. Hypertension. Renal dysfunction (10 per cent). Cryptorchidism in one third of males. Underdeveloped breasts and irregular menstrual cycles are frequent. Thin, dry hair. Sclerotic "ivory" epiphyses most obviously in the fingers. Small, "squared off" pelvis with hypoplastic iliac wings.

OCCASIONAL ABNORMALITIES.

Intrauterine growth retardation. Intracranial calcification, small sella turcica, micropenis, anhidrosis, basal cell carcinoma, cardiac arrhythmias, peripheral vascular disease, asymmetric fingers, short second toes, hepatomegaly, splenomegaly. Osteoporosis.

NATURAL HISTORY. Although prenatal growth deficiency occasionally has been documented, growth and development usually proceed at a normal rate in early infancy, and it is not until 2 to 4 years of age that the pattern of defect is clearly evident. Personality and behavior tend to correspond to the mental age, which is defective. No affected individual has fathered or given birth to a child. Photosensitivity of the skin may lead to problems with exposure to sunlight. Although only rare patients have developed basal cell carcinomas, a defect in DNA repair following ultraviolet irradiation similar to that seen in xeroderma pigmentosa has been documented. The average age at death is $12^{3}/_{12}$ years; the major contributing factor being pneumonia.

COMMENT. An early onset "severe form" of Cockayne syndrome has been reported in at least 20 patients. Prenatal onset growth deficiency, a lack of all neurologic development, early postnatal onset of congenital cataracts, and structural eye defects characterize this condition. Death usually occurs by 6 or 7 years of age. The relationship of this disorder, referred to as Cockayne syndrome II, to classical Cockayne syndrome is unknown. Results of ultraviolet sensitivity studies on fibroblasts from patients with the severe form suggest that they have a disorder of DNA metabolism similar to that seen in patients with the classical form.

ETIOLOGY. Autosomal recessive. A defect in DNA metabolism has been documented in fibroblasts that involves increased sensitivity of cells to ultraviolet light, decreased RNA synthesis following UV exposure, and normal excision repair.

References

Cockayne, E. A.: Dwarfism with retinal atrophy and deafness. Arch. Dis. Child., 21:52, 1946.

Neill, C. A., and Dingwall, M. M.: A syndrome resembling progeria: A review of two cases. Arch. Dis. Child., 25:213, 1950.

MacDonald, W. B., Fitch, K. D., and Lewis, I. C.: Cockayne's syndrome. An heredo-familial disorder of growth and development. Pediatrics, 25:997, 1960.

Lowry, R. B.: Invited editorial comment: Early onset of Cockayne syndrome. Am. J. Med. Genet., 13:209, 1982.

Rainbow, A. J., and Howes, M.: A deficiency in the repair of UV and γ-ray damaged DNA in fibroblasts from Cockayne's syndrome. Mutat. Res., 93:235, 1982.

Patton, M. A., et al.: Early onset Cockayne's syndrome: Case reports with neuropathological and fibroblast studies. J. Med. Genet., 26:154, 1989.

Nance, M. A., and Berry, S. A.: Cockayne syndrome: Review of 140 cases. Am. J. Med. Genet., 42:68, 1992.

Lehmann, A. R., et al.: Cockayne's syndrome: Correlation of clinical features with cellular sensitivity of RNA synthesis to UV irradiation. J. Med. Genet., 30:679, 1993.

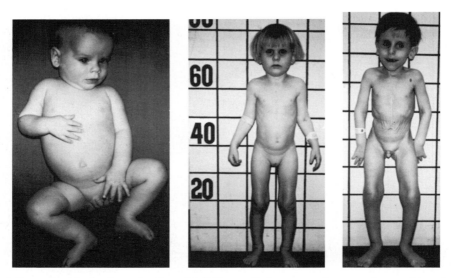

FIGURE 1. A 7-month-old who later developed full-blown Cockayne syndrome; a 4-year-old and a 2-year-old showing the dramatic changes that occur with age in this degenerative disorder. (Courtesy of Dr. Robert Summitt, University of Tennessee College of Medicine, Memphis, Tenn.)

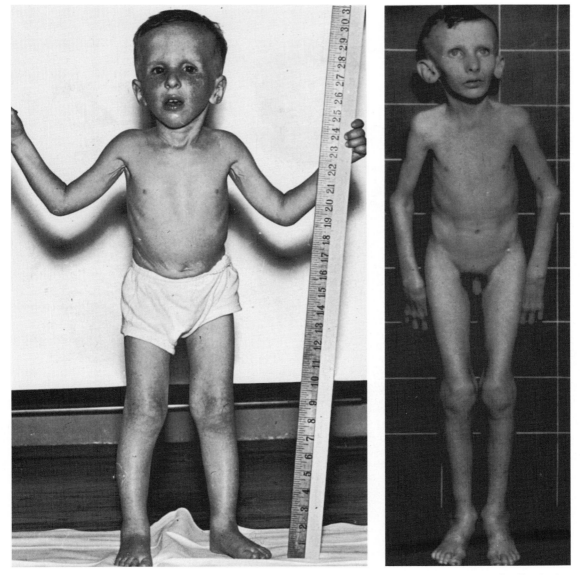

FIGURE 2. Cockayne syndrome. *Left*, Child, 6¹⁰/₁₂ years old. Height age, 16 months. (From Windmiller, J.: Am. J. Dis. Child., *105*:204, 1963, with permission.) *Right*, A 14⁶/₁₂-year-old. Height age, 3⁶/₁₂ years. Bone age, 16 years. (From Wilkins, L.: Diagnosis and Treatment of Endocrine Disorders in Childhood and Adolescence, 3rd ed. Springfield, Ill., Charles C Thomas, 1965. Courtesy of R. M. Blizzard.)

ROTHMUND-THOMSON SYNDROME

(Poikiloderma Congenitale Syndrome)

*Development of Poikiloderma, Cataract
With or Without Other Ectodermal Dysplasia*

This condition was first described in 1868 by Rothmund, a Munich ophthalmologist who discovered multiple cases among an inbred group of people living in the nearby Alps. An excellent review of over 200 cases has been published by Vennos et al.

ABNORMALITIES. Wide variance in expression, the most usual features being the following:

Growth. Small stature of prenatal onset in majority of cases.

Skin. Irregular erythema progressing to poikiloderma (i.e., telangiectasia, scarring, irregular pigmentation and depigmentation, atrophy). Although most marked in sun-exposed areas, skin changes frequently occur on buttocks. Hyperkeratotic lesions (33 per cent) may be warty or verrucous. Blister formation (20 per cent) occurs before onset of poikiloderma. Photosensitivity (35 per cent).

Hair. Sparse, prematurely gray, and occasionally alopecia (80 per cent). Thinning of brows and eyelashes occurs initially. Scalp, facial, and pubic hair are often only thin.

Eyes. Juvenile zonular cataract (52 per cent) in all cases bilateral; occasionally corneal dystrophy.

OCCASIONAL ABNORMALITIES

Skeletal. Small hands and feet (20 per cent), hypoplastic to absent thumbs, syndactyly, forearm reduction defects, absence of patella, club feet, osteoporosis, and/or areas of cystic or sclerotic change.

Facial. Frontal bossing, small saddle nose, prognathism.

Teeth. Microdontia and anodontia, ectopic eruption, dental caries (40 per cent).

Nails. Small, dystrophic (32 per cent).

Other Skin. Hyperkeratosis of palms and soles. Squamous cell carcinoma, basal cell carcinoma.

Other. Mental deficiency (5 to 13 per cent). Microcephaly. Hydrocephalus. Scoliosis. Osteogenic sarcoma in two patients. Hypogonadism or delayed sexual development (28 per cent). Cryptorchidism. Irregular menses. Anteriorly placed anus. Annular pancreas. Growth hormone deficiency. Anhidrosis.

NATURAL HISTORY. Although skin changes have been present in six patients at birth, they usually occur between 3 months and 1 year of age. The progression toward irregular "marbled" hypoplasia, termed poikiloderma, is mainly noted in the first few years. Cataract most commonly becomes evident between 2 and 7 years of age. Alopecia progresses and may be complete by the second or third decade. The principal problems for affected individuals are skin difficulties, sometimes photosensitivity; visual impairment requiring surgical intervention; and physical appearance, depending on the extent to which stature, hair, teeth, and/or nails are affected. Reduced fertility is frequent, although pregnancy has been reported on several occasions.

ETIOLOGY. Autosomal recessive.

References

Rothmund, A.: Ueber Cataracten in Verbindung mit einer eigenthümlichen Hautdegeneration. Arch. Ophthalmol., *14*:159, 1868.

Rook, A., Davis, R., and Stevanovic, D.: Poikiloderma congenitale. Rothmund-Thomson syndrome. Acta Derm. Venereol. (Stockh.), *39*:392, 1959.

Silver, H. K.: Rothmund-Thomson syndrome: An occulocutaneous disorder. Am. J. Dis. Child. *111*:182, 1966.

Oates, R. K., Lewis, M. B., and Walker-Smith, J. A.: The Rothmund-Thomson syndrome. Aust. Paediatr. J., *7*:103, 1971.

Hall, J. G., Pagon, R. A., and Wilson, K. M.: Rothmund-Thomson syndrome with severe dwarfism. Am. J. Dis. Child., *134*:165, 1980.

Starr, D. G., McClure, J. P., and Connor, J. M.: Nondermatological complications and genetic aspects of the Rothmund-Thomson syndrome. Clin. Genet., 27:102, 1985.

Kaufman, S., et al.: Growth hormone deficiency in the Rothmund-Thomson syndrome. Am. J. Med. Genet., 23:861, 1986.

Vennos, E. M., et al.: Rothmund-Thomson syndrome: Review of the world literature. J. Am. Acad. Dermatol., 27:750, 1992.

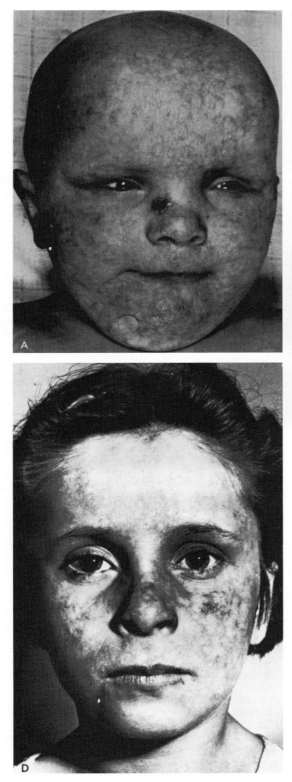

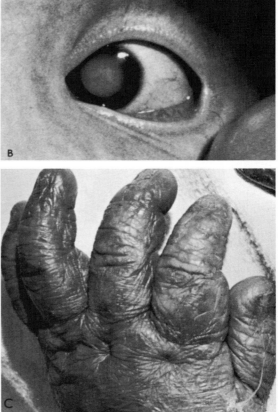

FIGURE 1. Rothmund-Thomson syndrome. *A*, A 15-month-old. (From Braun, W., and Unger, C.: Dermat. Wochenschr., *151*:11189, 1965, with permission.) *B*, A $2^6/_{12}$-year-old. Note absence of lashes and mature cataract. *C*, Patient shown in *B*. Note severe nail dysplasia. (*B* and *C* from Wahl, J. W., et al.: Am. J. Ophthalmol., *60*:722, 1965, with permission.) *D*, A 5-year-old. (From Rook, A. J., et al.: Acta Derm. Venereol. (Stockh.), *39*:392, 1959, with permission.)

E

E. EARLY OVERGROWTH WITH ASSOCIATED DEFECTS

FRAGILE X SYNDROME

(Martin-Bell Syndrome, Marker X Syndrome)

Mental Deficiency, Mild Connective Tissue Dysplasia, Macro-orchidism

This subgroup can now be differentiated from other types of X-linked mental retardation. In 1943, Martin and Bell published the first pedigree documenting a sex-linked form of mental retardation. Lubs in 1969 showed the presence of a fragile site on the long arm of the X chromosome in affected males and some carrier females in one family. Macro-orchidism without endocrinologic abnormalities was described by Turner et al. and Cantu et al. in the affected males of a number of families. However, it was not until Sutherland demonstrated that expression of the fragile site was dependent on the nature of the cell culture medium that the association between X-linked mental retardation, macro-orchidism, and the marker X chromosome was made.

The disorder appears to be common. Among populations of mentally handicapped individuals, fragile X–positive studies have been documented in up to 5.9 per cent of males and up to 0.3 per cent of females. The phenotype is most readily identified in the male.

ABNORMALITIES
Performance. Mild to profound mental retardation in males with I.Q.s of 30 to 55, but sometimes extending into the mildly retarded to borderline normal range. Hand flapping or biting (60 per cent) and poor eye contact (90 per cent). Cluttered speech in mildly retarded males, short bursts of repetitive speech in more severely retarded males, and complete lack of speech in severely and profoundly retarded males. Attention problems associated with hyperactivity are common. Autism (60 per cent). Approximately 50 per cent of females are mentally retarded or have educational difficulties.
Craniofacial. Macrocephaly in early childhood. Prognathism usually not noted until after puberty. Thickening of nasal bridge extending down to the nasal tip. Large ears with soft cartilage. Pale blue irides. Epicanthal folds. Dental crowding.

OCCASIONAL ABNORMALITIES. Nystagmus, strabismus, epilepsy, myopia, hypotonia, hyperextensible fingers, mild cutis laxa, torticollis, pectus excavatum, kyphoscoliosis, flat feet, submucous cleft palate, mitral valve prolapse, aortic dilation. Early features may suggest cerebral gigantism.

NATURAL HISTORY. Life span is normal. The patient's growth rate is slightly increased in the early years, with delayed motor milestones but no evidence of deterioration. Testicular size may be increased before puberty, but this increase becomes more obvious postpubertally. A characteristic speech pattern, referred to as "cluttering," is observed in higher functioning individuals. Psychologic profile is characterized by hyperkinetic behavior, emotional instability, hand biting, and other autistic features.

ETIOLOGY. X-linked inheritance. The marker on the X chromosome is a fragile site or nonstaining gap at Xq27.3. Within this locus is a region that contains a variable number of repeats of the trinucleotide CGG providing the basis for molecular diagnosis of this disorder. Normal individuals have from 6 to 54 repeats. Both male and female premutation carriers have 54 to 200 repeats, while affected individuals have greater than 200. Premutation carriers generally have no phenotypic manifestations but are at risk for affected offspring. Expansion of premutations to full mutations occurs only in female meiotic transmission and correlates with the size of the premutation. The risk that an individual will be affected clinically is dependent upon the position of that individual within the family. Thus the risk that the daughter of a phenotypically normal carrier male will be effected is zero. However, the risk that his daughter's son (his grandson) will be affected is 50 per cent. Most likely based on the phenomenon of X-inactivation, the risk that the daughter of a premutation carrier female will be clinically affected is smaller (approximately 15 to 30 per cent depending on the number of CGG repeats, i.e., the size of the premutation allele).

Although cytogenic analysis is a useful modality for detecting affected males, DNA-based molecular analysis allows both identification of full mutations and premutation carriers and, at the time of this writing, is the preferred laboratory adjunct to diagnosis.

References

Lubs, H. A.: A marker X chromosome. Am. J. Hum. Genet., 21:231, 1969.

Turner, G., et al.: X-linked mental retardation associated with macro-orchidism. J. Med. Genet., 12:367, 1975.

Cantu, J. M., et al.: Inherited congenital normofunctional testicular hyperplasia and mental deficiency. Hum. Genet., 33:23, 1976.

Sutherland, G. R.: Fragile sites on human chromosomes: Demonstration of their independence on the type of tissue culture medium. Science, 197:265, 1977.

Turner, G., et al.: Conference report: Second international workshop on the fragile X and on X-linked mental retardation. Am. J. Med. Genet., 23:11, 1986.

Chudley, A. E., and Hagerman, R. J.: Fragile X syndrome. J. Pediatr., 10:821, 1987.

Fu, Y., et al.: Variation of the CGG repeat at the fragile X site results in genetic instability: Resolution of the Sherman paradox. Cell, 67:1047, 1991.

Verkerk, A. J. M. H., et al.: Identification of a gene (FMR-1) containing a CGG repeat coincident with a breakpoint cluster region exhibiting length variation in fragile X syndrome. Cell, 67:905, 1991.

Erster, S. H., et al.: Polymerase chain reaction analysis of fragile X mutations. Hum. Genet., 90:55, 1992.

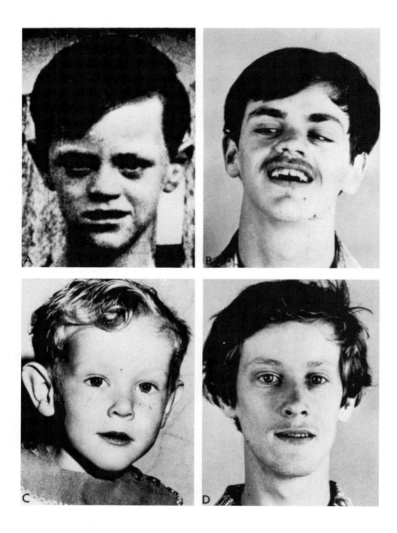

FIGURE 1. Fragile X syndrome. Increased head circumference with prominent forehead, prognathism, and big ears. *A* and *B* show the same patient at 8 and 21 years; *C* and *D* show the same patient at 3 and 22 years;

FIGURE 1. *Continued.* E shows a 2-year-old, and *F* shows a 4-year-old. (From Turner, G., et al.: J. Pediatr., *96*:837, 1980, with permission.)

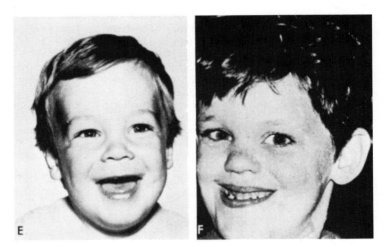

SOTOS SYNDROME
(Cerebral Gigantism Syndrome)

Large Size, Large Hands and Feet, Poor Coordination

Sotos et al. described five such patients in 1964, and at least 105 cases have subsequently been reported.

ABNORMALITIES
Performance. Variable mental deficiency. I.Q.s of 18 to 119, with a mean of 72. Poor coordination. Hypotonia. Hyperreflexia. Delayed gross motor function. Significant behavioral abnormalities.

Growth. Prenatal onset of excessive size. At birth, length more likely to be increased than weight. Mean full-term birth length 55.2 cm and birth weight 3.9 kg. Length increases rapidly, remains at or above 97th percentile throughout childhood and early adolescence, and is more significantly increased than weight. Final height often within normal range. Relatively large span. Large hands and feet (greater than 50th percentile even when plotted for height age). Advanced osseous maturation in childhood (84 per cent).

Craniofacial. Macrocephaly of prenatal onset in 50 per cent and by 1 year of age in 100 per cent. Mild dilatation of the cerebral ventricles. Prominent forehead (dolichocephalic). Sparse hair in frontoparietal region. Down-slanting palpebral fissures. Apparent hypertelorism not always confirmed by measurement. Prominent jaw. High, narrow palate with prominent lateral palatine ridges. Facial flushing frequently of nose but also cheeks and perioral region. Premature eruption of teeth.

Other. Orthopedic problems (60 per cent) primarily including pes planus and genu valgus. Thin, brittle fingernails.

OCCASIONAL ABNORMALITIES.
Seizures, EEG abnormalities, strabismus, cardiac defects, kyphoscoliosis, abnormal glucose tolerance test (14 per cent), malignancy (2.2 per cent) including Wilms (two patients), vaginal carcinoma (one), hepatocarcinoma (one), cavernous hemangioma (one), mixed parotid tumor (one), osteochondroma (one), neuroectodermal tumor (one), small cell lung carcinoma (one), neuroblastoma (one), acute lymphocytic leukemia (two) and non-Hodgkin lymphoma (one).

NATURAL HISTORY.
Neonatal problems have been frequent, including difficulties with respiration and feeding. Thereafter, appetite and fluid intake are frequently noted to be increased over normal and constipation is often a problem. An increased incidence of otitis media has been noted with conductive hearing loss and associated complications. Early developmental milestones are delayed. The median age of individuals at first sitting has been 9 months; walking, 17 months; and saying a few words, 25 months. However, these early assessments, which rely heavily on specific motor and verbal skills that are particularly delayed in Sotos syndrome, may well be poor predictors of ultimate intellectual performance. Even in those patients with normal intelligence, delay of expressive language and motor development is characteristically present in infancy. Behavior problems are significant. Excessive size, with poor coordination, leads to problems of social adjustment, often with undue aggressiveness and temper tantrums. Immaturity persisting into adulthood adds to the difficulties with socialization. A slightly increased risk for malignancy appears to exist. However, since the sites and types vary greatly, no routine screening with the exception of periodic clinical evaluation seems appropriate.

ETIOLOGY.
Unknown. Sporadic, with occasional exception. At least five families have been reported in which both parent and offspring are affected, raising the question of autosomal dominant inheritance. Under this hypothesis, the great majority would represent fresh mutational cases.

COMMENT.
Typical abnormalities have been noted on brain magnetic resonance imaging that can be helpful relative to diagnosis. These include abnormalities of the corpus callosum with complete or partial agenesis or hypoplasia, agenesis of the septum pellucidum and/or septum interpositum, wide or persistent cavum septi pellucidi, hypoplasia of the cerebellar vermi, and large cisterna magna.

References

Sotos, J. F., et al.: Cerebral gigantism in childhood. A syndrome of excessively rapid growth with acromegalic features and a nonprogressive neurologic disorder. N. Engl. J. Med., *271*:109, 1964.

Jaecken, J., van der Schueren-Lodeweyckx, and Eekels, R.: Cerebral gigantism syndrome. Z. Kinderheilkd., *112*:332, 1972.

Dodge, P. R., Holmes, S. J., and Sotos, J. F.: Cerebral gigantism. Dev. Med. Child Neurol., 25:248, 1983.

Rutter, S. C. and Cole, T. R. P.: Psychological characteristics of Sotos syndrome. Dev. Med. Child Neurol., 33:898, 1991.

Hersh, J. H., et al.: Risk of malignancy in Sotos syndrome. J. Pediatr., 120:572, 1992.

Schaefer, G. H., and Buehler, B. A.: Neuro-anatomic features of Sotos syndrome. Proc. Greenwood Genet. Center, 12:66, 1993.

Cole, T. R. P., and Hughes, H. E.: Sotos syndrome: A study of the diagnostic criteria and natural history. J. Med. Genet., 31:20, 1994.

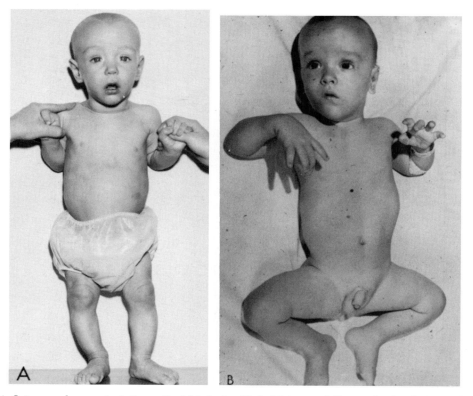

FIGURE 1. Sotos syndrome. *A,* A 7-month-old infant with height age of 15 months, head size at 2-year level and performance at 4½-month level. *B,* An 8½-month-old infant with height age at 21 months and borderline mental deficiency. (*B* from Sotos, J. F., et al.: N. Engl. J. Med., *271*:109, 1964, with permission.)

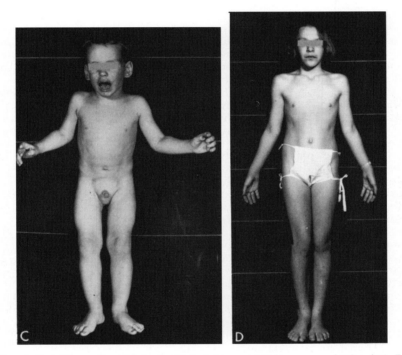

FIGURE 1. *Continued.* C, A 25-month-old infant with height age of 3⁶/₁₂ years and I.Q. of 70. D, An 11-year-old with height of 5 feet 8 inches and I.Q. of 70, (C and D are from Hook, E., and Reynolds, J. W.: J. Pediatr., *70*:900, 1967, with permission.)

WEAVER SYNDROME

Macrosomia, Accelerated Skeletal Maturation, Camptodactyly, Unusual Facies

Weaver et al. reported two strikingly similar boys with this pattern of overgrowth. Documentation of a number of additional cases indicates that this is a distinct disorder separate from Marshall-Smith syndrome.

ABNORMALITIES

Growth. Accelerated growth and maturation, of prenatal onset. Weight is more significantly increased than height.

Performance. Developmental delay or mental retardation, usually mild (81 per cent). Mild hypertonia, developmental lag, coarse low-pitched voice with slurred or dysarthric speech that is delayed in onset. Progressive spasticity. Strabismus.

Craniofacial. Macrocephaly (83 per cent). Large bifrontal diameter, flat occiput, ocular hypertelorism, epicanthal folds, depressed nasal bridge, down-slanting palpebral fissures, large ears, long philtrum, relative micrognathia.

Limbs. Camptodactyly, broad thumbs, thin deep-set nails, prominent fingertip pads. Limited elbow and knee extension, clinodactyly leading to overriding of toes. Flared metaphyses, especially distal femora and humeri, foot deformities including talipes equinovarus,. calcaneovalgus, and metatarsus adductus.

Other. Relatively loose skin, inverted nipples, thin hair. Umbilical hernia. Inguinal hernia. Cryptorchidism. Scoliosis. Kyphosis.

OCCASIONAL ABNORMALITIES.
Cardiac defects, short ribs, short fourth metatarsals. Hypotonia. Instability of the upper cervical spine. Seizures. Cyst in the septum pellucidum, cerebral atrophy, and enlarged vessels and hypervascularization in the areas of the middle and left posterior cerebral arteries. Neuroblastoma (one patient).

NATURAL HISTORY. These children are usually large at birth and show accelerated growth and markedly advanced skeletal maturation during infancy, with carpal centers more advanced than phalangeal centers. In a minority of patients, overgrowth does not develop until a few months of age. For the two well-documented adults, their final heights were 209.5 cm (+5 SD) and 187 cm (+3.5 SD), respectively. Behavioral problems, particularly poor concentration and temper tantrums, are common.

ETIOLOGY. Unknown. Most instances are sporadic. However, two instances have been reported of mildly affected mothers giving birth to severely affected sons, raising the possibility of either autosomal dominant inheritance with sex-limited expression or X-linked recessive inheritance.

References

Weaver, D. D., et al.: A new overgrowth syndrome with accelerated skeletal maturation, unusual facies, and camptodactyly. J. Pediatr., 84:547, 1974.

Fitch, N.: The syndromes of Marshall and Weaver. J. Med. Genet., 17:174, 1980.

Fitch, N.: Letter to the editor: Update on the Marshall-Smith-Weaver controversy. Am. J. Med. Genet., 20:559, 1985.

Ardinger, H. H., et al.: Further delineation of Weaver syndrome. J. Pediatr., 108:229, 1986.

Ramos-Arroyo, M. A., et al.: Weaver syndrome: A case without early overgrowth and review of the literature. Pediatrics, 88:1106, 1991.

Cole, T. R. P., et al.: Weaver syndrome. J. Med. Genet., 29:332, 1992.

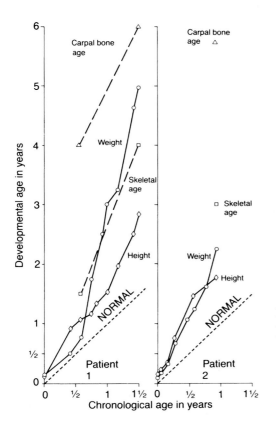

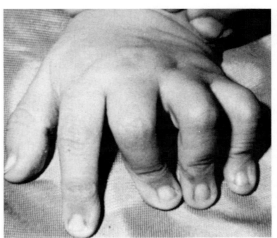

FIGURE 1. *Left*, Graph showing accelerated growth and maturation in two patients. *Right*, Hand showing camptodactyly.

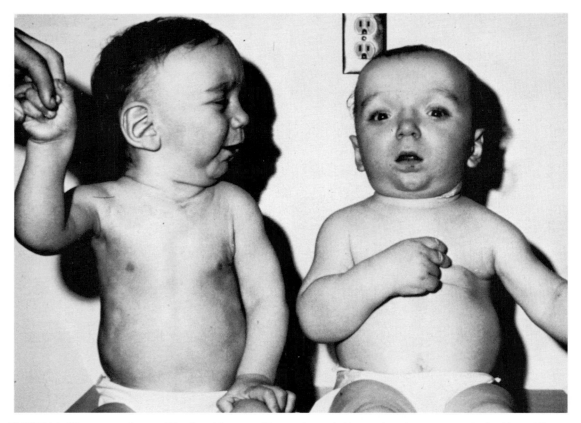

FIGURE 2. Weaver syndrome. Unrelated boys at 18 months and 11 months of age, respectively. (From Weaver, D. D., et al.: J. Pediatr., *84*:547, 1974, with permission.)

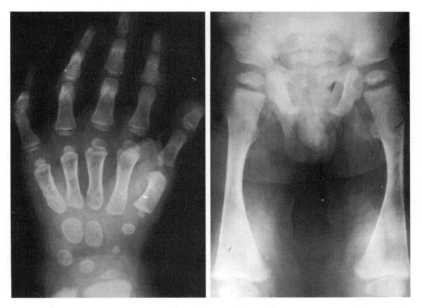

FIGURE 3. Weaver syndrome. Roentgenograms showing accelerated osseous maturation and broad distal splaying of femurs. (From Weaver, D. D., et al.: J. Pediatr., *84*:547, 1974, with permission.)

MARSHALL-SMITH SYNDROME

Accelerated Growth and Maturation,
Shallow Orbits, Broad Middle Phalanges

Initially described by Marshall and Smith in 1977, at least 19 patients with this disorder have been reported. Although categorized as an overgrowth syndrome, recent evidence suggests that this disorder involves an intrinsic structural or biochemical defect of cartilage, bone, and/or connective tissue, rather than generalized or localized cellular hyperplasia.

ABNORMALITIES

Growth. Accelerated linear growth and markedly accelerated skeletal maturation of prenatal onset. Underweight for length with failure to thrive in weight.

Performance. Motor and mental deficiency. Average I.Q. of 50. Hypotonia.

Craniofacial. Long cranium with prominent forehead, shallow orbits with prominent eyes, bluish sclerae, upturned nose, low nasal bridge, small mandibular ramus.

Limbs. Broad proximal and middle phalanges with narrow distal phalanges.

Other. Hypertrichosis. Umbilical hernia.

OCCASIONAL ABNORMALITIES.

Choanal atresia or stenosis or both. Abnormal larynx/laryngomalacia. Dysplastic teeth. Deafness and ear anomalies. Brain abnormalities including macrogyria, cerebral atrophy, and absent corpus callosum. Instability of the craniocervical junction with severe spinal stenoses. Short sternum. Scoliosis. Hypersegmented sacrococcyx. Rudimentary epiglottis. Omphalocele. Deep crease between hallux and second toe. Immunologic defect.

NATURAL HISTORY. These patients have failed to thrive in terms of weight. They have persistent respiratory difficulties manifested by stridor, hyperextension of the neck, and obstructing tongue. Although the majority die by 20 months with pneumonia, atelectasis, aspiration, and/or pulmonary hypertension, two children, 7 and 8 years of age, respectively, are being followed by Hoyme et al. Although neither can speak and both have a mild to moderate, conductive hearing loss, overall intellectual performance is in the lower range of normal. Aggressive management of respiratory difficulties is extremely important with respect to ultimate prognosis. The accelerated osseous maturation, of unknown cause, is of prenatal onset, as indicated by a wrist "bone age" of 3 to 4 years in one patient at 2 weeks of life.

ETIOLOGY. Unknown. Each has been a sporadic occurrence in the family.

COMMENT. Changes in the lower medulla secondary to the craniocervical instability may contribute to the respiratory distress leading to sudden early death in this disorder.

References

Marshall, R. E., et al.: Syndrome of accelerated skeletal maturation and relative failure to thrive: A newly recognized clinical growth disorder. J. Pediatr., 78: 95, 1971.

Visveshware, N., Rudolph, N., and Dragutsky, D.: Syndrome of accelerated skeletal maturation in infancy, peculiar facies and multiple congenital anomalies—an additional case. J. Pediatr., 84:553, 1974.

Fitch, N.: The syndromes of Marshall and Weaver. J. Med. Genet., 17:174, 1980.

Johnson, J. P., et al.: Marshall-Smith syndrome: Two case reports and a review of pulmonary manifestations. Pediatrics, 77:219, 1983.

Fitch, N.: Letter to the editor: Update on the Marshall-Smith-Weaver controversy. Am. J. Med. Genet., 20: 559, 1985.

Eich, G. F., et al.: Marshall-Smith Syndrome: New radiographic clinical and pathological observations. Radiology, 181:183, 1991.

Hoyme, H. E., et al.: The Marshall-Smith syndrome: Further evidence of osteochondrodysplasia in long-term survivors. Proc. Greenwood Genet. Clinic, 72: 70, 1993.

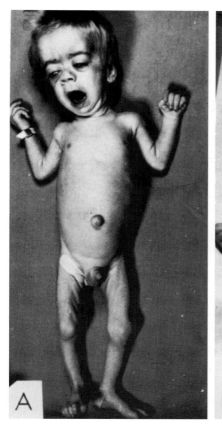

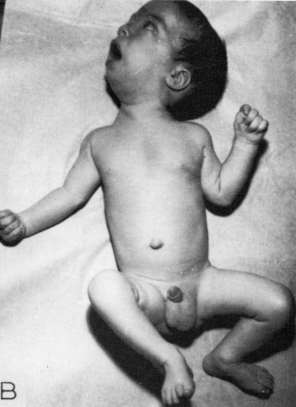

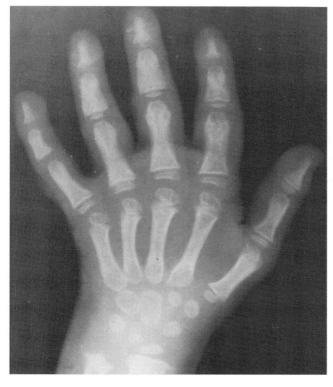

FIGURE 1. Marshall-Smith syndrome. *A* and *B*, 6- and 7-month-old patients. *Left*, Hand of one of them (patient *A*) at 16 months, showing a carpal bone age of 6 years and broad middle phalanges. (From Marshall, R. E., et al.: J. Pediatr., *78*:95, 1971, with permission.)

BECKWITH-WIEDEMANN SYNDROME

(Exomphalos-Macroglossia-Gigantism Syndrome)

Macroglossia, Omphalocele, Macrosomia, Ear Creases

Beckwith and Wiedemann first reported this distinct clinical entity, and about 200 cases have subsequently been reported.

ABNORMALITIES

Performance. Unknown incidence of mild to moderate mental deficiency; may be normal.

Growth. Macrosomia with large muscle mass and thick subcutaneous tissue. Accelerated osseous maturation. Metaphyseal flaring with overconstriction of diaphyses. Diminished tubulation of proximal humerus.

Craniofacial. Macroglossia. Prominent eyes with *relative* infraorbital hypoplasia. Capillary nevus flammeus, central forehead and eyelids. Metopic ridge. Large fontanels. Prominent occiput. Malocclusion with tendency toward mandibular prognathism and maxillary underdevelopment. Unusual linear fissures in lobule of external ear. Indentations on posterior rim of helix.

Hyperplasia and Dysplasia. Large kidneys with renal medullary dysplasia. Pancreatic hyperplasia, including excess of islets. Fetal adrenocortical cytomegaly—a *consistent feature*. Interstitial cell hyperplasia, gonads. Pituitary amphophil hyperplasia.

Other. Neonatal polycythemia. Hypoglycemia in early infancy (about one third to one half of cases). Omphalocele or other umbilical anomaly. Diastasis recti. Posterior diaphragmatic eventration. Cryptorchidism. Cardiovascular defects including isolated cardiomegaly.

OCCASIONAL ABNORMALITIES.
Hepatomegaly, mild microcephaly, hemihypertrophy, adrenal carcinoma, Wilms tumor, gonadoblastoma, hepatoblastoma, clitoromegaly, large ovaries, hyperplastic uterus and bladder, bicornuate uterus, hypospadias. Immunodeficiency. Cardiac hamartoma. Focal cardiomyopathy.

NATURAL HISTORY.
Hydramnios and a relatively high incidence of prematurity provide further indication of the rather profound prenatal alterations. Birth weight has averaged 4 kg, and length, 52.6 cm. Thereafter, length parallels the normal curve at or above the 95th percentile through adolescence. After 9 years of age, mean weight remains between the 75th and 95th percentile. Advanced bone age, most pronounced during the first 4 years, only rarely persists until maturity. Spontaneous pubertal development occurs at a normal time. Severe problems of neonatal adaptation may occur, with apnea, cyanosis, and seizures as symptoms. The large tongue may partially occlude the respiratory tract and lead to feeding difficulties. Placing the baby on the side or face down may help respiration, and a large, soft nipple may facilitate feeding. Infant mortality rate is estimated to be as high as 21 per cent. Detection and treatment of hypoglycemia in any neonate with features of this syndrome are critical. The hypoglycemia is responsive to hydrocortisone analogue therapy, which is usually required for only 1 to 4 months. Polycythemia might only merit therapeutic intervention during the early neonatal period. The frequency of tumor in this disorder is suggested to be 6.5 per cent. Obtaining ultrasonograms and measuring serum alpha fetoprotein every 6 months until the patient is 6 years of age to rule out Wilms tumor and hepatoblastoma, respectively, are warranted. An increased risk of malignancy seems to be associated with those children who have hemihypertrophy. Affected individuals who survive infancy generally are healthy. Growth may allow adequate oral room for the large tongue. Partial glossectomy has been performed successfully in a number of cases. Evidence suggests the prognathia and dental malocclusion are secondary to the large tongue.

ETIOLOGY.
Usually sporadic. The gene for Beckwith-Wiedemann syndrome (BWS) is located at 11p15.5. The characteristic phenotype occurs as a result of a variety of different genetic mechanisms, all of which result in a dosage imbalance of the gene. Currently it appears that the maternal copy of the gene is normally imprinted or inactivated. Therefore, there is normally only one active copy of the gene functioning at any given time (i.e., the paternal copy). Evidence in support of this is the following: Chromosomal abnormalities that cause duplication of the BWS location at 11p15.5 produce the BWS phenotype when they are paternally derived and thus associated with two active copies of the gene. Chromosomal inversions and translocations involving the BWS locus produce the phenotype if they are inherited from the mother. Presumably, disruption of the locus causes activation of a gene that is normally imprinted and thus in-

active. Also, the BWS phenotype has been seen in conjunction with paternal disomy, a situation in which both BWS loci are inherited from the father, giving two active copies of the gene. Because of the localization of the insulin-like growth factor 2 (IGF-2) gene to 11p, abnormalities in the insulin-like growth factors would seem to represent the most likely cause of the overgrowth.

References

Wiedemann, H. R.: Complexe malformatif familial avec hernie ombilicale et macroglossie—un "syndrome nouveau"? J. Genet. Hum., 13:223, 1964.

Beckwith, J. B.: Macroglossia, omphalocele, adrenal cytomegaly, gigantism, and hyperplastic visceromegaly. Birth Defects, 5(2):188, 1969.

Pettenati, M. J., et al.: Wiedemann-Beckwith syndrome: Presentation of clinical and cytogenetic data on 22 new cases and review of the literature. Hum. Genet., 74:143, 1986.

Sippell, W. G., et al.: Growth, bone maturation and pubertal development in children with the EMG syndrome. Clin. Genet., 35:20, 1989.

Normal, A. M., et al.: Recurrent Wiedmann-Beckwith syndrome with inversion of chromosome (11) (p11.2p15.5). Am. J. Med. Genet., 42:638, 1992.

Weksburg, R., et al.: Molecular characterization of cytogenetic alterations associated with the Beckwith-Wiedemann syndrome (BWS) phenotype refines the localization and suggests the gene for BWS is imprinted. Hum. Molec. Genet., 2:549, 1993.

Weksburg, R., et al.: Disruption of insulin-like growth factor 2 imprinting in Beckwith-Wiedemann syndrome. Nat. Genet., 5:143, 1993.

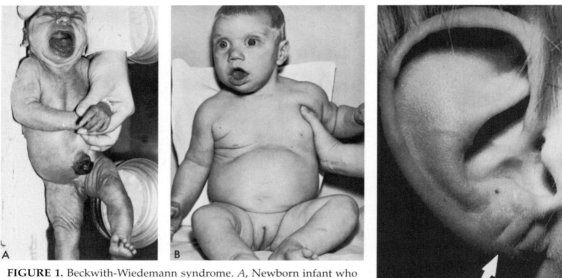

FIGURE 1. Beckwith-Wiedemann syndrome. *A*, Newborn infant who became hypoglycemic. Note clitoromegaly. *B*, A 6-month-old large infant. Note scar of repaired omphalocele. *C*, Unusual linear creases in the lobulus of the ear.

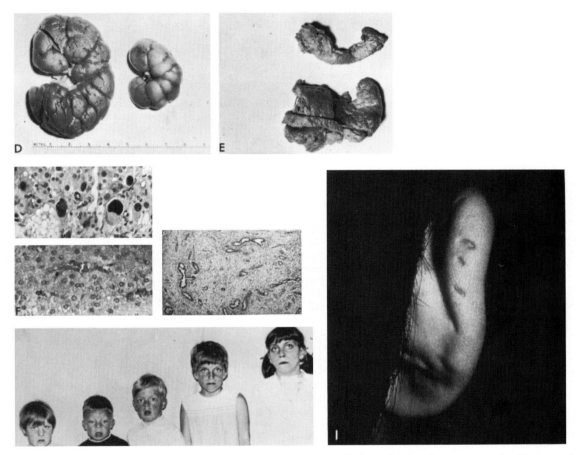

FIGURE 1. *Continued.* D and E, Kidney (D, left) and pancreas (E, lower) of patient compared with normal specimens. F and G, Fetal adrenal cytomegaly (above) compared with normal and renal medullary dysplasia (G). (F and G from Beckwith, J. B.: Birth Defects, 5[2]:188, 1969, with permission.) H, Similar facial appearance of five surviving children from 4 to 8 years of age, who tend to be large for age, with advanced skeletal maturation. (C and H from Irving, I. M.: J. Pediatr. Surg., 2:499, 1967, with permission.) I, Indentations on posterior rim of helix.

SIMPSON-GOLABI-BEHMEL SYNDROME

Neri et al. and Opitz et al. recognized in 1988 that the disorder initially reported by Simpson et al. in 1975 was the same as that described in 1984 by both Behmel et al. and by Golabi and Rosen. Marked inter- and intrafamilial variability in expression has been documented in this X-linked recessive disorder. Carrier females sometimes have mild manifestations.

ABNORMALITIES

Performance. Intelligence has varied from severely retarded to normal. Average I.Q. is approximately 1 SD below the mean. Hypotonia.

Growth. Prenatal onset of overgrowth. Birth weight as high as 5.9 kg. In seven out of eight affected adults, height was greater than the 97th percentile and ranged from 188 cm to 210 cm. Bone age, initially increased, becomes normal.

Craniofacial. Macrocephaly, present at birth, continues in childhood; coarse facies; downslanting palpebral fissures; ocular hypertelorism; broad flat nasal bridge with short nose; macrostomia; macroglossia; midline groove of lower lip; broad secondary alveolar ridge.

Limbs. Postaxial polydactyly of hands; syndactyly of second and third fingers and toes; nail hypoplasia (particularly of index finger); broad thumbs and great toes.

Skeletal. Vertebral segmentation defects including fusion of posterior elements of C2/C3, cervical ribs, six lumbar vertebrae, and sacral and coccygeal defects; pectus excavatum.

Other. Cardiac conduction defects; supernumerary nipples; cryptorchidism; spotty perioral or palatal pigmentation; thickened or dark skin; umbilical and/or inguinal hernias.

OCCASIONAL ABNORMALITIES.
Cleft lip and/or palate; indentations on posterior rim of helix; preauricular pits and tags; coloboma of optic disk; scoliosis; cleft of xiphisternum; preaxial polydactyly of feet; gastrointestinal anomalies including intestinal malrotation, pyloric ring, polysplenia, hepatosplenomegaly, and increased number of islets of Langerhans; genitourinary anomalies including large kidneys, cystic kidneys, duplication of renal pelvis, mild hydronephrosis with lobular cystic kidneys, and hypospadias; cardiac defects including ventricular septal defect, pulmonic stenosis, transposition of great vessels, and patent ductus arteriosus; central nervous system abnormalities including agenesis of corpus callosum, hypoplasia of cerebellar vermis, and hydrocephalus; embryonal tumors; diaphragmatic hernias.

NATURAL HISTORY. Approximately one half of reported patients have died of unknown causes prior to 6 months of age.

ETIOLOGY. X-linked recessive inheritance. Mutations in GPC3, a gene located at Xq26 which encodes a putative proteoglycan, glypican 3, have been identified. Glypican 3 is felt to play an important role in growth control in embryonic mesodermal tissue.

References

Simpson, J. L., et al.: A previously unrecognized X-linked syndrome of dysmorphia. Birth Defects, *XI*: 18, 1975.

Behmel, A., et al.: A new X-linked dysplasia gigantism syndrome: Identical with the Simpson dysplasia syndrome? Hum. Genet., *67*:409, 1984.

Golabi, M., and Rosen, L.: A new X-linked mental retardation-overgrowth syndrome. Am. J. Med. Genet., *17*:345, 1984.

Neri, G., et al.: Simpson-Golabi-Behmel syndrome: An X-linked encephalo-tropho-schisis syndrome. Am. J. Med. Genet., *30*:287, 1988.

Opitz, J. M., et al.: Simpson-Golabi-Behmel syndrome: Follow-up of the Michigan family. Am. J. Med. Genet., *30*:301, 1988.

Gargunta, C. L., and Bodurtha, J. N.: Report of another family with Simpson-Golabi-Behmel syndrome and a review of the literature. Am. J. Med. Genet., *44*: 129, 1992.

Hughes-Benzie, R. M., et al.: Simpson-Golabi-Behmel syndrome associated with renal dysplasia and embryonal tumor: Localization of the gene to Xqcen-q21. Am. J. Med. Genet., *43*:428, 1992.

Pilia, G., et al.: Mutations in GPC3, a glypican gene, cause the Simpson-Golabi-Behmel overgrowth syndrome. Nature Genet., *12*:1, 1996.

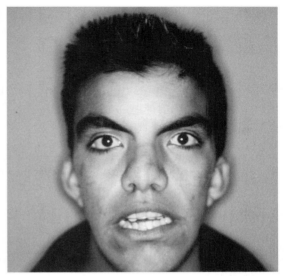

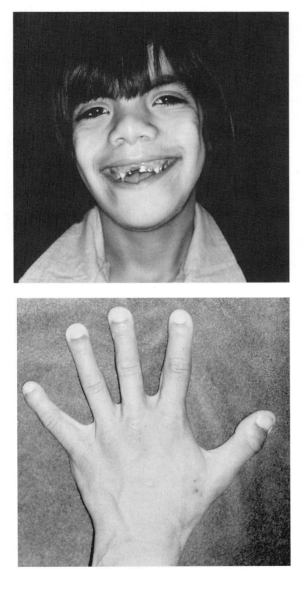

FIGURE 1. Affected male at 7 and 16 years of age. Note the ocular hypertelorism, broad flat nose, and nail hypoplasia. (From Golabi, M., and Rosen, L.: Am. J. Med. Genet., *17*:345, 1984, with permission.)

F

F. UNUSUAL BRAIN AND/OR NEUROMUSCULAR FINDINGS WITH ASSOCIATED DEFECTS

AMYOPLASIA CONGENITA DISRUPTIVE SEQUENCE

Arms Extended With Flexion of Hands and Wrists, Shoulders Internally Rotated With Decreased Muscle Mass, Bilateral Equinovarus, Variable Contractures of Other Major Joints

The first report with histopathologic studies was presented in 1907 by Howard. Over 500 cases have been reported in the literature since then. Hall reported 135 cases in 350 patients with congenital contractures of the joints. Usually the contractures are symmetric and involve all four extremities, although some cases involve only the upper limbs or the lower limbs.

ABNORMALITIES
Facies. Round face with micrognathia, small upturned nose, midline capillary hemangioma.
Shoulders. Rounded and sloping with decreased muscle mass, internally rotated.
Upper Limbs. Elbows usually in extension with wrists and hands flexed ("policeman tip" position). Severe flexion contractures at metacarpophalangeal joints with mild contractures at interphalangeal joints.
Lower Limbs. Hips, usually flexed, dislocated, adducted, or abducted. Knees, flexed or extended. Feet, usually equinovarus positioning bilaterally. Many combinations of hip and knee positions observed.
Other. Stiff, straight spine.

OCCASIONAL ABNORMALITIES. Cord wrapping of limb, amniotic bands, smashed digits, cryptorchidism, hypoplastic labia, dimples at contracture sites, torticollis, scoliosis, and hernias. Gastroschisis, nonduodenal intestinal atresia, and defects of muscular layer of trunk and abdominal musculature, Poland sequence, Moebius anomaly, hypoplasia of deltoids and biceps.

NATURAL HISTORY. Decreased movement in utero. Deliveries often difficult and breech presentation. Fractures of the limbs secondary to traumatic delivery. Intelligence normal unless birth trauma because of stiff joints. There is decreased bone growth of involved limbs, and there may be increased flexion and pterygium at development of the large joints with time. Patients almost always become ambulatory and self-supporting with good physical therapy. Multiple orthopedic procedures are usually necessary, with functional results. It is important to begin physical therapy early to mobilize any muscle tissue present (particularly intrinsic muscles), whereas casting and splinting may lead to muscle atrophy.

COMMENT. All four limbs are involved in 92 per cent of patients; the legs alone in 7 per cent and the arms alone in 1 per cent.

ETIOLOGY. Sporadic. Higher incidence than expected in identical twins, with only one affected. Based on the fact that many of the associated abnormalities have been shown to be caused by an intrauterine vascular accident, it is most likely that hypotension in the developing fetal spinal cord at a time when anterior horn cells are susceptible to insults is the mechanism responsible for the unique arthrogrypotic changes seen in this disorder. Prenatal diagnosis by serial real time ultrasonography, looking for abnormal movement, could be used to allay parental anxiety.

References

Howard, R.: A case of congenital defect of the muscular system and its association with congenital talipes equinovarus. Proc. Soc. Med., 1:157, 1907.
Hall, J. G., Reed, S. D., and Driscoll, E. P.: Part I. Amyoplasia: A common sporadic condition with congenital contractures. Am. J. Med. Genet., 15:571, 1983.
Hall, J. G., et al.: Part II: Amyoplasia—a specific type of arthrogryposis with an apparent excess of discordantly affected identical twins. Am. J. Med. Genet., 15:591, 1983.

Reid, C. O. M. V., et al.: Association of amyoplasia with gastroschisis, bowel atresia and defects of the muscular layer of the trunk. Am. J. Med. Genet., 24: 701, 1986.

Robertson, W. L., et al.: Further evidence that arthrogryposis multiple congenita in the human sometimes is caused by an intrauterine vascular accident. Teratology, 45:345, 1992.

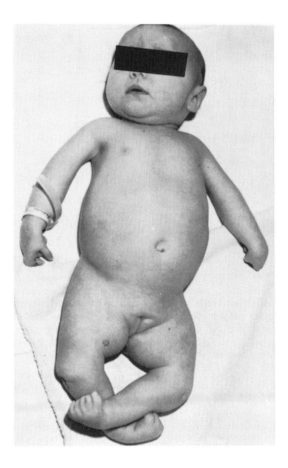

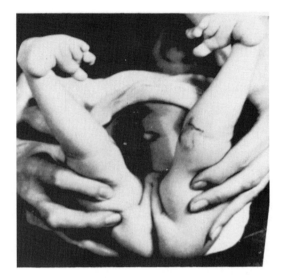

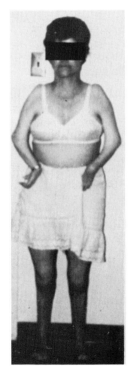

FIGURE 1. *Above*, Infant with amyoplasia. Note the "policeman tip" position of the arm and hand. *Right*, Adult with amyoplasia. (Courtesy of Dr. Judith Hall, University of British Columbia, Vancouver, British Columbia.)

DISTAL ARTHROGRYPOSIS SYNDROME

Distal Congenital Contractures, Clenched Hands With Medial Overlapping of the Fingers at Birth, Opening of Clenched Hands With Ulnar Deviation

In 1932, Lundblom described a mother and her son with congenital ulnar deviation and flexion of the fingers. In addition, the son had a calcaneovalgus positioning of the feet. Hall recognized this condition as an entity in 1982 in her report of 37 patients with congenital contractures of the distal joints. Two groups of patients were recognized: type I (typical)—14 probands—and type II (atypical)—23 probands. Atypical cases may have, in various combinations, cleft palate, cleft lip, small tongue, trismus, ptosis, mild epicanthal folds, short stature, scoliosis, and dull-normal intelligence. The distinct positioning of the hands at birth (as in trisomy 18) and the autosomal dominant inheritance pattern with variable expression are the most distinguishing features.

ABNORMALITIES

Hands. The neonate's hands are clenched tightly in a fist, with thumb adduction and medially overlapping fingers. Ulnar deviation and camptodactyly occur in the adult (98 per cent).

Feet. Position deformities (88 per cent): bilateral calcaneovalgus (33 per cent), bilateral equinovarus (25 per cent), combinations (30 per cent).

Hips. Hip involvement (38 per cent): congenital dislocations, decreased abduction, mild flexion, contracture deformities.

Knees. Mild flexion contractures (30 per cent).

Shoulders. Stiff at birth (17 per cent).

OCCASIONAL ABNORMALITIES. Trismus, mild scoliosis, dimples, cryptorchidism, hernias.

NATURAL HISTORY. "Trisomy 18 position" of hand at birth. Variable talipes involvement. Patients with atypical forms of the disorder may have trouble feeding. The hands eventually unclench and may have residual camptodactyly and ulnar deviation. Intelligence is normal. There is remarkably good response to treatment in all joints.

ETIOLOGY. Autosomal dominant with extensive intrafamilial and interfamilial variability. The parent of an affected child might possibly express the gene through mild hand contractures only. A gene for this disorder has been mapped to the pericentromeric region of chromosome 9. However, genetic heterogeneity is likely in that linkage has been excluded for at least one other family with this disorder.

Differential diagnosis includes whistling face syndrome, trismus-pseudocamptodactyly syndrome, and Beals syndrome.

COMMENT. Abnormal tendon attachments, attenuation, and tendon absence have been demonstrated in the hands and feet of some patients and may have been etiologic in producing contractures in utero. Prenatal diagnosis by serial real time ultrasonography, looking for normal movement should be considered.

References

Lundblom, A.: On congenital ulnar deviation of the fingers of familial occurrence. Acta Orthop. Scand., *8*:393, 1932.

Hall, J. G., Reed, S. D., and Greene, D.: The distal arthrogryposes. Delineation of new entities-Review and nosologic discussion. Am. J. Med. Genet., *11*: 185, 1982.

Bamshad, M., et al.: A gene for distal arthrogryposis type I maps to the pericentromeric region of chromosome 9. Am. J. Hum. Genet., *55*:1153, 1994.

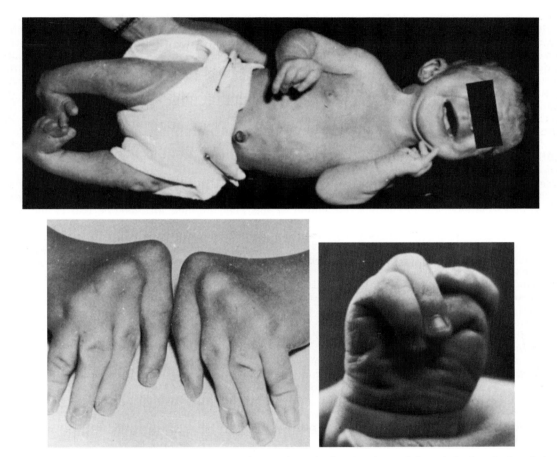

FIGURE 1. *Above*, Distal arthrogryposis in an infant. *Below*, The hands of an adult and the hand of an infant. (Courtesy of Dr. Judith Hall, University of British Columbia, Vancouver, British Columbia.)

PENA-SHOKEIR PHENOTYPE

(Fetal Akinesia/Hypokinesia Sequence)

Neurogenic Arthrogryposis, Pulmonary Hypoplasia, Hypertelorism

In 1974, Pena and Shokeir identified an early lethal disorder involving multiple joint contractures, facial anomalies, and pulmonary hypoplasia with an autosomal recessive mode of inheritance. Subsequently, a number of similar patients have been described. Hall recently suggested that this clinical phenotype is secondary to decreased in utero movement, no matter what the cause. As such, it is etiologically heterogeneous and is similar to the fetal akinesia deformation sequence, a pattern of structural defects described by Moessinger in rats who had been curarized in utero.

ABNORMALITIES

Growth. Prenatal onset growth deficiency. Head circumference is frequently spared.

Craniofacial. Rigid expressionless face; prominent eyes; hypertelorism; telecanthus; epicanthal folds; poorly folded, small, and posteriorly angulated ears; depressed nasal tip; small mouth; high arched palate; micrognathia.

Limbs. Multiple ankylosis (e.g., elbows, knees, hips, and ankles); ulnar deviation of the hands; rocker-bottom feet; talipes equinovarus, camptodactyly. Absent or sparse dermal ridges, with frequent absence of the flexion creases on the fingers and palms.

Lungs. Pulmonary hypoplasia.

Genitalia. Cryptorchidism.

Other. Apparent short neck; polyhydramnios; short-gut syndrome with malabsorption; small or abnormal placenta. Relatively short umbilical cord.

OCCASIONAL ABNORMALITIES. Cleft palate, cardiac defect.

NATURAL HISTORY. Some of these babies are born prematurely. Those born at term are invariably small for the estimated dates. Approximately 30 per cent are stillborn. Although the majority of those live-born die of the complications of pulmonary hypoplasia within the first month of life, it is important to recognize that the ultimate prognosis for children with this disorder depends on the cause of the decreased fetal movement.

COMMENT. The causes of this phenotype, as well as the pathogenetic mechanisms leading to it, are heterogeneous. Muscle histology was abnormal in 15 of 17 infants (predominately neurogenic atrophy); spinal cord histology was abnormal in 5 of 8 infants; and the cerebrum was abnormal in 11 of 16 infants studied. In one case, extensive prenatal exposure to cocaine leading to ischemic-anoxic brain damage including damage to motor neurons was documented. Whatever the cause, the common denominator is decreased fetal activity. Failure of normal deglutition results in polyhydramnios, and a neuromuscular deficiency in the function of the diaphragm and intercostal muscles leads to pulmonary hypoplasia. The short umbilical cord and multiple joint contractures are due to lack of normal fetal movement. The phenotype overlaps with that of trisomy 18, from which it needs to be distinguished in the neonatal period.

ETIOLOGY. Autosomal recessive inheritance has been implied in over one half of the published cases. However, recognition that this phenotype does not have a single etiology makes accurate recurrence risk counseling difficult. A 0 per cent or 25 per cent risk for recurrence seems most appropriate in a sporadic case.

References

Pena, S. D. J., and Shokeir, M. H. K.: Syndrome of camptodactyly, multiple ankyloses, facial anomalies and pulmonary hypoplasia: A lethal condition. J. Pediatr., *85*:373, 1974.

Pena, S. D. J., and Shokeir, M. H. K.: Syndrome of camptodactyly, multiple ankyloses, facial anomalies and pulmonary hypoplasia: Further delineation and evidence of autosomal recessive inheritance. *In* Bergsma, D., and Schimke, R. M. (eds.): Cytogenetics, Environment and Malformation Syndromes. Birth Defects Original Article Series, Vol. XII. New York, Alan R. Liss, Inc., 1976, p. 201.

Dimmick, J. E., et al.: Syndrome of ankylosis, facial anomalies and pulmonary hypoplasia: A pathologic analysis of one infant. *In* Bergsma, D., and Lowry, R. B. (eds.): Embryology and Pathogenesis and Prenatal diagnosis, Birth Defects Original Article Series, Vol. XIII. New York, Alan R. Liss, Inc., 1977, p. 133.

Chen, H., et al.: The Pena-Shokeir syndrome. Report of five cases and further delineation of the syndrome. Am. J. Med. Genet., *16*:213, 1983.

Moessinger, A. L.: Fetal akinesia deformation sequence: An animal model, Pediatrics, *72*:857, 1983.

Lindhout, D., Hageman, G., and Beemer, F. A.: The Pena-Shokeir syndrome: Report of nine Dutch cases. Am J. Med. Genet., *21*:655, 1985.

Hall, J. G.: Invited editorial comment: Analysis of Pena-Shokeir phenotype. Am. J. Med. Genet., 25:99, 1986.

Lavi, E., et al.: Fetal akinesia deformation sequence (Pena-Shokeir phenotype) associated with acquired intrauterine brain damage. Neurology, 47:1467, 1991.

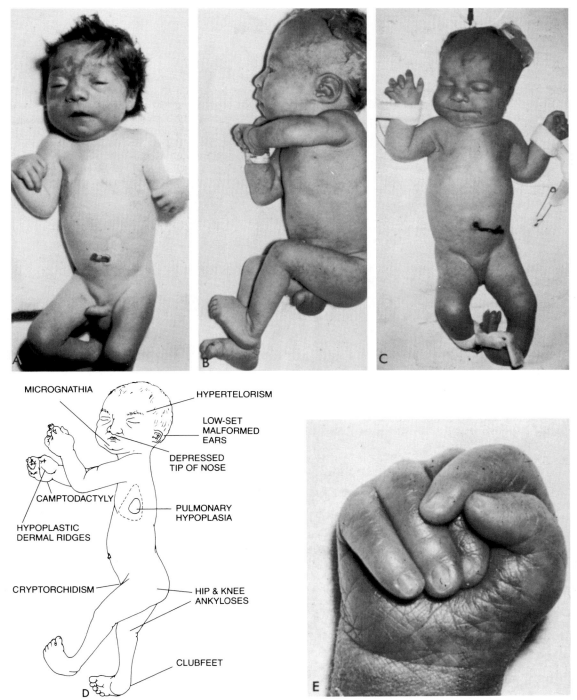

FIGURE 1. Pena-Shokeir phenotype. *A* to *C*, Affected infants. *D*, Predominant features of the disorder and, *E*, aberrant hand position, which can be similar to that of the 18 trisomy syndrome. (*A* appears courtesy of Dr. Hope Pewnett.)

CEREBRO-OCULO-FACIO-SKELETAL (COFS) SYNDROME

Neurogenic Arthrogryposis, Microcephaly, Microphthalmia and/or Cataract

Described initially by Pena and Shokeir in 1974, the disorder has been recognized as an autosomal recessive, apparently degenerative problem of the brain and spinal cord that is usually manifest before birth.

ABNORMALITIES

Brain and Neurologic. Reduced white matter of brain with gray mottling, subependymal focal gliosis of the third ventricle, focal microgyria, hypoplasia of temporal and hippocampal gyri, hypoplasia of optic tracts and chiasm, agenesis of corpus callosum, and intracranial calcification on CT scan in regions of lenticular nuclei and hemispheric white matter. Occasional infantile spasms. Generalized hypotonia and hyporeflexia or areflexia.

Craniofacial. Microcephaly, prominent root of the nose, large ear pinnae, upper lip overlapping lower lip, micrognathia (mild).

Eyes. Blepharophimosis with deep-set eyes, microphthalmia, cataracts, nystagmus.

Limbs. Camptodactyly, mild flexion contractures in the elbows and knees, rocker-bottom feet with vertical talus, posteriorly placed second metatarsal, longitudinal groove in the soles along the second metatarsal.

Other. Hirsutism, kyphoscoliosis, widely set nipples, shallow acetabular angles, coxa valga, longitudinal groove on soles, osteoporosis, renal defects.

NATURAL HISTORY. Babies with this disorder are usually born at term with normal birth weights. In the majority, the phenotype is evident at birth. However, in a few cases, the phenotype undergoes a dramatic evolution toward the full-blown picture in a matter of weeks to months. The course of the disorder in all cases is progressive, with downhill deterioration. It is characterized by virtually no growth and increasing cachexia despite apparently adequate caloric intake, ending in death, which is usually from pulmonary infections that complicate emaciation. Survival is usually under 5 years.

ETIOLOGY. Autosomal recessive.

References

Pena, S. D. J., and Shokeir, M. H. K.: Autosomal recessive cerebro-oculo-facio-skeletal (COFS) syndrome. Clin. Genet., 5:285, 1974.

Preus, M., and Fraser, F. C.: The cerebro-oculo-facio-skeletal syndrome. Clin. Genet., 5:294, 1974.

Scott-Emuakpor, A., Heffelfinger, J., and Higgins, J. V.: A syndrome of microcephaly and cataracts in four siblings. A new genetic syndrome? Am. J. Dis. Child., 131:167, 1977.

Surana, R. B., Fraga, J. R., and Sinkford, S. M.: The cerebro-oculo-facio-skeletal syndrome. Clin. Genet., 13:486, 1978.

Grizzard, W. S., O'Donnell, J. J., and Carey, J. C.: The cerebro-oculo-facial-skeletal syndrome. Am. J. Ophthalmol., 89:293, 1980.

Linna, S. L.: Intracranial calcifications in cerebro-oculo-facio-skeletal (COFS) syndrome. Pediatr. Radiol., 12:28, 1982.

Harden, C. L., et al.: Infantile spasms in COFS syndrome. Pediatr. Neurol., 7:302, 1991.

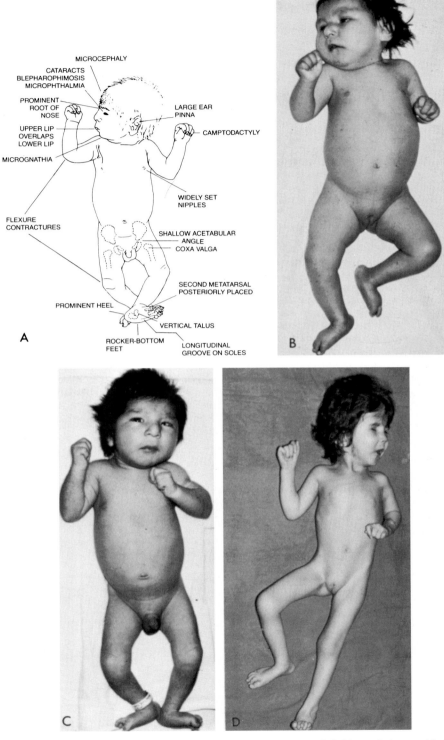

FIGURE 1. COFS syndrome. *A*, Predominant features of syndrome. *B* and *C*, Young infants with the syndrome. *D*, An 18-month-old affected infant with failure-to-thrive type of postnatal growth deficiency.

LETHAL MULTIPLE PTERYGIUM SYNDROME

Gillin and Pryse-Davis described three female siblings with this early lethal disorder in 1976. It was separated from other conditions associated with pterygia by Hall et al. in 1982. At least 40 cases have been reported.

ABNORMALITIES
Growth. Deficiency of prenatal onset.
Facies. Epicanthal folds. Ocular hypertelorism. Flat nose. Cleft palate. Small mouth. Micrognathia. Down-slanting palpebral fissures. Low-set, malformed ears.
Limbs. Flexion contractures involving elbows, shoulders, hips, knees, ankles, hands, and feet.
Pterygia. Present in the following areas: Chin to sternum, cervical, axillary, antecubital, crural, popliteal, and ankles.
Other. Small chest. Crytorchidism. Hypoplastic dermal ridges and creases. Neck edema and loose skin. Radiologic evidence of under-modeling of long bones and hypoplasia of vertebrae, sacrum, ileum, ischium, ribs, clavicles, and scapulae. Thin, gracile long bones.

OCCASIONAL ABNORMALITIES.
Short neck. Long philtrum. Midforehead hemangioma. Attenuated ascending and transverse colon. Intestinal malrotation. No appendix. Cardiac hypoplasia. Diaphragmatic hernia. Megaureter and hydronephrosis. Kyphoscoliosis. Posterior vertebral fusion. Fusion of long bones. Neuropathologic abnormalities including cerebellar and pontine hypoplasia with absence of pyramidal tracts. Decreased size of white matter tracts in spinal cord. Microcephaly.

NATURAL HISTORY.
All patients have been stillborn or have died in the immediate neonatal period, probably secondary to pulmonary hypoplasia. Polyhydramnios is present in about one third of cases and hydrops in greater than one half. Decreased fetal activity and an increased incidence of breech presentation have been documented.

ETIOLOGY.
Autosomal recessive in the majority of cases. However, a clinically indistinguishable X-linked recessive form has been reported. De Die-Smulders et al. have distinguished an "early" and a late form of the lethal multiple pterygium syndrome. The "early" form is characterized by intrauterine death in the second trimester and the presence of hydrops and/or cystic hygroma while fetuses with the late form survive into the third trimester and are not hydropic. The early group is genetically heterogeneous with both autosomal and X-linked recessive cases represented. Within the late group all familial cases have pedigrees consistent with autosomal recessive inheritance.

COMMENT.
In only a few cases has an autopsy been reported that provides adequate information regarding the neuromuscular system. However, enough variability exists to suggest that in some cases this disorder may be the result of an abnormal brain and spinal cord while others may be due to a primary muscle aplasia. The term lethal multiple pterygium phenotype might therefore be a more appropriate designation recognizing that the clinical features are secondary to decreased intrauterine movement from any cause beginning at an early stage of development.

References

Gillin, M. D., and Pryse-Davis, J.: Pterygium syndrome. J. Med. Genet., 13:249, 1976.
Hall, J. G., et al.: Limb pterygium syndromes. A review and report of eleven patients. Am. J. Med. Genet., 12:377, 1982.
De Die-Smulders, C. E. M., et al.: The lethal multiple pterygium syndrome. Genet. Couns., 1:13, 1990.
Spearritt, D. J., et al.: Lethal multiple pterygium syndrome: Report of a case with neurological anomalies. Am. J. Med. Genet., 47:45, 1993.

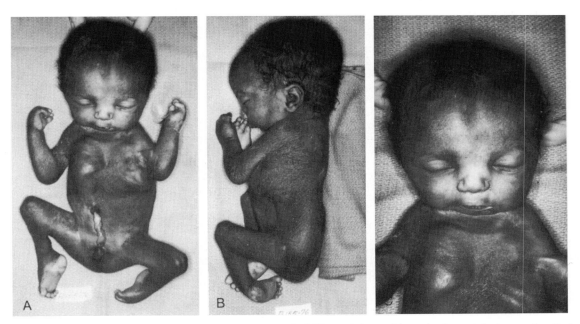

FIGURE 1. Lethal multiple pterygium syndrome. *A* to *C*, Stillborn infant with ocular hypertelorism, epicanthal folds, multiple joint contractures, and pterygia bridging virtually all joints.

NEU-LAXOVA SYNDROME

Microcephaly/Lissencephaly, Canine Facies With Exophthalmos, Syndactyly With Subcutaneous Edema

Neu et al. reported three siblings with microcephaly and multiple congenital abnormalities in 1971. An additional family with three affected siblings from a first-cousin mating was reported by Laxova et al. in 1972. At least 30 cases have been reported subsequently.

ABNORMALITIES
Growth. Prenatal onset of marked growth deficiency (100 per cent).
Central Nervous System. Microcephaly (84 per cent). Lissencephaly (83 per cent). Absence of corpus callosum (53 per cent). Hypoplasia of cerebrum, cerebellum (53 per cent), pons. Absence of olfactory bulbs.
Facies. Sloping forehead (100 per cent). Ocular hypertelorism (94 per cent). Protruding eyes with absent lids (40 per cent). Flattened nose. Round, gaping mouth and thick everted lips. Micrognathia (97 per cent). Large ears. Short neck.
Skin. Yellow subcutaneous tissue covered by thin, transparent, scaling skin and edema (85 per cent). Ichthyosis (50 per cent).
Limbs. Short limbs. Syndactyly of fingers and toes (60 per cent), extreme puffiness of hands and feet, overlapping of digits, calcaneovalgus, vertical talus, flexion contractures of major joints with pterygia (79 per cent). Poorly mineralized bones.
Other. Cataracts (25 per cent). Microphthalmia. Persistence of some embryonic structures of eye. Absent eyelashes and head hair. Muscular atrophy with hypertrophy of fatty tissue. Hypoplastic genitalia (50 per cent). Polyhydramnios. Short umbilical cord. Small placenta.

OCCASIONAL ABNORMALITIES.
Hydranencephaly. Spina bifida. Dandy-Walker malformation. Choroid plexus cysts. Hypodontia. Patent foramen ovale and ductus arteriosus. Atrial septal defect. Ventricular septal detect. Transposition of great vessels. Cleft lip. Cleft palate. Renal agenesis. Bifid uterus. Cryptorchidism.

NATURAL HISTORY. Most patients have been stillborn or have died in the immediate neonatal period. The oldest survivor died of pneumonia at 7 weeks.

ETIOLOGY. Autosomal recessive. Three families with two or more affected siblings born to normal parents have been reported. Consanguinity has been documented in one half of families.

References

Neu, R. L., et al.: A lethal syndrome of microcephaly with multiple congenital anomalies in three siblings. Pediatrics, 47:610, 1971.

Laxova, R., Ohdra, P. T., and Timothy, J. A. D.: A further example of a lethal autosomal recessive condition in siblings. J. Ment. Def. Res., 16:139, 1972.

Curry, C. J. R.: Letter to the editor: Further comments on the Neu-Laxova syndrome. Am. J. Med. Genet., 13:441, 1982.

Shved, I. A., Lazjuk, G. I., and Cherstovoy, E. D.: Elaboration of the phenotypic changes of the upper limbs in the Neu-Laxova syndrome. Am. J. Med. Genet., 20:1, 1985.

Ostrovskaya, T. I., and Lazjuk, G. I.: Cerebral abnormalities in the Neu-Laxova syndrome. Am. J. Med. Genet., 30:747, 1988.

Shapiro, I., et al.: Neu-Laxova syndrome: Prenatal ultrasonographic diagnosis, clinical and pathological studies, and new manifestations. Am. J. Med. Genet., 43:602, 1992.

FIGURE 1. Neu-Laxova syndrome. *A* and *B*, A 38-week-gestation infant with microcephaly, sloping forehead, protruding eyes with absent lids, flat nose, gaping mouth and thick lips, scaling skin with edema, and joint contractures. (From Mueller, R. F., et al.: Am. J. Med. Genet., *16*:645, 1983, with permission.)

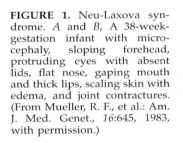
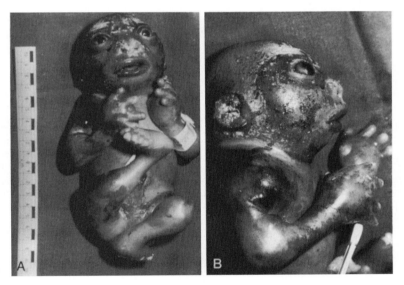

RESTRICTIVE DERMOPATHY

Initially described in two infants by Toriello et al. in 1983, this disorder has now been reported in 24 patients. Most of the features are constraint related, the result of restricted in utero movement secondary to the defective skin.

ABNORMALITIES

Growth. Intrauterine growth deficiency.

Craniofacies. Enlarged fontanels. Hypertelorism. Entropion. Small pinched nose. Small mouth with ankylosis of the temporomandibular joints. Micrognathia. Dysplastic ears.

Skin. Rigid and tense. Erosion may be present. Fissures often occur in groin, axilla, and neck. Superficial vasculature is prominent. Nails may be short or very long. Eyelashes, eyebrows, and lanugo are sparse or absent. Head hair may be normal. Histologically there is hyperkeratosis, delayed maturation of the pilosebaceous and eccrine sweat apparatus, and absence of elastin. The epidermis and subcutaneous fat layer are thickened. The dermis is thin with dense, thin collagen fibers in parallel with the epidermis.

Skeletal. Multiple joint contractures. Rocker-bottom feet. Thin, dysplastic, bipartite clavicles, ribbon-like ribs, overtubalated long bones of the arms, and a poorly mineralized skull are present radiographically.

Other. Polyhydramnios. Short umbilical cord. Increased anteroposterior diameter of chest. Pulmonary hypoplasia.

OCCASIONAL ABNORMALITIES. Natal teeth. Microcephaly. Short palpebral fissures. Choanal atresia. Submucous cleft palate. Cleft palate. Hypospadias. Ureteral duplication. Dorsal kyphoscoliosis. Adrenal hypoplasia. Patent ductus arteriosus. Atrial septal defect.

NATURAL HISTORY. Pregnancy is frequently abnormal with polyhydramnios and decreased fetal activity usually beginning at about 6 months' gestation. Prematurity is common. The majority of affected individuals are stillborn due to pulmonary hypoplasia. Intubation is extremely difficult due to the temporomandibular joint ankylosis. Most survivors die within the first week. The longest survival has been 120 days.

ETIOLOGY. Autosomal recessive.

References

Toriello, H. V., et al.: Autosomal recessive aplasia cutis congenita—report of two affected sibs. Am. J. Med. Genet., *15*:153, 1983.

Witt, D. R., et al.: Recessive dermopathy: A newly recognized autosomal recessive skin dysplasia. Am. J. Med. Genet., *24*:631, 1986.

Reed, M. H., et al.: Restrictive dermopathy. Pediatr. Radiol., *23*:617, 1992.

Verloes, A., et al.: Restrictive dermopathy, a lethal form of arthrogryposis multiplex with skin and bone dysplasias: Three new cases and review of the literature. Am. J. Med. Genet., *43*:539, 1992.

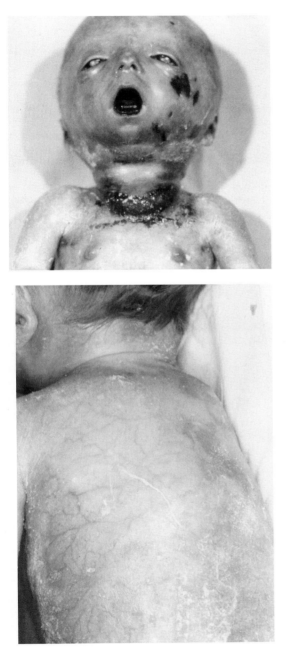

FIGURE 1. Two newborn infants. Note the small nose, translucent dermis, and flat helix with auricle attached to skin of scalp. (From Toriello, H. V., et al.: Am. J. Med. Genet., 15:153, 1983, with permission of Wiley-Liss, a division of John Wiley & Sons.)

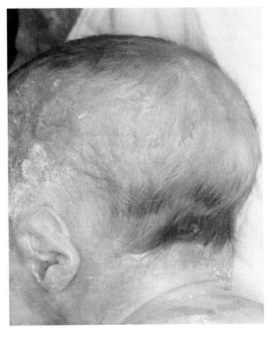

MECKEL-GRUBER SYNDROME

(Dysencephalia Splanchnocystica)

Encephalocele, Polydactyly, Cystic Dysplasia of Kidneys

Originally described by Meckel in 1822, later by Gruber, and more recently brought to recognition by Opitz and Howe, more than 200 cases of this severe disorder have been reported.

ABNORMALITIES

Growth. Variable prenatal growth deficiency.

Central Nervous System. Occipital encephalomeningocele. Microcephaly with sloping forehead, cerebral and cerebellar hypoplasia. Anencephaly. Hydrocephaly with or without an Arnold-Chiari malformation. Absence of olfactory lobes, olfactory tract, corpus callosum, and septum pellucidum.

Facial. Microphthalmia. Cleft palate. Micrognathia. Ear anomalies, especially slanting-type.

Neck. Short.

Limbs. Polydactyly (usually postaxial), talipes.

Kidney. Dysplasia with varying degrees of cyst formation.

Liver. Bile duct proliferation, fibrosis, cysts.

Genitalia. Cryptorchidism, incomplete development of external and/or internal genitalia.

OCCASIONAL ABNORMALITIES

Craniofacial. Craniosynostosis (possibly secondary). Coloboma of iris, hypoplastic optic nerve, hypotelorism or hypertelorism, hypoplastic to absent philtrum and/or nasal septum, cleft lip—sometimes midline.

Mouth. Lobulated tongue, cleft epiglottis, neonatal teeth.

Neck. Webbed.

Limbs. Relatively short bowed limbs, syndactyly, simian crease, clinodactyly.

Cardiac. Septal defect, patent ductus arteriosus, coarctation of aorta, pulmonary stenosis.

Lungs. Hypoplasia.

Other. Dandy-Walker malformation, single umbilical artery, patent urachus, omphalocele, intestinal malrotation, enlarged missing and/or accessory spleens, defects in laterality, adrenal hypoplasia, imperforate anus, missing or duplicated ureters, absence or hypoplasia of urinary bladder, enlarged placenta.

NATURAL HISTORY AND MANAGEMENT.

These patients seldom survive more than a few days to weeks. Death may be related to the severe central nervous system defects and/or renal defects.

COMMENT. Surprising variability of the clinical features exist. In a study of affected siblings of probands, 100 per cent had cystic dysplasia of the kidneys. However, 63 per cent had occipital encephaloceles and only 55 per cent had polydactyly; 18 per cent had no brain anomaly.

ETIOLOGY. Autosomal recessive, with no recognized expression in the presumed carriers of the gene. Prenatal diagnosis may be possible by an elevated alpha fetoprotein level when there is an encephalocele and/or a sonographic delineation of either the encephalocele or the dysplastic enlarged kidneys. The locus for the Meckel-Gruber syndrome has been mapped to 17q21-q24.

References

Meckel, J. R., Beschreibung zweier durch sehr úhnliche bildungsabweichung ensteller Geschwister. Dtsch. Arch. Physiol., 7:99, 1822.

Gruber, G. B.: Beiträge zur Frage "gekoppelter" missbildungen (Akrocephalosyndactylie und Dysencephalia splanchnocystica). Beitr. Pathol. Anat., 93: 459, 1934.

Opitz, J. M., and Howe, J. J.: The Meckel syndrome (dysencephalia splanchnocystica, the Gruber syndrome). Birth Defects, 5:167, 1969.

Hsia, Y. E., Bratu, M., and Herbordt, A.: Genesis of the Meckel syndrome (dysencephalia splanchnocystica). Pediatrics, 48:237, 1971.

Meckel, S., and Passarge, E.: Encephalocele, polycystic kidneys, and polydactyly as an autosomal recessive trait simulating certain other disorders: The Meckel syndrome. Ann. Genet. (Paris), 14:97, 1971.

Fraser, F. C., and Lytwyn, A.: Spectrum of anomalies in the Meckel syndrome, or "Maybe there is a malformation syndrome with at least one constant anomaly." Am. J. Med. Genet., 9:67, 1981.

Seppänen, U., and Herva, R.: Roentgenologic features of the Meckel syndrome. Pediatr. Radiol., 13:329, 1983.

Salonen, R.: The Meckel syndrome: Clinicopathological findings in 67 patients. Am. J. Med. Genet., 18: 671, 1984.

Nyberg, D. A., et al.: Meckel-Gruber syndrome. Importance of prenatal diagnosis. J. Ultrasound Med., 9:691, 1990.

Paavola, P., et al.: The locus for Meckel syndrome with multiple congenital anomalies maps to chromosome 17q21-q24. Nature Genetics, 11:213, 1995.

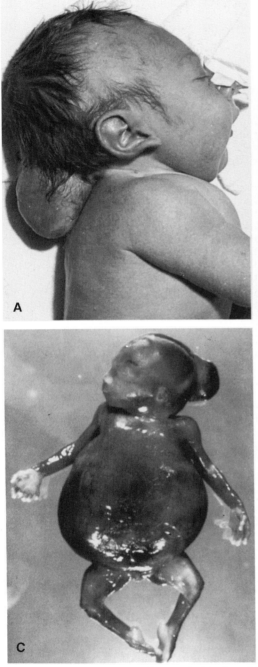

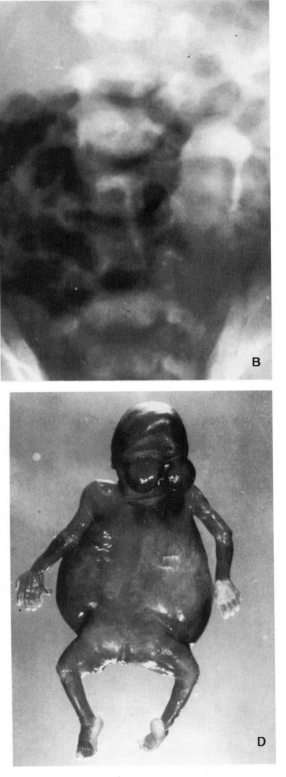

FIGURE 1. Meckel-Gruber syndrome. *A*, A 2-day-old male with palpable enlarged kidney who was having frequent seizures and other evidence of central nervous system abnormality. *B*, Intravenous pyelogram showed no visualization on one side and an aberrant calyceal system on the other side. The baby died at 4$^1/_2$ months of age, the oldest known survivor with this syndrome. (Patient of E. Hutton, Anchorage, Alaska.) *C* and *D*, Stillborn infant with posterior encephalocele, postaxial polydactyly, and flank masses caused by massively enlarged cystic kidneys.

185

PALLISTER-HALL SYNDROME

Hypothalamic Hamartoblastoma,
Hypopituitarism, Imperforate Anus, Postaxial Polydactyly

In 1980, Hall et al. described six unrelated newborn infants with this pattern of malformation. All died in the neonatal period. Culler and Jones subsequently described a similarly affected child, who died at the age of 19 months.

ABNORMALITIES
Growth. Mild intrauterine growth retardation.
Central Nervous System. Hypothalamic hamartoblastoma located on the inferior surface of the cerebrum, extending from the optic chiasma to the interpeduncular fossa, replacing the hypothalamus and other nuclei originating in the embryonic hypothalamic plate. Pituitary aplasia/dysplasia. Panhypopituitarism.
Craniofacial. Flat nasal bridge and midface with midline capillary hemangioma. Short nose. Anteverted nares. Bathrocephaly. External ear anomalies including posteriorly rotated, absent external auditory canals, microtia, malformed pinnae, simple auricles. Micrognathia.
Mouth. Multiple frenuli between alveolar ridge and buccal mucosa.
Respiratory. Laryngeal cleft. Bifid, hypoplasia or absence of epiglottis. Dysplastic tracheal cartilage. Absent lung. Abnormal lung lobation.
Limbs. Nail dysplasia, variable degrees of syndactyly and postaxial polydactyly involving both hands and feet. Oligodactyly. Small distally placed fourth metacarpal with one or two small fingers associated with it. Third metacarpal less frequently affected. Fourth metatarsal dysplastic. Distal shortening of limbs, particularly the arms.
Anus. Anal defects, including imperforate anus and variable degrees of rectal atresia.
Other. Renal ectopia/dysplasia. Congenital heart defects including endocardial cushion defect, patent ductus arteriosus, ventricular septal defect, mitral and aortic valve defects, and proximal aortic coarctation. Hypoplasia of adrenals.

OCCASIONAL ABNORMALITIES.
Holoprosencephaly with associated midline cleft lip and palate. Arrhinecephaly. Dandy-Walker malformation, polymicrogyria, occipital encephalocele. Cleft lip, palate, or uvula. Microphthalmia. Coloboma. Microglossia. Natal teeth. Narrow cervical vertebrae. Hemivertebrae, fused ribs, and multiple manubrial ossification centers. Subluxation of the radius. Congenital hip dislocation. Subluxation of knee. Simian crease. Camptodactyly. Hypoplasia of pancreas. Underdevelopment of thyroid. Testicular hypoplasia with micropenis.

NATURAL HISTORY. The majority of patients have died by 3 years of age. The major cause of death in the newborn period is hypoadrenalism. Most of the long-term survivors have required L-thyroxine, growth hormone, and corticosteroids from an early age as well as glucose infusions in the neonatal period. The complete spectrum of this disorder is unknown. However, it is now clear that hypothalamic hamartomas and neonatal death are not obligatory features; a number of affected individuals have reproduced, and normal mental capacity has been observed.

ETIOLOGY. At least five instances of parent-to-child transmission have been reported, indicating an autosomal dominant mode of inheritance with sporadic cases representing fresh gene mutations. Of interest, in most cases the gene was transmitted from the father to his offspring, suggesting a parent-of-origin effect. Sibling recurrence has been reported. However, the father of one of the sibling pairs was mildly affected.

References

Clarren, S. K., Alvord, E. C., and Hall, J. G.: Congenital hypothalamic hamartoblastoma, hypopituitarism, imperforate anus, and postaxial polydactyly: A new syndrome? Part II: Neuropathological considerations. Am. J. Med. Genet., 7:75, 1980.

Hall, J. G., et al.: Congenital hypothalamic hamartoblastoma, hypopituitarism, imperforate anus, and postaxial polydactyly. A new syndrome? Part I: Clinical, causal, and pathogenetic considerations. Am. J. Med. Genet., 7:47, 1980.

Culler, F. L., and Jones, K. L.: Hypopituitarism in association with postaxial polydactyly. J. Pediatr., 104: 881, 1984.

Iafolla, K., et al.: Case report and delineation of the congenital hypothalamic hamartoblastoma syndrome (Pallister-Hall syndrome). Am. J. Med. Genet., 33:489, 1989.

Finnigan, D. P., et al.: Extending the Pallister-Hall syndrome to include other central nervous system malformations. Am. J. Med. Genet., 40:395, 1991.

Topf, K. J., et al.: Autosomal dominant transmission of the Pallister-Hall syndrome. J. Pediatr., 23:943, 1993.

Thomas, H. M., et al.: Recurrence of Pallister-Hall syndrome in two sibs. J. Med. Genet., 31:145, 1994.

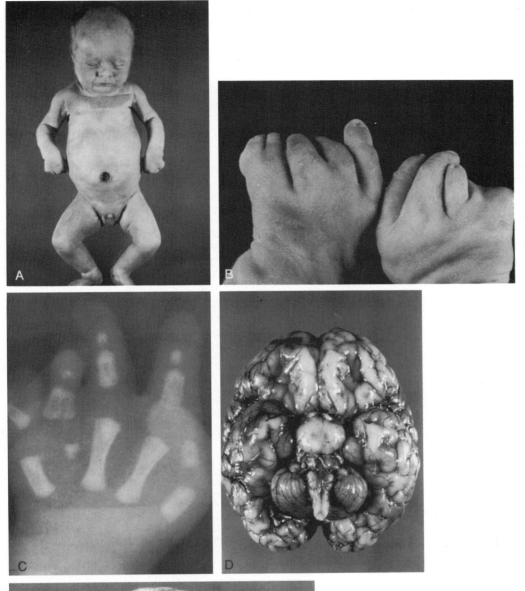

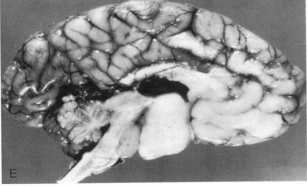

FIGURE 1. Pallister-Hall syndrome. *A* to *C*, Male infant who died at 7 days of age. He has camptodactyly, nail dysplasia, postaxial polydactyly, syndactyly, lack of ossification of distal phalanges, and a hypoplastic fourth metacarpal giving rise to two phàlanges. *D* and *E*, Note the hamartoblastoma apparent on the inferior cerebral surface and in the sagittal section. (From Hall, J. G., et al.: Am. J. Med. Genet., 7:47, 1980, with permission.)

X-LINKED HYDROCEPHALUS SPECTRUM

(X-Linked Hydrocephalus Syndrome, MASA Syndrome)

Hydrocephalus, Short Flexed Thumbs, Mental Deficiency

In 1949, Bickers and Adams first described X-linked recessive hydrocephalus associated with aqueductal stenosis. In 1974, Bianchine and Lewis delineated an X-linked recessive disorder referred to as MASA syndrome, an acronym for *m*ental retardation, *a*dducted thumbs, *s*huffling gait, and *a*phasia. Based on the similarities of their clinical phenotype as well as molecular studies that have placed the locus for both disorders at Xq28, it seems clear that the two conditions are phenotypic variations of mutations in the same gene.

ABNORMALITIES

Performance. Mental deficiency and spasticity, especially of lower extremities.
Brain. Aqueductal stenosis with hydrocephalus.
Hands. Thumb flexed over palm (cortical thumb.)

OCCASIONAL ABNORMALITIES.
Asymmetry of somewhat coarse facies; brain defects such as fusion of thalami, small pons, absence of septum pellucidum, hypoplasia of corticospinal tracts, porencephalic cyst, absence of corpus callosum.

NATURAL HISTORY.
Prenatal hydrocephalus may be severe enough to impede delivery. However, many of the affected males have no hydrocephalus. Such individuals often have a narrow scaphocephalic cranium with an I.Q. in the range of 30 and tend to have spasticity, a shuffling gait, and aphasia.

ETIOLOGY.
X-linked recessive. Several different mutations in the gene encoding for the neural cell adhesion molecule L1CAM located at Xq28 have been reported in X-linked hydrocephalus families and in MASA syndrome families. The carrier female is usually normal but may have dull intelligence and/or adducted thumbs.

COMMENT.
The gestational age at which hydrocephalus in this disorder can be diagnosed using prenatal ultrasonography is unknown. Ultrasonographic studies should be performed every 2 to 4 weeks from 16 through 28 weeks' gestation. However, it should be recognized that hydrocephalus might develop postnatally or might never occur.

References

Bickers, D. S., and Adams, R. D.: Hereditary stenosis of the aqueduct of Sylvius as a cause of congenital hydrocephalus. Brain, 72:246, 1949.

Edwards, J. H.: The syndrome of sex-linked hydrocephalus. Arch. Dis. Child., 36:486, 1961.

Holmes, L. B., et al.: X-linked aqueductal stenosis. Pediatrics, 51:697, 1973.

Bianchine, J. W., and Lewis, R. C., Jr.: The MASA syndrome: A new heritable mental retardation syndrome. Clin. Genet., 5:298, 1974.

Fryns, J. P., et al.: X-linked complicated spastic paraplegia, MASA syndrome, and X-linked hydrocephalus owing to congenital stenosis of the aqueduct of sylvius: Variable expression of the same mutation at Xq28. J. Med. Genet., 28:429, 1991.

Van Camp, G., et al.: A duplication in the L1CAM gene associated with X-linked hydrocephalus. Nat. Genet., 4:421, 1993.

Schrander-Stumpel, C., et al.: The spectrum of complicated spastic paraplegia, MASA syndrome and X-linked hydrocephalus. Contribution of DNA linkage analysis in genetic counseling of individual families. Genet. Couns., 5:1, 1994.

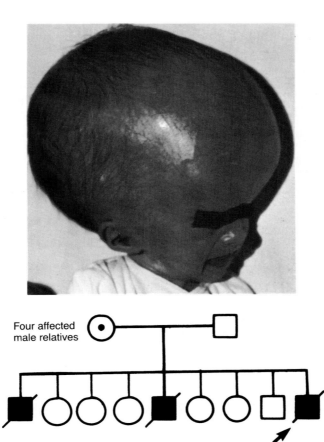

Four affected
male relatives

FIGURE 1. X-linked hydrocephalus spectrum. Male infant who later died and who was shown to have aqueductal stenosis as the cause for hydrocephalus. Note the family pedigree showing other affected males for whom
this X-linked condition was lethal. (Courtesy of J. M. Opitz, Helena, Mont.)

HYDROLETHALUS SYNDROME

Hydrocephalus, Micrognathia, Polydactyly

This disorder was described initially by Salonen et al. in 1981. Hydrolethalus refers to hydramnios, hydrocephalus, and lethality, three of the most common features of this condition. Of the approximately 65 cases reported, 56 have been from Finland.

ABNORMALITIES

Central Nervous System. Severe prenatal onset hydrocephalus. Absent corpus callosum and septum pellucidum. Abnormal gyrations. Cleft in the base of the skull. The resulting defect made up of the foramen magnum and the bony cleft extending posterior from it form a "key hole-shaped" opening in the base of the skull.

Craniofacies. Micrognathia. Cleft palate. Cleft lip that is lateral or midline. Broad nose especially at the root. Microphthalmia. Broad neck relative to the shoulders. Malformed low-set ears.

Limbs. Postaxial polydactyly of hands. Preaxial polydactyly of feet. Club feet.

Cardiac. Defects in 50 per cent, most commonly a large ventricular septal defect combined with an atrial septal defect to form an atrioventricular canal.

Respiratory. Defective lung lobation. Malformed or hypoplastic larynx. Trachea and/or bronchi are stenotic or rarely dilated.

Genitourinary. Duplicated uterus. Hypospadias. Malformations of vagina.

OCCASIONAL ABNORMALITIES. Absent pituitary. Arhinencephaly. Anencephaly. Clefts in the lower lip. Bifid nose. Agenesis of tongue. Hydronephrosis. Urethral atresia. Short arms. Syndactyly. Agenesis of diaphragm. Omphalocele.

NATURAL HISTORY. The gestation of most affected patients is complicated by polyhydramnios. Intrauterine growth deficiency is the rule. Seventy per cent of cases are stillborn. Liveborns survive for only a few minutes to a few hours.

ETIOLOGY. Autosomal recessive.

References

Salonen, R., et al.: The hydrolethalus syndrome: Delineation of a "new" lethal malformation syndrome based on 28 patients. Clin. Genet., *19*:321, 1981.

Salonen, R., and Herva, R.: Hydrolethalus syndrome. J. Med. Genet., *27*:756, 1990.

Toriello, H., and Bauserman, S. C.: Bilateral pulmonary agenesis: Association with the hydrolethalus syndrome and review of the literature from a developmental field perspective. Am. J. Med. Genet., *21*:93, 1985.

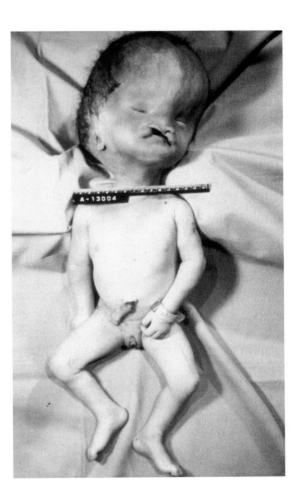

FIGURE 1. Newborn infant. Note the broad nasal root, cleft lip, and macrocephaly, which is due to hydrocephalus. (From Toriello, H. V., and Bauserman, S. C.: Am. J. Med. Genet., *21*:93, 1985, with permission of Wiley-Liss, a division of John Wiley & Sons.)

WALKER-WARBURG SYNDROME

(Hard With or Without E Syndrome, Warburg Syndrome)

Initially described by Walker in 1942, this disorder was first suggested as a distinct entity by Warburg in 1971. The first familial cases were reported by Chemke et al., and the full spectrum of associated defects was outlined by Pagon et al. and Whitley et al.

ABNORMALITIES

Brain. Type II lissencephaly (100 per cent) manifest by widespread argyria with scattered areas of macrogyria and/or polymicrogyria; abnormally thick cortex with absent white matter interdigitations; and absent or hypoplastic septum pallucidum and corpus callosum. Cerebellar malformation (100 per cent) including a polymicrogyric or smooth surface and hypoplasia of vermis. Occipital encephalocele which may be small (24 per cent). Dandy-Walker malformation (53 per cent). Hydrocephalus usually due to mechanical obstruction in the posterior fossa (53 per cent). Ventriculomegaly even in the absence of increased intracranial pressure (95 per cent).

Eye. Anterior chamber malformation (91 per cent) including cataract, corneal clouding usually secondary to Peters anomaly, and narrow iridocorneal angle with or without glaucoma. Retinal malformations (100 per cent) including microphthalmia (53 per cent), retrolental masses caused by hyperplastic primary vitreous, coloboma (24 per cent), retinal detachment secondary to retinal dysplasia.

Other. Congenital muscular dystrophy (100 per cent). Genital anomalies in males (65 per cent).

OCCASIONAL ABNORMALITIES. Cleft lip with or without cleft palate (14 per cent). Microcephaly (16 per cent). Slit-like ventricles (5 per cent). Mild renal dysplasia. Imperforate anus. Congenital contractures (43 per cent). Megalocornea. Microtia and absent auditory canals.

NATURAL HISTORY. The majority of affected children die within the first year of life secondary to the severe defect in brain development. Of those that survive, the majority have had profound mental retardation. Five to 10 per cent, especially those with less severe retardation, survive more than 5 years. For them rolling over and sitting should be expected to commence between 1 and 3 years. Seizures are common with increasing age.

ETIOLOGY. Autosomal recessive inheritance. Prenatal diagnosis at 20 weeks' gestation has been made on an affected fetus based on the presence of hydrocephalus.

COMMENT. Because of the wide spectrum of brain and eye defects, the diagnosis is frequently not considered. Postmortem examination of the brain and eyes is often necessary. Elevation of the serum creatine kinase (CK) and "myopathic" changes on electromyography can be helpful in documenting the presence of congenital muscular dystrophy, which is present in virtually all affected patients.

References

Warburg, M.: The hereogenicity of microphthalmia in the mentally retarded. Birth Defects, 7:136, 1971.

Chemke, J., et al.: A familial syndrome of central nervous system and ocular malformations. Clin. Genet., 7:1, 1975.

Pagon, R. A., et al.: Autosomal recessive eye and brain anomalies: Warburg syndrome. J. Pediatr., 102:542, 1983.

Whitley, C. B., et al.: Warburg syndrome. Lethal neurodysplasia with autosomal recessive inheritance. J. Pediatr., 102:547, 1983.

Dobyns, W. B., et al.: Diagnostic criteria for Walker-Warburg syndrome. Am. J. Med. Genet., 32:195, 1989.

Rodgers, B. L., et al.: Walker-Warburg syndrome: Report of three affected sibs. Am. J. Med. Genet., 49:198, 1994.

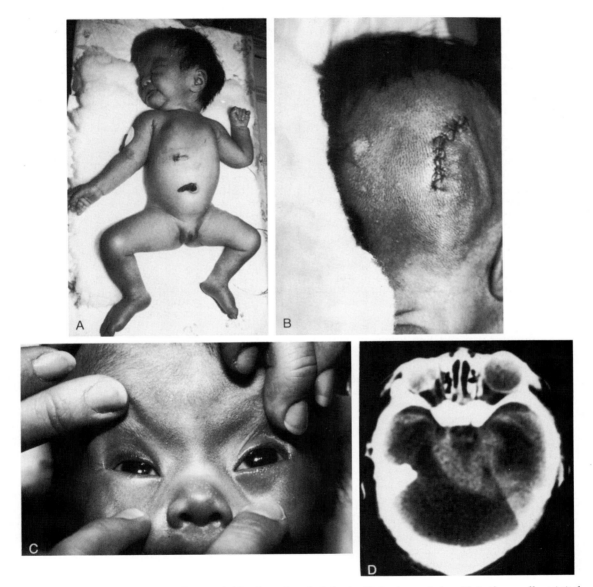

FIGURE 1. Walker-Warburg syndrome. *A*, Newborn female infant with hydrocephalus. Note the small occipital encephalocele (*B*) and unilateral microphthalmic eye (*C*), which is better demonstrated on the CT scan (*D*). (Courtesy of Dr. Marilyn C. Jones, Children's Hospital, San Diego, Calif.)

MILLER-DIEKER SYNDROME
(Lissencephaly Syndrome)

Miller in 1963 and later Dieker et al. described a specific pattern of malformation, one feature of which was lissencephaly (smooth brain). Jones et al. expanded the clinical phenotype and introduced the term Miller-Dieker syndrome to distinguish this disorder from other conditions associated with lissencephaly.

ABNORMALITIES

Brain and Performance. Incomplete development of brain, often with a smooth surface, although areas of pachygyria are often seen inferiorly. Heterotopias. Both frontal and temporal opercula fail to develop, leaving a wide-open Sylvian fossa and a figure-eight appearance on CT scan. Absent or hypoplastic corpus callosum (74 per cent) and large cavum septi pellucidi (77 per cent). Small midline calcifications in the region of third ventricle (45 per cent). Brain stem and cerebellum appear grossly normal. Severe mental deficiency with initial hypotonia, opisthotonos, spasticity, failure to thrive, seizures, occasionally hypsarrhythmia by EEG.

Craniofacies. Microcephaly with bitemporal narrowing. Variable high forehead, vertical ridging and furrowing in central forehead, especially when crying. Small nose with anteverted nostrils, up-slant to palpebral fissures, protuberant upper lip, thin vermilion border of upper lip, and micrognathia. Appearance of "low-set" and/or posteriorly angulated auricles. Wide secondary alveolar ridge. Late eruption of primary teeth.

Other. Crytorchidism, pilonidal sinus. Fifth finger clinodactyly. Transverse palmar crease. Polyhydramnios.

OCCASIONAL ABNORMALITIES.
Cardiac defect (tetralogy of Fallot, ventricular septal defect, valvular pulmonic stenosis). Intrauterine growth retardation. Decreased fetal activity. Omphalocele. Pelvic kidney. Cystic dysplasia of kidney. Lipomeningocele with tethered cord. Sacral tail. Cleft palate. Cataract.

NATURAL HISTORY.
Postnatal failure to thrive. Gastrostomy because of feeding problems, poor nutrition, and repeated aspiration pneumonia. Brief visual fixation, smiling, and nonspecific motor responses to stimulation are the only developmental skills usually acquired, although a few patients have rolled over occasionally. Death usually occurs before 2 years and often within the first 3 months. One child lived to 9 years of age.

ETIOLOGY.
A deletion at 17p13.3 has been documented in the majority of patients with this disorder. This defect has been found in association with ring chromosome 17, terminal deletion 17, unbalanced translocation inherited from a balanced reciprocal translocation carrier and a recombinant chromosome 17 due to crossover in a pericentric inversion carrier. For de novo abnormalities such as ring 17 or terminal deletions, the recurrence risk is negligible. In families with balanced rearrangements, the recurrence risk might be high. However, prenatal diagnosis is possible. In patients with highly suggestive phenotypes in which high-resolution chromosomal analysis is normal, the diagnosis can sometimes be established with fluorescent in situ hybridization using probes specific for the Miller-Dieker critical region on 17p. The gene for Miller-Dieker syndrome (LIS-1) in 17p13.3 has been identified. The gene product could be a human homologue of a subunit of bovine brain platelet-activating factor acetylhydrolase, which inactivates platelet-activating factor.

COMMENT.
At least two distinct types of lissencephaly exist: Type I lissencephaly, one feature of the Miller-Dieker syndrome, associated with microcephaly and a thickened cortex with four rather than six layers; and type II, associated with obstructive hydrocephalus and additional severe brain defects (see Walker-Warburg syndrome).

References

Miller, J. Q.: Lissencephaly in two siblings. Neurology, 13:841, 1963.

Dieker, H., et al.: The Lissencephaly syndrome. Birth Defects, 5:53, 1969.

Jones, K. L., et al.: The Miller-Dieker syndrome. Pediatrics, 66:277, 1980.

Dobyns, W. B., et al.: Miller-Dieker syndrome. Lissencephaly and monosomy 17p. J. Pediatr., 102:552, 1983.

Dobyns, W. B., Stratton, R. F., and Greenberg, F.: Syndromes with lissencephaly. I: Miller-Dieker and Norman-Roberts syndrome and isolated lissencephaly syndromes. Am. J. Med. Genet., 22:197, 1984.

Dobyns, W. B., et al.: Clinical and molecular diagnosis of Miller-Dieker syndrome. Am. J. Hum. Genet., 48:584, 1991.

Reiner, O., et al.: Isolation of a Miller-Dieker lissencephaly gene containing G protein B-subunit-like repeats. Nature, 364:717, 1993.

Alvarado, M., et al.: Miller-Dieker syndrome. Detection of a cryptic chromosome translocation using in situ hybridization in a family with multiple affected offspring. Am. J. Dis. Child., *147*:1291, 1993.

Hattori, M., et al.: Miller-Dieker syndrome gene encodes a subunit of brain platelet activating factor. Nature, *370*:216, 1994.

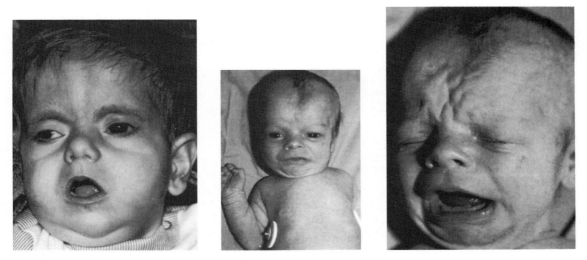

FIGURE 1. Facies of an infant with Miller-Dieker syndrome, showing high forehead with vertical soft tissue ridging and furrowing when crying, and small, anteverted nose.

ATAXIA-TELANGIECTASIA SYNDROME

(Louis-Bar Syndrome)

Ataxia, Telangiectasia, Lymphopenia, Immune Deficit

This disease was initially described by Louis-Bar in 1941. More recently it has received broader recognition, with many cases having been reported and its broader implications documented.

ABNORMALITIES

Growth. Deficiency, variable in age of onset.

Central Nervous System. Progressive ataxia and other evidence of degeneration of CNS function, including mental deficiency and posterior spinal column dysfunction.

Skin and Conjunctivae. Telangiectasia in bulbar conjunctivae and later over bridge of nose, auricles, and elsewhere.

Respiratory. Inflammation of mucous membranes, frequent respiratory infections; bronchiectasis.

Immune System. Deficiency in cellular immunity with thymic hypoplasia, hypoplasia of tonsil and adenoid lymphoid tissue, lymphopenia, low to absent serum and secretory IgA and serum IgE, and the presence of a low-molecular-weight IgM.

OCCASIONAL FEATURES

Skin and Hair. Areas of altered skin or hair pigmentation, including café au lait spots. Sclerodermatous changes.

Lymphoreticular System. Malignancy, including leukemia, sarcoma, and Hodgkin's disease, in about 10 per cent of patients.

Gonads. Hypogonadism with absent or hypoplastic ovaries. Ovarian dysgerminoma or hypoplasia.

Other. Endocrine abnormalities including hyperinsulinism, insulin resistance, and hyperglycemia. Hepatic abnormalities with increased alpha-fetoprotein. Hypersensitivity of fibroblasts and lymphocytes to ionizing radiation. Primary carcinomas of stomach, liver, ovary, salivary glands, oral cavity, breast, and pancreas have been reported infrequently.

NATURAL HISTORY. Growth deficiency, though it may be prenatal in onset, more commonly becomes evident in later infancy or in childhood. Progressive ataxia usually develops during infancy and is commonly accompanied by features of choreoathetosis and by dysrhythmic speech, drooling, aberrant ocular movements such as fixation nystagmus, stooped posture plus dull sad facies, and occasionally seizures. Instability, suggesting vestibular deficit, often becomes so severe that ambulation is no longer possible in later childhood. These children are usually affable and pleasant despite their progressive handicap. Mental deficiency, though difficult to assess, is considered a feature in about 50 per cent of cases, especially in later stages of this fatal disease. Telangiectasias usually appear between 2 and 8 years. The immune deficiency probably contributes to the frequent respiratory infections and bronchiectasis that become prominent after 3 years of age. The persistent inflammation and progressive generalized bronchiectasis are relatively unresponsive to antibiotic management, and there may be a basic problem in the mucous membranes besides the cellular immune deficit. Death is usually a consequence of lung infection, neurologic deficit, or malignancy. Patients seldom survive later childhood. The oldest survivor was 37 years old, and the disease had been quiescent for 20 years.

ETIOLOGY. Autosomal recessive. The gene has been localized to chromosomal region 11q23. Prenatal detection of an affected fetus has been performed successfully.

COMMENT. No common cellular metabolic defect has yet been detected. However, it has been suggested that there exists a defect in DNA repair. It is of interest to note certain common features among Fanconi syndrome, Bloom syndrome, and ataxia-telangiectasia. In each of these disorders, there is generalized growth deficiency, skin disorder, and a propensity to develop lymphoreticular malignancy, plus a high frequency of chromosomal breakage in cultured leukocytes.

In addition to patients who are homozygous for ataxia-telangiectasia, individuals who are heterozygous have an increased cancer risk, in particular breast cancer in women.

References

Louis-Bar, D.: Sur un syndrome progressif comprenant des télangiectasies capillaires cutanées et conjonctivales, à disposition naevoide et des troubles cérébelleux. Confin. Neurol., *4:*32, 1941.

McFarlin, D. W., Strober, W., and Waldmann, T. A.: Ataxia telangiectasia. Medicine, *51:*281, 1972.

Shaham, M., et al.: Prenatal diagnosis of ataxia-telangiectasia. J. Pediatr., *100:*134, 1982.

Swift, M., et al.: Breast and other cancers in families with ataxia-telangiectasia. N. Engl. J. Med., *316:*1289, 1987.

Gatti, R. A., et al.: Localization of an ataxia-telangiec-tasia gene to chromosome 11q22-23. Nature, *336*:577, 1988.

Swift, M., et al.: Incidence of cancer in 161 families affected by ataxia-telangiectasia. N. Engl. J. Med., *325*:1831, 1991.

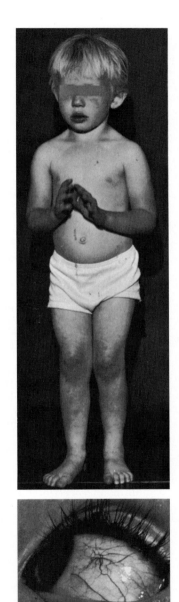

FIGURE 1. Ataxia-telangiectasia syndrome. *Top*, A $9^{6}/_{12}$-year-old. Height age, 8 years. *Bottom*, Bulbar conjunctiva. (From Smith, D. W.: J. Pediatr., *70*:487, 1967, with permission.)

MENKES SYNDROME

(Menkes Kinky Hair Syndrome)

Progressive Cerebral Deterioration
With Seizures, Twisted and Fractured Hair

Menkes et al. described five related male infants with this disease in 1962, and Danks et al. have subsequently indicated that all features of the disorder are the result of copper deficiency.

ABNORMALITIES

Growth. Deficiency, sometimes small at birth.

Central Nervous System. Severe degenerative process in cerebral cortex with gliosis and atrophy. Profound and progressive neurologic deficit beginning at from 1 to 2 months of age with hypertonia, irritability, seizures, intracranial hemorrhage, hypothermia, and feeding difficulties.

Facies. Lack of expressive movement, pudgy cheeks.

Hair. Sparse, stubby, and lightly pigmented; shows twisting and partial breakage by magnified inspection.

Skin. Occasionally thick and relatively dry. Unequal skin pigmentation at birth, particularly in darkly pigmented patients.

Skeletal. Wormian bones; metaphyseal widening, particularly of ribs and femur, with formation of lateral spurs that frequently fracture.

Other. Gastric polyps associated with gastrointestinal bleeding. Bladder diverticuli. Widespread arterial elongation and tortuosity noted on arteriograms and at autopsy most likely due to deficiency of copperdependent cross-linking in the internal elastic membrane of the arterial wall.

NATURAL HISTORY. Progressive deterioration beginning in early infancy, with death usually by 3 years, although in one child as late as 13 years. Hair is normal at birth but by 6 weeks begins to lose pigmentation. The skeletal changes have been confused with those occurring in the battered child syndrome.

COMMENT. The disease results from an abnormality in copper transport such that low levels of serum copper and ceruloplasmin have been found in all patients studied. The basic defect at least partially involves reduced ability to incorporate copper into certain enzymes that need it as a cofactor. The clinical phenotype is due to a deficiency of these enzymes. For example, hypopigmentation due to tyrosinase deficiency; vascular tortuosity and bladder diverticuli due to lysyl oxidase deficiency. Subcutaneous therapy with copper-histidine may be an effective treatment if started early.

ETIOLOGY. X-linked recessive. The gene responsible for this disorder encodes a coppertransporting ATPase and is located at Xq13. Manifestations in the carrier female include hair that is lighter than would be expected for the family, pili torti (180-degree twist of hair shaft), and increased fragility and breakage of hair. Prenatal diagnosis can be made in selected laboratories by demonstrating excessive copper uptake in cultured amniotic fluid cells.

References

Menkes, J. H., et al.: A sex-linked recessive disorder with retardation of growth, peculiar hair, and focal cerebral and cerebellar degeneration. Pediatrics, *29*: 764, 1962.

Danks, D. M., et al.: Menkes' kinky hair syndrome. An inherited defect in copper absorption with widespread effects. Pediatrics, *50*:188, 1972.

Danks, D. M., et al.: Menkes' kinky hair syndrome. Lancet, *1*:1100, 1972.

Horn, N.:Menkes X-linked disease: Prenatal diagnosis of hemizygous males and heterozygous females. Prenat. Diagn., *1*:121, 1981.

Kaler, S. G., et al.: Gastrointestinal hemorrhage associated with gastric polyps in Menkes disease. J. Pediatr., *122*:93, 1993.

Sarkar, B., et al.: Copper-histidine therapy for Menkes disease. J. Pediatr., *123*:828, 1993.

Vulpe, C., et al.: Isolation of a candidate gene for Menkes disease and evidence that it encodes a coppertransporting ATPase. Nat. Genet., *3*:7, 1993.

Bankier, A.: Menkes disease. J. Med. Genet., *32*:213, 1995.

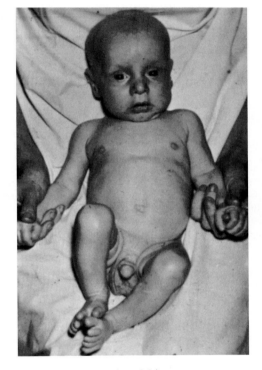

FIGURE 1. Menkes syndrome. (From Menkes, J. H., et al.: Pediatrics, *29*:764, 1962, with permission.)

2 months—2.6 kg

Scalp hair × 100

ANGELMAN SYNDROME

(Happy Puppet Syndrome)

"Puppet-Like" Gait, Paroxysms of Laughter, Characteristic Facies

This disorder, initially described in 1965 by Angelman in three unrelated children with severe mental deficiency, abnormal puppet-like gait, a characteristic facies, and frequent paroxysms of laughter, has been more completely delineated by Williams and Frias, who have documented the natural history of this disorder and have suggested that the term "happy puppet" is inappropriate.

ABNORMALITIES

Performance. Severe mental retardation with marked delay in attainment of motor milestones (100 per cent). Paroxysms of inappropriate laughter. Absent speech or less than six words (100 per cent).

Craniofacial. Microbrachycephaly. Blond hair (65 per cent). Ocular anomalies including decreased pigmentation of the choroid and iris, the latter resulting in pale blue eyes (88 per cent). Maxillary hypoplasia, deep-set eyes, a large mouth with tongue protrusion and widely spaced teeth. Prognathia.

Neurologic. Ataxia and jerky arm movements resembling a puppet gait (100 per cent). Characteristic position of arms which are upheld with flexion at wrists and elbows. Seizures varying from major motor to akinetic, beginning usually between 18 and 24 months (86 per cent). EEG abnormalities consisting of high-amplitude spike and slow waves at 2 to 3 Hz, posterior, large-amplitude slow waves mixed with spikes facilitated by eye closure, and generalized large-amplitude intermediate slow activity persisting for most of the record (92 per cent). Hypotonia and occasionally hyperreflexia. CT Scan showing cerebral atrophy (33 per cent). Left hand preference.

OCCASIONAL ABNORMALITIES.

Scoliosis. Hypopigmentation (39 per cent). Strabismus (42 per cent). Myopia and hypermetropia. Nystagmus.

NATURAL HISTORY.

The mental deficiency, although nonprogressive, is severe. Seizure activity most severe around 4 years, may stop by 10 years of age. The laughter is not apparently associated with happiness but rather is suggestive of a defect at the brain stem level. Decreased need for sleep particularly between 2 and 6 years.

Although severe problems exist with speech, the vast majority communicate in other ways such as sign language. Receptive ability may be sufficient to understand simple commands. Most individuals become toilet trained by day and some by night. None were capable of an independent living situation.

ETIOLOGY.

Between 60 and 80 per cent of affected individuals have an interstitial deletion of chromosome 15q11q13 by either cytogenetic or molecular analysis. Whereas the parental origin of the deleted chromosome 15 is paternal in Prader-Willi syndrome, it is always maternal in Angelman syndrome. The fact that the parent of origin of the deleted chromosome impacts the phenotype implies that genes located at 15q11q13 on the maternally inherited chromosome are expressed differently from those at the same locus on the paternally inherited chromosome, a phenomenon known as genomic imprinting.

Paternal uniparental disomy involving chromosome 15 is an infrequent cause of this disorder.

Except in rare cases in which a familial chromosomal rearrangement alters the Angelman locus, all cases are sporadic.

References

Angelman, H.: "Puppet" children: A report on three cases. Dev. Med. Child. Neurol., 7:681, 1965.

Williams, C. A., and Frias, J. L.: The Angelman ("happy puppet") syndrome. Am. J. Med. Genet., 11:453, 1982.

Boyd, S. G., et al.: The EEG in early diagnosis of the Angelman (happy puppet) syndrome. Eur. J. Pediatr., 147:508, 1988.

Clayton-Smith, J.: Clinical research on Angelman syndrome in the United Kingdom: Observations on 82 affected individuals. Am. J. Med. Genet., 46:12, 1993.

Knoll, J. H. M., et al.: Cytogenetic and molecular studies in the Prader-Willi and Angelman syndromes. Am. J. Med. Genet., 46:2, 1993.

Nicholls, R. D.: Genomic imprinting and uniparental disomy in Angelman and Prader-Willi syndrome: A review. Am. J. Med. Genet., 46:16, 1993.

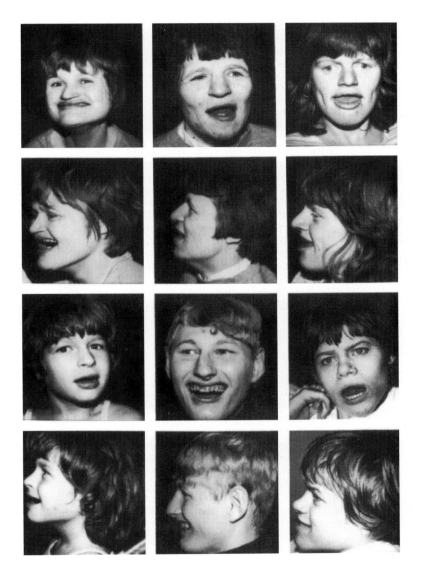

FIGURE 1. Angelman syndrome. Photographs of six affected individuals ranging from 11 to 33 years of age. (From Williams, C. A., and Frias, J. L.: Am. J. Med. Genet., *11*:453, 1982, with permission.)

PRADER-WILLI SYNDROME

Hypotonia, Obesity, Small Hands and Feet

Charles Dickens, in *The Pickwick Papers*, described "a fat and red-faced boy in a state of somnolency." The boy was subsequently addressed as "young dropsy," "young opium eater," and "boa constrictor," no doubt in reference to his obesity, somnolence, and excessive appetite, respectively. This may have been the first reported instance of Prader-Willi syndrome.

Prader et al. reported this pattern of abnormality in nine children in 1956. The prevalence has been estimated to be 1 in 15,000.

ABNORMALITIES. Variability in the extent and severity of features based particularly on age.

Growth. Normal birth length with deceleration in the first 2-months of life, steady linear growth rate during childhood, and fall-off in adolescence. Mean adult height in males is 155 cm and in females is 147 cm.

Obesity. Onset from 6 months to 6 years.

Craniofacial. Almond-shaped appearance to palpebral fissures, which may be up-slanting. Narrow bifrontal diameter. Strabismus. Thin upper lip.

Hair, Eye, and Skin. Blond to light brown hair with blue eyes and fair skin that is sun-sensitive. Picks excessively at sores.

Performance. Mental retardation is mild in 63 per cent, moderate in 31 per cent, and severe in the remainder. Almost three quarters of affected individuals receive special education and function at a six-grade level or below in reading and third-grade or below in math. Food-related behavior problems including excessive appetite, absent sense of satiation, obsession with eating. Speech articulation problems, particularly hypernasal speech. Hypotonia, severe in early infancy.

Hands and Feet. Small. Slowing in growth of hands and/or feet, usually becoming evident in midchildhood. One patient wore size 3 shoes at 23 years. Narrow hands with straight ulnar border.

Genitalia. Small penis and cryptorchidism. Hypoplastic labia minora and clitoris. Frequent hypogonadism secondary to hypogonadotropism.

Other. Scoliosis. Osteoporosis. Temperature instability. High pain threshold. Decreased vomiting.

OCCASIONAL ABNORMALITIES. Poor fine and gross motor coordination. Upsweep of frontal scalp hair. Microcephaly, seizures, clinodactyly, syndactyly, hypoplasia of auricular cartilage. Kyphosis. Early dental caries. Diabetes mellitus. Early adrenarche. Precocious puberty. Growth hormone deficiency.

NATURAL HISTORY. The mother may have noted feeble fetal activity, and the baby is often born in the breech position. The hypotonia is most severe in early infancy, when there may be respiratory tract and feeding problems, not uncommonly necessitating tube feeding. The degree of mental deficiency may appear to be greater in infancy than at a later age because of the severity of the hypotonia hindering developmental performance. Regarding behavior, these patients have been noted to be cheerful and good-natured. However, behavioral problems, including stubborness and rage-type responses, tend to become more frequent in later childhood. Verbal perseveration on favorite topics is common. Failure to thrive is frequent in early infancy, with obesity presenting at between 6 months and 6 years of age, especially over the lower abdomen, buttocks, and thighs. The obesity, which is due to excess intake and reduced activity, paradoxically develops at a time when the hypotonia is improving. Bizarre and binge-type eating are common. In order to control the progressive obesity, the number of calories consumed must be decreased dramatically and an exercise program should be instituted. One approach to obesity control has been to calculate calories per centimeter height (i.e., 7 to 8 cal/cm height for weight loss and 10 to 14 cal/cm height for weight maintenance). Another approach for adolescents and adults has been to determine the weight that would correspond to the 50th percentile for that individual's height and then add 14 to 20 pounds to set a realistic goal. This can usually be achieved only by full family cooperation and by making food inaccessible to the patient. The presence of a diabetic type of glucose tolerance curve relates to the severity of the obesity, and only an occasional patient develops diabetes mellitus during childhood. Hyperinsulinemia and blunted pituitary growth hormone responses also relate to the degree of obesity.

Reduced life expectancy appears to relate to complications of morbid obesity. In addition, the decline of I.Q. with age has been obviated with weight control. Early short-term testosterone therapy has resulted in enlargement of the micropenis to normal size for age. Any boy who is doing reasonably well at the age of adolescence should be considered for full testosterone replacement therapy, since his own production is usually inadequate. Sixty per cent of females have amenorrhea and the remaining begin to menstruate between 10 and 28 years with an average of 17 years.

ETIOLOGY. Approximately 70 per cent of affected individuals have a deletion of the long arm of chromosome 15 at q11q13 that is detectable either by high resolution chromosome analysis or fluorescent in situ hybridization (FISH) using specific probes. In all cases studied, the paternally derived chromosome has been deleted. The majority of the remainder are due to maternal disomy (i.e., two maternal copies and no paternal copies of 15q). Specific DNA testing is necessary to detect the latter. Except for the rare case involving a chromosome translocation, recurrence risk is negligible.

References

Prader, A., Labhart, A., and Willi, H.: Ein Syndrom von Adipositas, Kleinwuchs, Kryptorchismus und Oligophrenie nach myatonieartigem Zustand im Neugeborenenalter. Schweiz. Med. Wochenschr., *86*: 1260, 1956.

Hall, B. D., and Smith, D. W.: Prader-Willi syndrome. J. Pediatr., *81*:286, 1972.

Pipes, P. L., and Holm, V. A.: Weight control of children with Prader-Willi syndrome. J. Am. Diet. Assoc., *62*:520, 1973.

Clarren, S. K., and Smith, D. W.: Prader-Willi syndrome. Am. J. Dis. Child., *131*:798, 1977.

Ledbetter, D. H., et al.: Deletion of chromosome 15 as a cause of The Prader-Willi syndrome. N. Engl. J. Med., *304*:325, 1981.

Creel, D. J., et al.: Abnormalities of the central visual pathways in the Prader-Willi syndrome associated with hypopigmentation. N. Engl. J. Med., *314*:1606, 1986.

Nicholls, R. D., et al.: Genetic imprinting suggested by maternal heterodisomy in nondeletion Prader-Willi. Nature, *16*:281, 1989.

Butler, M. G., et al.: Prader-Willi syndrome: Current understanding of cause and diagnosis. Am. J. Med. Genet., *35*:319, 1990.

Hoffman, C. J., et al.: A nutrition study of and recommendations for individuals with Prader-Willi syndrome who live in group homes. J. Am. Diet. Assoc., *92*:823, 1992.

Holm, V. A., et al.: Prader-Willi syndrome: Consensus diagnostic criteria. Pediatrics, *91*:398, 1993.

Donaldson, M. D. C., et al.: The Prader-Willi syndrome. Arch. Dis. Child., *70*:58, 1994.

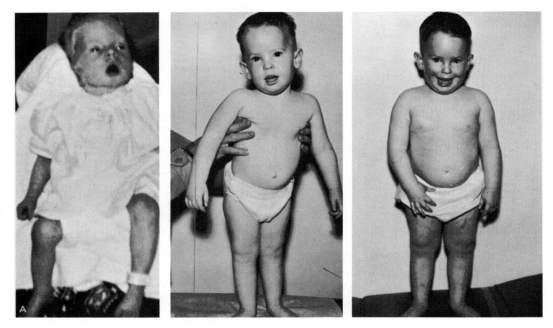

FIGURE 1. Prader-Willi syndrome. *A,* Same patient as neonate, at $1^{10}/_{12}$ years, and at $2^{10}/_{12}$ years (height age, $2^{4}/_{12}$ years; developmental quotient, 60.)

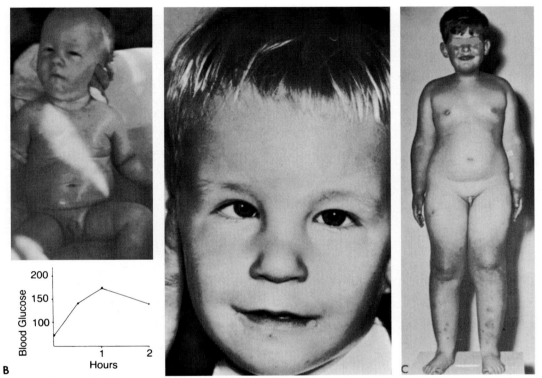

FIGURE 1. *Continued. B*, Same patient at 5 months and at $4^2/_{12}$ years, at which time height age was $3^2/_{12}$ years, developmental quotient was 50, and response to an oral glucose load was abnormal. *C*, A $9^6/_{12}$-year-old with height age of $7^6/_{12}$ years and mental age of 5 years. (Courtesy of Prof. A. Prader, University of Kinderspital, Zurich.)

COHEN SYNDROME

Hypotonia, Obesity, Prominent Incisors

This disorder was recognized in 1973 in two affected siblings and one isolated case by Cohen et al. In excess of 80 cases have subsequently been described.

ABNORMALITIES

Growth. Truncal obesity of midchildhood onset. Low birth weight. Postnatal growth deficiency.

Performance. Persisting hypotonia and weakness. Mental deficiency; I.Q.s of 30 to 70.

Craniofacial. Microcephaly. High nasal bridge, maxillary hypoplasia with mild down-slant to palpebral fissures, short philtrum, open mouth with prominent maxillary central incisors, high narrow palate, mild micrognathia, large ears.

Eyes. Decreased visual acuity, strabismus, defective vision in bright light, constricted visual fields, chorioretinal dystrophy with bull's-eye–like maculae, pigmentary deposits and optic atrophy.

Limbs. Narrow hands and feet with mild shortening of metacarpals and metatarsals, simian creases, hyperextensible joints, genu valgus, cubitus valgus.

Spine. Lumbar lordosis with mild scoliosis.

Other. Delayed puberty. Cryptorchidism.

OCCASIONAL ABNORMALITIES. Cardiac

defects. Microphthalmia, colobomata, mild cutaneous syndactyly, seizures, leukopenia, growth hormone deficiency, ureteropelvic obstruction, tall stature, mitral valve prolapse.

NATURAL HISTORY. Weakness and hypotonia persist beyond infancy, and obesity of moderate degree has developed in midchildhood. Motor milestones are delayed. All have developed speech, although to variable extent. Despite their moderate to severe degree of mental deficiency, the majority have a cheerful disposition.

ETIOLOGY. Autosomal recessive.

References

Cohen, M. M., Jr., et al.: A new syndrome with hypotonia, obesity, mental deficiency, and facial, oral, ocular, and limb anomalies. J. Pediatr., *83*:280, 1973.

Carey, J. C., and Hall, B. D.: Confirmation of the Cohen syndrome. J. Pediatr., *93*:239, 1978.

Kousseff, B. G.: Cohen syndrome: Further delineation and inheritance. Am. J. Med. Genet., *9*:25, 1981.

Norio, R., Christina, R., and Lindahl, E.: Further delineation of the Cohen syndrome; report on chorioretinal dystrophy, leukopenia, and consanguinity. Clin. Genet., *25*:1, 1984.

North, C., et al.: The clinical features of the Cohen syndrome. J. Med. Genet., *22*:131, 1985.

Young, I. D., and Moore, J. R.: Intrafamilial variation in Cohen syndrome. J. Med. Genet., *24*:488, 1987.

Massa, G., et al.: Growth hormone deficiency in a girl with the Cohen syndrome. J. Med. Genet., *28*:48, 1991.

Steinlein, O., et al.: Tapetoretinal degeneration in brothers with apparent Cohen syndrome: Nosology with Mirhosseini-Holmes-Walton syndrome. Am. J. Med. Genet., *41*:196, 1991.

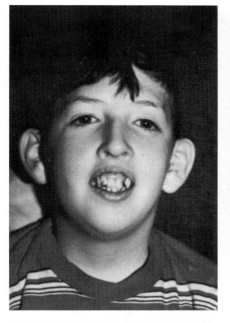
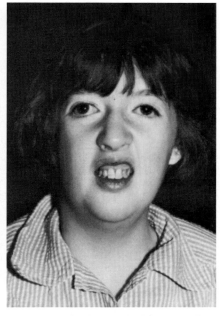
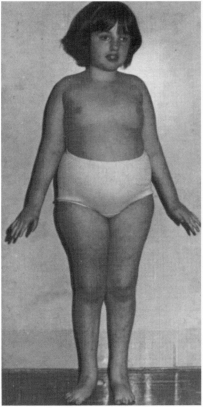
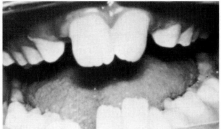
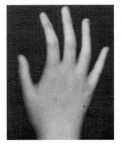

FIGURE 1. Cohen syndrome. *Above*, Brother and sister at 11 and 14 years of age, respectively. *Lower left*, An 8-year-old who developed obesity at 5 to 6 years. *Lower right*, Prominent central incisors and narrow hands with slim fingers. (From Cohen, M. M., Jr.: J. Pediatr., *83*:280, 1973, with permission.)

KILLIAN/TESCHLER-NICOLA SYNDROME

(Pallister Mosaic Syndrome, Tetrasomy 12p)

Teschler-Nicola and Killian described a 3-year-old female with this disorder in 1981. A second case was reported by Schroer and Stevenson in 1983. It was subsequently recognized that two adults with a similar phenotype and mosaicism for a marker chromosome reported by Pallister et al. in 1976 had the same condition. Recently, tetrasomy 12p, either mosaic or total, has been documented in skin fibroblasts from affected individuals, but not in peripheral blood.

ABNORMALITIES

Growth. Normal or increased birth length, weight, and head circumference, with postnatal deceleration of length and head circumference. Obesity frequently develops.

Performance. Profound mental deficiency with only minimal speech development. Seizures. Hypotonia with contractures developing with advancing age. Deafness.

Craniofacies. Sparse anterior scalp hair particularly in temporal areas in infancy, with sparse eyebrows and eyelashes. Prominent forehead. Coarsening of face over time. Upslanting palpebral fissures. Ocular hypertelorism. Ptosis. Strabismus. Epicanthal folds. Flat, broad nasal root and short nose with anteverted nostrils. Chubby cheeks. Long philtrum with thin upper lip and distinct cupid-bow shape. Protruding lower lip. Delayed dental eruption. Large ears with thick protruding lobules. Short neck.

Other. Streaks of hyper- and hypopigmentation. Broad hands with short digits. Accessory nipples. Disproportionate shortening of arms and legs.

OCCASIONAL ABNORMALITIES. Micro-
cephaly. Cataracts. Stenosis of external auditory canal. Macroglossia. Prominent lateral palatine ridges. Cleft palate. Bifid uvula. Micrognathia. Umbilical and inguinal hernias. Hypermobile joints. Kyphoscoliosis. Fifth finger clinodactyly. Distal digital hypoplasia. Postaxial polydactyly of hands and feet. Congenital hip dislocation. Simian crease. Sweating abnormalities. Lymphedema. Cardiac defect. Pericardial agenesis. Diaphragmatic hernia. Persistance of urogenital sinus/cloaca. Intestinal malrotation. Imperforate anus. Hypospadias. Sacral appendage. Renal defect. Omphalocele.

NATURAL HISTORY. A significant number of affected patients are stillborn or die in the neonatal period. Seizures usually begin in infancy. Survivors are frequently bedridden. Most will never talk. Physical characteristics change with age. Initially sparse, anterior scalp hair grows in by 2 to 5 years; a normal-size tongue becomes macroglossic; initial micrognathia progresses to prognathism, and contractures develop between 5 and 10 years after initial hypotonia. The face of adolescents and adults is coarse with thick lips, an everted lower lip, a broad nasal root, and high forehead. The oldest reported patient is a profoundly retarded, nonambulatory 45-year-old male with multiple joint contractures.

ETIOLOGY. Tetrasomy 12p, either mosaic or total, in skin fibroblasts. An older maternal age affect has been suggested. Although most patients tested have had normal karyotype in peripheral lymphocytes, at least five patients have had lymphocyte mosaicism for an isochromosome of 12 p. Fluorescent in situ hybridization (FISH) using chromosome 12–specific DNA probes has been successfully used to detect the isochromosome 12p in fibroblasts. Prenatal diagnosis is possible by amniocentesis and chorionic villus sampling.

References

Pallister, P. D., et al.: The Pallister mosaic syndrome. Birth Defects, 5XIII(3B):103, 1976.

Teschler-Nicola, M., and Killian, W.: Case report 72: Mental retardation, unusual facial appearance, abnormal hair. Synd. Ident., 7(1):6, 1981.

Buyse, M. L., and Korf, B. R.: Killian syndrome, Pallister mosaic syndrome, or mosaic tetrasomy 12p? An analysis. J. Clin. Dysmorph., 1(3):2, 1983.

Hall, B. D.: Teschler-Nicola/Killian syndrome: A sporadic case in an 11 year old male. J. Clin. Dysmorph., 1(3):14, 1983.

Schroer, R. J., and Stevenson, R. E.: Further clinical delineation of the syndrome of unusual facial appearance, abnormal hair and mental retardation reported by Teschler-Nicola and Killian. Proc. Greenwood Genet. Cntr., 2:3, 1983.

Reynolds, J. F., et al.: Isochromosome 12p mosaicism (Pallister mosaic aneuploidy or Pallister-Killian syndrome: Report of 11 cases. Am. J. Med. Genet., 27:257, 1987.

Wenger, S. L., et al.: Risk effect of maternal age in Pallister i(12p) syndrome. Clin. Genet., 34:181, 1988.

Schinzel, A.: Tetrasomy 12p (Pallister-Killian syndrome). J. Med. Genet., 28:122, 1991.

Bernert, J., et al.: Prenatal diagnosis of the Pallister-Killian mosaic aneuploidy syndrome by CVS. Am. J. Med. Genet., 42:747, 1992.

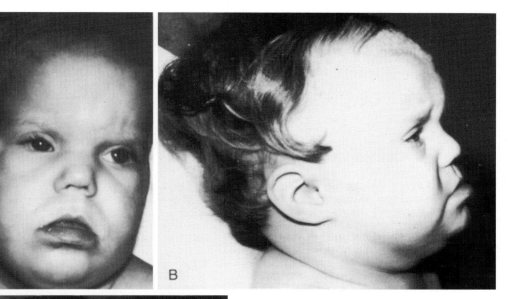

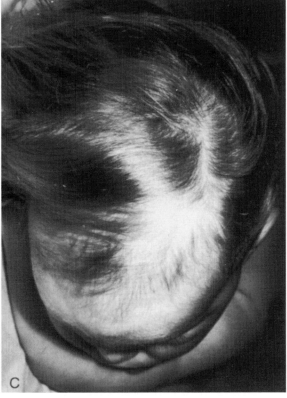

FIGURE 1. Killian/Teschler-Nicola syndrome. *A* to *C*, A 2-year-old with sparse anterior scalp hair, eyebrows, and eyelashes. Note the prominent forehead, long philtrum with thin upper lip, and distinct Cupid-bow configuration. (Courtesy of Dr. Robert Saul, Dr. Richard Schroer, and Dr. Roger Stevenson, Greenwood Genetic Center, Greenwood, S.C.)

FRYNS SYNDROME

Diaphragmatic Abnormalities,
Coarse Facies, Distal Digital Hypoplasia

This disorder was initially described in 1979 by Fryns et al. in two female siblings. Subsequently, 37 affected individuals have been reported.

ABNORMALITIES

Craniofacies. "Coarse" face (100 per cent). Abnormal ear shape (85 per cent). Cleft lip and/or palate (70 per cent). Large mouth (92 per cent). Microretrognathia (92 per cent). Broad nasal bridge (69 per cent). Anteverted nares (69 per cent).

Thorax. Diaphragmatic defects (89 per cent). Abnormal lung lobations (60 per cent).

Limbs. Distal digital hypoplasia (100 per cent) usually represented by hypoplastic to absent nails and short terminal phalanges.

Genitourinary. Anomalies of genital tract in 86 per cent including bicornuate uterus, uterus and vagina duplex, and/or uterine and cervical atresia in females and cryptorchidism, hypospadias, scrotalization of the phallus, and/or bifid scrotum in males. Cystic dysplasia of kidneys (54 per cent).

Central Nervous System. Malformation in 50 per cent including Dandy-Walker malformation, hypoplasia of optic or olfactory tracts, arrhinencephaly, and agenesis of corpus callosum.

Other. Intestinal malrotation and nonfixation. Ventricular septal defects. Broad medial ends of clavicles.

OCCASIONAL ABNORMALITIES. Large for gestational age. Microphthalmia. Cloudy corneas. Camptodactyly. Prominent fingertip pads.

Axial deviation of fingers. Single transverse palmar crease. Digitalization, proximal placement, wide or club-shaped and/or small thumbs. Omphalocele. Meckel diverticulum. Multiple accessory spleens. Duodenal atresia. Ectopic pancreatic tissue. Anterior or posterior placement and/or imperforate anus. Aganglionosis of colon and ureters.

NATURAL HISTORY. The vast majority of affected individuals have been stillborn or have died in the early neonatal period. The survivors, one of whom did not have a diaphragmatic hernia and the other who was maintained on extracorporeal membrane oxygenation therapy for 5 days followed by high-frequency oscillatory ventilation for 1 month, both have significant mental retardation.

ETIOLOGY. Autosomal recessive.

References

Fryns, J. P., et al.: A new lethal syndrome with cloudy corneae, diaphragmatic defects and distal limb deformities. Hum. Genet., 50:65, 1979.

Bamforth, J. S., et al.: Congenital diaphragmatic hernia, coarse facies, and acral hypoplasia: Fryns syndrome. Am. J. Med. Genet., 32:93, 1989.

Cunniff, C., et al.: Fryns syndrome: An autosomal recessive disorder associated with craniofacial anomalies, diaphragmatic hernia and distal digital hypoplasia. Pediatrics, 85:499, 1990.

Kershisnik, M. M., et al.: Osteochondrodysplasia in Fryns syndrome. Am. J. Dis. Child., 145:656, 1991.

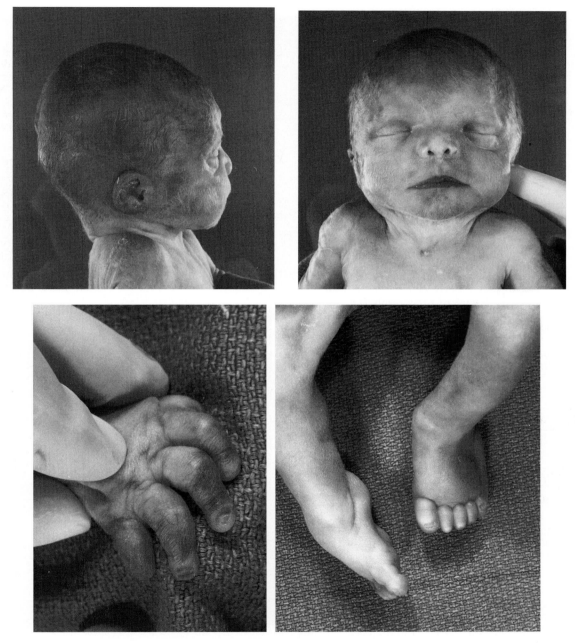

FIGURE 1. Postmortem photograph of newborn infant. Note the broad, depressed nasal bridge, anteverted nares, poorly formed auricles, and hypoplastic nails. (From Cunniff, C., et al.: Pediatrics, *85*:499, 1990, with permission.)

ZELLWEGER SYNDROME
(Cerebro-Hepato-Renal Syndrome)

Hypotonia, High Forehead With Flat Facies, Hepatomegaly

Bowen et al. and Smith et al. independently reported siblings with this pattern of malformation in 1964 and 1965. In 1973, Goldfischer et al. reported that peroxisomes, subcellular organelles that have been shown to play a role in lipid metabolism, were absent in the liver and kidneys of two affected children. Furthermore, lack of dihydroxyacetone phosphate acyltransferease (DHAP-AT), a peroxisomal enzyme with a major role in glycerol ether lipid synthesis, has been documented. Deficiency of this enzyme, as well as the observed increase in plasma and fibroblasts of very-long-chain fatty acids, provides a biochemical marker for the diagnosis of this disorder and for its potential treatment.

ABNORMALITIES
Growth. Postnatal growth deficiency; mean birth weight, 2740 g.
Performance. Hypotonia. Seizures. Poor suck. Severe mental retardation in survivors. Deafness.
Brain. Gross defects of early brain development including pachymicrogyria, heterotopias/abnormal migration, subependymal cysts, astrocytosis and gliosis, hypoplastic corpus callosum, hypoplastic olfactory lobes.
Craniofacial. Large fontanels. Flat occiput. High forehead with shallow supraorbital ridges and flat facies. Anteverted nares. Minor ear anomaly. Inner epicanthal folds. Brushfield spots. Mild micrognathia. Redundant skin of neck.
Eyes. Congenital cataracts. Pallid, hypoplastic optic disk. Retinal pigmentary changes.
Liver. Hepatomegaly with dysgenesis, including cirrhotic changes.
Kidneys. Albuminuria. Small cysts, chiefly of glomeruli.
Adrenals. Decreased weight. Striated adrenocortical cells.
Cardiac. Patent ductus arteriosus, septal defect.
Limbs. Variable contractures with camptodactyly, limited extension of knee, equinovarus deformity. Simian crease. Radiographic stippling of patellae, greater trochanters, and/or triradiate cartilages.
Other. Variable elevated serum iron level and evidence of excess iron storage, pipecolic acidemia (not always diagnostic in first weeks of life), abnormal bile acids, and absent liver peroxisomes.

OCCASIONAL ABNORMALITIES.
Prenatal growth deficiency, glaucoma, nystagmus, cubitus valgus, ulnar deviation of hands, deep sacral dimple, hypospadias, cryptorchidism, hypertrophied pylorus, single umbilical artery. Breech presentation.

NATURAL HISTORY. Most of these babies were born from the breech presentation and failed to thrive. Some developed icterus and some had bloody stools, possibly related to hypoprothrombinemia. The vast majority die within the first year of life. Survivors have severe mental retardation and seizures.

ETIOLOGY. Autosomal recessive. Two different loci have been identified, one at chromosome 7q11.23 and a second at 1p22-p21, the site of the peroxisomal membrane protein (PMP70) gene. This indicates the existence of nonallelic heterogeneity in this disorder. Diagnosis is based on a number of biochemical studies involving blood cells and fibroblasts including a decreased dihydroxyacetone phosphate acyltransferase (DHAP-AT) activity, a lowered plasmalogen content, impaired de novo plasmalogen biosynthesis, an accumulation of unmetabolized very-long-chain fatty acids,

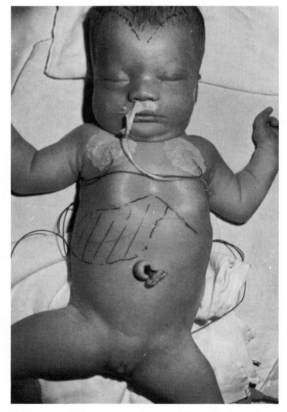

FIGURE 1. Zellweger syndrome. Affected infant showing hypotonia, enlarged fontanel, and enlarged liver.

and an absence of catalase-containing subcellular particles (peroxisomes) in fibroblasts. Prenatal diagnosis has been accomplished successfully.

COMMENT. Several of these babies were mistakenly identified initially as having Down syndrome.

References

Bowen, P., et al.: A familial syndrome of multiple congenital defects. Bull. Johns Hopkins Hosp., *114*:402, 1964.

Smith, D. W., Opitz, J. M., and Inhorn, S. L.: A syndrome of multiple developmental defects including polycystic kidneys and intrahepatic biliary dysgenesis in two siblings. J. Pediatr., *67*:617, 1965.

Opitz, J. M., et al.: The Zellweger syndrome. Birth Defects, *5*:144, 1969.

Goldfischer, S., et al.: Peroxisomal and mitochondrial defects in the cerebro-hepato-renal syndrome. Science, *182*:62, 1973.

Kelley, R. I.: Review: The cerebrohepatorenal syndrome of Zellweger. Morphologic and metabolic aspects. Am. J. Med. Genet., *16*:503, 1983.

Datta, N. S., Wilson, G. N., and Hajra, A. K.: Deficiency of enzymes catalyzing the biosynthesis of glycerol ether lipids in Zellweger syndrome. N. Engl. J. Med., *311*:1080, 1984.

Hajra, A. K., et al.: Prenatal diagnosis of Zellweger cerebrohepatorenal syndrome. N. Engl. J. Med., *312*:445, 1985.

Solish, J. I., et al.: The prenatal diagnosis of the cerebro-hepato-renal syndrome of Zellweger. Prenat. Diagn., *5*:27, 1985.

Wilson, G. N., et al.: Zellweger syndrome: Diagnostic assays, syndrome delineation, and potential therapy. Am. J. Med. Genet., *24*:69, 1986.

Lazarow, P. B., et al.: Zellweger syndrome amniocytes: Morphological appearance and a simple sedimentation method for prenatal diagnosis. Pediatr. Res., *24*:63, 1988.

Naritomi, K., et al.: Gene assignment of Zellweger syndrome to 7q11.23: Report of the second case associated with a pericentric inversion of chromosome 7. Hum. Genet., *84*:79, 1988.

Gartner, J., et al.: Mutations in the 70k peroxisomal membrane gene in Zellweger syndrome. Nat. Genet., *1*:16, 1992.

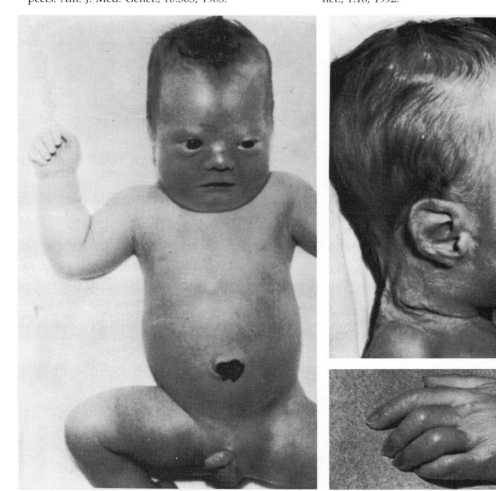

FIGURE 2. Zellweger syndrome. Affected siblings at 1 day of age (*left*) and postmortem at 10 weeks of age (*right*). Note camptodactyly of third, fourth, and fifth fingers. (From Smith, D. W., et al.: J. Pediatr., *67*:617, 1965, with permission.)

FREEMAN-SHELDON SYNDROME

(Whistling Face Syndrome)

Mask-like "Whistling" Facies,
Hypoplastic Alae Nasi, Talipes Equinovarus

This disorder was described by Freeman and Sheldon in 1938 and at least 60 cases have been reported.

ABNORMALITIES. Most of the features are secondary to increased muscle tone.

Facies. Full forehead and mask-like facies with small mouth giving a "whistling" appearance (100 per cent). Deep-set eyes, broad nasal bridge, telecanthus, epicanthal folds, strabismus, blepharophimosis, small nose, hypoplastic alae nasi with coloboma, long philtrum. H-shaped cutaneous dimpling on chin. High palate, small tongue, limited palatal movement with nasal speech.

Joints and Skeletal. Ulnar deviation of hands (91 per cent), cortical thumbs, flexion of fingers (88 per cent), thick skin over flexor surface of proximal phalanges. Equinovarus with contracted toes (59 per cent), vertical talus, kyphoscoliosis (84 per cent). Contracture of hips and/or knees (73 per cent). Contractures of shoulders. Steeply inclined anterior cranial fossa on radiographs.

Other. Postnatal growth deficiency (62 per cent). Inguinal hernia, incomplete descent of testes.

OCCASIONAL ABNORMALITIES. Microcephaly (44 per cent). Mental deficiency (31 per cent), seizures (19 per cent), flat face, ptosis, subcutaneous ridge across lower forehead, short neck, low birth weight, dislocation of hip, spina bifida occulta, prominent mental protuberance on radiographs of facial bones.

NATURAL HISTORY. These patients are not uncommonly born in the breech position, and/or delivery may be difficult. Vomiting and dysphagia may lead to failure to thrive in infancy. There may be early mortality, often related to aspiration. Eventual intelligence is in the normal range in the majority of patients. Difficulties with speech, oral hygiene, and dental treatment secondary to the small mouth can be a problem. Muscle rigidity following halothane anesthesia has been reported, giving credence to the theory that this disorder is the result of an underlying myopathy.

ETIOLOGY. Autosomal dominant. A clinically indistinguishable autosomal recessive type has been reported in three separate families.

References

Freeman, E. A., and Sheldon, J. H.: Craniocarpotarsal dystrophy. An undescribed congenital malformation. Arch. Dis. Child., 13:277, 1938.

Burian, F.: The "whistling face" characteristic in a compound cranio-facio-corporal syndrome. Br. J. Plast. Surg., 16:140, 1963.

Antley, R. M., et al.: Diagnostic criteria for the whistling face syndrome. Birth Defects, 11:161, 1975.

O'Connell, D. J., and Hall, C. M.: Cranio-carpotarsal dysplasia. A report of 7 cases. Radiology, 123:719, 1977.

Kousseff, B. G., McConnachie, P., and Hadro, T. A.: Autosomal recessive type of whistling face syndrome in twins. Pediatrics, 69:328, 1982.

Vanek, J., et al.: Freeman-Sheldon syndrome: A disorder of congenital myopathic origin? J. Med. Genet., 23:231, 1986.

Millner, M. M., et al.: Whistling face syndrome. A case report and literature review. Acta. Paediatr. Hung., 31:279, 1991.

Jones, R., and Dolcourt, J. L.: Muscle rigidity following halothane anesthesia in two patients with Freeman-Sheldon syndrome. Anesthesiology, 77:599, 1992.

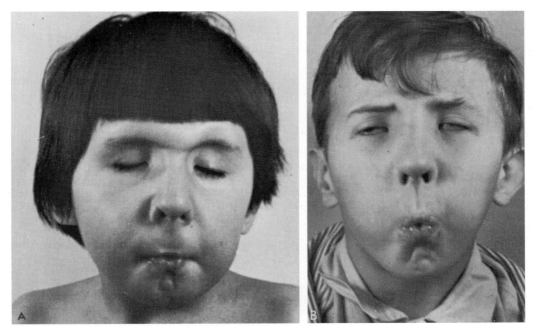

FIGURE 1. Freeman-Sheldon syndrome. *A*, A 5⁶/₁₂-year-old girl. Note crease pattern in chin. *B*, Older boy. Note the retraction of the alae nasi. (From Burian, F.: Br. J. Plast. Surg., *16*:140, 1963, with permission.)

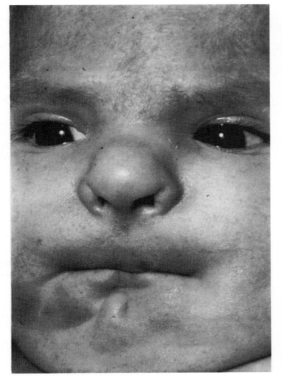

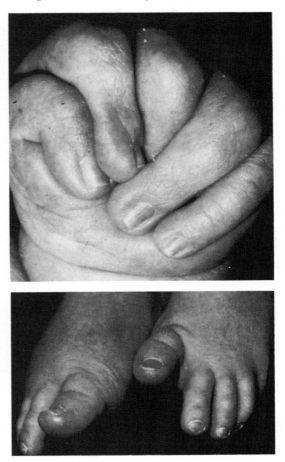

FIGURE 2. Freeman-Sheldon syndrome. Young infant showing characteristic facies and aberrant positioning in hands and feet. (Courtesy of Dr. Boris Koussef, University of South Florida, Tampa, Fla.)

STEINERT MYOTONIC DYSTROPHY SYNDROME

(Steinert Syndrome, Dystrophia Myotonica)

Myotonia With Muscle Atrophy, Cataract, Hypogonadism

The text by Caughey and Myrianthopoulos presents the manifold abnormalities that may occur as features of this single mutant gene. Approximately 1 in 8000 individuals are affected.

ABNORMALITIES

Muscle Degeneration. Myotonia (difficulty in relaxing a contracted muscle), often best appreciated in the hand or jaw or by tapping the tongue. Degeneration of swollen muscle cells giving way to thin and atrophic muscle fibers with weakness; ptosis of the eyelids is frequent. Myopathic facies.

Eyes. Cataract, often evident only as "myotonic dust" by slit lamp inspection.

Gonadal Insufficiency. Testicular atrophy (80 per cent) in males. Amenorrhea, dysmenorrhea, ovarian cyst in females.

Scalp. Premature frontal hair recession, especially in males.

Cardiac. Conduction defects with arrhythmias.

OCCASIONAL ABNORMALITIES. Hypotonia in infancy, mental deficiency, microcephaly, talipes, clinodactyly, hernia, cryptorchidism, kyphoscoliosis, hyperostotic cranial bones, atrophic thin skin, macular abnormality, blepharitis, keratitis sicca, goiter, thyroid adenomata, diabetes mellitus.

NATURAL HISTORY. The age of onset is from prenatal life to the sixth or seventh decade, with the average being between 20 and 25 years of age. Lens opacification is usually evident by slit lamp examination in the 20s. Initial signs of the disease are variable. Myotonia may be so mild as to be detected only when specifically tested for. Muscle wasting and weakness, occasionally asymmetric, most often involving the facial and temporal muscles, yielding the expressionless "myopathic facies." The most consistent evident weakness is in the orbicularis oculi muscles. Other involved muscles are the anterior cervical and those of the arms, thighs, and anterior lower leg, with progression from proximal to distal. Ptosis of the eyelids is frequent, and pseudo-hypertrophy is an occasional feature. One of the most sensitive early indicators of muscle dysfunction is the roentgenographic evidence of partial retention of radiopaque material in the pharynx after swallowing. Mental deterioration

may also be a feature. There is increasing debility, with death, usually by the fifth or sixth decade, as a consequence of pneumonia, cardiac failure, or intercurrent illness.

Congenital myotonic dystrophy is associated with polyhydramnios and decreased fetal activity. Severe hypotonia, difficulty in swallowing and sucking, a tented upper lip, talipes equinovarus (in some cases multiple joint contractures), cerebral ventricular enlargement, edema, and hematomas of the skin are all frequently present in the newborn period. Myotonia, muscle wasting, and cataracts are not seen initially. An infant mortality rate of about 25 per cent has been documented, the majority of deaths occurring in the neonatal period due to respiratory failure. For those that survive, the symptoms diminish. However, at adolescence, typical features of the adult variant develop. Although the vast majority of affected children walk by 3 years of age, psychomotor retardation is present in all survivors. With the exception of one case, congenital myotonic dystrophy has occurred only in the offspring of mothers who have myotonic dystrophy.

ETIOLOGY. Autosomal dominant with wide variability in expression. The disorder is caused by expansion in the number of trinucleotide repeats at chromosome region 19q13.3. With transmission of the disorder to family members in subsequent generations, the severity of clinical symptoms increases and their onset occurs earlier. This phenomenon, known as anticipation, is due to expansion of the repeat, which is estimated to have a 93 per cent chance of occurring when the altered allele is passed from parent to child. It is generally thought that the size of the triplet expansion correlates with the severity of the disease and the age of onset. Thus, newborns presenting with congenital myotonic dystrophy have on the average the largest repeat sizes.

COMMENT. DNA-based testing is indicated for evaluation of neonates with hypotonia and severe feeding problems, for confirmation of a clinical diagnosis, and for evaluation of at-risk asymptomatic individuals with a confirmed family history of myotonic dystrophy.

References

Caughey, J. E., and Myrianthopoulos, N. D.: Dystrophia Myotonica and Related Disorders. Springfield, Ill., Charles C Thomas, 1963.

Pruzanski, W.: Myotonic dystrophy—a multisystem disease; report of 67 cases and a review of the literature. Psychiatr. Neurol. Med. Pyschol. (Leipz.), 149:302, 1965.

Calderon, R.: Myotonic dystrophy: A neglected cause of mental retardation. J. Pediatr., 68:423, 1966.

Pruzanski, W.: Variants of myotonic dystrophy in preadolescent life (the syndrome of myotonic dysembryoplasia). Brain, 89:563, 1966.

Bell, D. B., and Smith, D. W.: Myotonic dystrophy in the neonate. J. Pediatr., 81:83, 1972.

Brook, J. D., et al.: Molecular basis of myotonic dystrophy: Expansion of a trinucleotide (CTG) repeat at the 3' end of a transcript encoding a protein kinase family member. Cell, 68:799, 1992.

Mahadevan, M., et al.: Myotonic dystrophy mutation: An unstable CTG repeat in the 3' untranslated region of the gene. Science, 255:1253, 1992.

Fu, Y. H., et al.: An unstable repeat in a gene related to myotonic dystrophy. Science, 255:1256, 1992.

Reardon, W., et al.: The natural history of congenital myotonic dystrophy: Mortality and long term clinical aspects. Arch. Dis. Child., 68:177, 1993.

Wieringa, B.: Commentary: Myotonic dystrophy reviewed: Back to the future? Hum. Mol. Genet., 3:1, 1994.

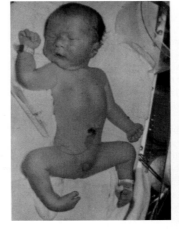

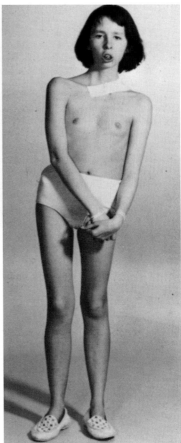

FIGURE 1. *Above*, Severely affected, almost immobile newborn baby of mother with myotonic dystrophy. (From Bell, D. B., and Smith, D. W.: J. Pediatr., *81*:83, 1972, with permission.) *Right*, A 14-year-old with relatively immobile facies, scoliosis, and an I.Q. of 58. *Below*, Correlation of protean features of myotonic dystrophy with age of onset, beginning with earliest age reported.

	FETAL-NEONATAL INFANCY	CHILDHOOD	ADULTHOOD
CNS	Mental deficiency – – – – – – – – – – – – – – – – – ➤		
OCULAR	Cataracts – – – – – – – – – – – – – – – – – – ➤ Ptosis – – – – – – – – – – – – – – – – – – – ➤		
SKELETAL	Clubfeet	Scoliosis/lordosis – – – – – – ➤ Cranial hyperostosis– – – – – – – ➤	
RESPIRATORY	Neonatal distress Recurrent infection – – – – – – – – – – – – – – – ➤		Chronic insufficiency
NEURO – MUSCULAR	Hypotonia/"floppy" Facial diplegia Weakness/atrophy – – – – – – – – – – – – – – – – ➤ Variable myotonia – – – – – – – – – – – – – – – – ➤	Dysarthria – – – – – – – – – – – ➤	
GI	Poor feeding Impaired deglutition – – – – – – – – – – – – – – – ➤		
GONADAL	Cryptorchidism – – – – – – – – – – – – – – – – ➤		Hypogonadism
CARDIAC	Disturbed conduction – – – – – – ➤		
MISC.	Frontal baldness – – – – – – – ➤ Decreased IgG and IgM – – – – – ➤		

SCHWARTZ-JAMPEL SYNDROME

(Chondrodystrophica Myotonia)

Myotonia, Blepharophimosis, Joint Limitation

Though Pinto and de Sousa were the first to report this disorder, this fact was only recently appreciated. Schwartz and Jampel described a brother and sister with this condition in 1962, and later Aberfeld et al. reported further observations on the same patients. At least 50 cases have been reported. Many, if not most, of the features appear to be secondary to a primary muscle disorder with myotonia.

ABNORMALITIES

Growth. Small stature, usually postnatal onset.

Muscle. Myotonia with sad, fixed facies, pursed lips, and narrowed palpebral fissures. Small mandible. Muscular hypertrophy in one half of patients. Hyporeflexia.

Joints. Limitation in hips, wrists, fingers, toes, and spine.

Other Skeletal. Vertical shortness of vertebrae (platyspondyly) with short neck. Fragmentation and flattening of femoral epiphyses. Diaphyses of leg bones bowed anteriorly. Hip dysplasia with acetabular flattening. Coxa valga/vara. Wide metaphyses. Osteoporosis. Pectus Carinatum.

Larynx. Small and high-pitched voice.

Eyes. Blepharophimosis, myopia, medial displacement of outer canthi. Long eyelashes in irregular rows.

Other. Low hairline, flat facies, small mouth, low-set ears, small testicles, umbilical and inguinal hernias.

OCCASIONAL ABNORMALITIES. Mental deficiency (25 per cent). Intrauterine growth deficiency, delayed bone age, equinovarus foot deformation, hip dislocation, cataract, microcornea.

NATURAL HISTORY. Onset of progressive myotonia, muscle wasting, and orthopedic problems during infancy, with slow linear growth. Myotonia, which usually reaches a plateau in midchildhood, is almost always recorded on electromyography, even when not present clinically. Light and electron microscopic and histochemical examinations of muscles show inconsistent myopathic abnormalities. Contractures are most severe by midadolescence and then re-main static. Anesthesia may constitute a serious risk due to difficulties with intubation and malignant hyperthermia. There is slowing of growth, and there are problems of motor function. Affected patients frequently have a waddling gait and crouched stance. Tiredness results from stiffness of joints. Intelligence is usually considered normal. However, myotonia may result in drooling and indistinct speech. Normal pubertal development occurs.

COMMENT. A more severe form of Swartz-Jampel syndrome has been reported with feeding, choking, and respiratory difficulties presenting in the neonatal period. Four out of 14 children reported with this form have died, primarily related to respiratory compromise.

ETIOLOGY. Autosomal recessive. It has been suggested that the hyperexcitability and muscle stiffness seen in this disorder are due to a sodium channel defect.

References

Pinto, L. M., and de Sousa, J. S.: Um caso de "doenca muscular" de dificil classificacao. Rev. Port. Pediatr. Pueric., *6*:1, 1961.

Schwartz, O., and Jampel, R. S.: Congenital blepharophimosis associated with a unique generalized myopathy. Arch. Ophthalmol., *68*:52, 1962.

Aberfeld, D. C., Hinterbuchner, L. P., and Schneider, M.: Myotonia, dwarfism, diffuse bone disease and unusual ocular and facial abnormalities (a new syndrome.) Brain, *88*:313, 1965.

Horan, F., and Beighton, P.: Orthopedic aspects of Schwartz syndrome. J. Bone Joint Surg., *57*:542, 1975.

Edward, W. C., and Root, A. W.: Chondrodystrophic myotonia (Schwartz-Jampel syndrome): Report of a new case and follow-up of patients initially reported in 1969. Am. J. Med. Genet., *13*:51, 1982.

Lehmann-Horn, F., et al.: Schwartz-Jampel syndrome: II. Na$^+$ channel defect causes myotonia. Muscle Nerve, *13*:528, 1990.

Viljoen, D., and Beighton, P.: Schwartz-Jampel syndrome (chondrodystrophic myotonia). J. Med. Genet., *29*:58, 1992.

Al Gazali, L. I.: The Schwartz-Jampel syndrome. Clin. Dysmorph., 2:47, 1993.

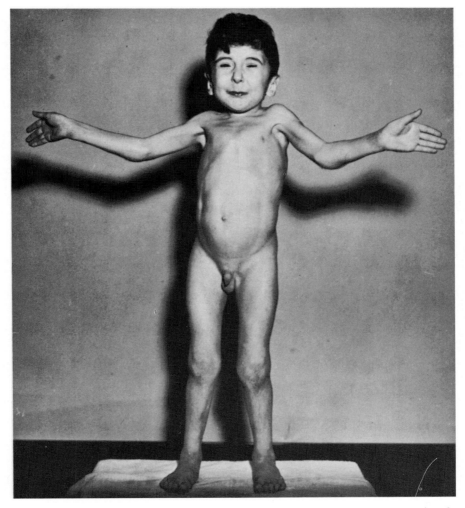

FIGURE 1. Schwartz-Jampel syndrome. A 6-year-old male with height age of 3⁶/₁₂ years. A female sibling had the same disorder, and the parents appeared normal. (From Schwartz, O., and Jampel, R. S.: Arch. Ophthalmol., *68*:52, 1962, with permission.)

MARDEN-WALKER SYNDROME

Blepharophimosis, Joint Contractures, Immobile Facies

This disorder was reported initially in 1966 by Marden and Walker, who described a female infant who died at 3 months of age. Subsequently, approximately 20 affected individuals have been reported.

ABNORMALITIES

Growth. Prenatal (35 per cent) and severe postnatal (88 per cent) growth deficiency.

Performance. Moderate to severe mental retardation (89 per cent). Hypotonia (86 per cent). Strabismus (69 per cent).

Craniofacies. Microcephaly (56 per cent). Large anterior fontanel. Fixed facial expression (100 per cent). Blepharophimosis (100 per cent). Cleft palate (38 per cent). High arched palate (88 per cent). Micrognathia (100 per cent). Small mouth (63 per cent).

Musculoskeletal. Multiple joint contractures present at birth (100 per cent). Camptodactyly (69 per cent). Arachnodactyly (71 per cent). Talipes equinovarus (63 per cent). Scoliosis/kyphosis (71 per cent). Pectus excavatum/carinatum (75 per cent). Decreased muscle mass (92 per cent).

OCCASIONAL ABNORMALITIES.

Seizures. EEG abnormalities. Microphthalmia. Ventricular dilatation. Agenesis of corpus callosum. Hypoplasia of cerebellum and inferior vermis. Hypoplastic brain stem. Dandy-Walker malformation with vertebral anomalies. Short neck. Cardiac defect. Hypospadias. Cryptorchidism. Micropenis. Microcystic or hypoplastic kidneys. Inguinal hernia. Radioulnar synostosis. Zollinger-Ellison syndrome. Pyloric stenosis and duodenal bands. Absent clavicle. Hypoplastic lung. Patent omphalomesenteric duct.

NATURAL HISTORY. Death has occurred at about 3 months of age due to aspiration, sepsis, and/or cardiac failure in 19 per cent. The vast majority of survivors have been significantly mentally retarded.

ETIOLOGY. Autosomal recessive. The primary abnormality in this disorder is most likely related to a major defect in CNS development. Muscle biopsies performed on some affected individuals have revealed nonspecific changes that are most likely secondary to the primary CNS process.

References

Marden, P. M., and Walker, W. A.: A new generalized connective tissue syndrome. Am. J. Dis. Child., *112*: 225, 1966.

Ramer, J. C., et al.: Marden-Walker phenotype: Spectrum of variability in three infants. Am. J. Med. Genet., *45*:285, 1993.

Schrander-Stumple, C., et al.: Marden-Walker syndrome: Case report, literature review and nosologic discussion. Clin. Genet., *43*:303, 1993.

Williams, M. S., et al.: Marden-Walker syndrome: A case report and a critical review of the literature. Clin. Dysmorph., 2:211, 1993.

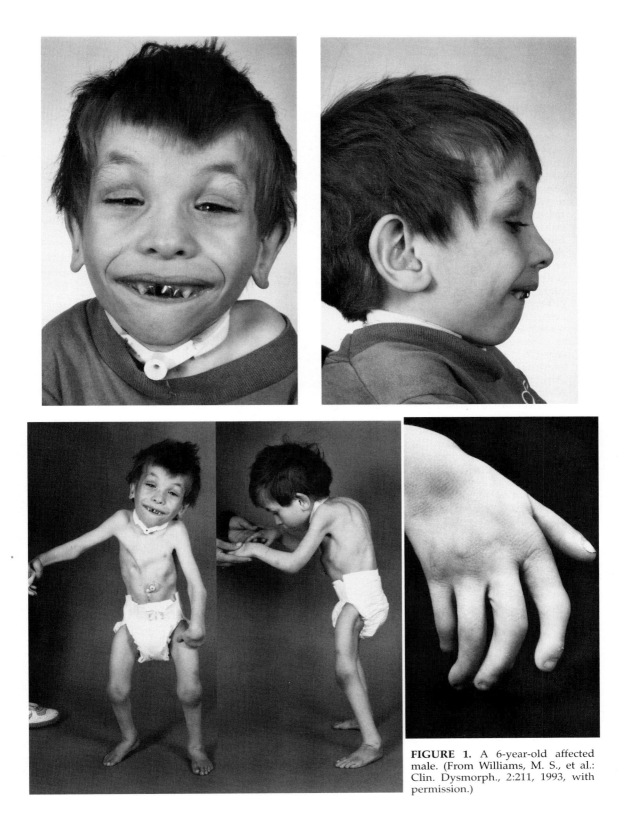

FIGURE 1. A 6-year-old affected male. (From Williams, M. S., et al.: Clin. Dysmorph., 2:211, 1993, with permission.)

SCHINZEL-GIEDION SYNDROME

A brother and sister with this disorder were described in 1978 by Schinzel and Giedion. Sixteen cases have been reported.

ABNORMALITIES

Growth. Postnatal growth deficiency.

Performance. Profound mental deficiency. Seizures, Opisthotonus. Spasticity. Hypsarrhythmia. Ventriculomegaly secondary to cerebral atrophy in four of five cases in which CT scan or MRI were performed.

Craniofacies. Coarse face. Widely patent fontanels and sutures (100 per cent) with metopic suture extending anteriorly to nasal root. High, protruding forehead (100 per cent). Short nose with low nasal bridge and anteverted nares (83 per cent). Shallow orbits with apparent proptosis (100 per cent). Ocular hypertelorism. Midface hypoplasia (100 per cent). Choanal stenosis (45 per cent). Attached helix with protruding lobules of low-set ear (91 per cent).

Limbs. Moderate shortening of forearms and legs (70 per cent). Talipes equinovarus. Hyperconvex nails (75 per cent). Hypoplastic dermal ridges (100 per cent). Simian crease (70 per cent).

Genital. Anomalies in 100 per cent including hypospadias, short penis, hypoplastic scrotum in males. Deep interlabial sulcus, hypoplasia of labia majora or minora, hymenal atresia, and a short perineum in females.

Renal. Anomalies in 92 per cent including hydronephrosis, vesicoureteric junction dysplasia, ureteric stenosis, hydroureter, and megacalyces.

Radiologic. Steep short base of skull (60 per cent), sclerotic skull base (80 per cent), wide occipital synchondrosis (60 per cent), multiple wormian bones (63 per cent), hypoplastic first ribs, broad ribs (90 per cent), long clavicles, hypoplastic/aplastic pubic bones (36 per cent), hypoplasia of distal phalanges (78 per cent), short metacarpals of thumbs (56 per cent). Broad cortex and increased density of long bones. Widening of distal femurs. Tibial bowing. Mesomelic brachymelia.

Other. Hypertrichosis (91 per cent). Short neck with redundant skin. Hypoplastic nipples.

OCCASIONAL ABNORMALITIES. Macroglossia, facial hemangiomata (27 per cent), postaxial polydactyly, cardiac defect (30 per cent), fifth toe overlapping fourth, short sternum. Bicornuate uterus. Embryonal tumors (14 per cent) including a hepatoblastoma and a malignant sacrococcygeal teratoma.

NATURAL HISTORY. Severe postnatal growth deficiency and profound mental retardation and seizures as well as visual and hearing problems have occurred in all patients who have survived. Death prior to 2 years of age in 55 per cent of cases. Although no specific cause of death has been determined, it is most likely related to the severe alteration in CNS function.

ETIOLOGY. Autosomal recessive inheritance is likely based on documentation of one instance of affected siblings born to unaffected parents.

References

Schinzel, A., and Giedion, A.: A syndrome of severe midface retraction, multiple skull anomalies, clubfeet, and cardiac and renal malformations in siblings. Am. J. Med. Genet., 1:361, 1978.

Donnai, D., and Harris, R.: A further case of a new syndrome including midface retraction, hypertrichosis and skeletal anomalies. J. Med. Genet., 16:483, 1979.

Kelley, R. I., Zackai, E. H., and Charney, E. G.: Congenital hydronephrosis, skeletal dysplasia, and severe developmental retardation: The Schinzel-Giedion syndrome. J. Pediatr., 100:943, 1982.

Al-Gazali, L. I., et al.: The Schinzel-Giedion syndrome. J. Med. Genet., 27:42, 1990.

Robin, N. H., et al.: New findings of Schinzel-Giedion syndrome. A case with a malignant sacrococcygeal teratoma. Am. J. Med. Genet., 47:852, 1993.

Labrune, P., et al.: Three new cases of Schinzel-Giedion syndrome and review of the literature. Am. J. Med. Genet., 50:90, 1994.

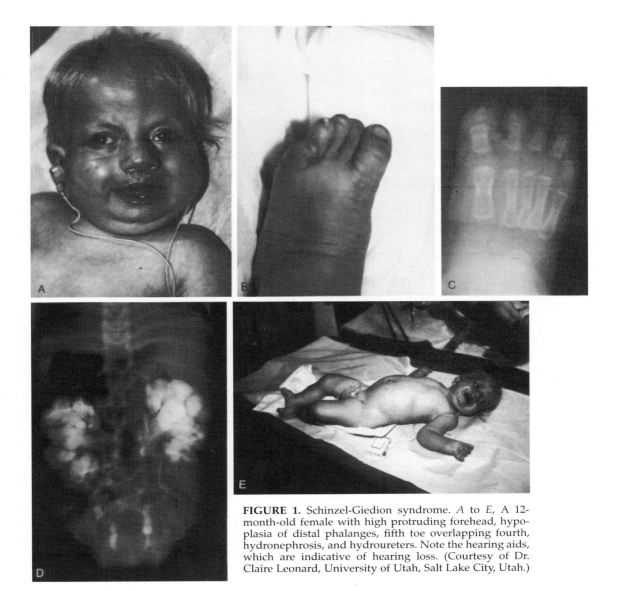

FIGURE 1. Schinzel-Giedion syndrome. *A* to *E*, A 12-month-old female with high protruding forehead, hypoplasia of distal phalanges, fifth toe overlapping fourth, hydronephrosis, and hydroureters. Note the hearing aids, which are indicative of hearing loss. (Courtesy of Dr. Claire Leonard, University of Utah, Salt Lake City, Utah.)

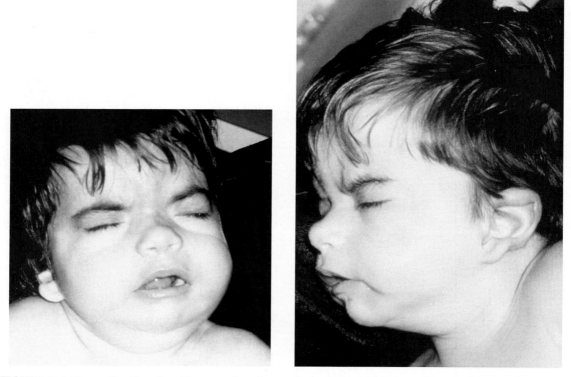

FIGURE 2. A 13-month-old male with coarse face, hypertelorism, attached helix with protruding lobule, and on the radiographs the broad ribs, long clavicles, hypoplastic distal phalanges, and short metacarpals of thumbs. (From Robin, N. H., et al.: Am. J. Med. Genet., 47:852, 1993, with permission of Wiley-Liss, a division of John Wiley & Sons.)

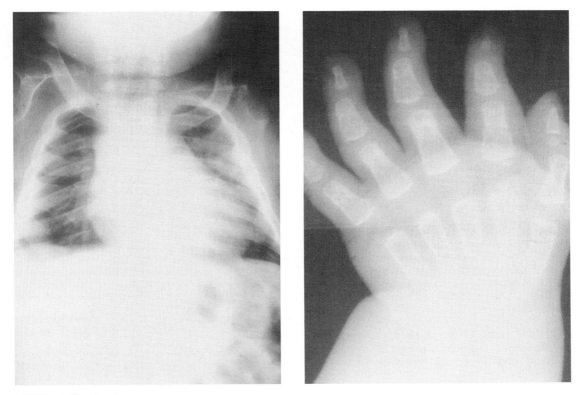

FIGURE 2. *Continued.*

ACROCALLOSAL SYNDROME

Hypoplastic or Absent Corpus Callosum,
Postaxial Polydactyly of Hands and Feet, Hallux Duplication

Since the initial description of this disorder by Schinzel in 1979, approximately 26 cases have been reported.

ABNORMALITIES

Neurologic. Hypoplastic or absent corpus callosum. Severe mental retardation. Seizures. Strabismus. Hypotonia.

Craniofacial. Macrocephaly. Prominent forehead. Large anterior fontanel. Hypertelorism. Epicanthal folds. Down-slanting palpebral fissures. Small nose with broad nasal bridge. Malformed ears. Short philtrum.

Limbs. Postaxial polydactyly of hands and feet. Preaxial polydactyly of feet. Syndactyly of toes. Tapered fingers. Fifth finger clinodactyly.

Other. Eye findings including optic atrophy, and decreased retinal pigmentation. Cardiac defects, primarily septal defects and abnormalities of the pulmonary valves. Umbilical hernia.

OCCASIONAL ABNORMALITIES.

Micropolygyria. Prominent occiput. Hyperreflexia. Nystagmus. Cleft lip. Cleft palate. Supernumerary nipples. Rib hypoplasia. Preaxial polydactyly of hands. Syndactyly of fingers. Cryptorchidism. Prenatal overgrowth. Postnatal growth deficiency.

NATURAL HISTORY.

Marked retardation in the attainment of developmental milestones. Neonatal respiratory distress and intercurrent infection leading to early death occur in approximately 15 per cent of patients. Family data documenting an increased incidence of spontaneous abortions suggests an apparent increased lethality of the gene.

ETIOLOGY.

Autosomal recessive.

COMMENT.

Three affected children have had siblings with anencephaly, two of which had polydactyly, suggesting that anencephaly may be the severe end of the spectrum of brain defects in the acrocallosol syndrome.

References

Schinzel, A.: Postaxial polydactyly, hallux duplication, absence of the corpus callosum, macrencephaly and severe mental retardation: A new syndrome? Helv. Paediatr. Acta, *34*:141, 1979.

Schinzel, A., and Schmid, W.: Hallux duplication, postaxial polydactyly, absence of the corpus callosum, severe mental retardation, and additional anomalies in two unrelated patients: A new syndrome. Am. J. Med. Genet., *6*:241, 1980.

Schinzel, A.: The acrocallosal syndrome in first cousins: Widening of the spectrum of clinical features and further support for autosomal recessive inheritance. J. Med. Genet., *25*:332, 1988.

Casamassima, A. C., et al.: Acrocallosal syndrome: Additional manifestations. Am. J. Med. Genet., *32*: 311, 1989.

Lurie, I. W., et al.: The acrocallosal syndrome: Expansion of the phenotypic spectrum. Clin. Dysmorph., *3*:31, 1994.

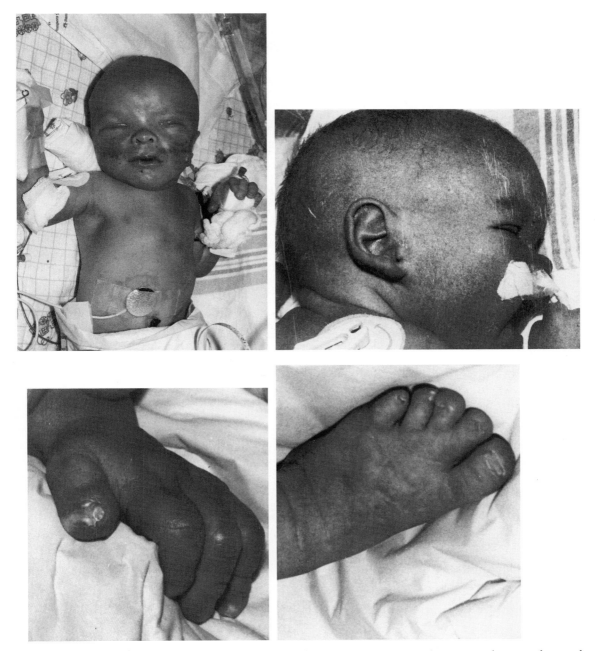

FIGURE 1. Newborn boy with broad forehead, hypertelorism, broad nose with anteverted nares, abnormal auricles, and redundant nuchal skin. In addition, note the broad thumbs and great toes with partial duplication of the thumb, nail hypoplasia, and syndactyly of the feet. (From Casamassima, A. C., et al.: Am. J. Med. Genet., *32*:11, 1989, with permission of Wiley-Liss, a division of John Wiley & Sons.)

HECHT SYNDROME

(Trismus Pseudocamptodactyly Syndrome)

This disorder of muscle development and function was first described by Hecht and Beals and by Wilson et al. in 1968. It was more recently well delineated by Mabry et al. in a huge kindred in which the initial United States case was a young Dutch girl who arrived in this country with "crooked hands and a small mouth."

ABNORMALITIES. Appear to be based on short muscles and especially tendons.

Muscles and Tendons. Limited opening of mouth, sometimes with an enlarged coronoid process. Short flexor tendons, so that when the hand is dorsiflexed, the fingers are partially flexed. Occasionally, short flexor muscles to the feet cause such problems as downturning toes, talipes equinovarus, metatarsus adductus, and short gastrocnemius.

NATURAL HISTORY. The newborn baby may have tightly fisted hands and later usually crawls on the knuckles. These patients may have feeding problems because of the small mouth, and they tend to eat slowly. Tonsillectomy and/or intubation may present serious problems. There can be occupational handicaps relative to the military service, typing, or other situations requiring high levels of hand dexterity.

ETIOLOGY. Autosomal dominant, with an unexplained 2:1 excess of affected females.

References

Hecht, F., and Beals, R. K.: Inability to open the mouth fully. *In* Bergsma, D. (ed.): Birth Defects Original Article Series, Part III, Limb Malformation, Vol. V. New York, The National Foundation March of Dimes, 1968, p. 96.

Wilson, R. V., et al.: Autosomal dominant inheritance of shortening of flexor profundus muscle tendon. *In* Bergsma, D. (ed.): Birth Defects Original Article Series, Part III, Limb Malformation, Vol. V. New York, The National Foundation March of Dimes, 1968, p. 99.

Mabry, C. C., et al.: Trismus camptomelic syndrome. J. Pediatr., *85*:503, 1974.

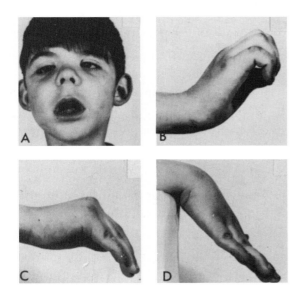

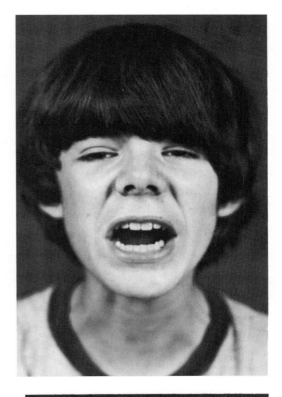

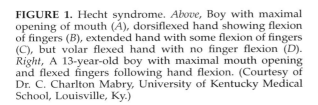

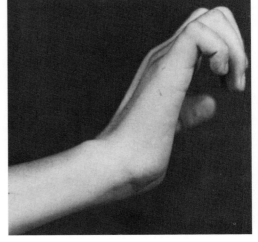

FIGURE 1. Hecht syndrome. *Above,* Boy with maximal opening of mouth (*A*), dorsiflexed hand showing flexion of fingers (*B*), extended hand with some flexion of fingers (*C*), but volar flexed hand with no finger flexion (*D*). *Right,* A 13-year-old boy with maximal mouth opening and flexed fingers following hand flexion. (Courtesy of Dr. C. Charlton Mabry, University of Kentucky Medical School, Louisville, Ky.)

G

G. FACIAL DEFECTS AS MAJOR FEATURE

MOEBIUS SEQUENCE

Sixth and Seventh Nerve Palsy

The basic features of Moebius sequence are mask-like facies with sixth and seventh nerve palsy, usually bilaterally. The necropsy cases implicate at least four modes of developmental pathology in the genesis of the problem. These are (1) hypoplasia to absence of the central brain nuclei; (2) destructive degeneration of the central brain nuclei (most common type); (3) peripheral nerve involvement; and (4) a myopathy. Thus, the Moebius sequence is but a sign and is quite nonspecific. Micrognathia, a frequent feature, may be interpreted as secondary to a neuromuscular deficit in early movement of the mandible. Some patients have more extensive cranial nerve involvement, including the third, fourth, fifth, ninth, tenth, and twelfth nerves. In the latter cases, the tongue may be limited in mobility and/or small. There may be ocular ptosis and/or a protruding auricle. About one third of the patients have talipes equinovarus, which might be the consequence of neurologic deficiency relative to early foot movement. About 15 per cent of patients have mental deficiency as a more obvious indication that in some cases the CNS defect involves more than the cranial nerve nuclei alone. Feeding difficulties and problems of aspiration often lead to failure to thrive during infancy. The expressionless facies and speech impediments create problems in acceptance and social adaptation. Associated non–CNS-related defects have included limb reduction defects, syndactyly, the Poland sequence, and occasionally the Klippel-Feil anomaly.

The Moebius sequence is most commonly a sporadic occurrence in an otherwise normal family. In the majority of those cases, insufficient blood supply to structures supplied by the developing primitive subclavian artery lead to the variable features seen in this disorder. Evidence that a number of affected individuals have been born to women who experienced events during pregnancy that could cause transient ischemic/hypoxic insults to the fetus suggests that this disorder may be due to any event that interferes with the uterine/fetal circulation.

The association of seventh nerve palsy with or without sixth nerve palsy but without limb reduction defects may be familial with an autosomal dominant mode of inheritance in some cases.

References

Moebius, P. J.: Ueber engeborene doppelseitige Abducens-Facialis-Laehmung. Munch. Med. Wochenschr., 35:91, 1888.

Henderson, J. L.: The congenital facial diplegia syndrome. Clinical features, pathology, and aetiology. A review of sixty-one cases. Brain, 62:381, 1939.

Sugarman, G. I., and Stark, H. H.: Möbius anomaly with Poland's anomaly. J. Med. Genet., 10:192, 1973.

Baraitser, M.: Genetics of Möbius syndrome. J. Med. Genet., 14:415, 1977.

Meyerson, M. D., and Foushee, D. R.: Speech, language and hearing in Moebius syndrome. Dev. Med. Child. Neurol., 20:357, 1978.

Bouwes-Bavinck, J. N., and Weaver, D. D.: Subclavian artery supply disruption sequence: Hypothesis of a vascular etiology for Poland, Klippel-Feil, and Mobius anomalies. Am. J. Med. Genet., 23:903, 1986.

Lipson, A. H., et al.: Moebius syndrome: Animal model–human correlations and evidence for a brainstem vascular etiology. Teratology, 40:339, 1989.

Kumar, D.: Moebius syndrome. J. Med. Genet., 27:122, 1990.

St. Charles, S., et al.: Mobius sequence: Further in vivo support for the subclavian artery supply disruption sequence. Am. J. Med. Genet., 47:289, 1993.

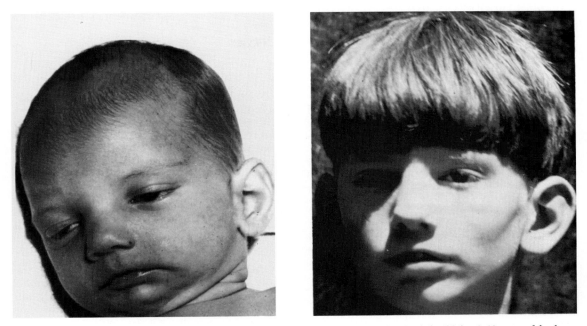

FIGURE 1. *Left,* A 5-week-old with Moebius sequence, including ptosis of the eyelids. *Right,* A 12-year-old whose facial appearance had improved since early childhood. Note the protruding auricle.

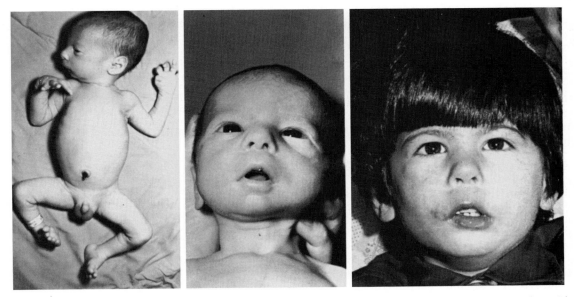

FIGURE 2. *Left* and *Middle,* A newborn with Moebius sequence, showing high nasal bridge, micrognathia with limited mandibular movement, small mouth with downturned corners, expressionless facies with deficit of lateral gaze, mild ptosis, mild talipes, and mild alteration in finger positioning. These clinical findings were interpreted as being the secondary neurologic consequence of a single primary defect in CNS development, especially of the nuclei of the sixth and seventh nerves. *Right,* Same patient at 3 years of age. He had achieved limited ability to open his mouth, was responding well to speech training, and was interpreted as having normal intelligence.

BLEPHAROPHIMOSIS SYNDROME

(Familial Blepharophimosis Syndrome)

Inner Canthal Fold, Lateral
Displacement of Inner Canthi, Ptosis

This entity, predominantly a dysplasia of the eyelids, was described by Vignes in 1889, and more than 150 families have been reported. The existence of two types has recently been suggested: type I, associated with infertility in affected females and complete penetrance of the altered gene, and type II, transmitted by both males and females and associated with incomplete penetrance.

ABNORMALITIES

Eyes. Inverted inner canthal fold between upper and lower lid, short palpebral fissures with lateral displacement of inner canthi, low nasal bridge and ptosis of eyelids, and hypoplasia, and fibrosis of the levator palpebrae muscle. Strabismus. Amblyopia. The eyebrows are increased in their vertical height and are arched.

Ears. Incomplete development, cupping.

Genitalia. Menstrual irregularity and infertility in females with type I. Primary hypogonadism has been documented occasionally in females with type I; in most cases the cause is unknown.

Other. Variable hypotonia in early life.

OCCASIONAL ABNORMALITIES. Mental deficiency. Cardiac defect. Ocular abnormalities including microphthalmia, microcornea, hypermetropia, trichiasis, colobomas of the optic disk, trabecular dysgenesis, congenital optic nerve hypoplasia, nystagmus.

NATURAL HISTORY. Plastic surgery is indicated both for cosmetic reasons and for improvement of ocular function. Amblyopia, which occurs in greater than one half of patients, is most frequently associated with asymmetrical ptosis, although it also occurs when the ptosis is bilateral.

ETIOLOGY. Autosomal dominant for both type I and type II. A similar interstitial deletion in the long arm of chromosome 3 has been documented in a number of affected individuals, suggesting that the gene for this disorder is located at 3q22.3-q23. The importance of distinguishing between the types relates to reproductive capabilities and menstrual irregularities, including amenorrhea in females with type I. With the exception of infertility in females, the two types are indistinguishable clinically. Therefore, separating the two types can be accomplished only through a careful family history. If the affected individual, either male or female, is a member of a family in which the disorder has been transmitted only through males, it is most likely type I, whereas if transmission has occurred through both males and females, it is type II.

COMMENT. The facial appearance may initially suggest a condition with associated mental retardation; however, the affected individuals are not generally mentally deficient. Sacrez et al. reported I.Q.s from 75 to 100, with a mean value of 86.

References

Vignes: Epicanthus héréditaire. Rev. Gen. Ophthalmol. (Paris), 8:438, 1889.

Sacrez, R., et al.: Le blépharophimosis compliqué familial. Étude des membres de la famille Blé. Ann. Pediatr. (Paris), 10:493, 1963.

Kohn, R., and Romano, P. E.: Blepharoptosis, blepharophimosis, epicanthus inversus, and telecanthus— a syndrome with no name. Am. J. Ophthalmol. 72: 625, 1972.

Zlotogora, J., Sagi, M., and Cohen, T.: The blepharophimosis, ptosis and epicanthus inversus syndrome: Delineation of two types. Am. J. Hum. Genet., 35:1020, 1983.

Jones, C. A., and Collin, J. R. D.: Blepharophimosis and its association with female infertility. Br. J. Ophthalmol., 68:533, 1984.

Oley, C., and Baraister, M.: Blepharophimosis, ptosis, epicanthus inversus syndrome (BPES syndrome). J. Med. Genet., 25:47, 1988.

Beaconsfield, M., et al.: Visual development in the blepharophimosis syndrome. Br. J. Ophthalmol., 75: 746, 1991.

Jewett, T., et al.: Blepharophimosis, ptosis and epicanthus inversus syndrome (BPES) associated with interstitial deletion of band 3q22: Review and gene assignment to the interface of band 3q22.3 and 3q23. Am. J. Med. Genet., 47:1147, 1993.

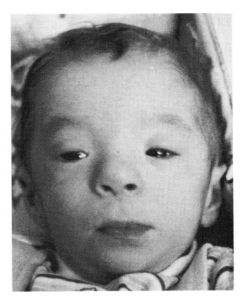

FIGURE 1. Infant with blepharophimosis syndrome.

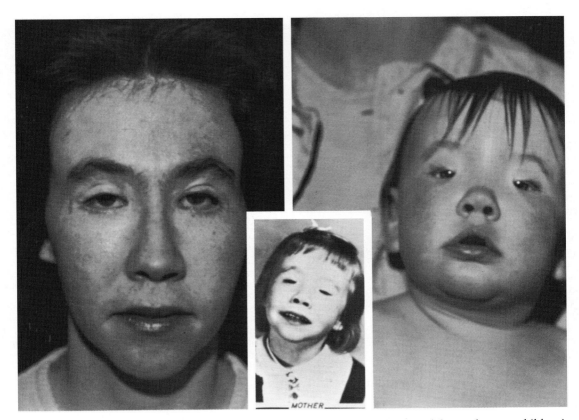

MOTHER

FIGURE 2. Blepharophimosis syndrome. Mother and infant daughter, with inset of the mother as a child, prior to surgical repair.

ROBIN SEQUENCE

(Pierre Robin Syndrome)

Micrognathia, Glossoptosis, Cleft Soft
Palate; Primary Defect—Early Mandibular Hypoplasia

The single initiating defect of this disorder may be hypoplasia of the mandibular area prior to 9 weeks in utero, allowing the tongue to be posteriorly located and thereby impairing the closure of the posterior palatal shelves that must "grow over" the tongue to meet the midline. The mode of pathogenesis is depicted to the right. The rounded contour of the "cleft" palate in some of these patients (see illustration) is compatible with this mode of developmental pathology and differs from the usual inverted V shape of most palatal clefts. Latham's study of

a 17-week-old fetus with the Robin sequence led him to the same conclusion: that early mandibular retrognathia is the primary anomaly. The posterior airway obstruction may require in order of increasing invasiveness prone positioning, nasal pharyngeal airway, nasal esophageal intubation, lip-tongue adhesion, and tracheostomy. Airway obstruction can lead to hypoxia, cor pulmonale, failure to thrive, and cerebral impairment. Mortality rates as high as 30 per cent have been reported. Significant airway obstruction may develop over the first 1 to 4 weeks of life. Therefore, affected children should be monitored carefully during that period, focusing on the obstruction pathogenesis of the apnea and airway concerns in the condition. In that significant hypoxia may occur without obvious clinical signs of obstruction, serial polysomnographic studies may be helpful over the first month in order to identify infants at significant risk. Although the Robin sequence often occurs in otherwise normal individuals, in whom the prognosis is very good if they survive the early period of respiratory obstruction, this disorder commonly occurs as one feature in a multiple malformation syndrome, such as the trisomy 18 syndrome, the Stickler syndrome, or a number of other disorders. It may also be a result of early in utero mechanical constraint, with the chin compressed in such a manner as to limit its growth prior to palatine closure.

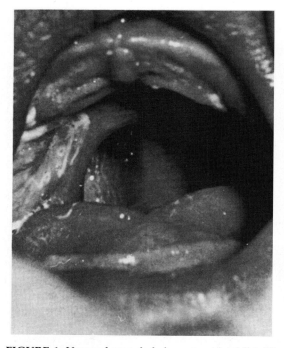

FIGURE 1. Unusual rounded shape to palatal "cleft" in a patient with the Robin sequence compatible with the incomplete closure of the palate having been secondary to the posterior displacement of the tongue.

References

Dennison, W. M.: The Pierre Robin syndrome. Pediatrics, *36*:336, 1965.

Latham, R. A.: The pathogenesis of cleft palate associated with the Pierre Robin syndrome. Br. J. Plast. Surg., *19*:205, 1966.

Hanson, J. W., and Smith, D. W.: U-shaped palatal defect in the Robin anomalad: Developmental and clinical relevance. J. Pediatr., *87*:30, 1975.

Bull, M. J., et al.: Improved outcome in Pierre Robin sequence: Effect of multidisciplinary evaluation and management. Pediatrics, *86*:294, 1990.

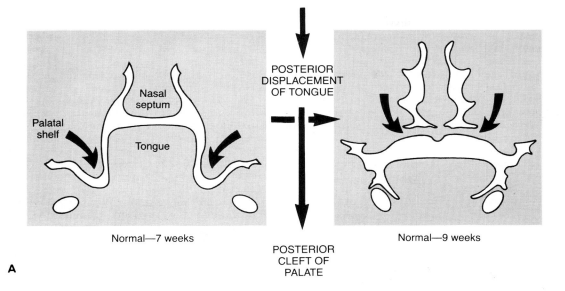

A PRIMARY ANOMALY IN MANDIBULAR DEVELOPMENT HYPOPLASIA
OF MANDIBLE PRIOR TO 9 WEEKS

POSTERIOR
DISPLACEMENT
OF TONGUE

POSTERIOR
CLEFT OF
PALATE

Normal—7 weeks

Normal—9 weeks

A

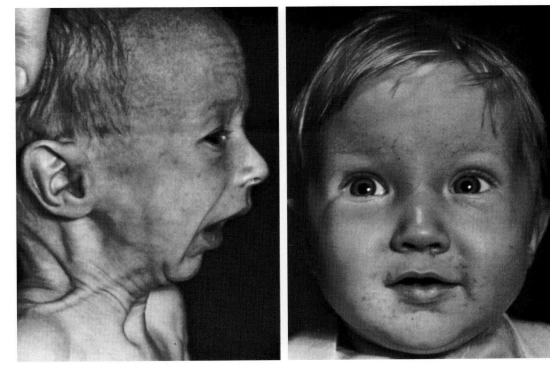

B

C

FIGURE 2. *A*, Mode of pathogenesis of the Robin sequence. *B*, Robin sequence with upper respiratory obstruction and failure to thrive in a 3-week-old (weight, 4.9 pounds [2.2 kg]). *C*, Same patient at 13 months, showing catch-up in mandibular growth. Patient thriving with normal growth (weight, 14.8 pounds [6.6 kg]).

CLEFT LIP SEQUENCE

Primary Defect—Closure of Lip

By 35 days of uterine age, the lip is normally fused, as illustrated in the figure. A failure of lip fusion, as shown, may impair the subsequent closure of the palatal shelves, which do not completely fuse until the eighth to ninth week. Thus, cleft palate is a frequent association with cleft lip. Other secondary anomalies include defects of tooth development in the area of the cleft lip and incomplete growth of the ala nasi on the side of the cleft. There may be mild ocular hypertelorism, the precise reason for which is undetermined. Tertiary abnormalities can include poor speech and repeated otitis media as a consequence of palatal incompetence and conductive hearing loss.

ETIOLOGY AND RECURRENCE RISK COUNSELING. Usually unknown. It is more likely to occur in the male. The more severe the defect, the higher the recurrence risk for future siblings. For a unilateral defect, the recurrence risk is 2.7 per cent; for bilateral, it is 5.4 per cent. The following are the general risk figures: unaffected parents with one affected child, 4 per cent for future siblings; unaffected parents with two affected children, 10 per cent for future siblings. If either the mother or father is affected, the risk for offspring is 4 per cent. An affected parent with one affected child has a 14 per cent risk for future offspring.

COMMENT. Recent reports have documented that as many as 35 per cent of newborns with cleft lip, with or without cleft palate, have the defect as part of a broader pattern of altered morphogenesis. One should identify such individuals prior to using the above figures for recurrence risk counseling. In addition, the underlying diagnosis may well have an impact on prognosis.

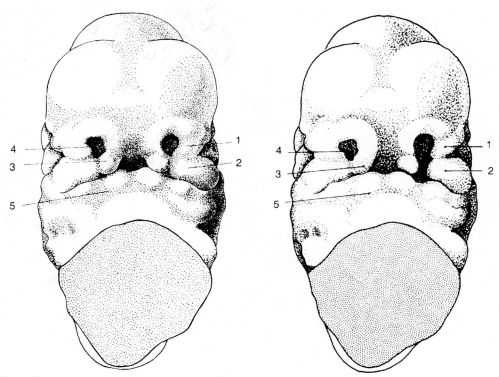

FIGURE 1. Cleft lip sequence. *Left,* Normal embryo of 35 days. *Right,* Spontaneously aborted 35-day embryo with hypoplasia of the left lateral nasal swelling and, therefore, a cleft lip. *1,* Lateral nasal swelling; *2,* maxillary swelling; *3,* medial nasal swelling; *4,* nares; *5,* mandibular swelling. (Courtesy of Prof. G. Töndury, University of Zurich, Zurich.)

References

Bixler, D.: Heritability of clefts of the lip and palate. J. Prosthet. Dent., *33*:100, 1975.

Carter, C. O., et al.: A three generations family study of cleft lip with or without cleft palate. J. Med. Genet., *19*:246, 1982.

Shprintzen, R. J., et al.: Anomalies associated with cleft lip, cleft palate, or both. Am. J. Med. Genet., *20*:585, 1985.

Jones, M. C.: Facial clefting: Etiology and developmental pathogenesis. Clin. Plast. Surg., *20*:599, 1993.

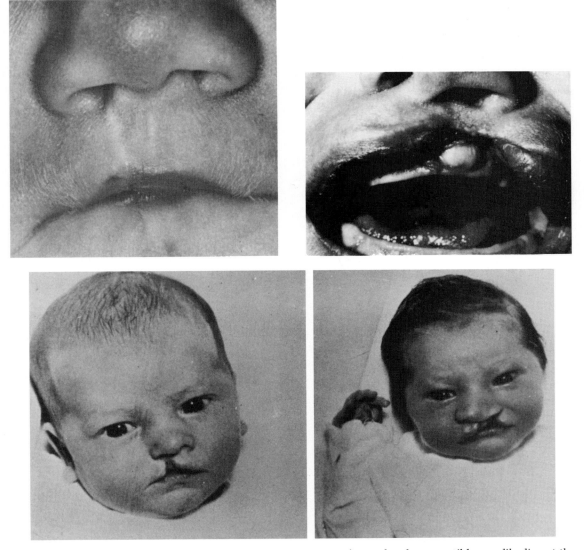

FIGURE 2. All gradations of cleft lip and its consequences occur, from a barely perceptible scar-like line at the site of closure on the right side (*above left*) to a widely open cleft with secondary consequences of cleft palate, flared ala nasi, and mild ocular hypertelorism (*lower right*). (Upper left photo courtesy of University of Arizona Medical School, Tucson, Ariz.)

VAN DER WOUDE SYNDROME

(Lip Pit–Cleft Lip Syndrome)

Lower Lip Pit(s), With or Without Cleft Lip, With or Without Missing Second Premolars

Originally reported by Van der Woude in 1954.

ABNORMALITIES

Oral. Lower lip pits (80 per cent). Hypodontia, missing central and lateral incisors, canines, and/or bicuspids. Cleft lip with or without cleft palate, cleft palate, cleft uvula.

NATURAL HISTORY. Surgical removal of the fistulas, which represent small accessory salivary glands, is recommended because they may produce a watery mucoid discharge that can be embarrassing for the individual.

ETIOLOGY. Autosomal dominant. The gene responsible for this disorder has been mapped to the long arm of chromosome 1 at q32-41.

References

Van der Woude, A.: Fistula labii inferioris congenita and its association with cleft lip and palate. Am. J. Hum. Genet., 6:244, 1954.

Cervenka, J., Gorlin, R. J., and Anderson, V. E.: The syndrome of pits of the lower lip and cleft lip or cleft palate. Genetic considerations. Am. J. Hum. Genet., 19:416, 1967.

Janku, P., et al.: The van der Woude syndrome in a large kindred: variability, penetrance, genetic risks. Am. J. Med. Genet., 5:117, 1980.

Sander, A., et al.: Evidence for a microdeletion in 1q32-41 involving the gene responsible for Van der Woude syndrome. Hum. Mol. Genet., 3:575, 1994.

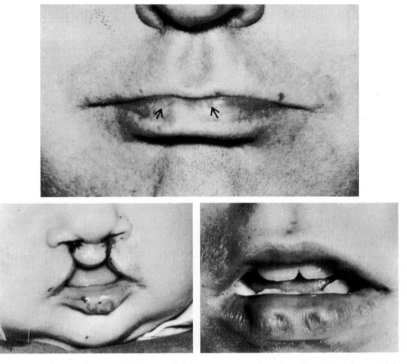

FIGURE 1. Van der Woude syndrome. Father and his two sons showing lip pits (denoted by *arrows* for the father), with cleft lip expression in the infant son.

FRONTONASAL DYSPLASIA SEQUENCE

(Median Cleft Face Syndrome)

*Unknown Primary Defect in Midfacial Development
With Incomplete Anterior Appositional Alignment of Eyes*

DeMyer recognized the transitional gradations in severity of this presumed single primary localized defect in 33 cases and termed the pattern of anomaly the median facial cleft syndrome. Sedano et al. subsequently extended these observations and recommended frontonasal dysplasia as a more appropriate designation for this defect. The accompanying figure sets forth a crude interpretation of the developmental pathogenesis and gradations of the sequence.

ABNORMALITIES Defects that may occur in the more severe cases; the milder cases may have only a few of the defects.
Eyes. Ocular hypertelorism. Lateral displacement of inner canthi.
Forehead. Widow's peak. Deficit in midline frontal bone (cranium bifidum occultum).
Nose. Variability from notched broad nasal tip to completely divided nostrils with hypoplasia to absence of the prolabium and premaxilla with a median cleft lip. Variable notching of alae nasi. Broad nasal root. Lack of formation of nasal tip.

OCCASIONAL ABNORMALITIES. Accessory nasal tags. Microphthalmia. Anomalies of optic disk, optic nerve, retina, or iris. Preauricular tags, low-set ears, conductive deafness. Mental deficiency. Frontal cutaneous lipoma or lipoma of corpus callosum. Agenesis of the corpus callosum. Anterior basal encephalocele. Tetralogy of Fallot

NATURAL HISTORY. Depending on the severity of the defect, radical cosmetic surgery is usually merited. The majority of affected individuals are of normal intelligence. DeMyer noted 8 per cent severe mental deficiency and 12 per cent mild impairment of intelligence.

ETIOLOGY. Unknown. Generally a sporadic occurrence; it may occasionally be familial. Frontonasal dysplasia can occur as one feature of a multiple malformation syndrome, in which case recurrence risk is for the overall pattern of malformation.

References

DeMyer, W.: The median cleft face syndrome. Differential diagnosis of cranium bifidum occultum, hypertelorism, and median cleft nose, lip, and palate. Neurology [Minneap.], *17*:961, 1967.

Sedano, H. O., et al.: Frontonasal dysplasia. J. Pediatr., *76*:906, 1970.

Pascual-Castroviejo, I., Pascual-Pascual, S. I., and Perez-Hiqueras, A.: Fronto-nasal dysplasia and lipoma of the corpus callosum. Eur. J. Pediatr., *144*: 66, 1985.

Sedano, H. O., and Gorlin, R. J.: Frontonasal malformation as a field defect and in syndromic associations. Oral Surg. Oral Med. Oral Pathol., *65*:704, 1988.

Grubben, C., et al.: Anterior basal encephalocele in the median cleft face syndrome. Comments on nosology and treatment. Genet. Couns., *38*:103, 1990.

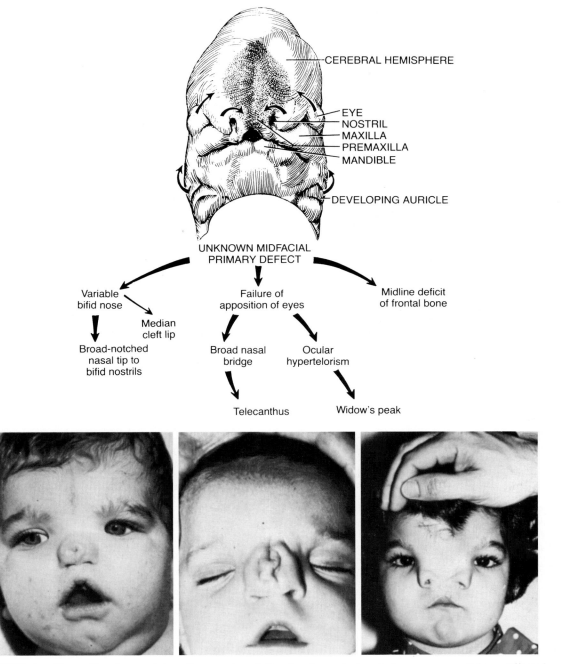

FIGURE 1. *Above*, Developmental pathogenesis of the frontonasal dysplasia sequence. *Below*, Affected individuals.

FRASER SYNDROME
(Cryptophthalmos Syndrome)

Cryptophthalmos,* Defect of Auricle, Genital Anomaly

The association of other multiple malformations in patients with the rare anomaly of cryptophthalmos had been appreciated prior to 1962, when a rather distinctive syndrome found in two sets of siblings was set forth by Fraser. Over 100 patients have been reported. Since cryptophthalmos is not an obligate feature of this disorder, it is more appropriately termed Fraser syndrome.

ABNORMALITIES
Facial. Cryptophthalmos (93 per cent), usually bilateral and frequently with defect of eye. Hair growth on lateral forehead extending to lateral eyebrow (34 per cent), often associated with a depression of underlying frontal bone. Hypoplastic notched nares. Broad nose with depressed bridge. Ear anomalies (44 per cent), most commonly atresia of external auditory canal and cupped ears.
Performance. Mental deficiency in approximately 50 per cent of survivors.
Limbs. Partial cutaneous syndactyly (57 per cent).
Genitalia. Incomplete development (49 per cent). Male: hypospadias, cryptorchidism. Female: bicornuate uterus, vaginal atresia, clitoromegaly.
Other. Laryngeal stenosis or atresia (21 per cent). Renal hypoplasia or agenesis (37 per cent).

OCCASIONAL ABNORMALITIES.
Microcephaly, abnormal gyral pattern, meningomyelocele, midline groove toward nasal tip. Unilateral absence of a nostril. Cleft lip, with or without cleft palate (4 per cent), and cleft palate (3 per cent). Tongue tie (6 per cent). Dental malocclusion and crowding. Bony skull defects. Hypertelorism, lacrimal duct defect (9 per cent), coloboma of upper lid (6 per cent), partial midfacial cleft, defect of middle ear, fusion of superior helix to scalp, microtia, low-set ears, widely spaced nipples, abnormalities of ureters or bladder, umbilical anomaly, anal atresia, malformation of small bowel, cardiac defects, thymic aplasia/hypoplasia, diastasis of symphysis pubis, partial absence of sternum, absent phalanges, hypoplastic or absent thumb.

NATURAL HISTORY. This disorder should be considered in stillborn babies with renal agenesis. Because the defect of eyelid development is frequently accompanied by ocular anomaly, the likelihood of achieving adequate visual perception is small, although early surgical intervention was of value in one case. Hearing is usually normal. Twenty-five per cent of affected individuals are stillborn and an additional 20 per cent die before 1 year of age. Death is related primarily to the renal or laryngeal defects. No affected individual has been reported to have reproduced.

ETIOLOGY. Autosomal recessive. There is etiologic heterogeneity for the cryptophthalmos anomaly. A number of individuals with isolated cryptophthalmos who do not have the Fraser syndrome have been reported.

---

*Cryptophthalmos (hidden eye) fundamentally means absence of the palpebral fissure but usually includes varying absence of eyelashes and eyebrows and defects of the eye, especially the anterior part.

References

Fraser, C. R.: Our genetical "load." A review of some aspects of genetical variation. Ann. Hum. Genet., 25:387, 1962.

Gupta, S. P., and Saxena, R. C.: Cryptophthalmos. Br. J. Ophthalmol., 46:629, 1962.

Azvedo, E. S., Biondi, J., and Ramaldo, L. M.: Cryptophthalmos in two families. J. Med. Genet., 10:389, 1973.

Mortimer, G., McEwen, H. P., and Yates, J. R. W.: Fraser syndrome presenting as monozygous twins with bilateral renal agenesis. J. Med. Genet., 22:76, 1985.

Thomas, I. T., et al.: Isolated and syndromic cryptophthalmos. Am. J. Med. Genet., 25:85, 1986.

Gattuso, J., et al.: The clinical spectrum of the Fraser syndrome: Report of three new cases and review. J. Med. Genet., 24:549, 1987.

Ford, G. R., et al.: ENT manifestations of Fraser syndrome. J. Laryngol. Otol., 106:1, 1992.

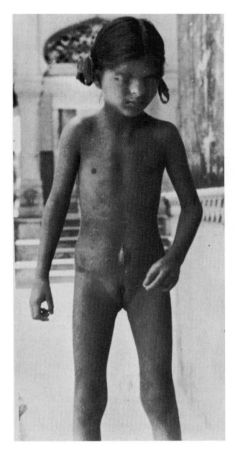

FIGURE 1. Fraser syndrome. A genetic male with cryptophthalmos, malformed ears with atresia of external auditory canals,
aberrant umbilicus, and incomplete development of external
genitalia. (Courtesy of S. P. Gupta, University of Lucknow,
India.)

MELNICK-FRASER SYNDROME

(Branchio-Oto-Renal (BOR) Syndrome)

The association of branchial arch anomalies (preauricular pits, branchial fistulas), hearing loss, and renal hypoplasia constitutes the branchio-oto-renal syndrome first described by Melnick et al. in 1975 and further delineated by Fraser et al. The prevalence is roughly 1 in 40,000. The syndrome occurs in about 2 per cent of profoundly deaf children.

ABNORMALITIES

Hearing loss	89%
Preauricular pits	77%
Branchial fistulas or cysts	63%
Anomalous pinna	41%
Malformed middle and/or inner ear	—
Lacrimal duct stenosis/aplasia	—
Renal dysplasia	66%

OCCASIONAL ABNORMALITIES. Long, narrow face, "constricted palate," deep overbite, cleft palate, bifid uvula, facial paralysis, gustatory lacrimation (the shedding of tears during eating due to misdirected growth of seventh cranial nerve fibers).

NATURAL HISTORY. The ear pits or branchial clefts may go unnoticed until the hearing loss appears, or they may become infected and require surgery. The hearing loss may be sensorineural (25 per cent), conductive (25 per cent), or mixed (50 per cent) and ranges from mild to severe. Age of onset can be from early childhood to young adulthood, and hearing loss is occasionally precipitous. There may be malformations of the middle ear, vestibular system, and cochlea, including displaced, malformed, or fused ossicles and the Mondini malformation of the cochlea. Defects of the external ear range from severe microtia to minor anomalies of the pinna, which is variously described as cup- or loop-shaped, flattened, or hypoplastic. The external canal can be narrow, slanted upward, or malformed, making otoscopic examination difficult.

The renal anomalies range from minor dysplasia (sharply tapered superior poles, blunting of calyces, duplication of the collecting system) to bilateral renal agenesis with renal failure in about 6 per cent of patients.

ETIOLOGY. An autosomal dominant gene with high penetrance and variable expression. The gene has been localized to a rather small region on the long arm of chromosome 8.

COMMENTS. The probability that a newborn child with a preauricular pit will have profound hearing loss is about 1 in 200. A preauricular pit or branchial cleft in a deaf child is a strong indication for renal investigation, and since renal dysplasia can be detected prenatally, carriers, of the BOR gene are candidates for prenatal diagnosis.

References

Melnick, M., et al.: Autosomal dominant branchio-oto-renal dysplasia. Birth Defects, *XI*(5):121, 1975.

Fraser, F. C., et al.: Genetic aspects of the BOR syndrome—branchial fistulas, ear pits, hearing loss, and renal anomalies. Am. J. Med. Genet., 2:241, 1978.

Fraser, F. C., Sproule, J. R., and Halal, F.: Frequency of the branchio-oto-renal (BOR) syndrome in children with profound hearing loss. Am. J. Med. Genet., 7: 341, 1980.

Heimler, A., and Lieber, E.: Branchio-oto-renal syndrome: Reduced penetrance and variable expressivity in four generations of a large kindred. Am. J. Med. Genet., 25:15, 1986.

Wang, Y., et al.: Localization of branchio-oto-renal (BOR) syndrome to a 3 Mb region of chromosome 8q. Am. J. Med. Genet., *51*:169, 1994.

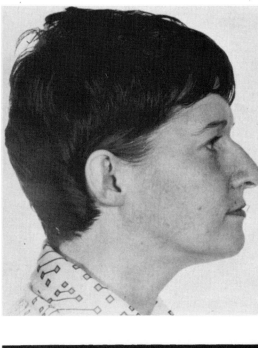

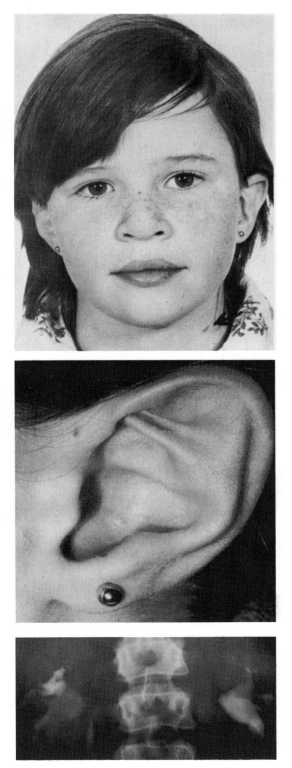

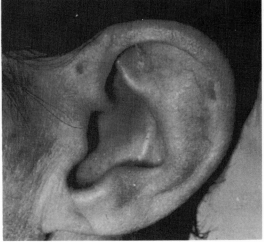

FIGURE 1. Melnick-Fraser syndrome. *Upper left*, Note mildly altered auricle. *Upper right*, Note small branchial fistula (*arrow*). *Middle*, Preauricular pits and mildly altered ear form. *Lower right*, Roentgenographic evidence of renal dysplasia. (Courtesy of Dr. F. Clarke Fraser, McGill Center for Human Genetics, Montreal, Quebec.)

BRANCHIO-OCULO-FACIAL SYNDROME

Branchial Defects, Lacrimal Duct
Obstruction, Pseudocleft of Upper Lip

Individuals with this disorder were initially described in 1982 by Lee et al. and in 1983 by Hall et al. The designation branchio-oculo-facial syndrome was introduced by Fujimoto et al. Over 30 cases have been described.

ABNORMALITIES

Performance. Mental retardation (25 per cent) in most cases mild.

Growth. Prenatal growth deficiency (27 per cent). Postnatal growth deficiency (50 per cent).

Branchial. Sinus/fistulous tract (45 per cent). Atrophic skin lesion/aplasia cutis congenita/scarring (57 per cent). Hemangiomatous lesion (36 per cent).

Ocular. Lacrimal duct obstruction (78 per cent). Colobomata (47 per cent). Microphthalmia/anophthalmia (44 per cent). Up-slanting palpebral fissures (48 per cent). Telecanthus (58 per cent). Myopia (46 per cent).

Auricular. Low-set, posteriorly rotated, over-folded and/or malformed ears (85 per cent). Hypoplastic superior helix (43 per cent). Conductive hearing loss (71 per cent). Supra-auricular sinuses (15 per cent).

Oral. Abnormal upper lip (90 per cent), which includes pseudocleft (appearance of repaired cleft lip), incomplete and/or complete cleft lip. Dental abnormalities (56 per cent). Micrognathia (50 per cent).

Other. Premature graying of hair (67 per cent).

OCCASIONAL ABNORMALITIES. Microcephaly. Ptosis. Orbital cyst. Cataract. Strabismus. Preauricular pit. Posterior auricular pit. Microtia. Cleft palate. Lip pits. Broad or divided nasal tip. Subcutaneous cysts of the scalp. Renal agenesis. Hand anomalies including polydactyly, clinodactyly and a single transverse palmar crease. Agenesis of cerebellar vermis.

NATURAL HISTORY. Hypernasal speech with conductive hearing loss is common. Premature graying of scalp hair normally begins around 18 years but has been seen as early as 10 years. Intelligence is usually normal. Reduced reproductive fitness in both males and females has been suggested.

ETIOLOGY. Autosomal dominant.

References

Lee, W. K., et al.: Bilateral branchial cleft sinuses associated with intrauterine and postnatal growth retardation, premature aging, and unusual facial appearance: A new syndrome with dominant transmission. Am. J. Med. Genet., 11:345, 1982.

Hall, B. D., et al.: A new syndrome of hemangiomatous branchial clefts, lip pseudoclefts, and unusual facial appearance. Am. J. Med. Genet., 14:135, 1983.

Fujimoto, A., et al.: New autosomal dominant branchio-oculo-facial syndrome. Am. J. Med. Genet., 27:943, 1987.

McCool, M., and Weaver, D.: Branchio-oculo-facial syndrome: Broadening the spectrum. Am. J. Med. Genet., 49:414, 1994.

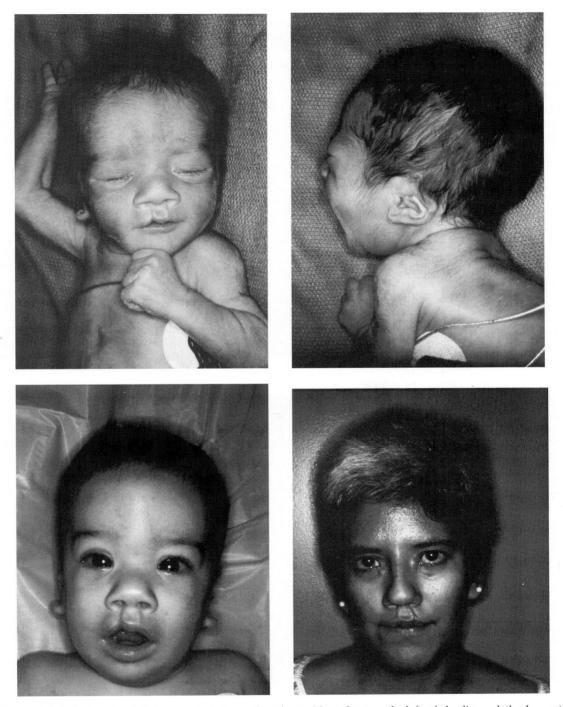

FIGURE 1. Infant male at 3 days and at 8 months of age. Note the pseudocleft of the lip and the low-set, posteriorly rotated ears with hypoplastic superior helix. Note the pseudocleft lip and premature graying of scalp hair in his 24-year-old mother. (From Fujimoto, A., et al.: Am. J. Med. Genet., 27:943, 1987, with permission.)

WAARDENBURG SYNDROME, TYPES I AND II

Lateral Displacement of Medial Canthi, Partial Albinism; Deafness

Waardenburg set forth this pattern of malformation in 1951. He found this syndrome in 1.4 per cent of congenitally deaf children and from these data estimated the incidence to be about 1 in 42,000 in Holland. Among the more than 1000 cases that have been reported, Hageman and Delleman have distinguished two different disorders; in type I, there is lateral displacement of the inner canthi, whereas in type II, there is not.

ABNORMALITIES. Lateral displacement of inner canthi with short palpebral fissures. Broad and high nasal bridge with hypoplastic alae nasi. Medial flare of bushy eyebrows, which may meet in midline. Partial albinism manifest by hypopigmented ocular fundus, white forelock, premature graying, hypopigmented skin lesions, hypochromic iridis. Deafness. Aplasia of the posterior semicircular canal is commonly noted on tomography or CT scan. Broad mandible.

OCCASIONAL ABNORMALITIES. Rounded tip of nose, full lips with accentuated "Cupid's bow" to upper lip, smooth philtrum, cleft lip and palate, cardiac anomaly (ventricular septal defect), upper limb defect. Hirschsprung aganglionosis, esophageal atresia, and anal atresia. Sprengel anomaly, supernumerary vertebrae and ribs, neural tube closure defects, scoliosis. Absence of vagina and adnexa uteri.

NATURAL HISTORY. The partial albinism is most commonly expressed as a white forelock and/or isochromic beautiful pale blue eyes with hypoplastic iridic stroma; however, it may be present as heterochromia of the iris, areas of vitiligo on the skin, patches of white hair other than the forelock, and/or mottled peripheral pigmentation of the retina. The white forelock may be present at birth only to become pigmented early in life; the hair may become prematurely gray or white.

Deafness is the most serious feature, and if present, is usually bilateral and severe. The defect appears to be in the organ of Corti, with atrophic changes in the spiral ganglion and nerve. Deafness is a feature in 25 per cent of type I cases (with lateral displacement of inner canthi) and in about 50 per cent of type II cases.

ETIOLOGY. Autosomal dominant for both type I and type II. Type I is caused by loss of function mutations in the PAX3 gene at chromosomal location 2q35. Type II is caused by mutations in the human microphthalmia gene at chromosome 3p12.3-p14.1. Older paternal age has been a factor in the fresh mutation cases.

COMMENTS. It has previously been suggested that Waardenburg syndrome type III (Klein-Waardenburg) is a genetically distinct disorder, the principal features of which include upper limb defects including hypoplasia of muscles and bones, flexion contractures and syndactyly, in addition to the oculoauditory and pigmentary abnormalities characteristic of type I. Evidence that mutations in the PAX3 gene also cause type III indicates that type I and type III have a common molecular basis.

References

Waardenburg, P. J.: A new syndrome combining developmental anomalies of the eyelids, eyebrows and nose root with pigmentary defects of the iris and head hair and with congenital deafness. Am. J. Hum. Genet., 3:195, 1951.

DiGeorge, A. M., Olmsted, R. W., and Harley, R. D.: Waardenburg's syndrome. J. Pediatr., 57:649, 1960.

Hageman, M. J., and Delleman, J. W.: Heterogeneity in Waardenburg syndrome. Am. J. Hum. Genet., 29: 468, 1977.

Klein, D.: Historical background and evidence for dominant inheritance of the Klein-Waardenburg syndrome (type III). Am. J. Med. Genet., 14:231, 1983.

Tassabehji, M., et al., Waardenburg's syndrome patients have mutations in the human homologue of the PAX-3 paired box gene. Nature, 355:635, 1992.

Hoth, C. F., et al.: Mutations in the paired domain of the human PAX3 gene cause Klein-Waardenburg syndrome (WS-III) as well as Waardenburg syndrome type I (WS-I). Am. J. Hum. Genet., 52:455, 1993.

Tassabehji, M., et al.: Waardenburg syndrome type II caused by mutations in the human microphthalmia (MITF) gene. Nat. Genet., 8:251, 1994.

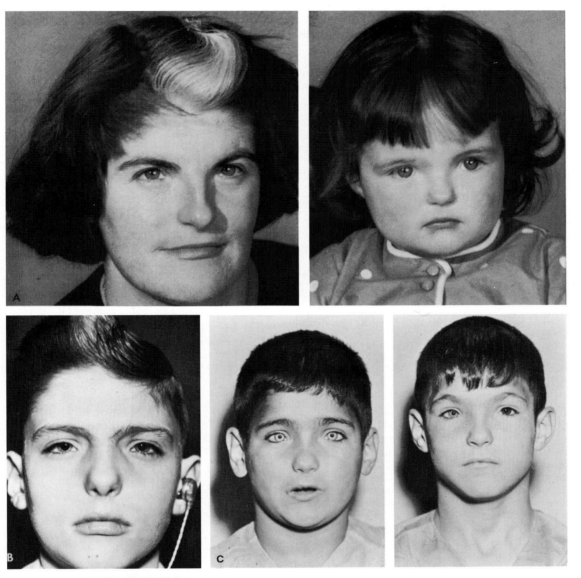

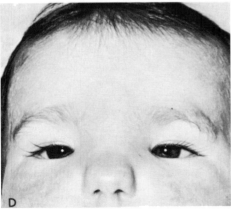

FIGURE 1. Waardenburg syndrome. *A,* Mother and daughter. Note the isochromic light iris. (From Partington, M. W.: Arch. Dis. Child., *34*:154, 1959, with permission.) *B,* A 10-year-old with congenital deafness. Note prominent nasal root, small alae nasi. (From DiGeorge, A. M., et al.: J. Pediatr., *57*:649, 1960, with permission.) *C,* Brothers, only one of whom has deafness. Note the lack of a white forelock. *D,* A 4-month-old infant who had a white forelock at birth that is now pigmented. Note heterochromia of irises, lateral placement of inner canthi, and small alae nasi.

TREACHER COLLINS SYNDROME

(Mandibulofacial Dysostosis, Franceschetti-Klein Syndrome)

Malar Hypoplasia With Down-Slanting Palpebral
Fissures, Defect of Lower Lid, Malformation of External Ear

Although Thomson reported the first case in 1846, the syndrome has been associated with Treacher Collins, who described two cases in 1900. Franceschetti and Klein made extensive reports on this condition and called it mandibulofacial dysostosis (1940s).

ABNORMALITIES

Antimongoloid slanting palpebral fissures	89%
Malar hypoplasia, with or without cleft in zygomatic bone	81%
Mandibular hypoplasia	78%
Lower lid coloboma	69%
Partial to total absence of lower eyelashes	53%
Malformation of auricles	77%
External ear canal defect	36%
Conductive deafness	40%
Visual loss	37%
Cleft palate	28%
Incompetent soft palate	32%
Projection of scalp hair onto lateral cheek	26%

OCCASIONAL ABNORMALITIES. Pharyngeal hypoplasia. Coloboma of the upper lid. Dacrostenosis. Microphthalmia. Strabismus. Ptosis. Macrostomia. Microstomia. Choanal atresia. Blind fistulas and skin tags between auricle and angle of the mouth. Absence of the parotid gland. Congenital heart defect. Cryptorchidism. Mental deficiency has been reported in only 5 per cent of the cases.

NATURAL HISTORY. These patients can develop early respiratory problems as a result of having a narrow airway and may occasionally require temporary tracheostomy. The narrow airway may make intubation difficult. As the great majority of these patients are of normal intelligence, the early recognition of deafness and its correction with hearing aids or surgery (when possible) are of great importance for development. Amblyopia secondary to refractive errors, anisometropia, strabismus, and/or ptosis is the most common cause of visual loss and should be carefully sought for in all cases. The growth of the facial bones during infancy and childhood results in some cosmetic improvement that may be enhanced by plastic surgery.

ETIOLOGY. Autosomal dominant, 60 per cent of the cases representing presumed fresh mutations. Mutations in a gene of unknown function referred to as Treacle which maps to 5q32-33.1 are responsible for at least some cases of Treacher Collins syndrome. There is wide variability in expression.

COMMENTS. Despite the marked variability in expression, a careful clinical and radiologic examination to rule out such subtle features as hypoplasia of the zygomatic arch on the occipitomental radiographs are usually diagnostic even in the most mildly affected individual. In the case of a large family in which linkage analysis has suggested that the gene is linked to markers in the region 5q32-33.2, linkage analysis can be used to identify affected individuals even in the absence of clinical and radiologic evidence of Treacher Collins syndrome.

References

Thomson, A.: Notice of several cases of malformation of the external ear, together with experiments on the state of hearing in such persons. Month. J. Med. Sci., 7:420, 1846.

Treacher Collins, E.: Case with symmetrical congenital notches in the outer part of each lower lid and defective development of the malar bones. Trans. Ophthalmol. Soc. U. K., 20:90, 1900.

Franceschetti, A., and Klein, D.: The Mandibulofacial Dysostosis, A New Hereditary Syndrome. Copenhagen, E. Munksgaard, 1949.

Peterson-Falzone, S., and Pruzansky, S.: Cleft palate and congenital palatopharyngeal incompetency in mandibulofacial dysostosis. Cleft Palate J., 13:354, 1976.

Shprintzen, R. J., and Berkman, M. D.: Pharyngeal hypoplasia in Treacher Collins syndrome. Arch. Otolaryngol., 105:127, 1979.

Dixon, M. J., et al.: Narrowing the position of the Treacher Collins syndrome locus to a small interval between three new microsatellite markers at 5q32-33.1. Am. J. Hum. Genet., 52:907, 1993.

Hertle, R. W., et al.: Ophthalmic features and visual prognosis in the Treacher Collins syndrome. Br. J. Ophthalmol., 77:642, 1993.

Dixon, M. J., et al.: Treacher Collins syndrome: Correlation between clinical and genetic linkage studies. Clin. Dysmorph., 3:96, 1994.

The Treacher Collins Syndrome Collaborative Group: Positional cloning of a gene involved in the pathogenesis of Treacher Collins syndrome. Nature Genet., 12:130, 1996.

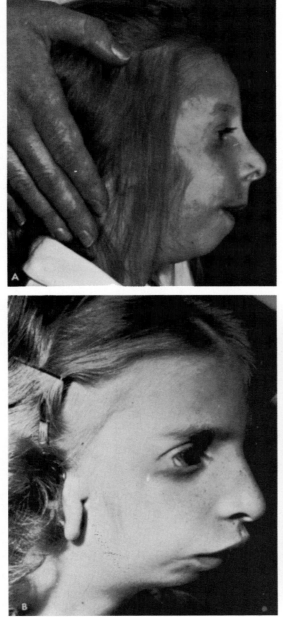

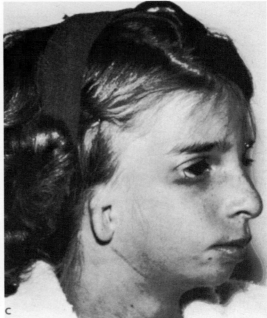

FIGURE 1. Treacher-Collins syndrome. *A*, A 6-year-old. Note the hair extending onto the lateral cheek. *B*, Preadolescent girl. Note the defect of lower eyelid and the malar hypoplasia. *C*, Same as *B*, postadolescent. Note the improvement in cosmetic appearance after a sliding osteotomy to the mandible and plastic surgery to the rudimentary auricle.

MARSHALL SYNDROME

In 1958, Marshall described seven family members in three generations with a disorder characterized by cataracts, sensorineural deafness, and an extremely short nose with a flat bridge. Subsequently, more than 20 cases have been reported.

ABNORMALITIES

Growth. Short stature.

Facies. Short depressed nose with flat nasal bridge and anteverted nares. Appearance of large eyes. Flat midface. Prominent, protruding upper incisors. Thick lips.

Eyes. Myopia. Cataracts. Esotropia.

Hearing. Sensorineural deafness.

Skeletal. Calvarial thickening. Absent frontal sinuses. Falx, tentorial, and meningeal calcifications. Spondyloephiphyseal abnormalities including mild platyspondyly, slightly small and irregular distal femoral and proximal tibial epiphyses, outward bowing of radius and ulna, and wide tufts of distal phalanges.

OCCASIONAL ABNORMALITIES. Mental deficiency. Retinal detachment. Cleft palate.

NATURAL HISTORY. The cataracts may spontaneously resorb, leading to glaucoma and/or lens dislocation.

ETIOLOGY. Autosomal dominant.

References

Marshall, D.: Ectodermal dysplasia. Report of a kindred with ocular abnormalities and hearing defect. Am. J. Ophthalmol., *45*:143, 1958.

Zellweger, H., Smith, J. K., and Grützner, P.: The Marshall syndrome: Report of a new family. J. Pediatr., *84*:868, 1974.

O'Donnell, J. J., Sirkin, S., and Hall, B. D.: Generalized osseous abnormalities in the Marshall syndrome. Birth Defects, *XII*(5):299, 1976.

Aymé, S., and Preus, M.: The Marshall and Stickler syndromes: Objective rejection of lumping. J. Med. Genet., *21*:34, 1984.

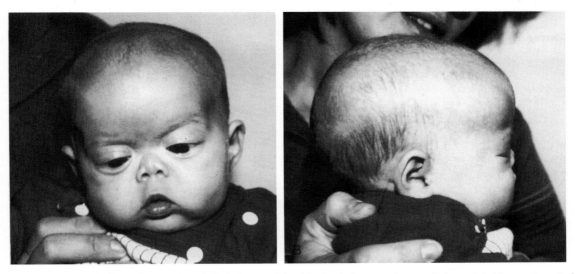

FIGURE 1. Marshall syndrome. *A* and *B*, A 1-year-old with short depressed nose, flat nasal bridge, anteverted nares, and the appearance of large eyes.

CERVICO-OCULO-ACOUSTIC SYNDROME

(Wildervanck Syndrome)

Klippel-Feil Anomaly, Abducens Paralysis
With Retracted Globes, Sensorineural Deafness

Initially described by Wildervanck in 1952, this disorder was further characterized by the same investigator, who summarized the clinical features of 62 affected patients in 1978.

ABNORMALITIES

Craniofacies. Asymmetry with a short neck and low hairline. Preauricular skin tags and pits.

Eyes. Duane anomaly (abducens paralysis with retraction of the globe and narrowing of the palpebral fissure of the affected eye on adduction). Epibulbar dermoids.

Hearing. Sensorineural, conductive, or mixed loss. A malformed vestibular labyrinth is usually present. The cochlea is sometimes altered.

Skeletal. Klippel-Feil anomaly (fusion of two or more cervical and sometimes thoracic vertebrae). Torticollis. Sprengel deformity.

OCCASIONAL ABNORMALITIES. Mental retardation. Occipital meningocele. Psuedopapilledema. Hydrocephalus. Growth deficiency. Cleft palate. Ear anomalies. Cardiac defects. Cervical ribs. Absent kidney. Cholelithiases.

NATURAL HISTORY. Severe deformations of the craniofacies can progress in cases with significant degrees of torticollis.

Intelligence in the vast majority of cases is normal. Computed tomography should be performed to document any abnormality of the inner ear.

ETIOLOGY. Unknown. All cases have been sporadic. The vast majority of affected individuals have been females.

References

Wildervanck, L. S.: The cervico-oculo-acusticus syndrome. *In* Vinken, P. J., and Bruyn, G. W. (eds.): Handbook of Clinical Neurology. Congenital Malformations of the Spine and Spinal Cord, Vol. 32. Elsevier/North-Holland Biomedical Press. Amsterdam, N.Y., 1978.

West, P. D. B., et al.: Wildervanck's syndrome: Unilateral Mondini dysplasia identified by computed tomography. J. Laryngol. Otol., *103*:408, 1989.

Gupte, G., et al.: Wildervanck syndrome (cervico-oculo-acoustic syndrome). J. Postgrad. Med., *38*:180, 1992.

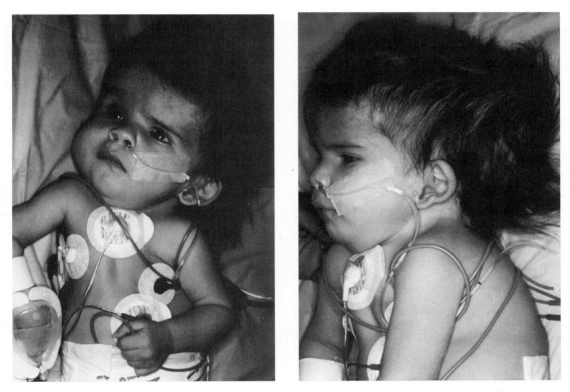

FIGURE 1. Note the short neck with low hairline, preauricular skin tag, and ear anomalies.

H

H. FACIAL-LIMB DEFECTS AS MAJOR FEATURE

MILLER SYNDROME
(Postaxial Acrofacial Dysostosis Syndrome)

*Treacher Collins—like Facies,
Limb Deficiency, Especially Postaxial*

In 1979, Miller et al. brought together six cases, four of which were from the literature, and recognized this disorder as a concise entity. The facies is similar to that of Treacher Collins syndrome and, in combination with limb defects, resembles Nager syndrome. The severity of the postaxial deficiencies distinguishes it from the latter syndrome.

ABNORMALITIES.
Craniofacial. Malar hypoplasia, sometimes with radiologic evidence of a vertical bony cleft, with down-slanting palpebral fissures. Colobomata of eyelids and ectropion. Micrognathia. Cleft lip and/or cleft palate. Hypoplastic, cup-shaped ears.
Limbs. Absence of fifth digits of all four limbs with or without shortening and in-curving of forearms with ulnar and radial hypoplasia. Syndactyly.
Other. Accessory nipple(s).

OCCASIONAL ABNORMALITIES. Postnatal growth deficiency, choanal atresia, conductive hearing loss, thumb hypoplasia, low arch dermal pattern, pectus excavatum, radioulnar synostosis, supernumerary vertebrae, rib defects, congenital hip dislocation, heart defects, absence of hemidiaphragm, pyloric stenosis, renal anomalies, cryptorchidism, midgut malrotation.

NATURAL HISTORY. These individuals are usually of normal intelligence. Hearing evaluation is indicated in all cases.

Craniofacial appearance sometimes changes with increasing age with a progressively greater degree of ectropian and facial asymmetry as well as a more triangular facial appearance with thin lips.

ETIOLOGY. Autosomal recessive inheritance.

References

Genée, E.: Une forme extensive de dysostose mandibulofaciale. J. Genet. Hum., *17*:45, 1969.

Smith, D. W., Pashayan, H., and Wildervanck, L. S.: Case report 28. Syndrome Identification, *3*(1):7, 1975.

Miller, M., Fineman, R., and Smith, D. W.: Postaxial acrofacial dysostosis syndrome. J. Pediatr., *95*:970, 1979.

Ogilvy-Stuart, A. L., and Parsons, A. C.: Miller syndrome (postaxial acrofacial dysostosis): Further evidence for autosomal recessive inheritance and expansion of the phenotype. J. Med. Genet., *28*:695, 1991.

Chrzanowska, K., and Fryns, J. P.: Miller postaxial acrofacial dysostosis: The phenotypic changes with age. Genet. Couns., *4*:131, 1993.

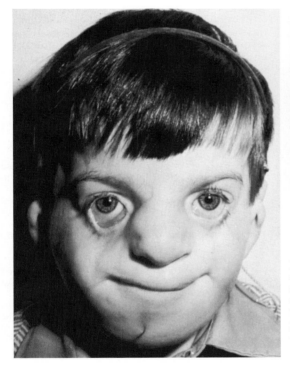

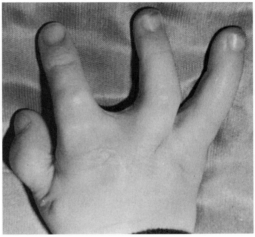

FIGURE 1. Miller syndrome. Affected individual showing striking malar and maxillary hypoplasia and lower lid defects. Note the hearing aid, required for middle ear deafness. The deficiency in the hand is complete for the fifth ray and incomplete for the other digits. (From Miller, M., et al.: J. Pediatr., *95*:970, 1979, with permission.)

NAGER SYNDROME

(Nager Acrofacial Dysostosis Syndrome)

Radial Limb Hypoplasia, Malar Hypoplasia, Ear Defects

Nager and deReynier described a Treacher Collins syndrome–like patient with radial limb defects in 1948, and subsequently over 75 cases have been recognized.

ABNORMALITIES

Performance. Intelligence normal. Conductive deafness usually bilateral and problems with articulation.

Craniofacial. Malar hypoplasia with down-slanting palpebral fissures. High nasal bridge. Micrognathia. Partial to total absence of lower eyelashes. Low-set, posteriorly rotated ears. Preauricular tags. Atresia of external ear canal. Cleft palate.

Limbs. Hypoplasia to aplasia of thumb, with or without radius. Proximal radioulnar synostosis and limitation of elbow extension. Short forearms.

OCCASIONAL ABNORMALITIES. Mental retardation. Postnatal growth deficiency. Lower lid coloboma. Projection of scalp hair onto lateral cheek. Cleft lip. Velopharyngeal insufficiency. Hypoplasia of larynx or epiglottis. Temporomandibular joint fibrosis and ankylosis. Syndactyly, clinodactyly, and/or camptodactyly of hands. Duplicated and triphalangeal thumbs. Missing or hypoplastic toes. Overlapping toes. Syndactyly of toes. Posteriorly placed hypoplastic halluces, hallux valgus, broad hallux. Absent distal flexion creases on toes. Limb reduction defects. Hip dislocation. Clubfeet. Hypoplastic first rib. Scoliosis. Cervical vertebral anomalies. Cardiac defects. Microcephaly. Hydrocephalus secondary to aqueductal stenosis. Polymicrogyria. Genitourinary anomalies. Hirschsprung disease. Urticaria pigmentosa.

NATURAL HISTORY. The recommendations for early detection of deafness, hearing aid augmentation, and plastic surgery are similar to those for Treacher Collins syndrome. Delays in speech and language development are related primarily to hearing loss. Early respiratory and feeding problems frequently occur. Gastrostomy or gavage feeding is often necessary. The incidence of prematurity is high. Perinatal mortality is approximately 20 per cent and is related to respiratory distress secondary to micrognathia and palatal anomalies. Management should be the same as for the Robin sequence.

ETIOLOGY. Most cases have been sporadic. However, seven cases of parent-to-child transmission have been documented, suggesting autosomal dominant inheritance for some cases; and six families in which unaffected parents have given birth to more than one affected child have been reported, suggesting autosomal recessive inheritance for others.

References

Nager, F. R., and deReynier, J. P.: Das Gehörogan bei den angeborenen Kopfmissbildungen. Pract. Otorhinolaryngol. (Basal), *10*(Suppl. 2):1, 1948.

Bowen, P., and Harley, F.: Mandibulofacial dysostosis with limb malformations (Nager's acrofacial dysostosis). Birth Defects, *X*(5):109, 1974.

Walker, F.: Apparent autosomal recessive inheritance of Treacher-Collins syndrome. Birth Defects, *X*(8): 135, 1974.

Meyerson, M. D., et al.: Nager acrofacial dysostosis: Early invention and long-term planning. Cleft Palate J., *14*:35, 1977.

Halal, F., et al.: Differential diagnosis of Nager acrofacial dysostosis syndrome: Report of four patients with Nager syndrome and discussion of other related syndromes. Am. J. Med. Genet., *14*:209, 1983.

Krauss, C. M., Hassell, L. A., and Gang, D. L.: Brief clinical report: Anomalies in an infant with Nager acrofacial dysostosis. Am. J. Med. Genet., *21*:761, 1985.

Aylsworth, A. L., et al.: Nager acrofacial dysostosis: Male-to-male transmission in 2 families. Am. J. Med. Genet., *41*:83, 1991.

McDonald, M. T., and Gorski, J. L.: Nager acrofacial dysostosis. J. Med. Genet., *30*:779, 1993.

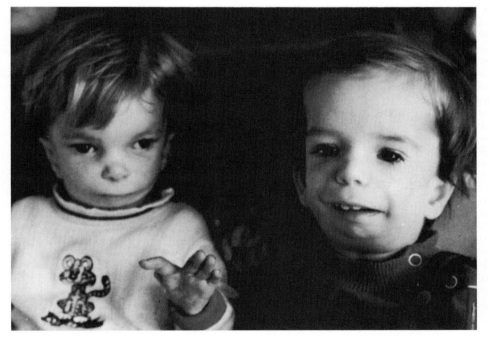

FIGURE 1. Nager syndrome. Unrelated young girl and boy showing the facies and hypoplasia of the thumb. (From Meyerson, M. D., et al.: Cleft Palate J., *14*:35, 1977, with permission.)

TOWNES-BROCKS SYNDROME

Thumb Anomalies, Auricular Anomalies, Anal Anomalies

Townes and Brocks first described this disorder in 1972, and at least 50 affected individuals have been reported.

ABNORMALITIES

Craniofacial. Auricular anomalies including overfolding of the superior helix and large ears. Variable features of hemifacial microsomia, especially preauricular tags.

Limbs. Hand anomalies including hypoplastic, broad, bifid, or triphalangeal thumb. Preaxial polydactyly. Distal ulnar deviation of thumb. Pseudoepiphysis of second metacarpals. Fusion of triquetrum and hamate. Absence of triquetrum and navicular bones. Fusion and/or short metatarsals. Prominence of distal ends of lateral metatarsals. Absent or hypoplastic third toe. Clinodactyly of fifth toe.

Anus. Anal defects including imperforate anus, anterior placement, and stenosis. Rectovaginal or rectoperineal fistula.

Renal. Anomalies, from renal hypoplasia to ureterovesical reflux to urethral valves.

OCCASIONAL ABNORMALITIES. Deafness.
Mental retardation. Microcephaly. Microtia. Preauricular pit. Cardiac defect. Duodenal atresia. Cystic ovary. Prominent perineal raphe. Hypospadius. 2–3 and 3–4 syndactyly of fingers. Abnormalities of toes including fifth toe clinodactyly, absence or hypoplasia of third toe, 3–4 syndactyly of toes, overlapping second, third, and fourth toes.

ETIOLOGY. Autosomal dominant with marked variability in the severity of expression for each feature.

COMMENT. It is of interest that this single gene disorder encompasses many of the features of both the VATER association and the facio-auriculo-vertebral malformation sequence.

References

Townes, P. L., and Brocks, E. R.: Hereditary syndrome of imperforate anus with hand, foot and ear anomalies. J. Pediatr., *81*:321, 1972.

Reid, I. S., and Turner, G.: Familial anal abnormality. J. Pediatr., *88*:992, 1976.

Kurnit, D. M., et al.: Autosomal dominant transmission of a syndrome of anal, ear, renal and radial congenital malformations. J. Pediatr., *93*:270, 1978.

Walpole, I. R., and Hockey, A.: Syndrome of imperforate anus, abnormalities of hands and feet, satyr ears, and sensorineural deafness. J. Pediatr., *100*:250, 1982.

Monteiro de Pino-Neto, J.: Phenotypic variability in Townes-Brocks syndrome. Am. J. Med. Genet., *18*: 147, 1984.

O'Callaghan, M., and Young, I. D.: The Townes-Brocks syndrome. J. Med. Genet., *27*:457, 1990.

Cameron, T. H., et al.: Townes-Brocks syndrome in two mentally retarded youngsters. Am. J. Med. Genet., *41*:1, 1991.

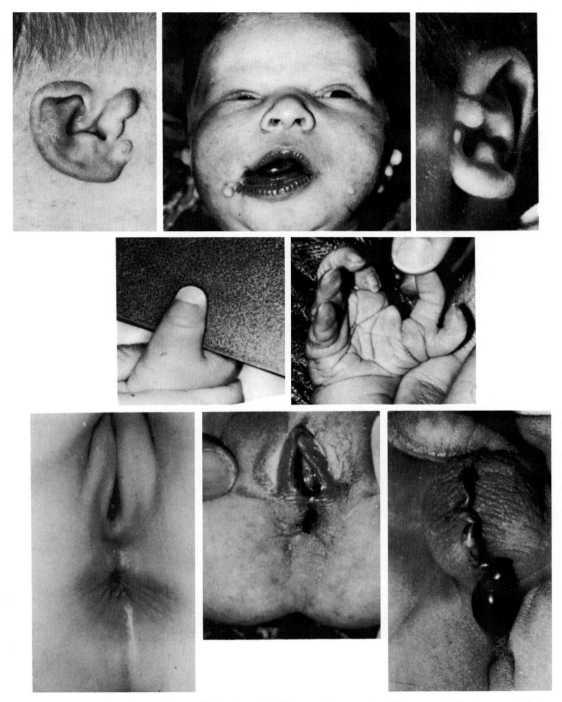

FIGURE 1. Townes-Brocks syndrome. Variation of facial morphogenesis with preauricular tags and features resembling facio-auriculo-vertebral sequence (hemifacial microsomia Goldenhar syndrome). Note the alterations of thumb development, from hypoplasia to supernumerary and finger-like thumb, and of anal development, from altered placement to imperforate anus. (Left side and lower right side photos are courtesy of Dr. Gillian Turner, Prince of Wales Hospital, Sydney, Australia.)

ORAL-FACIAL-DIGITAL SYNDROME

(OFD Syndrome, Type I)

Oral Frenula and Clefts,
Hypoplasia of Alae Nasi, Digital Asymmetry

Papillon-Léage and Psaume set this condition forth as a clinical entity in 1954. More than 160 cases have been reported. Nine different oral-facial-digital syndromes have been delineated. Only types I and II have been set forth in detail in this text.

ABNORMALITIES

Oral. Multiple and/or hyperplastic frenuli between the buccal mucous membrane and alveolar ridge. Median cleft lip. Lobated/bifid tongue with nodules. Cleft of alveolar ridge (at area of lateral incisors, which may be missing). Cleft palate. Dental caries and anomalous anterior teeth.

Facial. Hypoplasia of alar cartilages, lateral placement of inner canthi. Milia of ears and upper face in infancy.

Digital. Asymmetric shortening of digits with clinodactyly, syndactyly, and/or brachydactyly of hands and unilateral polydactyly of feet.

Scalp. Dry, rough, sparse hair and dry scalp.

Central Nervous System. Variable mental deficiency in about 57 per cent, with average I.Q. of 70. Brain malformation, including absence of corpus callosum and heterotopia of gray matter, in about 20 per cent of patients.

Cranium. Increased naso-sella-basion angle at base of cranium.

Renal. Adult polycystic kidney disease.

OCCASIONAL ABNORMALITIES

Oral. Enamel hypoplasia, supernumerary teeth, hamartoma of tongue, fistula in lower lip. Choanal atresia.

Facial. Frontal bossing. Hypoplastic mandibular ramus and zygoma.

Skeletal. Nonprogressive metaphyseal rarefaction.

Central Nervous System. Trembling, hydrocephalus, seizures, berry aneurysm.

Hair. Alopecia.

Skin. Granular seborrheic skin.

NATURAL HISTORY. Patients may do poorly in early infancy; as many as one third die during this period. Management is directed toward plastic surgical correction of oral clefts and dental care, including dentures when indicated. Psychometric evaluation is merited because about one half of the reported patients have mental deficiency. Renal function should be monitored.

ETIOLOGY. X-linked dominant with lethality in the vast majority of affected males.

COMMENT. Toriello has set forth the major features that distinguish types III through IX. With the exception of type V, all have similar oral, facial, and digital abnormalities. Significant overlap exists between the nine types, making it difficult to provide appropriate counseling relative to prognosis.

Type III (Sugarman syndrome), an autosomal recessive disorder, is distinguished clinically by polydactyly that is only postaxial, a bulbous nose, extra, small teeth, and macular red spots associated with see-saw winking of eyelids and/or myoclonic jerks.

Type IV (Buru-Baraister syndrome), an autosomal recessive disorder, is distinguished by short tibiae, pre- and/or postaxial polydactyly of hands and feet, cerebral atrophy, porencephaly, and short stature.

Type V (Thurston syndrome), an autosomal recessive condition, includes midline cleft lip, duplicated frenulum, and postaxial polydactyly of hands and feet.

Type VI (Varadi-Papp syndrome), an autosomal recessive condition, is distinguished by preaxial polysyndactyly of toes and postaxial polydactyly of fingers, a forked metacarpal, cerebellar anomalies (vermis hypoplasia/aplasia or Dandy-Walker anomaly). Occasional features include growth hormone deficiency, hypogonadotrophic hypogonadism, and a hypothalamic hamartoma.

Type VII (Whelan syndrome). Reported in a mother-daughter pair, features that distinguish this condition include congenital hydronephrosis, coarse hair, facial asymmetry, facial weakness, and preauricular tags.

Type VIII, an X-linked recessive disorder distinguished from type I by pre- and postaxial polydactyly of hands and bilateral duplication of halluces, abnormal tibiae, short stature, hypoplasia of the epiglottis, absent/abnormal central incisors, broad/bifid nasal tip, and metacarpal forking.

Type IX. Reported in three males, the features that distinguish this condition are retinal abnormalities consisting of atrophic areas of colobomatous origin.

References

Papillon-Léage, Mme., and Psaume, J.: Une malformation héréditaire de la muqueuse buccale: Brides et freins anormaux. Rev. Stomatol. (Paris), 55:209, 1954.

Gorlin, R. J., and Psaume, J.: Orodigitofacial dysostosis—a new syndrome. J. Pediatr., 61:520, 1962.

Doege, T. C., et al.: Studies of a family with the oral-facial-digital syndrome. N. Engl. J. Med., 271:1073, 1964.

Majewski, F., et al.: Das oro-facio-digitale Syndrom. Symptome und Prognose. Z. Kinderheilkd., 112:89, 1972.

Whelan, D. T., Feldman, W., and Dost, I.: The oro-facial-digital syndrome. Clin. Genet., 8:205, 1975.

Donnai, D., et al.: Familial orofaciodigital syndrome type I presenting as adult polycystic kidney disease. J. Med. Genet., 24:84, 1987.

Gillerot, Y., et al.: Oral-facial-digital syndrome type I in a newborn male. Am. J. Med. Genet., 46:335, 1993.

Toriello, H. V.: Oral-facial-digital syndromes, 1992. Clin. Dysmorphol., 2:95, 1993.

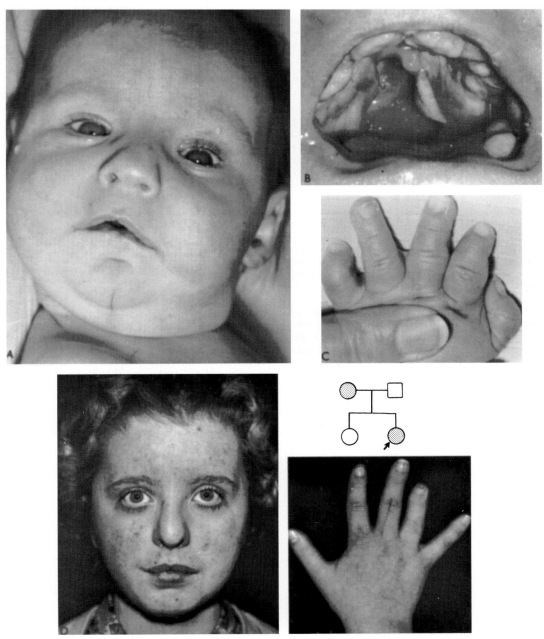

FIGURE 1. Oral-facial-digital syndrome type I. *A,* Young infant of a normal mother. *B,* Irregular clefts in alveolar ridge, palate, and tongue. *C,* Short third finger; partial syndactyly of third and fourth fingers. *D,* A 17-year-old daughter of affected mother.

MOHR SYNDROME

(OFD Syndrome, Type II)

*Cleft Tongue, Conductive
Deafness, Partial Reduplication of Hallux*

Mohr described this pattern in several male siblings in 1941. Subsequently, a number of cases have been reported.

ABNORMALITIES

General. Mild shortness of stature. Conductive deafness due apparently to defect of incus.

Facies and Mouth. Low nasal bridge with lateral displacement of inner canthi. Broad nasal tip, sometimes slightly bifid. Midline partial cleft of lip. Hypertrophy of usual frenula. Midline cleft of tongue, nodules on tongue. Flare to alveolar ridge. Hypoplasia of zygomatic arch, maxilla, and body of mandible.

Limbs. Partial reduplication of hallux and first metatarsal, cuneiform and cuboid bones. Relatively short hands with clinodactyly of fifth finger. Bilateral postaxial polydactyly of hands. Bilateral polysyndactyly of feet (occasionally only unilateral). Metaphyseal flaring and irregularity.

OCCASIONAL ABNORMALITIES.
Wormian cranial bones, missing central incisors, cleft palate, multiple frenula, pectus excavatum, scoliosis, mental deficiency, porencephaly, hydrocephaly.

NATURAL HISTORY. These patients apparently have normal intelligence, and plastic surgery is indicated for the clefts, frenula, and partial reduplication of the hallux. A surgical attempt to reconstruct the auditory ossicles was unsuccessful in one case.

ETIOLOGY. Autosomal recessive.

References

Mohr, O. L.: A hereditary sublethal syndrome in man. Skr. Norske Vidensk. Akad., I. Mat. Naturv. Klasse, *14*:3, 1941.

Rimoin, D. L., and Edgerton, M. T.: Genetic and clinical heterogeneity in the oral-facial-digital syndromes. J. Pediatr., *71*:94, 1967.

Pfeiffer, R. A., Majewski, F., and Mannkopf, H.: Das syndrome von Mohr und Classen. Klin. Paediatr., *184*:224, 1972.

Levy, E. P., Fletcher, B. D., and Fraser, F. C.: Mohr syndrome with subclinical expression of the bifid great toe. Am. J. Dis. Child, *128*:531, 1974.

Baraitser, M.: The orofacial digital (OFD) syndromes. J. Med. Genet., 23:116, 1986.

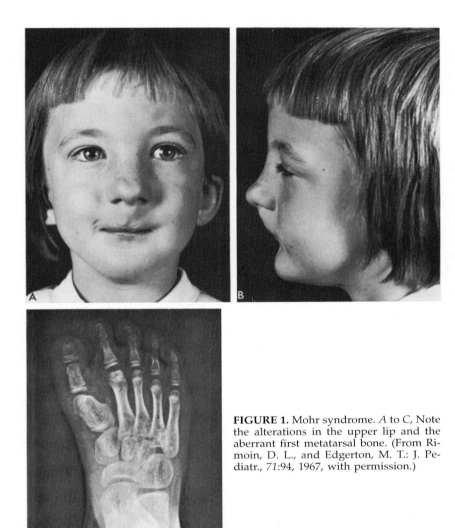

FIGURE 1. Mohr syndrome. *A* to C, Note the alterations in the upper lip and the aberrant first metatarsal bone. (From Rimoin, D. L., and Edgerton, M. T.: J. Pediatr., *71*:94, 1967, with permission.)

SHPRINTZEN SYNDROME

(Velo-Cardio-Facial Syndrome)

This syndrome was recognized by Shprintzen et al. in 1978. Well over 100 cases subsequently have been reported. Since the patients were predominantly evaluated at craniofacial centers, there is a bias toward those with palatal defects.

ABNORMALITIES

Performance. Learning disabilities; mild intellectual impairment (approximately 40 per cent); I.Q. generally ranges from 70 to 90, with some slightly higher. Psychiatric disorders in approximately 10 per cent of cases.

Growth. Postnatal onset short stature (33 per cent).

Ears and Hearing. Conductive hearing loss secondary to cleft palate; minor auricular anomalies.

Craniofacial. Cleft of the secondary palate, either overt or submucous; velopharyngeal incompetence; small or absent adenoids; prominent nose with squared nasal root and narrow alar base; narrow palpebral fissures; abundant scalp hair; deficient malar area; vertical maxillary excess with long face; retruded mandible with chin deficiency; microcephaly (40 to 50 per cent).

Limbs. Slender and hypotonic with hyperextensible hands and fingers (63 per cent).

Cardiac. Defects present in 85 per cent, the most common being ventricular septal defect (62 per cent); right aortic arch (52 percent); tetralogy of Fallot (21 per cent); aberrant left subclavian artery.

OCCASIONAL ABNORMALITIES.

Robin malformation sequence; enlargement, medial displacement, tortuosity or other abnormalities of internal carotid arteries (25 per cent); other types of cardiac defect; scoliosis; umbilical or inguinal hernia; cryptorchidism; hypospadias; laryngeal web. Tortuosity of retinal vessels (30 per cent). Small optic disks. Ocular coloboma. Cataracts. Holoprosencephaly. Hypothyroidism. Abnormal T cell function and absent thymic tissue.

NATURAL HISTORY.

Hypotonia in infancy is frequent (70 to 80 per cent). Transient neonatal hypocalcemia occurs in 20 per cent of cases. Speech development is often delayed, and language is impaired. Speech is almost always hypernasal, with the pharyngeal musculature being hypotonic. Socialization skills may surpass intellectual skills. Personality may tend toward perseverative behavior, with concrete thinking secondary to intellectual impairment or learning disorders. Approximately 10 per cent of affected individuals have developed psychiatric disorders, primarily chronic schizophrenia and paranoid delusions with onset varying between 10 and 21 years of age. Obstructive sleep apnea has been noted following pharyngeal surgery to improve speech in several patients. The abnormalities of the internal carotid arteries can be diagnosed by the demonstration of visible pulsations in the posterior pharyngeal wall musculature using fiberoptic nasopharyngoscopy and by MRI of the pharynx.

ETIOLOGY.

Autosomal dominant. Affected individuals have an interstitial deletion of chromosome 22q11.21-q11.23 and are thus monosomic for that chromosomal region. Cytogenetic analysis will detect only 20 per cent of the deletions in the region. Therefore, fluorescent in situ hybridization (FISH) needs to be used to demonstrate the deletion.

COMMENT.

Chromosome 22q11 is the same region that is deleted in some cases of the DiGeorge sequence. Based on a number of clinical studies in which a child with the DiGeorge sequence was born to a parent with velo-cardio-facial syndrome, it is now believed that the two disorders represent different manifestations of the same genetic defect.

References

Shprintzen, R. J., et al.: A new syndrome involving cleft palate, cardiac anomalies, typical facies, and learning disabilities; velo-cardio-facial syndrome. Cleft Palate J., 15:56, 1978.

Young, D., Shprintzen, R. J., and Goldberg, R. B.: Cardiac malformations in the velo-cardio-facial syndrome. Am. J. Cardiol., 46:643, 1980.

Shprintzen, R. J., et al.: The velo-cardio-facial syndrome: A clinical and genetic analysis. Pediatrics, 67:167, 1981.

Fitch, N.: Velo-cardio-facial syndrome and eye abnormality. Am. J. Med. Genet., 15:699, 1983.

Williams, M. A., Shprintzen, R. J., and Goldberg, R. B.: Male-to-male transmission of the velo-cardio-facial syndrome: A case report and review of 60 cases. J. Craniofac. Genet. Dev. Biol., 5:175, 1985.

Driscoll, D. A., et al.: Deletions and microdeletions of 22q11.2 in velo-cardio-facial syndrome. Am. J. Med. Genet., 44:261, 1992.

Scrambler, P. J., et al.: The velo-cardio-facial syndrome is associated with chromosome 22 deletions which encompass the DiGeorge syndrome locus. Lancet, 339:1138, 1992.

Goldberg, R., et al.: Velo-cardio-facial: A review of 120 patients. Am. J. Med. Genet., 45:313, 1993.

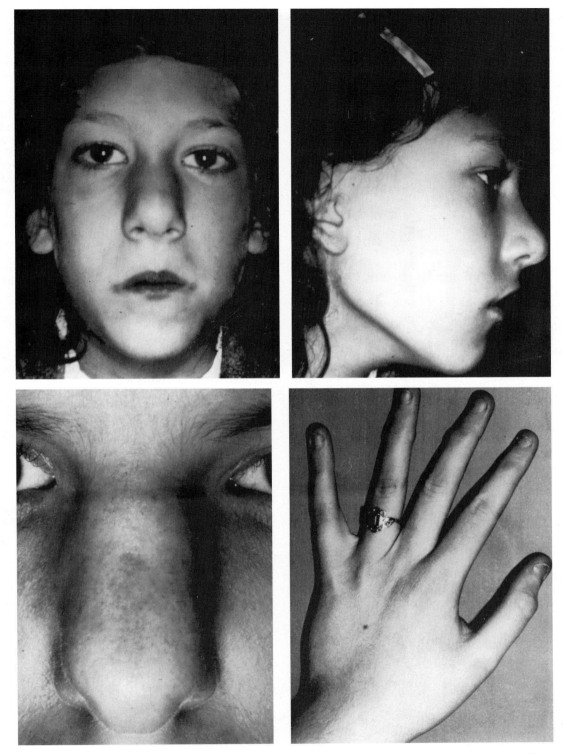

FIGURE 1. Facies, emphasizing the nasal configuration, and relatively slender hands in Shprintzen syndrome.

OCULODENTODIGITAL SYNDROME

(Oculodentodigital Dysplasia)

Microphthalmos, Enamel Hypoplasia, Camptodactyly of Fifth Fingers

Originally described in 1920 by Lohmann, this pattern was more fully characterized by Gorlin, Meskin, and St. Geme in 1963.

ABNORMALITIES

Eyes. Microphthalmos, microcornea, fine porous iris. Short palpebral fissures and epicanthal folds.

Nose. Thin, hypoplastic alae nasi with small nares.

Teeth. Enamel hypoplasia.

Hands and Feet. Syndactyly of fourth and fifth fingers, third and fourth toes. Camptodactyly of fifth fingers. Midphalangeal hypoplasia or aplasia of one or more fingers and/or toes.

Hair. Fine, dry, and/or sparse and slow growing.

Other Skeletal. Broad tubular bones and mandible with wide alveolar ridge.

OCCASIONAL ABNORMALITIES.
Mental retardation. Microcephaly. Glaucoma, cataract, bony orbital hypotelorism with normal inner canthal distance, partial anodontia, microdontia, premature loss of teeth, cleft lip and palate, conductive hearing impairment, cubitus valgus, hip dislocation, osteopetrosis, poor posture. Skull and vertebral hyperostosis. Neurologic dysfunction, including hyperactive deep tendon reflexes, paraparesis, quadriparesis, ataxia, spasticity and dysarthria. Abnormal CNS white matter on MRI scan. Calcification of basal ganglia.

NATURAL HISTORY. Intellectual performance is usually normal. In some cases progressive neurologic dysfunction develops secondary either to spinal cord compression from presumed hyperostosis at the skull base or cerebral white matter abnormalities. Facial features become more obvious after the first 3 to 4 years of life. Because open angle glaucoma has been reported as a late complication, periodic ophthalmic evaluation is recommended.

ETIOLOGY. Autosomal dominant with variable expression; many cases represent fresh mutations.

References

Lohmann, W.: Beitrag zur Kenntnis des reinen Mikrophthalmus. Arch. Augenh., *86*:136, 1920.

Gorlin, R. J., Meskin, L. H., and St. Geme, J. W.: Oculodentodigital dysplasia. J. Pediatr., *63*:69, 1963.

Eidelman, E., Chosack, A., and Wagner, M. L.: Orodigitofacial dysostosis and oculodentodigital dysplasia. Two distinct syndromes with some similarities. Oral Surg., *23*:311, 1967.

Judisch, G. F., et al.: Oculodentodigital dysplasia. Arch. Ophthalmol., *97*:878, 1979.

Traboulsi, E. I., Faris, B. M., and Der Kaloustian, V. M.: Persistent hyperplastic primary vitreous and recessive oculo-dento-osseous dysplasia. Am. J. Med. Genet., *24*:95, 1986.

Gutmann, D. H., et al.: Oculodentodigital dysplasia syndrome associated with abnormal cerebral white matter. Am. J. Med. Genet., *41*:18, 1991.

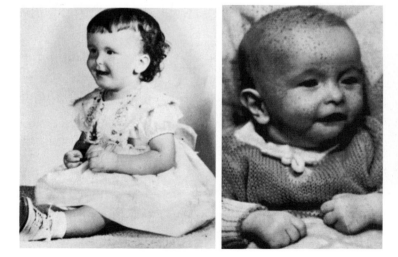

FIGURE 1. Infants with oculodentodigital syndrome. Note the small alae nasi, small mandibles, and 4–5 cutaneous syndactyly. (Courtesy of Teresa Hadro, Southern Illinois University School of Medicine [left photo] and Dr. David R. Cox [right photo].)

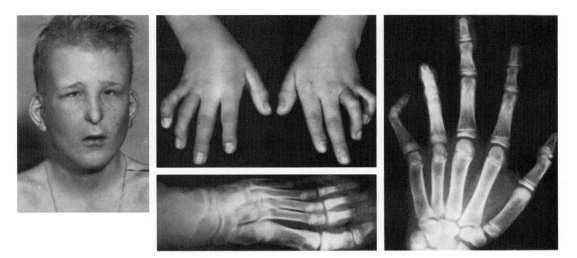

FIGURE 2. Oculodentodigital syndrome. A 12-year-old. Note the microcornea, small eyes, hypoplasia of the alae nasi, camptodactyly, repaired syndactyly of the fourth and fifth fingers, and bony abnormalities. (From Gorlin, R. J., et al.: J. Pediatr., 63:69, 1963, with permission.)

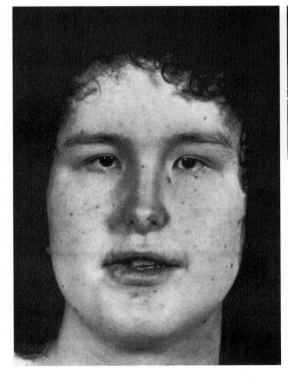

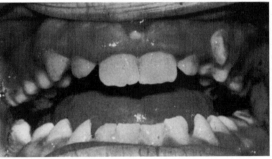

FIGURE 3. Oculodentodigital syndrome. Young woman who had shunted hydrocephalus in early childhood. Note the similar facial features and the small melanomata also present in the upper photo. (Courtesy of Dr. Boris G. Kousseff, University of South Florida, Tampa, Fla.)

OTO-PALATO-DIGITAL SYNDROME, TYPE I

(Taybi Syndrome)

Deafness, Cleft Palate, Broad Distal Digits With Short Nails

Initially described by Taybi in 1962, many cases have been recognized subsequently.

ABNORMALITIES
Performance. Mild mental deficiency; I.Q.s of 75 to 90.
Growth. Small stature. Below tenth percentile for age.
Hearing. Moderate conductive deafness.
Cranium. Frontal and occipital prominence with thick frontal bone and thick base of skull, having a steep naso-basal angulation. Absence of frontal and sphenoid sinuses.
Facies. Facial bone hypoplasia and hypertelorism with small nose and mouth but lateral fullness of the supraorbital ridges.
Mouth. Partial anodontia, impacted teeth, or both. Cleft soft palate, small tonsils.
Midskeletal. Small trunk, pectus excavatum, failure of neural arch fusion, small iliac crests.
Limbs. Limited elbow extension, inward-bowing tibiae. Short, broad distal phalanges of thumbs and toes, to a lesser extent for other digits, with short nails. Relatively short third, fourth, fifth metacarpals. Fusion of hamate and capitate bones. Accessory ossification center at the base of the second metatarsal.

OCCASIONAL ABNORMALITIES. Delayed closure of anterior fontanel, hip dislocation, limited knee flexion, syndactyly of toes, hallucal nail dystrophy, scoliosis.

NATURAL HISTORY. Speech development is retarded on the basis of hearing impairment, mental deficiency, or both.

ETIOLOGY. X-linked transmission with intermediate expression in females and complete expression in males. The altered gene has been mapped to Xq28. Features in females include fullness of the lateral supraorbital ridges, short nails, clinodactyly of toes, and roentgenographic abnormalities in limbs and skull.

References

Taybi, H.: Generalized skeletal dysplasia with multiple anomalies. Am. J. Roentgenol. Radium Ther. Nucl. Med., *88*:450, 1962.

Dudding, B. A., Gorlin, R. J., and Langer, L. O.: The oto-palato-digital syndrome. A new symptom-complex consisting of deafness, dwarfism, cleft palate, characteristic facies, and a generalized bone dysplasia. Am. J. Dis. Child., *113*:214, 1967.

Gorlin, R. J., Poznanski, A. K., and Hendon, I.: The oto-palato-digital (OPD) syndrome in females. Oral Surg., *35*:218, 1973.

Biancalana, V., et al.: Oto-palato-digital syndrome type I: Further evidence for assignment of the locus to Xq28. Hum. Genet., *88*:228, 1991.

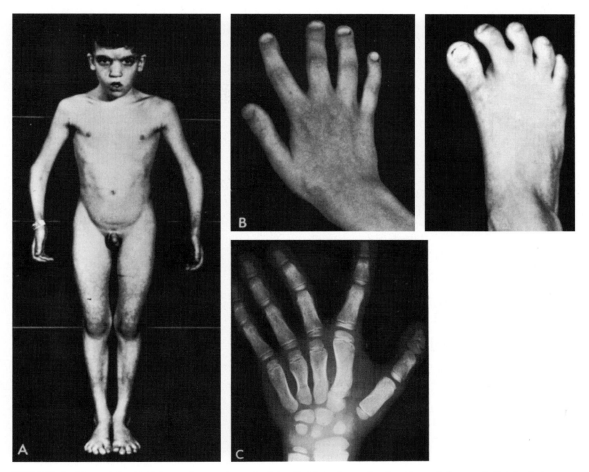

FIGURE 1. Oto-palato-digital syndrome, type I. *A* to *C*, Note irregular length and form of distal phalanges, especially thumb. (From Dudding, B. A., Gorlin, R. J., and Langer, L. O.: Am. J. Dis. Child., *113*:214, 1967, with permission. Copyright 1967, American Medical Association.)

OTO-PALATO-DIGITAL SYNDROME, TYPE II

Fitch et al. and later Kozlowski et al. each described this pattern of malformation in two half-brothers. Approximately 20 cases have been reported.

ABNORMALITIES

Growth. Postnatal growth deficiency in survivors.

Craniofacies. Late closure of large anterior fontanel. Wide sutures. Prominent forehead. Low-set malformed ears. Ocular hypertelorism. Antimongoloid slant to palpebral fissures. Flat nasal bridge. Small mouth. Micrognathia. Cleft palate. Radiographic evidence of dense fontanels, supraorbital ridge, and skull base with undermineralization of cranial vault. Small mandible with obtuse angle.

Limbs. Flexed, overlapping fingers. Short broad thumbs and great toes. Polydactyly. Variable syndactyly of hands and feet. Clinodactyly of second finger. Bowing of radius, ulna, femur, and tibia. Small to absent fibula. Hypoplastic, irregular metacarpals. Nonossified fifth metatarsal. Short, absent, and/or poorly ossified phalanges of fingers and toes. Subluxed elbows, wrists, and knees. Congenital hip dislocation. Rocker-bottom feet.

Other. Conductive hearing loss. Pectus excavatum. A narrow chest with thin, wavy clavicles and ribs. Flattened vertebral bodies. Hypoplastic ilia. Widened lumbosacral canal. Mental deficiency.

OCCASIONAL ABNORMALITIES. Dental abnormalities, transverse capitate bone, clinodatyly of second finger, retarded carpal bone age and advanced phalangeal bone age, absent halluces, omphalocele, cryptorchidism, hypospadias, absent adrenal.

NATURAL HISTORY. The majority of affected individuals have been stillborn or died prior to 5 months of age because of, in most cases, respiratory difficulties. The incidence of mental deficiency in survivors is unknown. Although significant developmental delay has been documented, one 18-month-old and one 6-year-old affected male are developmentally normal. The facial appearance as well as the bone curvatures tend to normalize with age.

ETIOLOGY. X-linked, with mild manifestations in heterozygous females such as broad face, antimongoloid slant of palpebral fissures, and cleft palate or bifid uvula.

References

Fitch, N., Jequier, S., and Papageorgiou, A.: A familial syndrome of cranial, facial, oral and limb anomalies. Clin. Genet., 10:226, 1976.

Kozlowski, K., et al.: Oto-palato-digital syndrome with severe x-ray changes in two half brothers. Pediatr. Radiol., 6:97, 1977.

Fitch, N., Jequier, S., and Gorlin, R.: The oto-palato-digital syndrome, proposed type II. Am. J. Med. Genet., 15:655, 1983.

Brewster, T. G., et al.: Oto-palato-digital syndrome, type II—an X-linked skeletal dysplasia. Am. J. Med. Genet., 20:249, 1985.

Blanchet, P., et al.: Multiple congenital anomalies associated with an oto-palatal-digital syndrome type II. Genet. Couns., 4:289, 1993.

Holder, S. E., and Winter, R. M.: Otopalatodigital syndrome type II. J. Med. Genet., 30:310, 1993.

Preis, S., et al.: Oto-palato-digital syndrome type II in two unrelated boys. Clin. Genet., 45:154, 1994.

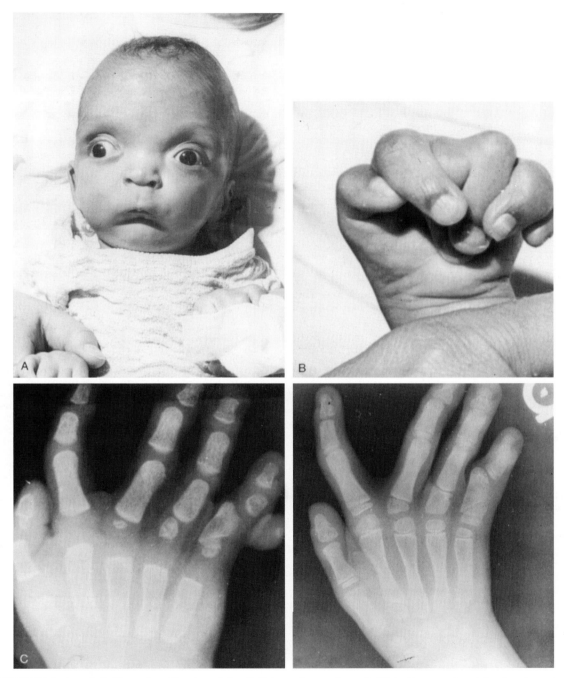

FIGURE 1. *A* and *B*, Neonate with oto-palato-digital syndrome, type II. Note the prominent forehead, ocular hypertelorism, flat nasal bridge, small mouth, micrognathia, and the flexed overlapping fingers. *C*, Radiographs of the hand at 1 and 5 years of age reveal hypoplastic irregular metacarpals, abnormal epiphyses of proximal phalanges 4 and 5, and postaxial polydactyly. (From Fitch, N., et al.: Am. J. Med. Genet., *15*:655, 1983, with permission.)

COFFIN-LOWRY SYNDROME

Down-Slanting Palpebral Fissures,
Bulbous Nose, Tapering Fingers

Coffin et al. in 1966 and Lowry et al. in 1971 independently described a mental retardation syndrome associated with coarse facies, short stature, and thick, soft hands with tapering fingers. Temtamy recognized the similarity between the two and referred to the disorder as the Coffin-Lowry syndrome. The facies may appear similar to that of the Williams syndrome.

ABNORMALITIES

Growth. Mild to moderate growth deficiency, apparently of postnatal onset.

Performance. Mental deficiency, usually severe. Relative weakness. Hypotonia.

Facies. Coarse appearance, with down-slanting palpebral fissures and maxillary hypoplasia, mild hypertelorism, prominent brow, and short, broad nose with thick alae nasi and septum, and anteverted nares. Large open mouth with thick, everted lower lip. Prominent ears.

Dental. Hypodontia, malocclusion, wide-spaced teeth, and large medial incisors.

Thorax. Short bifid sternum with pectus carinatum, and excavatum.

Spine. Anterior superior marginal vertebral defects, thoracolumbar scoliosis, and kyphosis.

Limbs. Large, soft hands with tapering fingers and tufted drumstick appearance to distal phalanges on roentgenogram. Small fingernails. Accessory transverse hypothenar crease. Flat feet. Lax ligaments.

OCCASIONAL ABNORMALITIES.

Microcephaly. Thick calvarium, dilated lateral ventricles. Seizures. Hypoplastic sinuses and mastoids. Simian crease. Forearm fullness. Delayed closure of anterior fontanel. Inguinal hernia. Rectal prolapse. Uterine prolapse. Mitral insufficiency. Sensorineural hearing loss. Premature loss of primary teeth.

NATURAL HISTORY. The mental deficiency is usually of severe degree, leaving the patient without speech. Although the face coarsens with age, and the vertebral dysplasia and kyphoscoliosis generally do not develop until after 6 years, there is no evidence of progressive mental deterioration.

ETIOLOGY. X-linked inheritance is implied, with striking similarity between the severely affected hemizygous males. Clinical findings in carrier females include slight to moderate mental deficiency, mild facial changes, tapered fingers, and short stature, although some obligate carriers are completely normal. Linkage analysis has suggested that the locus of the gene is at Xp22.1-p22.2.

References

Coffin, G. S., Siris, E., and Wegienka, L. C.: Mental retardation with osteocartilaginous anomalies. Am. J. Dis. Child., 112:205, 1966.

Lowry, B., Miller, J. R., and Fraser, F. C.: A new dominant gene mental retardation syndrome. Am. J. Dis. Child., 121:496, 1971.

Temtamy, S. A., et al.: The Coffin-Lowry syndrome. A simply inherited trait comprising mental retardation, facio-digital anomalies and skeletal anomalies. Birth Defects, XI(6):133, 1975.

Hunter, A. G. W., Partington, M. W., and Evans, J. A.: The Coffin-Lowry syndrome. Experience from four centres. Clin. Genet., 21:321, 1982.

Vles, J. S. H., et al.: Early signs in Coffin-Lowry syndrome. Clin. Genet., 26:448, 1984.

Gilgenkrautz, S., et al.: Coffin-Lowry syndrome: A multicenter study. Clin. Genet., 34:230, 1988.

Hartsfield, J. K., et al.: Pleiotrophy in Coffin-Lowry syndrome: Sensorineural hearing deficit and premature tooth loss as early manifestations. Am. J. Med. Genet., 45:552, 1993.

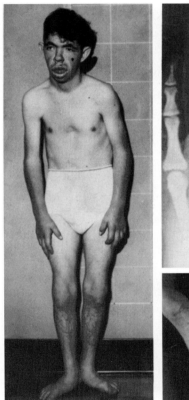
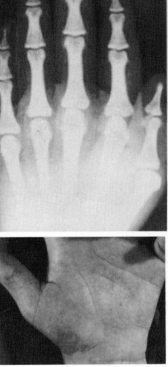
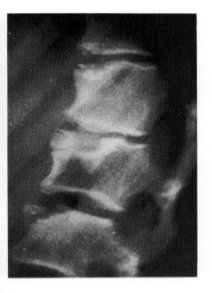

FIGURE 1. Coffin-Lowry syndrome. Seriously mentally deficient young adult patient. Note stooped posture, facies, vertebral changes, tufted terminal phalanges, and accessory transverse hypothenar crease. (Courtesy of Dr. Selma Myhre, Rainier State Training School, Buckley, Wash.)

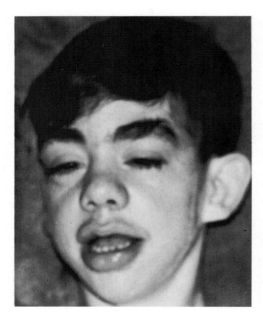

FIGURE 2. Coffin-Lowry syndrome. A 15-year-old mentally deficient boy with height of 4 feet 9 inches, ptosis of eyelids, pectus excavatum, scoliosis, and clinodactyly of the fifth finger, in addition to the obvious facial features. (Courtesy of Dr. Selma Myhre, Rainier State Training School, Buckley, Wash.)

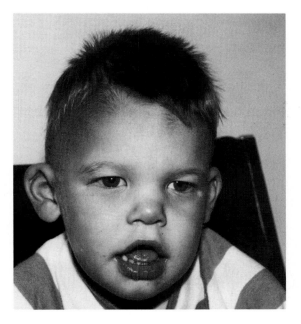

FIGURE 3. Coffin-Lowry syndrome. A 3-year-old boy showing aberrant facies with short nose and thick everted lower lip.

X-LINKED α-THALASSEMIA/MENTAL RETARDATION (ATR-X) SYNDROME

Severe Mental Retardation,
Characteristic Face, Genital Abnormalities

First described in 1990 by Wilkie et al., this disorder was further characterized by Gibbons et al. in 1991. More than 40 affected individuals have been identified.

ABNORMALITIES

Performance. Severe mental retardation. Initial hypotonia frequently followed by spasticity. Seizures.

Growth. Postnatal growth deficiency sometimes not evident until adolescence.

Craniofacies. Microcephaly. Telecanthus. Epicanthal folds. Low nasal bridge. Small, triangular nose with anteverted nares. Midface hypoplasia. Large "carp-like" mouth that is frequently held open. Full lips. Large, protruding tongue. Wide-spaced incisors. Small, simple, deformed, low-set, and/or posteriorly rotated ears.

Limbs. Tapering fingers. Fifth finger clinodactyly.

Genitalia. Cryptorchidism. Testicular dysgenesis. Shawl and/or hypoplastic scrotum. Small penis. Hypospadias.

Hematologic. Mild hypochromic microcytic anemia. Mild form of hemoglobin H disease (a type of α-thalassemia). The hemoglobin H that can be detected electrophoretically in this disorder ranges from 0 to 6.7 per cent. In almost all cases, by using 1 per cent brilliant cresyl blue (BCB), hemoglobin H forms inclusions which can be detected in from 0.01 to 40 per cent of red cells.

OCCASIONAL ABNORMALITIES. Cerebral atrophy. Kyphoscoliosis. Hemivertebra. Missing rib. Talipes equinovarus. Coxa valga. Ovoid vertebral bodies. Small or drumstick appearing terminal phalanges. Absent frontal sinuses. Flexion deformity of index finger. Umbilical hernia. Perimembranous ventricular septal defect. Renal agenesis. Hydronephrosis.

NATURAL HISTORY. Severe mental retardation with lack of expressive speech, limited comprehension, and the development of only partial bladder and bowel control is the rule. Regurgitation of food often induced by putting fingers down throat, gastroesophageal reflux, and constipation are also common.

ETIOLOGY. X-linked recessive. Mutations involving XH2, a gene mapped to Xq13.3, are responsible for this disorder. XH2 when mutated, down-regulates expression of several genes and as such could be a global transcriptional regulator. The most sensitive diagnostic test is the demonstration of hemoglobin H inclusions in red blood cells after incubation with BCB. The inability to demonstrate hemoglobin H electrophorectically should not exclude the diagnosis. Carrier females frequently have rare cells containing hemoglobin H in their peripheral blood after incubation with 1 per cent BCB. A faint band of hemoglobin H is sometimes visible on electrophoresis.

COMMENT. A disorder referred to as α-thalassemia/mental retardation (ATR-16) syndrome is due to deletions involving chromosome 16p13.3. In that disorder the clinical phenotype is nonspecific, the mental retardation is milder than in ATR-X (I.Q. ranges from 48 to 76), and the features of hemoglobin H disease are more severe than in ATR-X, usually including anemia, severe hypochromia, hemoglobin H on electrophoresis, and hemoglobin H inclusions in red cells. In ATR-16, the phenotype is explained by deletions including the α-globin locus in chromosome band 16p13.3 while in ATR-X the α-globin complex is normal, suggesting that the mutation may encode a *trans*-acting factor involved in the normal regulation of α globin expression.

References

Wilkie, A. O. M., et al.: Clinical features and molecular analysis of the α thalassemia/mental retardation syndromes. II. Cases due to deletions involving chromosome band 16p13.3. Am. J. Hum. Genet., 46:1112, 1990.

Wilkie, A. O. M., et al.: Clinical features and molecular analysis of the α thalassemia/mental retardation syndromes. II. Cases without detectable abnormality of the α globin complex. Am. J. Hum. Genet., 46:1127, 1990.

Gibbons, R. J., et al.: A newly defined X linked mental retardation syndrome with α thalassemia. J. Med. Genet., 28:729, 1991.

Gibbons, R. J., et al.: X linked α thalassemia/mental retardation (ATR-X) syndrome: Localization to Xq12-q21.31 by X inactivation and linkage analysis. Am. J. Hum. Genet., 51:1136, 1992.

Logie, L. J., et al.: Alpha thalassemia mental retardation (ATR-X): a typical family. Arch. Dis. Child., 70:439, 1994.

Gibbons, R. J., et al.: Mutations in a putative global transcriptional regulator cause X-linked mental retardation with α-thalassemia (ATR-X syndrome). Cell, 80:837, 1995.

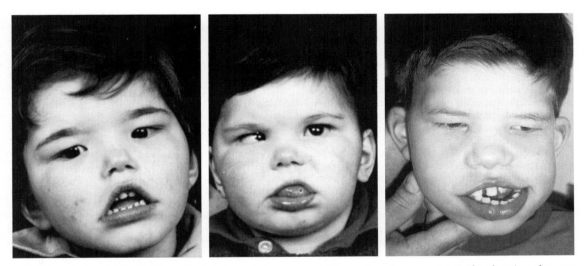

FIGURE 1. *Left and Middle*, Two affected boys at 3 years and 15 months of age, respectively, showing aberrant facies with short noses. (Courtesy of Dr. Marcus Pembrey, Institute of Child Health, University of London.) *Right*, A 15-year-old boy. Note the characteristic facies.

FG SYNDROME

Imperforate Anus, Hypotonia, Prominent Forehead

Initially described by Opitz and Kaveggia in three brothers and two of their male first cousins, over 50 cases of this X-linked recessive disorder now have been documented.

ABNORMALITIES
Performance. Mental deficiency (97 per cent). Delayed motor development and/or hypotonia (90 per cent). EEG disturbances with seizures (70 per cent). Strabismus (52 per cent). Hyperactive behavior with short attention span (70 per cent). Affable, extroverted personality with occasional temper tantrums when frustrated (54 per cent).
Growth. Postnatal onset of short stature.
Craniofacies. Postnatal onset of macrocephaly (74 per cent). Large anterior fontanel (77 per cent). Prominent forehead (95 per cent). Frontal hair upsweep (91 per cent). Ocular hypertelorism (83 per cent). Prominent lower lip (44 per cent). Small ears with simple structure (66 per cent). Facial skin wrinkling. Fine, sparse hair (66 per cent). Epicanthal folds. Short down-slanting palpebral fissures (85 per cent). Narrow palate. Large-appearing cornea (75 per cent).
Gastrointestinal. Anal anomalies including stenosis, imperforate anus, and anteriorly placed anus (38 per cent). Constipation (69 per cent).
Skeletal. Broad thumbs and great toes (81 per cent). Clinodactyly (53 per cent). Camptodactyly (55 per cent). Multiple joint contractures. Syndactyly (54 per cent). Simian crease (60 per cent). Minor vertebral defects (64 per cent). Abnormal sternum (69 per cent).
Other. Sacral dimple. Cryptorchidism (36 per cent). Low total dermal ridge count. Persistent fetal fingertip pads (50 per cent).

OCCASIONAL ABNORMALITIES. Craniosynostosis. Cleft palate. Cleft lip. Choanal atresia. Hydrocephalus. Stenotic ear canal. Short neck. Absence of corpus callosum. Defects of neuronal migration. Malrotation of cecum. Absence of mesentery. Pyloric stenosis. Dilatation of urinary tract. Hypospadias. Cardiac defect. Sensorineural deafness. High-pitched voice.

NATURAL HISTORY. Death prior to 2 years of age occurred in one third of the patients primarily because of complications of the cardiac defect or imperforate anus. Although mental deficiency has been severe in the survivors, their generally affable personality has led to an adequate social adjustment in most cases.

ETIOLOGY. X-linked recessive inheritance. In one study, five out of eight mothers of affected patients showed normal features.

References

Opitz, J. M., and Kaveggia, E. G.: Studies of malformation syndromes of man XXXIII: The FG syndrome. An X-linked recessive syndrome of multiple congenital anomalies and mental retardation. Z. Kinderhlkd., *117*:1, 1974.

Keller, M. A., et al.: A new syndrome of mental deficiency with craniofacial, limb and anal abnormalities. J. Pediatr., *8*:589, 1976.

Opitz, J. M., et al.: FG syndrome update 1988: Note of 5 new patients and bibliography. Am. J. Med. Genet., *30*:309, 1988.

Romano, C., et al.: A clinical follow-up of British patients with FG syndrome. Clin. Dysmorphol., *3*:104, 1994.

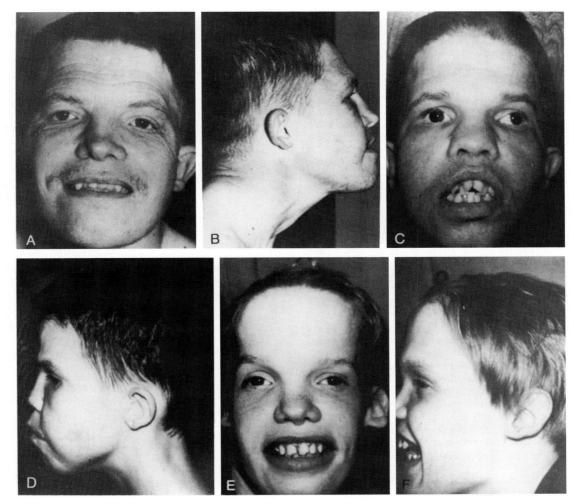

FIGURE 1. FG syndrome. Three affected male siblings; 29 (*A* and *B*), 27 (*C* and *D*), and 17 (*E* and *F*) years old. Note the frontal upsweep, lateral displacement of the medial canthi, and small ears.

STICKLER SYNDROME

(Hereditary Arthro-ophthalmopathy)

Flat Facies, Myopia, Spondyloepiphyseal Dysplasia

In 1965, Stickler et al. reported the initial observations on affected individuals in five generations of one family; the skeletal aspects have been further documented by Spranger, and the total spectrum of the disorder has been set forth by Herrmann et al.

ABNORMALITIES

Orofacial. Flat facies with depressed nasal bridge, prominent eyes, epicanthal folds, a short nose and anteverted nares; midfacial or mandibular hypoplasia, clefts of hard and/or soft palate and occasionally of uvula, Robin sequence, deafness (both sensorineural and conductive), dental anomalies.

Ocular. Myopia (8 to 18 diopters) usually present before the age of 10; chorioretinal degeneration that can occur independently of myopia; retinal detachment and/or cataracts.

Musculoskeletal. Hypotonia, hyperextensible joints, talipes equinovarus. Prominence of large joints may be present at birth. Severe arthropathy can occur in childhood. Lesser joint pains simulate juvenile rheumatoid arthritis. Subluxation of hip. Roentgenographic findings beginning in childhood include mild to moderate spondyloepiphyseal dysplasia (i.e., flat vertebrae with anterior wedging, underdevelopment of the distal tibial epiphyses, and flat irregular femoral epiphyses). Long bones show disproportionately narrow shafts relative to their metaphyseal width. Secondary degeneration of articular surfaces occurs in adulthood.

Other. Mitral valve prolapse (46 per cent).

OCCASIONAL ABNORMALITIES. Scoliosis, kyphosis, and increased lumbar lordosis. Arachnodactyly with marfanoid habitus. Pectus excavatum. Thoracic disk herniation. Thoracic myelopathy. Pes planus. Genu valgus. Mental deficiency. Short stature. Lens dislocation. Glaucoma.

COMMENT. The Stickler syndrome should be considered in any neonate with the Robin sequence, particularly in those with a family history of cleft palate and in patients with dominantly inherited myopia, nontraumatic retinal detachment, and/or mild spondyloepiphyseal dysplasia.

NATURAL HISTORY. Arthritis, if present, most commonly becomes a problem after 30 years of age. Symptoms become more severe with advancing years, leading in some cases to total hip replacement. Progressive myopia may give rise to retinal detachment and lead to blindness, the most severe complication of this disorder. Although 40 per cent develop myopia prior to 10 years of age and 75 per cent by age 20, it does not occur in some patients until after age 50. Retinal detachment can occur in childhood but usually not until after 20 years of age. It is to be hoped that the detachment can be corrected surgically if recognized early. Affected individuals with mitral valve prolapse should be evaluated periodically and should receive antibiotic prophylaxis for certain surgical procedures.

ETIOLOGY. Autosomal dominant inheritance. Although highly variable expression of this disorder has been documented, the variability is mostly between families. Within individual families, similarity in the clinical phenotype from patient to patient is the rule.

Mutations of the type II collagen gene, COL2AI, located on chromosome 12q13.11-q13.2, are responsible for the Stickler syndrome. Type II collagen is a major component of cartilage, vitreous, and nucleus pulposus, all of which are abnormal in this disorder.

References

Stickler, G. B., et al.: Hereditary progressive arthro-ophthalmopathy. Mayo Clin. Proc., 40:433, 1965.

Stickler, G. B, and Pugh, D. G.: Hereditary progressive arthro-ophthalmopathy. II. Additional observations on vertebral abnormalities, a hearing defect, and a report of a similar case. Mayo Clin. Proc., 42:495, 1967.

Spranger, J.: Arthro-ophthalmopathia hereditaria. Ann. Radiol. (Paris), 11:359, 1968.

Herrmann, J., et al.: The Stickler syndrome (hereditary arthroophthalmopathy). Birth Defects, 11(2):76, 1975.

Liberfarb, R. M., Hirose, T., and Holmes, L. B.: The Wagner-Stickler syndrome. A study of 22 families. J. Pediatr., 99:394, 1981.

Liberfarb, R. M., and Goldblatt, A.: Prevalence of mitral-valve prolapse in the Stickler syndrome. Am. J. Med. Genet., 24:387, 1986.

Francomano, C. A., et al.: The Stickler syndrome: Evidence for close linkage to the structural gene for type II collagen. Genomics, 1:293, 1987.

Temple, I. K.: Stickler's syndrome. J. Med. Genet., 26:119, 1989.

Lewkonia, R. A.: The arthropathy of hereditary arthroophthalmopathy (Stickler syndrome). J. Rheumatol., 19:1271, 1992.

Zlotogora, J., et al.: Variability of Stickler syndrome. Am. J. Med. Genet., 42:337, 1992.

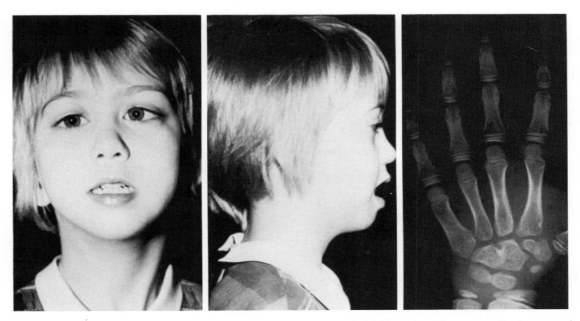

FIGURE 1. Stickler syndrome. Girl showing flat facies, inner canthal folds, relatively narrow diaphyses, and hamate-capitate carpal synostosis. (Courtesy of Dr. Judith Hall, University of British Columbia, Vancouver, British Columbia.)

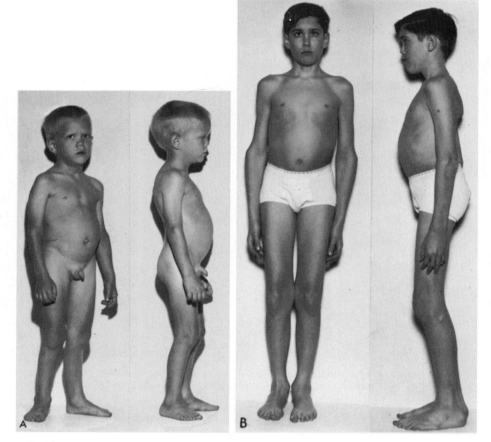

FIGURE 2. Stickler syndrome. *A* and *B,* Child and adolescent from a large affected kindred. Note relative arachnodactyly in adolescent boy. (From Stickler, G. B., et al.: Mayo Clin. Proc., *40*:433, 1965, with permission.)

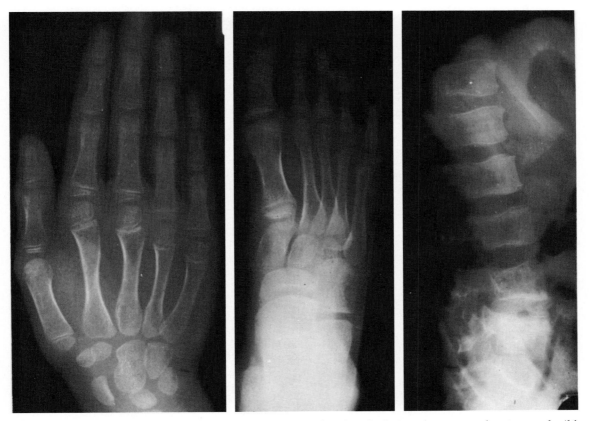

FIGURE 3. Stickler syndrome. Roentgenograms showing arachnodactyly, fusion of some carpal centers, and mild spondyloepiphyseal dysplasia.

LARSEN SYNDROME

Multiple Joint Dislocation, Flat Facies, Short Fingernails

Larsen, Schottstaedt, and Bost described six sporadic cases of this condition in 1950.

ABNORMALITIES

Facies. Flat, with depressed nasal bridge and prominent forehead, hypertelorism. Cleft palate.

Joints. Dislocations of elbows, hips, knees, and wrists, with dysplastic epiphyseal centers developing in childhood.

Hands. Long, nontapering fingers with spatulate thumbs, short nails, short metacarpals, and multiple carpal ossification centers.

Feet. Talipes equinovalgus or varus. Delayed coalescence of the two calcaneal ossification centers.

Spine. Dysraphism manifest by spina bifida and hypoplastic bodies of cervical vertebrae; scoliosis, wedged vertebrae, lordosis, and anomalies of posterior elements of thoracic spine; dysraphism, spondylolysis, and scoliosis of lumbar spine; and dysraphism of sacral spine manifest by spina bifida occulta.

OCCASIONAL ABNORMALITIES. Mental retardation. Cleft lip. Hypodontia. Conductive and sensorineural hearing loss. Hypoplastic humerus. Entropion of lower eyelids. Anterior cortical lens opacities. Simian crease. Cardiovascular defect. Mobile, infolding arytenoid cartilage. Tracheomalacia. Bronchomalacia. Tracheal stenosis. Cryptorchidism.

NATURAL HISTORY. Recent evaluations of adults in four generations of one family indicate that prognosis is relatively good following aggressive orthopedic management. Many patients begin walking late. Osteoarthritis involving large joints and progressive kyphoscoliosis are potential complications. Airway obstruction due to tracheomalacia and bronchomalacia may be life-threatening. All affected individuals should be evaluated for cervical spine instability. Particular care should be exercised during anesthesia because of the mobile arytenoid cartilage as well as the potentially dangerous spinal anomalies.

ETIOLOGY. Unknown. Autosomal dominant is the most commonly reported mode of inheritance. Presumed autosomal recessive inheritance also has been suggested based on documentation of two affected children born to clinically normal parents. However, it is equally possible that one of the clinically normal parents is a germ-line mosaic for what is actually an autosomal dominant rather than a recessive disorder.

COMMENT. A rare lethal form of this disorder has been described. The principal features include a flat facies, cleft soft palate, redundant neck skin, multiple joint dislocations, rhizomelic shortening of the upper limbs, hypoplasia of the fibula, and hypoplastic vertebral bodies. Death is secondary to pulmonary hypoplasia.

References

Larsen, L. J., Schottstaedt, E. R., and Bost, F. C.: Multiple congenital dislocations associated with characteristic facial abnormality. J. Pediatr., *37*:574, 1950.

Latta, R. J., et al.: Larsen's syndrome: A skeletal dysplasia with multiple joint dislocations and unusual facies. J. Pediatr., *78*:291, 1971.

Silverman, F. N.: Larsen's syndrome: Congenital dislocation of the knees and joints, distinctive facies, and frequently, cleft palate. Ann. Radiol. (Paris), 15: 297, 1972.

Striscinglio, P., et al.: Severe cardiac anomalies in sibs with Larsen syndrome. J. Med. Genet., *20*:422, 1983.

Bowen, J. R., et al.: Spinal deformities in Larsen's syndrome. Clin. Orthop., *197*:159, 1985.

Stanley, D., and Seymoor, N.: The Larsen syndrome occurring in four generations of one family. Int. Orthop., *8*:267, 1985.

Clayton-Smith, J., and Donnai, D.: A further patient with the lethal type of Larsen syndrome. J. Med. Genet., *25*:499, 1988.

Patrella, R., et al.: Long-term follow-up of two sibs with Larsen syndrome possibly due to parental germ-line mosaicism. Am. J. Med. Genet., *47*:187, 1993.

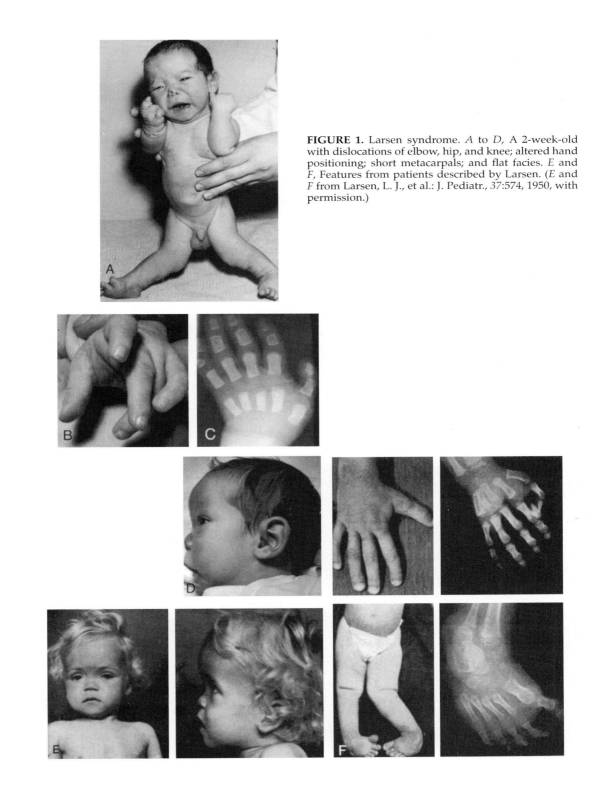

FIGURE 1. Larsen syndrome. *A* to *D*, A 2-week-old with dislocations of elbow, hip, and knee; altered hand positioning; short metacarpals; and flat facies. *E* and *F*, Features from patients described by Larsen. (*E* and *F* from Larsen, L. J., et al.: J. Pediatr., *37*:574, 1950, with permission.)

CATEL-MANZKE SYNDROME

Micrognathia, Cleft Palate, Hyperphalangy of Index Finger

First reported by Catel in 1961 in a patient who was reevaluated by Manzke in 1966, approximately 20 patients have been described with this condition.

ABNORMALITIES

Growth. Postnatal growth deficiency (75 per cent).

Facies. Cleft palate (78 per cent). Micrognathia (72 per cent). Malformed ears (33 per cent).

Limbs. Hyperphalangy of index finger in 100 per cent (an accessory bone between proximal phalanges of fingers 2 and 3). Fifth finger clinodactyly (39 per cent). Single palmar crease (40 per cent).

Other. Cardiac defects (39 per cent), primarily septal defects accompanied by overriding aorta, aortic coarctation, and/or dextrocardia.

OCCASIONAL ABNORMALITIES.

Developmental delay. Seizures. Prenatal growth deficiency. Short neck. Cleft lip. Vertebral/rib anomalies. Pectus excavatum/carinatum. Talipes equinovarus. Joint laxity/dislocation. Camptodactyly. Cryptorchidism. Umbilical and inguinal hernias. Facial paresis.

NATURAL HISTORY. Careful observation to recognize upper airway obstruction secondary to the Robin sequence should be part of routine care of newborns with this disorder. Failure to thrive is related to respiratory or cardiac problems. The vast majority of cases have normal intelligence. With advancing age, the accessory bone fuses to the proximal phalangeal epiphysis.

ETIOLOGY. Unknown. The majority of cases have been sporadic and all but two have been males.

References

Catel, W.: Differentialdiagnose von Krankheitssymptomen bei kindern und jugendlichten, Vol. 1, Ed. 3. Stuttgart, G. Thieme, 1961, p. 218.

Manzke, V. H.: Symmetrische hyperphalangie des zweiten fingers durch ein akzessorisches metacarpale. Fortschr. Roentgenstr., *105*:425, 1966.

Skinner, S. A., et al.: Catel-Manzke syndrome. Proc. Greenwood Genet. Center, *8*:60, 1989.

Wilson, G. N., et al.: Index finger hyperphalangy and multiple anomalies: Catel-Manzke syndrome? Am. J. Med. Genet., *46*:176, 1993.

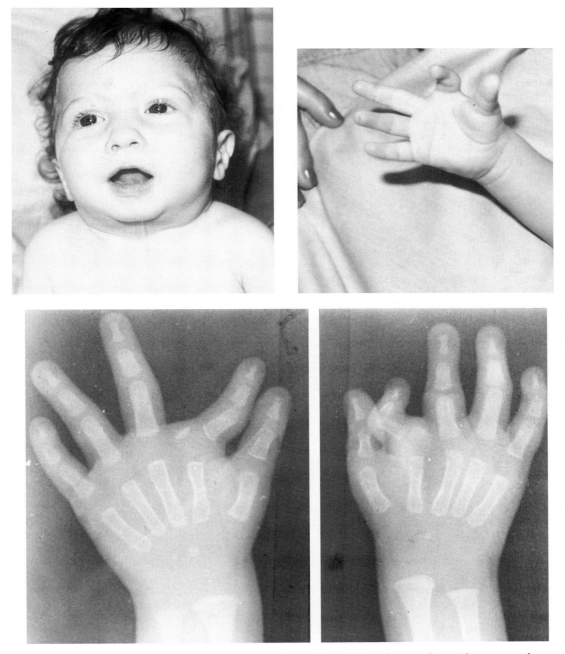

FIGURE 1. A 15-month-old male. Note the micrognathia and typical hand anomalies with accessory bones at the base of the index finger and hypoplasia of the second metacarpal. (From Stevenson, R. E., et al.: J. Med. Genet., *17*:238, 1980, with permission.)

LANGER-GIEDION SYNDROME

(Tricho-Rhino-Phalangeal Syndrome, Type II, TRP II)

*Multiple Exostoses, Bulbous Nose
With Peculiar Facies, Loose Redundant Skin in Infancy*

Hall et al. in 1974 reported five new cases of this disorder and included two further sporadic cases from the literature. An extensive review of the literature, including data from over 30 patients, has been published by Langer et al. Although the facies of these patients resemble that of tricho-rhino-phalangeal syndrome type I, other features allow for separation of the two syndromes.

ABNORMALITIES

Growth. Postnatal onset of mild growth deficiency.

Performance. Mild to severe mental deficiency in 70 per cent, with the remaining patients in the normal to dull-normal range. Delayed onset of speech. Hearing deficit.

Cranium. Microcephaly.

Facies. Large laterally protruding ears; heavy eyebrows; deep-set eyes; large bulbous nose with thickened alae nasi and septum, dorsally tented nares, and broad nasal bridge; simple philtrum, which is prominent and elongated; thin upper lip; recessed mandible.

Hair. Sparse scalp hair.

Skin. Redundancy and/or looseness in infancy, which regresses with age. Maculopapular nevi about the scalp, facies, neck, upper trunk, and upper limbs.

Hands. Cone-shaped epiphyses, which become radiologically evident at about 3 to 4 years of age; lack of normal modeling in metaphyseal regions; poor funnelization at proximal ends of phalanges; metaphyseal hooking over the lateral edges of the cone-shaped epiphyses; exostosis. Brittle nails.

Bones. Multiple exostoses of long tubular bones, with onset and distribution similar to the autosomal dominant variety of multiple cartilaginous exostoses. Exostoses can involve other areas, such as the ribs, scapulae, and pelvic bones.

Other. Perthes-like changes in capital femoral epiphysis, segmentation defects of vertebrae with scoliosis, narrow posterior ribs. Winged scapulae. Syndactyly. Lax joints. Hypotonia. Exotropia. Recurrent upper respiratory tract infections. Malocclusion. Dental abnormalities.

OCCASIONAL ABNORMALITIES. Tendency toward fractures, thin hypomineralized bones, clinobrachydactyly, simian crease, bowed femora, ocular hypotelorism, ptosis, prominent eyes, epicanthal folds, iris coloboma, abducens palsy, tragal skin tag, cardiac defects, inguinal and umbilical hernia, ureteral reflux, widely spaced nipples, delayed sexual development, small phallus, cryptorchidism, premature thelarche and pubarche, hydrometrocolpos, abnormal EEG, seizures. Hypochromic anemia.

NATURAL HISTORY. Some of these children have such redundancy and/or looseness to their skin at birth that they are misdiagnosed as having the Ehlers-Danlos syndrome. Recurrent respiratory tract infections during the first 4 to 5 years. General health is usually good after that except for a tendency toward fractures and the usual problems of multiple exostoses with their variable effects on bone growth.

ETIOLOGY. A deletion in the region 8q24.11-q24.13. In most cases the deletion is visible cytogenetically. A few cases of vertical transmission have been described. However, the vast majority have been sporadic. Langer-Giedion syndrome (TRP II) and TRP I result from different sized deletions in 8q and thus may be considered contiguous gene syndromes. Deletion of 8q24.12 is responsible for the features common to TRP I and II; deletion of 8q24.13 accounts for the development of exostosis; and the mental retardation is expected when larger pieces of 8q are deleted.

References

Hall, B. D., et al.: Langer-Giedion syndrome. Birth Defects, 10(12):147, 1974.

Langer, L. O., et al.: The tricho-rhino-phalangeal syndrome with exostosis (or Langer-Giedion syndrome): Four additional patients without mental retardation and review of the literature. Am. J. Med. Genet., 19:81, 1984.

Bühler, E. M., et al.: A final word on the tricho-rhino phalangeal syndromes. Clin. Genet., 31:273, 1987.

Ludecke, H-J., et al.: Molecular definition of the shortest region of overlap in the Langer-Giedion syndrome. Am. J. Hum. Genet. 49:1197, 1991.

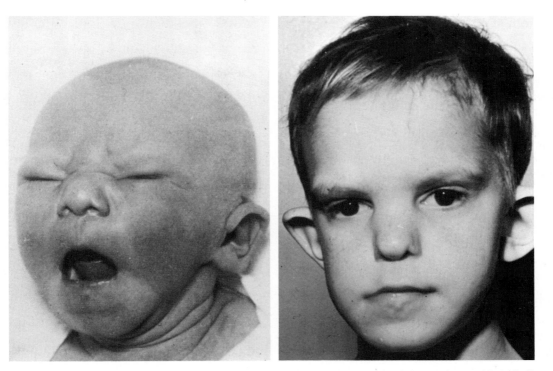

FIGURE 1. Langer-Giedion syndrome. Patient as neonate and at 7 years. Note the sparseness of hair, bulbous nose, simple but prominent philtrum, redundant folds of skin on the neck, superiorly tented nares, thin upper lip, and prominent ears.

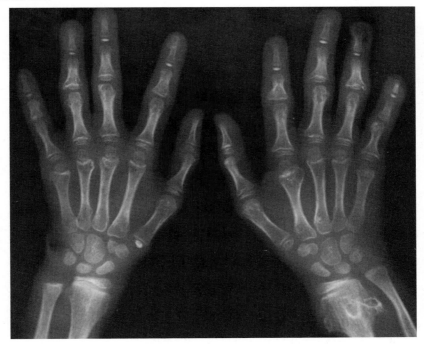

FIGURE 2. Langer-Giedion syndrome. An 11⁶/₁₂-year-old, showing exostoses, cone-shaped epiphyses, and metaphyseal hooking at the proximal ends of a number of the middle phalanges.

TRICHO-RHINO-PHALANGEAL SYNDROME, TYPE I

(TRP I)

Bulbous Nose, Sparse Hair, Epiphyseal Coning

Klingmuller reported two siblings with this pattern of malformation in 1956. Giedion further established the syndrome and set forth the tricho-rhino-phalangeal designation for it.

ABNORMALITIES

Growth. Mild growth deficiency (third to tenth percentiles).

Facial. Pear-shaped nose, prominent and long philtrum, narrow palate, with or without micrognathia, large prominent ears. Small, carious teeth with dental malocclusion. Horizontal groove on chin.

Hair. Sparse, thin hair with relative hypopigmentation.

Nails. Thin.

Skeletal. Short metacarpals and metatarsals, especially the fourth and fifth. Development of broadened middle phalangeal joint with cone-shaped epiphyses, especially the second through fourth fingers and toes. Split distal radial epiphyses. Winged scapulae.

OCCASIONAL ABNORMALITIES. Coxa plana and coxa magna, flattening of capital femoral epiphysis, partial syndactyly, pectus carinatum, pes planus, short stature, mental deficiency, craniosynostosis, deep voice, hypotonia during infancy.

NATURAL HISTORY. The hair is usually sparse at birth. Osseous changes such as the cone-shaped epiphyses may develop in early childhood and become worse until adolescent growth is complete. Increased frequency of upper respiratory tract infections has been noted in some cases. A form of degenerative hip disease often develops in young adulthood or later life.

ETIOLOGY. A deletion in chromosome region 8q24.12. Because 8q24.12 is a very narrow dark band, chromosome analysis is normal in the majority of affected individuals. Autosomal dominant inheritance has been described frequently.

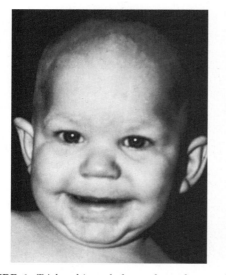

FIGURE 1. Tricho-rhino-phalangeal syndrome. A 1-year-old, showing sparse, fine hair and slight bulbous change in the nasal tip. The facial and digital aberrations change with age. (Courtesy of Dr. Jaime L. Frias, University of South Florida, Tampa, Fla.)

References

Klingmuller, G.: Über eigentumliche Konstitutionsanomalien bei 2 Schwestern und ihre Beziehungen zu neuerenentwicklungspathologischen Befunden. Hautarzt, 7:105, 1956.

Giedion, A.: Das tricho-rhino-phalangeale Syndrom. Helv. Paediatr. Acta, 21:475, 1966.

Gorlin, R. J., Cohen, M. M., and Wolfson, J.: Tricho-rhino-phalangeal syndrome. Am. J. Dis. Child., 118:585, 1969.

Fontaine, G., et al.: Le syndrome trichorhinophalangien. Arch. Fr. Pediatr., 27:635, 1970.

Felman, A. H., and Frias, J. L.: The tricho-rhino-phalangeal syndrome: Study of 16 patients in one family. Am. J. Roentgenol., 129:631, 1977.

Goodman, R. M., et al.: New clinical observations in the trichorhinophalangeal syndrome. J. Craniofac. Genet. Dev. Biol., 1:15, 1981.

Buhler, E. M., et al.: A final word on the tricho-rhino-phalangeal syndromes. Clin. Genet., 31:273, 1987.

Morchau, F. E., et al.: Tricho-rhino-phalangeal syndrome type I (TRP I) due to an apparently balanced translocation involving 8q24. Am. J. Med. Genet., 45:450, 1993.

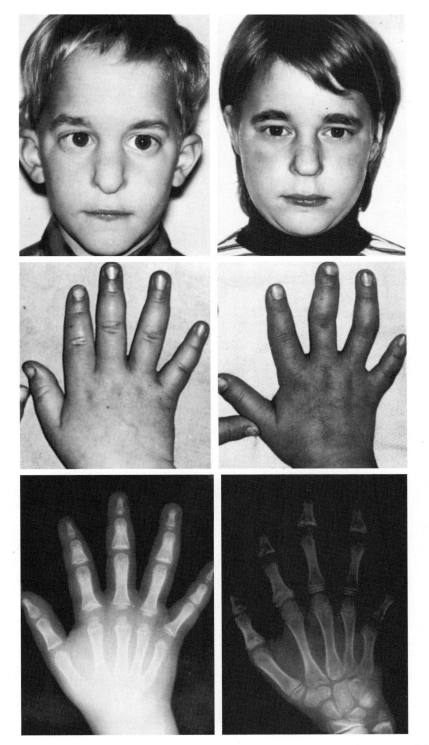

FIGURE 2. Tricho-rhino-phalangeal syndrome. A 6-year-old son (*left*) and 9-year-old daughter (*right*) of an affected father who became bald at 21 years of age. The children have fine, slow-growing hair. Note the tented hypoplastic nares, prominent philtrum, and the asymmetric length of fingers related to radiographic evidence of irregular metaphyseal cupping with cone-shaped epiphyses. (Courtesy of D. Weaver, University of Indiana, Indianapolis, Ind.)

ECTRODACTYLY–ECTODERMAL DYSPLASIA–CLEFTING SYNDROME

(EEC Syndrome)

Ectrodactyly, Ectodermal Dysplasia, Cleft Lip-Palate

Although the association of ectrodactyly and cleft lip had been noted, it was not until 1970 that Rüdiger et al. appreciated that at least some of these patients also had features of ectodermal dysplasia and named the disorder the EEC syndrome. Bixler et al. added two additional cases and summarized the past observations. Well over 100 cases have been reported.

ABNORMALITIES. All features are variable.
Skin. Fair and thin, with mild hyperkeratosis. Hypoplastic nipples.
Hair. Light-colored, sparse, thin, wiry hair on all hair-bearing areas. Distortion of the hair bulb and longitudinal grooving of hair shaft is seen on scanning electron microscopic observation.
Teeth. Partial anodontia, microdontia, caries.
Eyes. Blue irides, photophobia, blepharophimosis, defects of lacrimal duct system (84 per cent), blepharitis, dacryocystitis.
Face. Cleft lip, with or without cleft palate (72 per cent), maxillary hypoplasia, mild malar hypoplasia.
Limbs. Defects in midportion of hands and feet, varying from syndactyly to ectrodactyly (84 per cent). Mild nail dysplasia.
Genitourinary. Anomalies in 52 per cent including megaureter, duplicated collecting system, vesicoureteral reflux, ureterocele, bladder diverticuli, renal agenesis/dysplasia, hydronephrosis, micropenis, cryptorchidism, transverse vaginal septum.

OCCASIONAL ABNORMALITIES. Deafness (14 per cent), mental retardation (7 per cent), small or malformed auricles, choanal atresia, semilobar holoprosencephaly, growth hormone deficiency, hypogonadotropic hypogonadism, central diabetes insipidus.

NATURAL HISTORY. These individuals are usually of normal intelligence and adapt reasonably well with surgical closure of the facial clefts plus (as needed) limb surgery, dentures, and wigs. Early and continued ophthalmologic evaluation and management for the defective lacrimal duct system are imperative, since chronic dacryocystitis with corneal scarring can be the major debilitating problem in this disorder.

ETIOLOGY. Autosomal dominant inheritance is implied, with variable expression. No single feature, including ectrodactyly, is obligatory. Two reports have described affected individuals with cytogenetic abnormalities of the long arm of chromosome 7, suggesting that the EEC syndrome may result from disruption of the same gene or genes responsible for the autosomal dominant split hand/split foot syndrome, which maps to 7q21-q22.

References

Cockayne, E. A.: Cleft palate, hare lip, dacryocystitis and cleft hand and feet. Biometrika, 28:60, 1936.
Walker, J. C., and Clodius, L.: The syndromes of cleft lip, cleft palate and lobster-claw deformities of hands and feet. Plast. Reconstr. Surg., 32:627, 1963.
Rüdiger, R. A., Haase, W., and Passarge, E.: association of ectrodactyly, ectodermal dysplasia, and cleft lip-palate. Am. J. Dis. Child., 120:160, 1970.
Bixler, D., et al.: The ectrodactyly-ectodermal dysplasia-clefting (EEC) syndrome. Clin. Genet., 3:43, 1972.
Rodini, E. S. O., and Richieri-Costa, A.: EEC syndrome: Report on 20 new patients, clinical and genetic considerations. Am. J. Med. Genet., 37:42, 1990.
Naardi, A. C., et al.: Urinary tract involvement in EEC syndrome: A clinical study in 25 Brazilian patients. Am. J. Med. Genet., 44:803, 1992.
Scherer, S. W., et al.: Fine mapping of the autosomal dominant split hand/split foot locus on chromosome 7, band q21.3-q22.1. Am. J. Hum. Genet., 55:12, 1994.

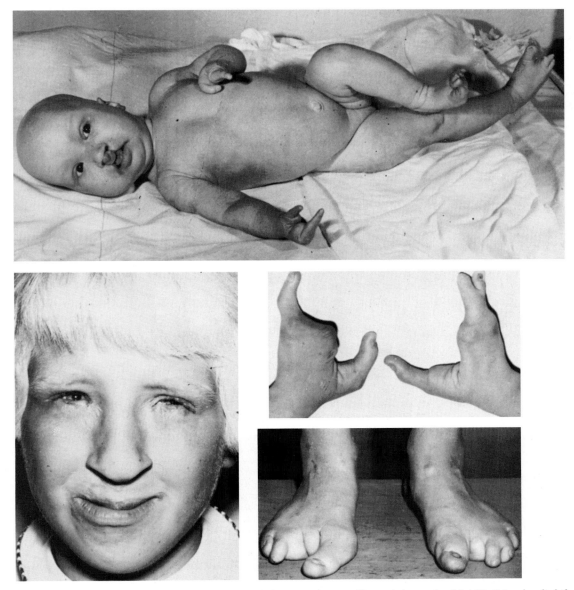

FIGURE 1. Ectrodactyly–ectodermal dysplasia–clefting syndrome. *Above*, A 6-month-old with thin, dry, lightly pigmented skin; sparse, fine hair; photophobia with inflammation of conjunctiva; facial cleft; and small ears. Note the intraindividual variability of anomaly in the feet. (From Rüdiger, R. A., et al.: Am. J. Dis. Child., *120*: 160, 1970. Courtesy of E. Passarge.) *Below*, An 18-year-old (wearing a wig) with coarse, sparse hair who has photophobia and blepharophimosis and only five poorly developed teeth. Note the small melanomata in the thin skin, which shows patchy areas of dermatitis. Studies revealed absence of the right kidney, with a double collecting system on the left.

HAY-WELLS SYNDROME OF ECTODERMAL DYSPLASIA

(Ankyloblepharon–Ectodermal Dysplasia–Clefting Syndrome, AEC Syndrome)

Ankyloblepharon, Ectodermal Dysplasia, Cleft Lip-Palate

In 1976, Hay and Wells described a specific type of ectodermal dysplasia associated with cleft lip or cleft palate and congenital filiform fusion of the eyelids. The association of facial clefting with ankyloblepharon filiforme adnatum had previously been documented in several case reports.

ABNORMALITIES

Craniofacies. Oval face. Broadened nasal bridge. Maxillary hypoplasia. Cleft lip, cleft palate, or both. Conical, widely spaced teeth. Hypodontia to partial anodontia. Ankyloblepharon filiforme adnatum.

Skin. Palmar and plantar keratoderma. Peeling erythematous, eroded skin at birth from limited to high percentage of body surface area. Hyperkeratosis. Patchy, partial deficiency of sweat glands. Partial anhidrosis. Hyperpigmentation.

Nails. Absent or dystrophic.

Hair. Wiry and sparse to alopecia.

OCCASIONAL ABNORMALITIES.
Deafness. Atretic external auditory canal. Cup-shaped auricles. Lacrimal duct atresia. Supernumerary nipples. Soft-tissue syndactyly. Rarely, ventricular septal defect or patent ductus arteriosus. Hypospadias. Micropenis. Vaginal dryness or erosions.

NATURAL HISTORY.
Surgical excision of the ankyloblepharon filiforme adnatum is required during the early neonatal period. Anomalies of the eye are not associated with these tissue bands. However, photophobia is common. Surgical closure of facial clefting and early ophthalmologic evaluation of the lacrimal duct system are required. Otitis media occurs frequently. Severe chronic granulomas of the scalp, which begin as infections, have been a serious problem and in one case have required multiple skin grafts. Although these patients have a partial capacity to produce sweat from fewer glands, so that hyperthermia is not a serious threat, heat intolerance is common. Intelligence is normal.

ETIOLOGY.
Autosomal dominant with marked variability of expression. Ankyloblepharon filiforme adnatum is not a simple failure of eyelid separation. The eyelid fusion bands histologically are composed of a central core of vascular connective tissue entirely surrounded by epithelium. Muscle fibers may be observed as well. These bands may represent abnormal proliferation of mesenchymal tissue at certain points on the lid margin or an ectodermal deficit allowing mesodermal union. The associated anomalies of this syndrome, with the exception of cleft lip, originate at 8 to 9 weeks of fetal life and can be explained as an abnormality in ectodermal development or defective ectodermal-mesodermal interaction.

References

Duke-Elder, S.: Textbook of Ophthalmology, Vol. 5. London, Kimpton, 1952, p. 4665.

Khanna, V. N.: Ankyloblepharon filiforme adnatum. Am. J. Ophthalmol., 43:774, 1957.

Rogers, J. W.: Ankyloblepharon filiforme adnatum. Arch. Ophthalmol., 65:114, 1961.

Long, J. C., and Blandford, S. E.: Ankyloblepharon filiforme adnatum with cleft lip and palate. Am. J. Ophthalmol., 53:126, 1962.

Hay, R. J., and Wells, R. S.: The syndrome of ankyloblepharon, ectodermal defects, and cleft lip and palate: An autosomal dominant condition. Br. J. Dermatol., 94:277, 1976.

Spiegel, J., and Colton, A.: AEC syndrome: Ankyloblepharon, ectodermal defects, and cleft lip and palate. J. Am. Acad. Dermatol., 12:810, 1985.

Vanderhooft, S. L., et al.: Severe skin erosions and scalp infections in AEC syndrome. Pediatr. Dermatol., 10:334, 1993.

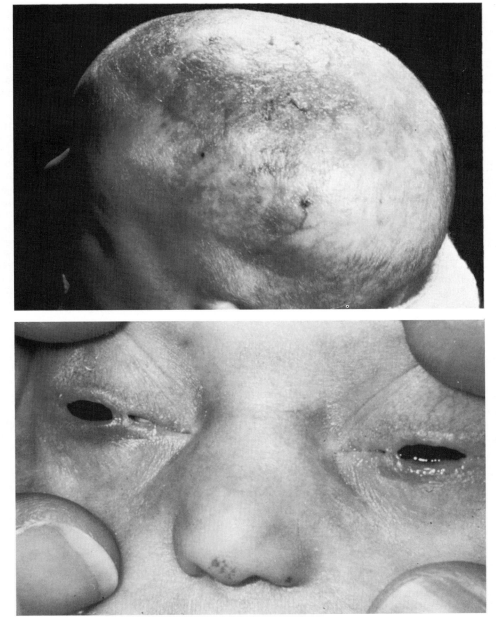

FIGURE 1. Ectodermal dysplasia with folliculitis of scalp, adhesions between eyelids, and cleft palate. (Courtesy of Dr. Mark Stephan, Madigan General Hospital, Tacoma, Wash.)

ROBERTS-SC PHOCOMELIA
(Pseudothalidomide Syndrome,
Hypomelia-Hypotrichosis–Facial Hemangioma Syndrome)

Hypomelia, Midfacial Defect, Severe Growth Deficiency

This disorder was initially described by Roberts in 1919 and more recently by Appelt et al. Freeman et al. reported five cases and reviewed the features in the 17 previously recognized patients. The cases reported by Herrmann et al. as "pseudothalidomide or SC syndrome" and the case reported by Hall and Greenberg as "hypomelia-hypotrichosis–facial hemangioma syndrome" are most likely examples of this disorder.

ABNORMALITIES
Performance. Microcephaly (80 per cent). Severe mental defect in some and borderline to mild mental deficiency in others.
Growth. Profound growth deficiency of prenatal onset. Birth weight in full-term infants 1.5 to 2.2 kg (88 per cent) and birth length frequently less than 40 cm. Mild or severe postnatal growth deficiency.
Facial. Cleft lip with or without cleft palate and prominent premaxilla, hypertelorism (87 per cent), midfacial capillary hemangioma (78 per cent), thin nares, shallow orbits and prominent eyes (69 per cent), bluish sclerae, corneal clouding (68 per cent), micrognathia. Malformed ears with hypoplastic lobules.
Hair. Sparse, may be silvery blond in some survivors.
Limbs. Hypomelia, more severe in upper limbs, varying from tetraphocomelia to lesser degrees of limb reduction, often including reduction in length or absence of the humerus (77 per cent), radius (98 per cent), or ulna (96 per cent). Reduction in numbers or length of fingers (75 per cent), syndactyly (42 per cent), or clinodactyly. Reduction or absence of femur (65 per cent), tibia (74 per cent), or fibula (80 per cent). Reduction in number of toes (27 per cent). Incomplete development of dermal ridges. Flexion contractures of knees, ankles, wrists, and/or elbows.
Genitalia. Cryptorchidism. Phallus may *appear* relatively large in relation to body size.

OCCASIONAL ABNORMALITIES.
Frontal encephalocele, hydrocephalus, brachycephaly, craniosynostosis, microphthalmia, cataract, lid coloboma, cranial nerve paralysis, short neck, nuchal cystic-hygroma, cardiac anomaly (atrial septal defect), renal anomaly (polycystic and/or horseshoe kidney). Bicornuate uterus. Rudimentary gallbladder. Accessory spleen. Polyhydramnios. Thrombocytopenia. Hypospadias.

NATURAL HISTORY.
Most individuals born at term with birth length less than 37 cm and severe defects in midfacial and limb development have been stillborn or have died in early infancy. The survivors have had marked growth deficiency, and some have had severe mental deficiency as well. Birth length greater than 37 cm, less severe limb defects, absence of cleft palate, and presence of thin nares have been associated with a better prognosis.

ETIOLOGY.
Autosomal recessive with great variability of expression within families.

COMMENT.
Approximately 80 per cent of tested individuals have had premature separation of centrometric heterochromatin of many chromosomes. Included have been a number of patients exhibiting phenotypic overlap between the Roberts syndrome and the SC phocomelia syndrome, suggesting that the two represent variable severity of the same genetic condition. Only one patient has been reported who had premature centromere separation but did not have Roberts-SC phocomelia.

References

Roberts, J. B.: A child with double cleft of lip and palate, protrusion of the intermaxillary portion of the upper jaw and imperfect development of the bones of the four extremities. Ann. Surg., 70:252, 1919.

Appelt, H., Gerken, H., and Lenz, W.: Tetraphokomelie mit Lippen-Kiefer-Gaumenspalte und Clitorishypertrophie—Ein Syndrom. Paediatr. Paedol., 2:119, 1966.

Herrmann, J., et al.: A familial dysmorphogenetic syndrome of limb deformities, characteristic facial appearance and associated anomalies: The pseudothalidomide or SC-syndrome. Birth Defects, 5:81, 1969.

Freeman, M. V. R., et al.: Roberts syndrome. Clin. Genet., 5:1, 1974.

Grosse, F. R., Pandel, C., and Wiedemann, H. R.: Tetraphocomelia–cleft palate syndrome. Humangenetik, 28:353, 1975.

Herrmann, J., and Opitz, J. M.: The SC phocomelia and the Roberts syndrome: Nosologic aspects. Eur. J. Pediatr., 125:117, 1977.

Waldenmaier, C., Aldenhoff, P., and Klemm, T.: The Roberts syndrome. Hum. Genet., 40:345, 1978.

Parry, D. M., et al.: SC phocomelia syndrome, premature centromere separation, and congenital cranial nerve paralysis in two sisters, one with malignant melanoma. Am. J. Med. Genet., 24:653, 1986.

Holmes-Siedle, M., et al.: A sibship with Roberts/SC phocomelia syndrome. Am. J. Med. Genet., 37:18, 1990.

Van Den Berg, D. J., and Francke, U.: Roberts syndrome: A review of 100 cases and a new rating syndrome for severity. Am. J. Med. Genet., 47:1104, 1993.

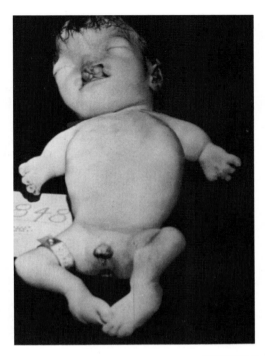

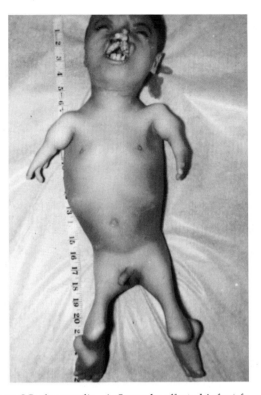

FIGURE 1. Roberts-SC phocomelia. *A,* Severely affected infant female at autopsy and, *B,* her severely growth deficient and mentally deficient 10-year-old brother. (From Freeman, M. V., et al.: Clin. Genet., *5:*1, 1974, with permission.)

FIGURE 2. *C,* An 8-year-old severely mentally deficient boy with silvery blond hair and a height age of 3^6/$_{12}$ years. (From S. Jurenka, St. Amant Wards, Winnipeg, Manitoba.) *D,* Same patient as an infant and at 8 years of age. Note capillary hemangioma on forehead in infancy and sparse scalp hair as a child. (From Hall, B. D., and Greenberg, M. H.: Am. J. Dis. Child., *123:*602, 1972, with permission.)

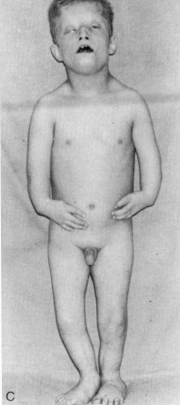

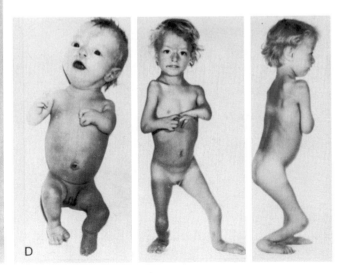

I. LIMB DEFECT AS MAJOR FEATURE

GREBE SYNDROME

Marked Distal Limb Reduction, Polydactyly, Normal Facies

Grebe described this disorder in 1952, Quelce-Salgado reported 47 cases in five kindreds in an inbred Brazilian population, and Scott more recently summarized the findings. Over 50 cases have been described.

ABNORMALITIES

Growth. Small stature due to limb deficiency.

Limbs. Reduction, most striking distally, with very short digits. Fingers resemble toes. Missing or hypoplastic bones. Legs shorter than arms. Valgus position of feet. Obese limbs. Polydactyly.

Radiographic. Short radii and ulnae, the latter most severe. Rudimentary carpal bones and phalanges. Short tibiae, with increased severity from proximal to distal segments. Short feet in valgus, with rudimentary phalanges.

NATURAL HISTORY. Many of the patients have been stillborn or have died in infancy. Survivors are said to be of normal intelligence, develop normal secondary sexual characteristics, and walk without difficulty.

ETIOLOGY. Autosomal recessive.

References

Grebe, H.: Die Achondrogenesis. Ein einfach rezessives Erbmerkmal. Folia Hered. Pathol. (Milano), 2: 23, 1952.

Quelce-Salgado, A.: A new type of dwarfism with various bone aplasias and hypoplasia of the extremities. Acta Genet., *14*:63, 1964.

Scott, C. I.: Skeletal dysplasias. Birth Defects, *5*(3):14, 1969.

Garcio-Castro, J. M., and Pereze-Comas, A.: Nonlethal achondrogenesis in two Puerto Rican sibships. J. Pediatr., *87*:948, 1975.

Romeo, G., et al.: Heterogeneity of non-lethal severe short-limb dwarfism. J. Pediatr., *91*:918, 1977.

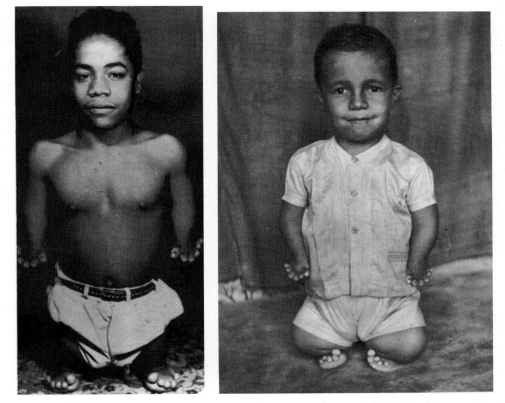

FIGURE 1. Grebe syndrome. (From Quelco-Salgado, A.: Acta Genet., *14*:63, 1964, with permission.)

POLAND SEQUENCE

Unilateral Defect of Pectoralis Muscle, Syndactyly of Hand

In 1841, Poland reported unilateral absence of the pectoralis minor and the sternal portion of the pectoralis major muscles in an individual who also had cutaneous syndactyly of the hand on the same side. This unique pattern of defects has subsequently been noted in numerous cases and has an incidence of about 1 in 20,000. It has been estimated that 10 per cent of patients with syndactyly of the hand have the Poland sequence.

ABNORMALITIES. Variable *unilateral* features from among the following:

Thorax. Hypoplasia to absence of the pectoralis major muscle, nipple, and areola. Rib defects.

Upper Limbs. Hypoplasia distally with varying degrees of syndactyly, brachydactyly, oligodactyly, and occasionally, more severe reduction deficiency.

Other. Occasional hemivertebrae, renal anomaly, Sprengel anomaly, dextrocardia in left-sided Poland sequence.

NATURAL HISTORY. Generally an otherwise normal individual.

ETIOLOGY. Unknown. It is three times as common in the male as in the female and is 75 per cent right-sided. Bouvet et al. have presented evidence of diminished blood flow to the affected side and have suggested that the primary defect may be in the development of the proximal subclavian artery, with early deficit of blood flow to the distal limb and the pectoral region, yielding partial loss of tissue in those regions. Bavinck and Weaver have proposed that early interruption of blood flow in the subclavian artery occurs proximal to the origin of the internal thoracic artery but distal to the origin of the vertebral artery. Although the vast majority of cases are sporadic and recurrence risk is negligible, there are several reports of parent-to-child transmission as well as affected siblings born to un-

affected parents. Marked variability in expression has been documented including two sibships in which the propositus had the "full" Poland sequence, whereas a sibling in one instance had only absence of the pectoral muscle and, in the other instance, only syndactyly of the hand.

COMMENT. Bavinck and Weaver suggested that the Poland, Klippel-Feil, and Moebius sequences, all of which may occur in various combinations in the same individual, should be grouped together based on a similar developmental pathogenesis into a single category referred to as the subclavian artery disruption sequence. They hypothesized that these conditions are the result of diminished blood flow in the subclavian artery, vertebral artery, and/or their branches during or around the sixth week of development. The pattern of defects depends on the specific area of diminished blood flow.

References

Poland, A.: Deficiency of the pectoral muscles. Guy's Hosp. Rep., 6:191, 1841.

Clarkson, P.: Poland's syndactyly. Guy's Hosp. Rep., 111:335, 1962.

David, T. J.: Nature and etiology of the Poland anomaly. N. Engl. J. Med., 287:487, 1972.

Mace, J. W., et al.: Poland's syndrome. Clin. Pediatr. (Phila.), 11:98, 1972.

Bouvet, J., Maroteaux, P., and Briard-Guillemot, M.: Poland's syndrome: Clinical and genetic studies— physiopathology. Nouv. Presse Med., 5:185, 1976.

Bavinck, J. N. B., and Weaver, D. D.: Subclavian artery supply disruption sequence: Hypothesis of a vascular etiology for Poland, Klippel-Feil and Möebius anomalies. Am. J. Med. Genet., 23:903, 1986.

Fraser, F. C., et al.: Pectoralis major defect and Poland sequence in second cousins: Extension of the Poland sequence spectrum. Am. J. Med. Genet., 33:468, 1989.

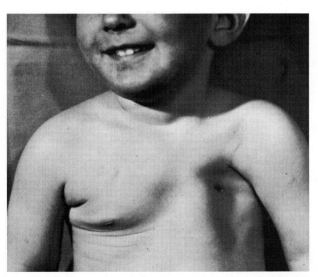

FIGURE 1. Poland sequence. The absence of the pectoralis minor and the sternal portion of the pectoralis major plus the ipsilateral syndactyly of the hand are the more usual features of this complex sequence. The bony thoracic anomaly and the hypoplasia of the hand, as noted in this otherwise normal boy, are more severe expressions of this defect.

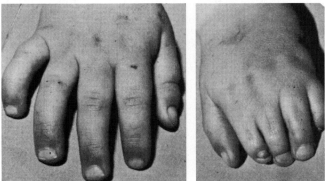

POPLITEAL PTERYGIUM SYNDROME

(Facio-Genito-Popliteal Syndrome)

Popliteal Web, Cleft Palate, Lower Lip Pits

This disorder was first reported by Trelat in 1869; greater than 80 cases have been recorded.

ABNORMALITIES

Oral. Cleft palate with or without cleft lip (90 per cent). Salivary lower lip pits (46 per cent). Intraoral fibrous band connecting maxillary and mandibular alveolar ridges (43 per cent).

Limbs. Popliteal web, in extreme form from heel to ischium (90 per cent). Toenail dysplasia, pyramidal skinfold extending from base to tip of great toe (33 per cent), syndactyly of toes.

Genitalia. Anomalies in 51 per cent including hypoplastic labia majora, scrotal dysplasia, cryptorchidism.

OCCASIONAL ABNORMALITIES. Unusual oral frenula, hypodontia, cutaneous webs between eyelids (20 per cent), atresia of external ear canal, intercrural pterygium (9 per cent), syndactyly of fingers most commonly 3–4, hypoplasia or aplasia of digits, reduction defect of thumb, fusion of distal interphalangeal joints, valgus deformity of feet, hypoplasia of tibia, bifid or absent patella, posterior dislocation of fibulae, low acetabular angle, spina bifida occulta, other vertebral anomalies, bifid ribs, short sternum, scoliosis, ambiguous external genitalia, penile ectopia and/or torsion, ectopic testes, underdevelopment of vagina and/or uterus, inguinal hernia, abnormal scalp hair.

NATURAL HISTORY. There is usually a dense fibrous cord in the posterior portion of the popliteal pterygium, and extreme care must be exercised in the surgical repair because this cord may contain the sciatic nerve and popliteal artery. There may be associated defects of muscle in the lower extremities, with limitation of function despite repair of the pterygium. The genital anomalies are most likely due to distortion by intercrural webs that often run from medial thigh to the base of the phallus. Other webbing across the eyelids or in the mouth may require excision. Although a number of cosmetic and orthopedic corrective procedures are frequently required, normal intelligence and good ambulation should be anticipated in the majority of affected individuals.

ETIOLOGY. Autosomal dominant inheritance has been implied, with wide variability in severity. No single defect including the popliteal web represents an invariable feature of this disorder.

References

Trelat, U.: Sur un vice conformation trés-rare de la lèvre-inférieure. J. Med. Chir. Prat., *40*:442, 1869.

Hecht, F., and Jarvinen, J. M.: Heritable dysmorphic syndrome with normal intelligence. J. Pediatr., *70*: 927, 1967.

Escobar, V., and Weaver, D.: The facio-genito-popliteal syndrome. Birth Defects, *14*:185, 1978.

Raithel, H., Schweckendiek, W., and Hillig, U.: The popliteal pterygium syndrome in three generations. Z. Kinderchir., *26*:56, 1979.

Hall, J. G., et al.: Limb pterygium syndromes: A review and report of eleven patients. Am. J. Med. Genet., *12*:377, 1982.

Froster-Iskenius, U. G.: Popliteal pterygium syndrome. J. Med. Genet., *27*:320, 1990.

Hunter, A.: The popliteal pterygium syndrome: Report of a new family and review of the literature. Am. J. Med. Genet., *36*:196, 1990.

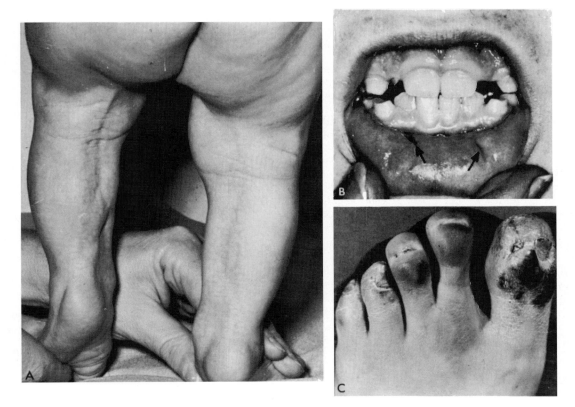

FIGURE 1. *A,* Infant with popliteal web. Note rod-like taut core. *B,* Boy with lower lip pits (*arrows*). *C,* Toenail dysplasia, a variable feature. (From Hecht, F., and Jarvinen, J. M.: J. Pediatr., *70:*927, 1967, with permission.)

ESCOBAR SYNDROME
(Multiple Pterygium Syndrome)

Multiple Pterygia, Camptodactyly, Syndactyly

Originally described by Bussiere in 1902, this disorder was fully delineated as a distinct entity by Escobar et al. in 1978. About 50 cases have been noted.

ABNORMALITIES
Growth. Small stature.

Facies. Ptosis of eyelids with antimongoloid slant of palpebral fissures; inner canthal folds; hypertelorism; micrognathia with downturning corners of mouth; difficulty opening mouth widely; long philtrum; cleft palate; sad, flat, emotionless face. Low-set ears.

Pterygia. Pterygia of neck, axillae, antecubital, popliteal, and intercrural areas.

Limbs. Pterygia plus camptodactyly, syndactyly, equinovarus, and/or rocker-bottom feet.

Genitalia. Cryptorchidism, absence of labia majora.

Other. Scoliosis, kyphosis, fusion of vertebrae and/or fused laminae, rib anomalies, absent or dysplastic patella.

OCCASIONAL ABNORMALITIES. Anterior clefts of vertebral bodies, tall vertebral bodies with decreased anteroposterior diameter, failed fusion of posterior neural arches. Rib fusions. Long clavicles with lateral hooks, modeled scapulae, dislocated radial head, distal radioulnar separation. Dislocation of hip, hypoplastic nipples, conductive hearing loss, abnormal ossicles, diaphragmatic hernia, hypospadias, cardiac defects.

NATURAL HISTORY. The majority of affected individuals become ambulatory. Intelligence is normal. Respiratory problems including pneumonia plus episodes of dyspnea and apnea presumably secondary to the kyphoscoliosis and small chest size lead to significant morbidity as well as death in the first year of life in approximately 6 per cent of patients.

The pterygia may become more obvious with time, leading to fixed contractures. Early, vigorous physical therapy is indicated to retain the greatest joint mobility. Scoliosis occurs prior to 5 years of age in the majority of patients and frequently requires surgical fusion. Formal hearing evaluation is indicated in all individuals.

ETIOLOGY. Autosomal recessive.

References

Escobar, V., et al.: Multiple pterygium syndrome. Am. J. Dis. Child., *132*:609, 1978.

Hall, J. G., et al.: Limb pterygium syndromes: A review and report of eleven patients. Am. J. Med. Genet., *12*:377, 1982.

Thompson, E. M., et al.: Multiple pterygium syndrome: Evolution of the phenotype. J. Med. Genet., *24*:733, 1987.

Ramer, J. C., et al.: Multiple pterygium syndrome. An overview. Am. J. Dis. Child., *142*:794, 1988.

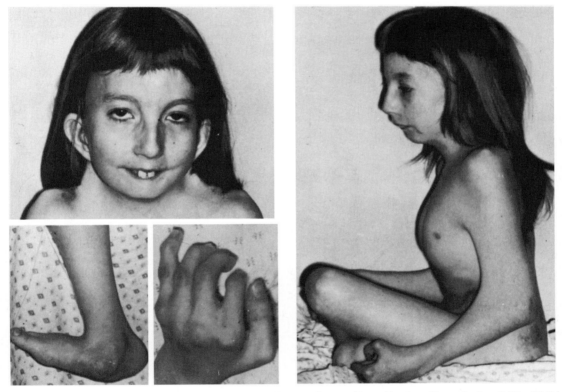

FIGURE 1. A 12-year-old girl showing features of Escobar syndrome. (From Escobar, V., et al.: Am. J. Dis. Child., *132*:609, 1978, with permission.)

CHILD SYNDROME

Unilateral Hypomelia and Skin Hypoplasia, Cardiac Defect

Falek et al. reported two female siblings with this unique pattern of malformation in 1968, and Shear noted a comparable case. At least 30 cases have now been reported. The term CHILD is an acronym for *c*ongenital *h*emidysplasia with *i*chthyosiform erythroderma and *l*imb *d*efects.

ABNORMALITIES

Growth. Mild prenatal growth deficiency.

Limbs. Unilateral hypomelia varying from absence of a limb to hypoplasia of some metacarpals and phalanges. Webbing at elbows and knees. Joint contractures.

Skin. Unilateral erythema and scaling, with sharp midline demarcation anteriorly and posteriorly. Unilateral alopecia, hyperkeratosis, and nail destruction.

Other Skeletal. Ipsilateral hypoplasia of bones involving any part of the skeleton, including mandible, clavicle, scapula, ribs, and vertebrae. Ipsilateral punctate epiphyseal calcifications.

Other. Cardiac septal defects. Single coronary ostium. Single ventricle. Unilateral renal agenesis.

OCCASIONAL ABNORMALITIES.
Ipsilateral hypoplasia of brain, cranial nerves, spinal cord, lung, thyroid, adrenal gland, ovary, and fallopian tube. Mild mental deficiency. Mild contralateral anomalies of skin, bone, and/or viscera. Scoliosis. Cleft lip. Umbilical hernia. Hearing loss. Meningomyelocele.

NATURAL HISTORY.
The erythema and scaling usually present at birth may develop during the first few weeks of life. New areas of involvement may occur as late as 9 years. The face is spared. Early death is due primarily to cardiac defects. The right side of the body has been involved in 14 cases, the left side in six. Treatment with etretinate, an aromatic retinoid, has been successful in management of the skin problems in some cases.

COMMENT.
CHILD syndrome is clinically similar to Conradi-Hünermann syndrome and rhizomelic chondrodysplasia punctata, disorders which exhibit a deficiency of peroxisomal function. The activity of two peroxisomal enzymes were decreased and fewer peroxisomes were present in fibroblasts from a child with CHILD syndrome, suggesting that these three disorders may be related pathogenetically.

ETIOLOGY.
Unknown. All but one affected individual has been a female, raising the possibility of X-linked dominant inheritance; lethal in the hemizygous male.

References

Falek, A., et al.: Unilateral limb and skin deformities with congenital heart disease in twin siblings. A lethal syndrome. J. Pediatr., *73*:910, 1968.

Shear, C. S., et al.: Syndrome of unilateral ectromelia, psoriasis, and central nervous system anomalies. Birth Defects, *7*:197, 1971.

Happle, R., Koch, H., and Lenz, W.: The CHILD syndrome. Eur. J. Pediatr., *134*:27, 1980.

Christiansen, J. R., Petersen, H. O., and Søgaard, H.: The CHILD syndrome—congenital hemidysplasia with ichthyosiform erythroderma and limb defects. A case report. Acta Derm. Venereol. (Stockh.), *64*:165, 1984.

Hebert, A., et al.: The CHILD syndrome: Histologic and ultrastructural studies. Arch. Dermatol., *123*:503, 1987.

Emami, S., et al.: Peroxisomal abnormality in fibroblasts from involved skin of CHILD syndrome. Case study and review of peroxisomal disorders in relation to skin disease. Arch. Dermatol., *128*:1213, 1992.

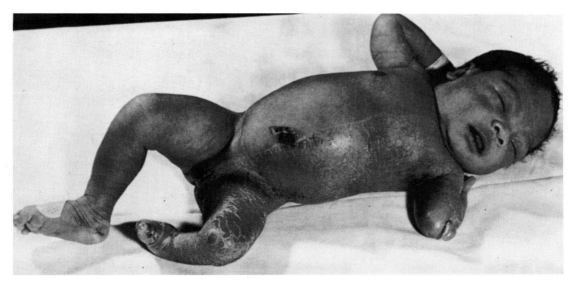

FIGURE 1. CHILD syndrome. One of two affected siblings, both with left-sided involvement. (From Falek, A., et al.: J. Pediatr., 73:910, 1968, with permission.)

FEMORAL HYPOPLASIA– UNUSUAL FACIES SYNDROME

Femoral Hypoplasia, Short Nose, Cleft Palate

Following single case reports in 1961 and 1965 by Franz and O'Rahilly and by Kucera et al., Daentl et al. recognized four additional patients and set forth this unique syndrome in 1975.

ABNORMALITIES

Growth. Small stature, predominantly the result of short lower limbs.

Facial. Short nose with hypoplastic alae nasi, long philtrum, and thin upper lip. Micrognathia, cleft palate. Up-slanting palpebral fissures. Low-set, poorly formed pinnae.

Limbs. Bilateral, usually asymmetrical involvement. Hypoplastic to absent femora and variable asymmetric involvement of fibula and tibia. Variable hypoplasia of humeri with restricted elbow movement, including radioulnar and radiohumeral synostosis and limited shoulder movement. Sprengel deformity. Talipes equinovarus.

Pelvis. Hypoplastic acetabulae, constricted iliac base with vertical ischial axis, and large obturator foramina.

Spine. Dysplastic sacrum. Missing vertebrae and/or hemivertebrae. Sacralization of lumbar vertebrae. Scoliosis.

Genitourinary. Cryptorchidism. Inguinal hernia. Small penis, testes, or labia majora. Polycystic kidneys, absent kidneys, abnormal collecting system.

OCCASIONAL ABNORMALITIES. Astigmatism; esotropia; short third, fourth, and fifth metatarsals; preaxial polydactyly of feet; tapered, fused, or missing ribs; inguinal hernia. Cardiac defects including ventricular septal defect, pulmonary stenosis, and truncus arteriorus. Craniosynostosis.

NATURAL HISTORY. Though there may be problems in speech development, the patients have been of normal intelligence. Most of them have been ambulatory.

ETIOLOGY. Unknown. Although the vast majority of cases are sporadic, an affected male whose daughter is similarly affected raises the possibility of autosomal dominant inheritance. Maternal diabetes has been documented frequently.

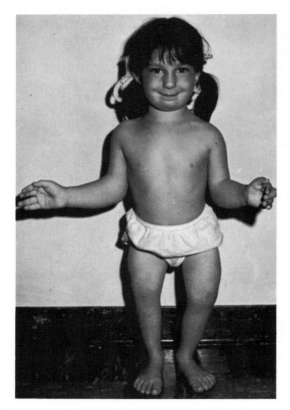

FIGURE 1. Femoral hypoplasia–unusual facies syndrome. Girl showing short humeri with synostosis at the elbow, in addition to femoral shortness.

References

Franz, C. H., and O'Rahilly, R.: Congenital skeletal limb deficiencies. J. Bone Joint Surg. [Am.], *43*:1202, 1961.

Kucera, V. J., Lenz, W., and Maier, W.: Missbildungen der Beine und der Kaudalen Wirbelsaeule bei Kindern diabetischer Muetter. Dtsch. Med. Wochenschr., *90*:901, 1965.

Daentl, D. L., et al.: Femoral hypoplasia–unusual facies syndrome. J. Pediatr., *86*:107, 1975.

Lampert, R. P.: Dominant inheritance of femoral hypoplasia–unusual facies syndrome. Clin. Genet., *17*:255, 1980.

Johnson, J. P., et al.: Femoral hypoplasia–unusual facies syndrome in infants of diabetic mothers. J. Pediatr., *102*:866, 1983.

Baraitser, M., et al.: Femoral hypoplasia unusual facies syndrome with preaxial polydactyly. Clin. Dysmorphol., *3*:40, 1994.

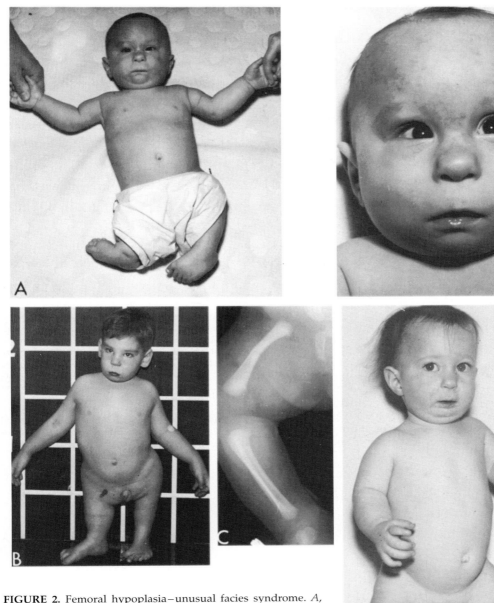

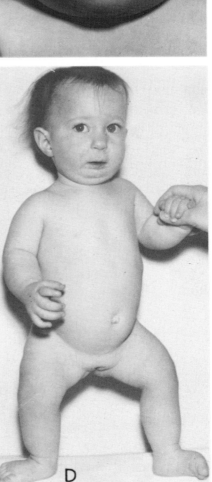

FIGURE 2. Femoral hypoplasia–unusual facies syndrome. *A*, Female infant. *B*, A 5-year-old boy. *C* and *D*, Roentgenogram and female infant, showing hypoplastic fibula and lag in mineralization of secondary centers at the knee. Note the short nose, small mandible, variable and asymmetric hypoplasia of the femurs and humeri, and inability to extend the elbow fully. (From Daentl, D. L., et al.: J. Pediatr., *86*:107, 1975, with permission.)

TIBIAL APLASIA-ECTRODACTYLY SYNDROME

Split-Hand/Split-Foot,
Absence of Long Bones of Arms and Legs

A single patient with this pattern of malformation was described in 1575 by Ambroise Paré. Subsequently, more than 100 affected individuals have been reported. The complete spectrum of this condition has been set forth by Majewski et al. and by Hoyme et al.

ABNORMALITIES

Hands. Abnormalities in 68 per cent, most commonly ectrodactyly (split hand). Absence of multiple fingers.

Feet. Abnormalities in 64 per cent, most commonly variable absence of tarsals, metatarsals, and toes.

Limbs. Absence of long bone of legs in 55 per cent, most commonly tibial aplasia. Tibial hypoplasia. Fibular hypoplasia or aplasia.

OCCASIONAL ABNORMALITIES. Cup-shaped ears. Aplasia of ulna, radius, or humerus. Monodactyly. Absence of multiple fingers. Syndactyly. Proximally placed thumbs. Ectrodactyly of feet. Metatarsus adductus. Talipes equinovarus. Supernumerary preaxial digit. Postaxial polydactyly. Absence of entire leg. Bifid or hypoplastic femur. Contracted knee joint with patellar hypoplasia. Hypoplasia of great toe. Craniosynostosis. Bifid xiphoid.

ETIOLOGY. Autosomal dominant with widely variable expression and frequent examples of nonpenetrance in structurally normal obligate carriers.

COMMENT. Because of the frequency of clinically normal individuals who carry the gene for this disorder, prenatal ultrasonographic studies should be performed in all pregnancies in affected families.

References

Majewski, F., et al.: Aplasia of tibia with split-hand/split-foot deformity. Report of six families with 35 cases and considerations about variability and penetrance. Hum. Genet., 70:136, 1985.

Hoyme, H. E., et al.: Autosomal dominant ectrodactyly and absence of long bones of upper or lower limbs: Further clinical delineation. J. Pediatr., 111: 538, 1987.

Richieri-Costa, A., et al.: Tibial hemimelia: Report on 37 new cases. Clinical and genetic considerations. Am. J. Med. Genet., 27:867, 1987.

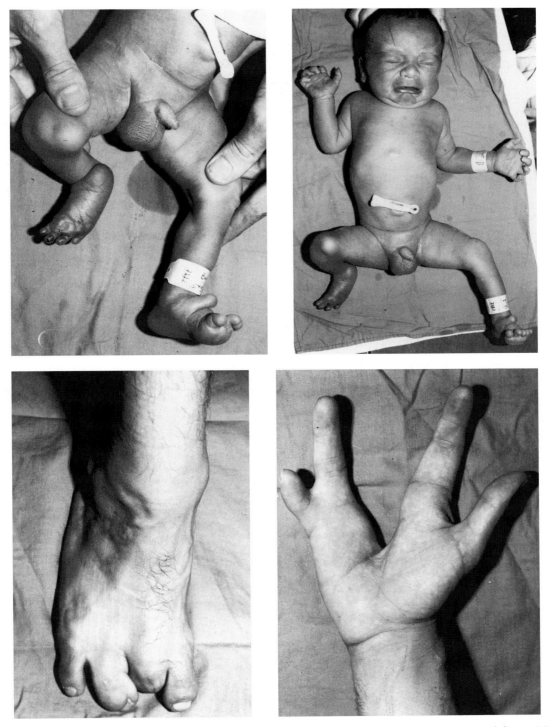

FIGURE 1. *Above*, Newborn infant with absent right tibia and great toe and supernumerary preaxial digit arising from dorsum of right foot. *Below*, Father of newborn infant pictured above. Note the typical split hand. Ectrodactyly of the foot has been surgically repaired. (From Hoyme, H. E., et al.: Pediatr., *111*:538, 1987, with permission.)

ADAMS-OLIVER SYNDROME

Aplasia Cutis Congenita,
Terminal Transverse Defects of Limbs

Adams and Oliver described eight members of a family with this disorder in 1945. More than 80 affected individuals have been reported.

ABNORMALITIES
Growth. Mild growth deficiency (third to tenth percentile).
Scalp. Aplasia cutis congenita over posterior parietal region, with or without an underlying defect of bone. In older individuals, solitary or multiple, round-oval hairless scars are found in the parietal region. Tortuous veins over posterior scalp.
Limbs. Variable degrees of terminal transverse defects, including those of lower legs, feet, hands, fingers, toes, and/or distal phalanges. Short fingers. Small toenails.
Skin. Cutis marmorata.

OCCASIONAL ABNORMALITIES. Encephalocele. Acrania. Microcephaly. Arrhinencephaly. Esotropia. Microphthalmia. Mental retardation. Cleft lip. Cleft palate. Cardiac defect. Syndactyly. Talipes equinovarus. Accessory nipples. Duplicated collecting system. Imperforate vaginal hymen. Aplasia cutis congenita on trunk and limbs. Thin, hyperpigmented skin. Poland sequence. Chylothorax.

NATURAL HISTORY. Although prognosis is excellent in the vast majority of cases, larger scalp defects are more likely to be associated with underlying defects of bone and, where the superior sagittal sinus or dura are exposed, an increased risk of hemorrhage and/or meningitis. For those cases, early surgical intervention with grafting is indicated. For the usual case in which the sagittal sinus and/or dura are not exposed, healing without need for grafting virtually always occurs.

ETIOLOGY. Autosomal dominant with marked variability in expression and lack of penetrance in some cases. A careful physical examination and radiographs of hands and feet are indicated in first-degree relatives of affected individuals.

References

Adams, F. H., and Oliver, C. P.: Hereditary deformities in man due to arrested development. J. Hered., *36*:3, 1945.
Scribanu, N., and Tamtamy, S. A.: The syndrome of aplasia cutis congenita with terminal transverse defects of limbs. J. Pediatr., *87*:79, 1975.
Bonafede, R. P., and Beighton, P.: Autosomal dominant inheritance of scalp defects with ectrodactyly. Am. J. Med. Genet., *3*:35, 1979.
Kuster, W., et al.: Congenital scalp defects with distal limb anomalies (Adams-Oliver syndrome): Report of ten cases and review of the literature. Am. J. Med. Genet., *31*:99, 1988.
Toriello, H. W., et al.: Scalp and limb defects with cutis marmorata telangiectatica congenita: Adams-Oliver syndrome? Am. J. Med. Genet., *29*:269, 1988.
Der Kaloustian, V. M., et al.: Possible common pathogenetic mechanisms for Poland sequence and Adams-Oliver syndrome. Am. J. Med. Genet., *38*:69, 1991.
Whitely, C. B., and Gorlin, R. J.: Adams-Oliver syndrome revisited. Am. J. Med. Genet., *40*:319, 1991.
Bamforth, J. S., et al.: Adams-Oliver syndrome: A family with extreme variability in clinical expression. Am. J. Med. Genet., *49*:393, 1994.

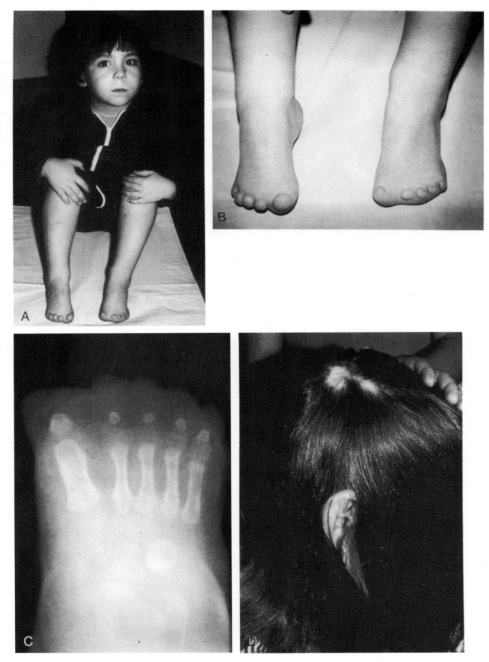

FIGURE 1. Adams-Oliver syndrome. *A* to *D*, Boy, 3⁹/₁₂ years old, and his mother's sister. Note the terminal transverse defects involving the toes (*A* to *C*) and the area of aplasia cutis congenita over his maternal aunt's posterior scalp (*D*). She was otherwise normal.

HOLT-ORAM SYNDROME

(Cardiac-Limb Syndrome)

Upper Limb Defect, Cardiac Anomaly, Narrow Shoulders

This syndrome of skeletal and cardiovascular abnormalities was first described by Holt and Oram in 1960. Over 200 cases have been reported.

ABNORMALITIES

Skeletal. All gradations of defect in the upper limb and shoulder girdle. The thumbs may be absent, hypoplastic, triphalangeal, or bifid. Syndactyly often occurs between thumb and index finger. Phocomelia (10 per cent). Asymmetric involvement is frequently seen. Hypoplasia to absence of first metacarpal and radius. Defects of ulna, humerus, clavicle, scapula, sternum. Decreased range of motion at elbows and shoulders, which are often narrow and sloping. Carpal anomalies particularly involving the scaphoid, which is often hypoplastic and/or has a bipartite ossification. Proximal as well as distal epiphyses of metacarpals, particularly the first.

Cardiovascular. Ostium secundum atrial septal defect, sometimes with arrhythmia, and ventricular septal defect have been the most common defects, and about one third of the patients have had other types of congenital heart defects. Hypoplasia of distal blood vessels.

OCCASIONAL ABNORMALITIES.
Hypertelorism. Patent ductus arteriosus, pulmonic stenosis. Absent pectoralis major muscle. Pectus excavatum, thoracic scoliosis. Vertebral anomalies. Absence of one or more ossification centers in the wrist. Sprengel deformity. Postaxial and central polydactyly.

ETIOLOGY. Autosomal dominant with variable expression. The gene responsible for some cases of Holt-Oram syndrome is located on the long arm of chromosome 12 (12q2). However, at least two phenotypically indistinguishable families have been analyzed that did not show linkage to 12q2, indicating genetic heterogeneity for this disorder.

COMMENT. There is no correlation between the severity of the limb defect and the cardiac defect. Because of the marked variability in expression, at-risk individuals with a normal physical exam should have radiographs of wrists, arms, and hands and an echocardiogram.

References

Holt, M., and Oram, S.: Familial heart disease with skeletal malformations. Br. Heart J., 22:236, 1960.

Poznauski, A., et al.: Objective evaluation of the hand in the Holt-Oram Syndrome. Birth Defects, 8:125, 1972.

Kaufman, R. L., et al.: Variable expression of the Holt-Oram syndrome. Am. J. Dis. Child., 127:21, 1974.

Hurst, J. A., et al.: The Holt-Oram syndrome. J. Med. Genet., 28:406, 1991.

Moens, P., et al.: Holt-Oram syndrome: Postaxial and central polydactyly as variable manifestations in a four generation family. Genet. Couns., 4:277, 1993.

Basson, C. T., et al.: The clinical and genetic spectrum of the Holt-Oram syndrome (heart-hand syndrome). N. Engl. J. Med., 330:885, 1994.

Terrett, J. A., et al.: Holt-Oram syndrome is a genetically heterogeneous disease with one locus mapping to human chromosome 12q. Nat. Genet., 6:401, 1994.

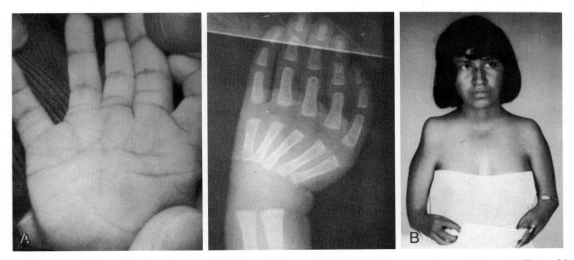

FIGURE 1. *A*, Finger-like thumb (to right) in an infant with the Holt-Oram syndrome. (From M. Feingold, National Birth Defects Center, Brighton, Mass.) *B*, A 15-year-old with auricular septal defect. Note severe forearm hypoplasia, absence of thumbs, and altered shoulder girdle.

LEVY-HOLLISTER SYNDROME

(Lacrimo-Auriculo-Dento-Digital Syndrome,
LADD Syndrome)

Although Levy described the first affected patient in 1967, this disorder was first delineated by Hollister et al. in 1973. At least 20 cases have been reported.

ABNORMALITIES

Lacrimal Anomalies. Nasolacrimal duct obstruction; aplasia or hypoplasia of lacrimal puncta (45 per cent). Alacrima due to hypoplasia or aplasia of lacrimal glands (40 per cent).

Ears. Simple, cup-shaped ears with short helix and underdeveloped antihelix (70 per cent).

Hearing. Mild to severe mixed conductive and sensorineural hearing loss (55 per cent).

Dental. Abnormalities in 90 per cent including hypodontia, peg-shaped incisors, enamel hypoplasia of both deciduous and permanent teeth. Delayed eruption of primary teeth.

Limb. Digital abnormalities in 95 per cent including digitalization of thumb; deficiency of bone and soft tissue of thumb and index finger; preaxial polydactyly; triphalangeal thumb; duplication of distal phalanx of thumb; thenar muscle hypoplasia; syndactyly between index and middle fingers; clinodactyly of third and fifth fingers; absent radius and thumb, and broad first toe. Shortening of radius and ulna.

OCCASIONAL ABNORMALITIES. Absence of parotid glands and Stensen ducts. Nasolacrimal fistulae. Hypertelorism or telecanthus; down-slanting palpebral fissures; renal agenesis; coronal hypospadias. Nephrosclerosis. 2–3 and 3–4 syndactyly of toes. Cystic ovarian disease.

NATURAL HISTORY. A persistent dry mouth with eating difficulties and a propensity to develop inflammation of the oral mucosa and candidiasis frequently occur early in life. Because of decreased salivation and enamel hypoplasia, severe dental caries occur. A lack of tears and chronic dacryocystitis results from hypoplasia of the nasolacrimal duct system. A decreased tear production also can occur. Although the hearing loss is usually mild to moderate, it has been severe in a few cases.

ETIOLOGY. Autosomal dominant.

References

Levy, W. J.: Mesoectodermal dysplasia. Am. J. Ophthalmol., *63*:978, 1967.

Hollister, D. W., et al.: The lacrimo-auriculo-dento-digital syndrome. J. Pediatr., *83*:438, 1973.

Shiang, E. L., and Holmes, L. B.: The lacrimo-auriculo-dento-digital syndrome. Pediatrics, *59*:927, 1977.

Thompson, E., Pembrey, M., and Graham, J. M.: Phenotypic variation in LADD syndrome. J. Med. Genet., *22*:382, 1985.

Wiedemann, H. R., and Drescher, J.: LADD syndrome: Report of new cases and review of the clincal spectrum. Eur. J. Pediatr., *144*:579, 1986.

Heinz, G. W., et al.: Ocular manifestations of the lacrimo-auriculo-dento-digital syndrome. Am. J. Ophthalmol., *115*:243, 1993.

Horn, D., and Witkowski, R.: Phenotype and counseling in lacrimo-auriculo-dento-digital (LADD) syndrome. Genet. Couns., *4*:305, 1993.

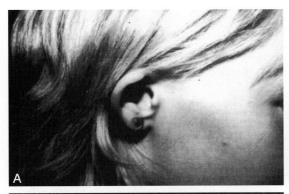

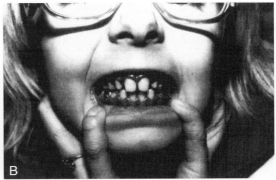

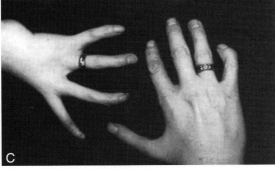

FIGURE 1. Levy-Hollister syndrome. A 9-year-old female showing small, cupped ears (*A*), small, peg-shaped teeth with enamel dysplasia (*B*), and (*C*) the digitalized thumb plus fifth finger clinodactyly on the hand at the right of the photograph and a long tapering thumb with absent creases and surgically removed index finger on the hand at the left of the photograph. (Courtesy of Dr. H. E. Hoyme, University of Arizona, Tucson, Ariz.)

FANCONI PANCYTOPENIA SYNDROME

Radial Hypoplasia, Hyperpigmentation, Pancytopenia

Since Fanconi's original description of three affected siblings in 1927, numerous cases have been reported. Glanz and Fraser as well as Giampietro et al. have documented the marked variability of the clinical phenotype. Since 25 per cent of affected individuals are structurally normal, the importance of considering this diagnosis in any anemic child with chromosome breaks, even in the absence of dysmorphic features on the physical examination, has been emphasized. Conversely, since the median age of onset of the hematologic abnormalities is 7 years (range, birth to 31 years), this diagnosis should be considered in all children with the characteristic dysmorphic features even in the absence of hematologic abnormalities.

ABNORMALITIES
Growth. Short stature, frequently of prenatal onset.
Performance. Microcephaly (25 to 37 per cent). Mental deficiency in 25 per cent.
Eye. Anomalies in 41 per cent including ptosis of eyelid, strabismus, nystagmus, and microphthalmus.
Skeletal. Radial ray defect in 49 per cent including hypoplasia to aplasia of thumb, with supernumerary thumbs in some cases and/or hypoplastic or aplastic radii.
Urogenital. Renal and urinary tract anomalies in 34 per cent including hypoplastic and/or malformed kidneys and double ureters. Abnormalities in males including hypospadias, small penis, small testes, and/or cryptorchidism in 20 per cent.
Hematologic. Pancytopenia manifested by poikilocytosis, anisocytosis, reticulocytopenia, thrombocytopenia, and leukopenia. Decreased bone marrow cellularity. Leukemia. Myelodysplastic syndrome.
Skin. Brownish pigmentation (64 per cent).

OCCASIONAL ABNORMALITIES
Central Nervous System. Abnormalities in 8 per cent including hydrocephalus, absent septum pellucidum, absent corpus callosum, neural tube closure defect, migration defect, Arnold-Chiari malformation, and/or single ventricle.
Gastrointestinal. Abnormalities in 14 per cent, including anorectal, duodenal atresia, tracheoesophageal fistula with or without esophageal atresia, annular pancreas, intestinal malrotation, intestinal obstruction, and duodenal web.

Other Skeletal. Defects occurring in 22 per cent, including congenital hip dislocation, scoliosis, rib anomalies, talipes equinovarus, broad base of proximal phalanges, sacral agenesis and/or hypoplasia, Perthes disease, Sprengel deformity, genu valgum, leg length discrepancy, and kyphosis.
Other. Cardiac defect (13 per cent). Auricular anomaly (15 per cent). Deafness (11 per cent). Syndactyly.

NATURAL HISTORY. The majority of patients are relatively small at birth. Respiratory tract infections may be a frequent problem. The uneven brownish pigmentation of the skin tends to increase with age, being most evident in the anogenital area, groin, axillae, and trunk. Development of bleeding, pallor, and/or recurring infection usually appears between 5 and 10 years of age, although pancytopenia may occur in infancy or as late as the third decade. Although the majority of patients get hematologic improvement from high-dose androgen therapy, bone marrow transplant is the only treatment offering an actual cure.

Batturini et al. have analyzed data from 388 affected individuals reported to the International Fanconi Anemia Registry. One hundred thirty-five (35 per cent) died at a median age of 13 years, the majority (120) secondary to hematologic abnormalities. Forty-nine of the hematologic-related deaths were from bone marrow failure, 37 from treatment-related complications after transplant, and 34 from myelodysplastic syndrome or acute myelogenous leukemia.

ETIOLOGY. Autosomal recessive. Four complementation groups (A, B, C, and D) have been identified, indicating that this disorder is genetically heterogeneous. A gene for group A has been linked to the distal region of chromosome 20q. A gene for complimentation group C has been cloned and mapped to 9q22.3.

COMMENT. Successful prenatal and postnatal diagnoses of this disorder can now be accomplished by demonstrating a high frequency of diepoxy-butane–induced chromosomal breakage in peripheral blood lymphocytes as well as in cultured amniotic fluid cells.

References

Fanconi, G.: Familiäre infantile pernizosaaritige anämie. Z. Kinderheilkd., *117*:257, 1927.

Garriga, S., and Crosby, W. H.: The incidence of leukemia in families of patients with hypoplasia of the marrow. Blood, *14*:1008, 1959.

Nilsson, L. R.: Chronic pancytopenia with multiple congenital abnormalities (Fanconi's anaemia). Acta Paediatr., *49*:518, 1960.

Schmid, W. K., et al.: Chromosomenbrueihigkeit bei der familiären Panmyelopathie (Typus Fanconi). Schweiz. Med. Wochenschr., *95*:1461, 1965.

Glanz, A., and Fraser, F. C.: Spectrum of anomalies in Fanconi anemia. J. Med. Genet., *19*:412, 1982.

Mann, W. R., et al.: Fanconi anemia: Evidence for linkage heterogeneity on chromosome 20q. Genomics, *9*:329, 1991.

Strathdee, C. A., et al.: Evidence for at least four Fanconi anaemia genes including FACC on chromosome 9. Nat. Genet., *1*:196, 1992.

Strathdee, C. A., et al.: Cloning of CDNAs for Fanconi anaemia by functional complimentation. Nature, *356*:763, 1992.

Giampietro, P. F., et al.: The need for more accurate and timely diagnosis in Fanconi anemia: A report from the International Fanconi Anemia Registry. Pediatrics, *91*:1116, 1993.

Butturini, A., et al.: Hematologic abnormalities in Fanconi anemia: An International Fanconi Anemia Registry Study. Blood, *84*:1650, 1994.

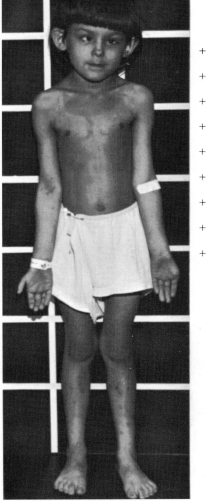

+ PIGMENTATION (BROWN) OF SKIN

+ SHORT STATURE

+ SMALL CRANIUM

+ MENTAL RETARDATION

+ STRABISMUS

+ ABNORMAL EARS

+ ABNORMAL THUMBS

+ RENAL ANOMALY

+ HYPOPLASIA OF MARROW, WITH TIME

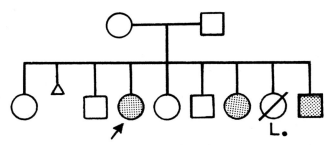

FIGURE 1. Fanconi pancytopenia syndrome. A 7-year-old with a height age of $3^6/_{12}$ years who has the anomalies listed above. The pedigree notes two affected siblings and one otherwise normal brother who died of leukemia during infancy. (From Smith, D. W.: J. Pediatr., *70*:479, 1967, with permission.)

RADIAL APLASIA–THROMBOCYTOPENIA SYNDROME

(TAR Syndrome)

Gross, Groh, and Weippl described this entity in siblings in 1956; subsequently, well over 100 cases have been reported.

ABNORMALITIES

Hematologic. Most severe in early infancy. Thrombocytopenia with absence or hypoplasia of megakaryocytes (absent in 66 per cent, decreased in 12 per cent, inactive in 12 per cent). "Leukemoid" granulocytosis in 62 per cent of patients, especially during bleeding episodes. Eosinophilia in 53 per cent. Anemia, often out of proportion to apparent blood loss.

Limbs. Arms: Bilateral absence of radius (100 per cent). Abnormalities of ulna including hypoplasia (100 per cent), bilateral absence (20 per cent) and/or unilateral absence (10 per cent). Abnormal humerus (50 per cent) with bilateral absence in 5 to 10 per cent. Shoulder joint may be abnormal. The thumbs are always present.

Legs: Abnormalities in 50 per cent, including hip dislocation, subluxation of knees, coxa valga, dislocation of patella, femoral and tibial torsion, abnormal tibiofibular joint, ankylosis of knee, small feet, abnormal toe placement. Absence of fibula.

OCCASIONAL ABNORMALITIES.
Congenital heart defect (33 per cent), primarily tetralogy of Fallot and atrial septal defect, small stature, nevus flammeus of forehead, strabismus, ptosis, dysseborrheis dermatitis, excessive perspiration, pedal dorsal edema, renal anomaly, spina bifida, brachycephaly, micrognathia, lateral clavicular hook, pancreatic cyst, Meckel diverticulum. Hypogammaglobulinemia. Mental deficiency (7 per cent) that is usually related to intracranial bleed. Delayed myelination, hypoplasia of cerebellum, particularly the vermis and a cavum septum pellucidum on MRI of brain (one patient).

NATURAL HISTORY.
About 40 per cent of the patients have died, usually as a result of hemorrhage during early infancy. Thrombocytopenia during that time is precipitated by viral illness, particularly gastrointestinal. With advancing age, the severity of the hematologic disorder usually becomes less profound, and therefore, vigorous early management is indicated. With the exception of menorrhagia, affected adults usually have no problem. Intracranial bleeding, when present, almost always occurs before 1 year of age. Delayed motor development is due to the skeletal abnormalities. Bracing, splinting, or stabilization of the wrist centrally should be considered. Arthritis of wrist and knees is a late complication. Cow's milk allergy or intolerance is common and can be a significant problem with introduction of cow's milk precipitating thrombocytopenia, eosinophilia, and/or leukamoid reactions.

ETIOLOGY.
Autosomal recessive. Prenatal diagnosis can be made by demonstrating the defect of the upper limb on sonography.

References

Gross, H., Groh, C., and Weippl, G.: Congenitale hypoplastische Thrombopenie mit Radialaplasie. Neue Osterr. Z. Kinderheilkd., 1:574, 1956.

Shaw, S., and Oliver, R. A. M.: Congenital hypoplastic thrombocytopenia with skeletal deformities in siblings. Blood, 14:374, 1956.

Hall, J. G., et al.: Thrombocytopenia with absent radius (TAR). Medicine, 48:441, 1969.

Anyane-Yeboa, K., et al.: Brief clinical report: Tetraphocomelia in the syndrome of thrombocytopenia with absent radii (TAR syndrome). Am. J. Med. Genet., 20:571, 1985.

Hall, J. G.: Thrombocytopenia and absent radius (TAR) syndrome. J. Med. Genet., 24:79, 1987.

Mac Donald, M. R., et al.: Hypoplasia of the cerebellar vermis and corpus callosum in thrombocytopenia with absent radius syndrome on MRI studies. Am. J. Med. Genet., 50:46, 1994.

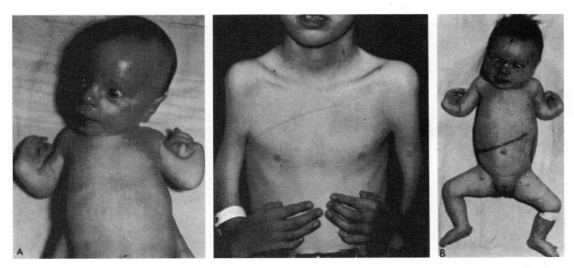

FIGURE 1. Radial aplasia–thrombocytopenia syndrome. *A,* Same patient, as infant and young boy. *B,* Young infant with serious bleeding and hepatosplenomegaly. Patient also had a cardiac defect. (Courtesy of J. M. Opitz, Helena, Mont., and R. Hunter, University of Washington, Seattle, Wash.)

AASE SYNDROME

Triphalangeal Thumb, Congenital Anemia

Aase and Smith described this disorder in two male siblings in 1969. At least ten additional cases have been recognized.

ABNORMALITIES. Based on eight cases.
Growth. Mild growth deficiency, about third percentile.
Hematologic. Hypoplastic anemia that tends to improve with age.
Skeletal. Triphalangeal thumbs, mild radial hypoplasia, narrow shoulders, late closure of fontanels.

OCCASIONAL ABNORMALITIES. Downslanting palpebral fissures, cleft lip, cleft palate, retinopathy, webbed neck, 11 pairs of ribs, bifid thoracic vertebra, agenesis of clavicle, underdeveloped ilia, distal sacrum and coccygeal vertebrae, dysplastic middle phalanx of fifth finger.

NATURAL HISTORY. The anemia, which has been responsive to prednisone therapy, tends to improve with age.

ETIOLOGY. Unknown. Occurrence in siblings and in both sexes makes autosomal recessive inheritance most likely. However, a report of a mother with congenital hypoplastic anemia whose son has the same anemia plus bilateral radial hypoplasia raises the possibility of autosomal dominant inheritance.

References

Aase, J. M., and Smith D. W.: Congenital anemia and triphalangeal thumbs: A new syndrome. J. Pediatr., *74*:417, 1969.

Murphy, S., and Lubin, B.: Triphalangeal thumbs and congenital erythroid hypoplasia: Report of a case with unusual features. J. Pediatr., *81*:987, 1972.

Higginbottom, M. C., et al.: Case report: The Aase syndrome in a female patient. J. Med. Genet., *15*:484, 1978.

Muis, N., et al.: The Aase syndrome: Case report and review of the literature. Eur. J. Pediatr., *145*:153, 1986.

Hurst, J. A., et al.: Autosomal dominant transmission of congenital erythroid hypoplastic anemia with radial abnormalities. Am. J. Med. Genet., *40*:482, 1991.

Hing, A. V., and Dowton, S. B.: Aase syndrome: Novel radiographic features. Am. J. Med. Genet., *45*:413, 1993.

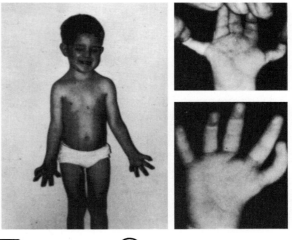

FIGURE 1. Aase syndrome. Affected boy who had been seriously anemic in infancy, during which time the anemia responded to prednisone therapy. He is now mildly anemic without therapy. His brother, whose hand is also shown, is similarly affected. (From Aase, J. M., and Smith, D. W.: J. Pediatr., 74:417, 1969, with permission.)

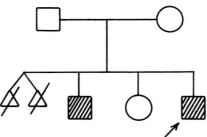

J

J. OSTEOCHONDRODYSPLASIAS

ACHONDROGENESIS, TYPES IA AND IB

Low Nasal Bridge, Very Short Limbs,
Incomplete Ossification of Lower Spine

This early lethal disorder was described in 1925 by Donath and Vogl and termed achondrogenesis by Fraccaro in 1952. More than 20 cases have been reported. Recent studies by Borochowitz et al. indicate that achondrogenesis type I (previously referred to as Parenti-Fraccaro type) represents two radiographically and histopathologically distinct disorders, referred to as types IA and IB. In the classification set forth by Whitley and Gorlin, type I is synonymous with type IA and type II with type IB.

ABNORMALITIES

Growth. Extremely small stature, 22 to 30 cm.
Craniofacies. Cranium large for gestational age. Low nasal bridge, micrognathia.
Limbs. Severe micromelia.
Radiographs. In both types, the skull, vertebral bodies, fibula, talus, and calcaneus are poorly ossified; the ilia are crenated; the long bones are stellate; and the ribs are extremely short. In type IA, multiple rib fractures are present, and the proximal femurs have metaphyseal spikes. Conversely, in type IB, rib fractures do not occur, and the distal femurs have metaphyseal irregularities.

NATURAL HISTORY AND COMMENT.

The defect in the development of cartilage and bone is severe. In type IA, normal-appearing but hypervascular cartilage matrix is present with increased cellular density. Large lacuna surround the chondrocytes, which contain round cytoplasmic inclusion bodies. In type IB, sparse interterritorial cartilaginous matrix is present, with a marked deficiency of collagen fibers. The chondrocytes are large, have a central round nucleus, and are surrounded by a dense collagenous ring. Developmental pathology beyond the skeletal system is implied by the frequent findings of polyhydramnios, hydrops, and early lethality. Most infants are stillborn or die shortly after birth.

ETIOLOGY. Autosomal recessive. It is now recognized that achondrogenesis, type IB is due to mutations in the gene for diastrophic dysplasia which has been shown to encode a sulfate transporter (DTDST). Thus achondrogenesis, type IB and diastrophic dysplasia are allelic disorders.

References

Donath, J., and Vogl, A.: Untersuchungen über den chondrodystrophischen Zwergwuchs. Wien. Arch. Intern. Med., *10*:1, 1925.

Fraccaro, M.: Contributo allo studies delle malattie del mesenchima osteopoietico. L'achondrogenesi. Folia Hered. Pathol. (Milano), *1*:190, 1952.

Maroteaux, P., and Lamy, M.: Le diagnostic des nanismes chondrodystrophiques chez les nouveaunés. Arch. Fr. Pediatr., *25*:241, 1968.

Whitley, C. B., and Gorlin, R. J.: Achondrogenesis: New nosology with evidence of genetic heterogeneity. Radiology, *148*:693, 1983.

Borochowitz, Z., et al.: Achondrogenesis type I—further heterogeneity. J. Pediatr., *112*:23, 1988.

Freisinger, P., et al.: Achondrogenesis type IB (Fraccaro): Study of collagen in the tissue and in chondrocytes cultured in agarose. Am. J. Med. Genet., *49*:439, 1994.

Superti-Furga, A., et al.: Achondrogenesis type IB is caused by mutations in the diastrophic dysplasia sulfate transporter gene. Nature Genet., *12*:100, 1996.

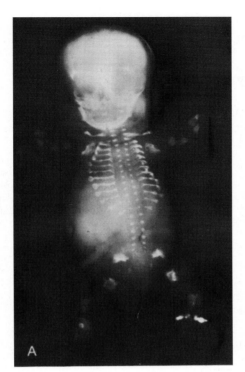

TYPE	ACHONDROGENESIS IA	ACHONDROGENESIS IB
Skull	Poorly ossified	Poorly ossified
Ribs	Short & fractured	Short, no fractures, cupped ends
Spine	Completely unossified	Posterior pedicles only
Ilium	Arched	Crenated
Ischium	*Ossified-hypoplastic	Unossified
Femur	Wedged with metaph. spike	Trapezoid
Tibia Fibula	Short with metaph. flare	Crenated Unossified
	*Unossified 30 weeks' gestation	

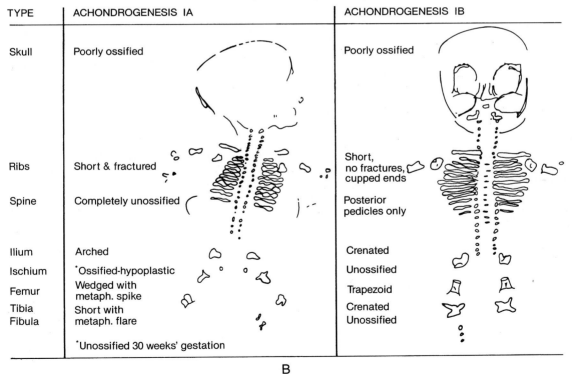

B

FIGURE 1. *A,* Stillborn infant at 30 weeks' gestation with acrondrogenesis, type IA. *B,* Radiographic features that differentiate type IA from type IB are delineated on the drawings. (Courtesy of Dr. R. Lachman, Harbor-UCLA Medical Center, and Dr. D. Rimoin, Cedars-Sinai Medical Center, Los Angeles, Calif.)

TYPE II ACHONDROGENESIS-HYPOCHONDROGENESIS

(Langer-Saldino
Achondrogenesis, Hypochondrogenesis)

Initially described by Langer et al. and Saldino, this early lethal disorder has recently been more completely delineated by Chen et al. and Borochowitz et al.

ABNORMALITIES

Growth. Extremely short stature (27 to 36 cm).

Craniofacies. Large calvarium with large anterior and posterior fontanels, flat nasal bridge, small anteverted nostrils, micrognathia.

Limbs. Short.

Radiographs. Normal cranial ossification. Short ribs without fractures. Short, broad long bones with disproportionately long fibula and metaphyseal irregularity of distal ulna. Variable degrees of failure of ossification of lumbar spine, cervical spine, sacrum, ischial and pubic bones, and calcaneus and talus.

Other. Polyhydramnios.

OCCASIONAL ABNORMALITIES. Cleft soft palate. Cystic hygroma. Hydrops.

NATURAL HISTORY. Although one child survived to 3 months, the majority are stillborn or die in the first few hours of life due to pulmonary hypoplasia.

ETIOLOGY. The vast majority of cases are sporadic. Molecular studies have documented mutations of COL2A1, the gene encoding type II collagen. In all cases where mutations have been identified, they have been heterozygous, indicating an autosomal dominant mode of inheritance. However, autosomal recessive inheritance cannot be ruled out in all cases, particularly those with the most severe radiographic and pathologic features.

COMMENT. Hypochondrogenesis previously thought to be a distinct disorder, and achondrogenesis type II represent a spectrum of the same disorder referred to as type II achondrogenesis-hypochondrogenesis. Patients with the most severe radiographic and pathologic features have been labeled achondrogenesis type II, while those with less severe, although similar features, hypochondrogenesis.

References

Langer, L. O., et al.: Thanatophoric dwarfism: A condition confused with achondroplasia in the neonate, with brief comments on achondrogenesis and homozygous achondroplasia. Radiology, 92:285, 1969.

Saldino, R. M.: Lethal short-limbed dwarfism: Achondrogenesis and thanatophoric dwarfism. Am. J. Roentgenol., 112:185, 1971.

Chen, H., Lin, C. T., and Yang, S. S.: Achondrogenesis: A review with special consideration of achondrogenesis type II (Langer-Saldino). Am. J. Med. Genet., 10:379, 1981.

Borochowitz, Z., et al.: Achondrogenesis II-hypochondrogenesis: variability versus heterogeneity. Am. J. Med. Genet., 24:273, 1986.

Godfrey, M., and Hollister, D. W.: Type II achondrogenesis-hypochondrogenesis: Identification of abnormal type II collagen. Am. J. Hum. Genet., 43:904, 1988.

Horton, W. A.: Characterization of a type II collagen gene (COL2A1) mutation identified in cultured chondrocytes from human hypochondrogenesis. Proc. Natl. Acad. Sci. U. S. A., 89:4583, 1992.

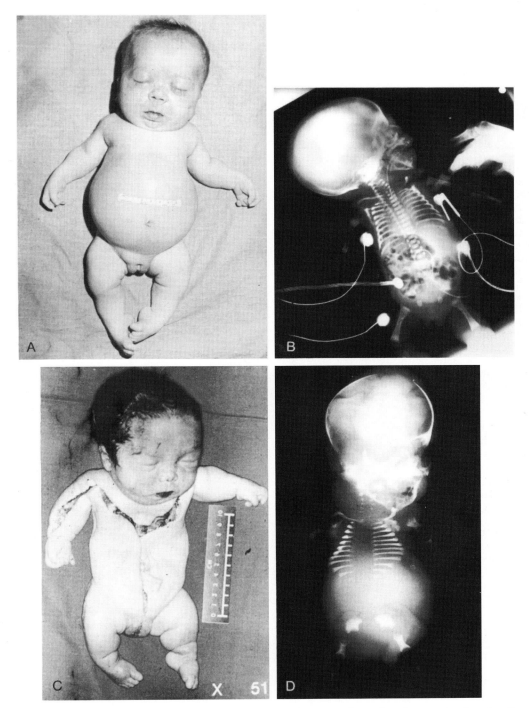

FIGURE 1. *A* to *D*, Two stillborn infants with type II achondrogenesis-hypochondrogenesis, showing the variation in severity of the disorder. Note the relatively normal cranial ossification, short ribs, and variable degrees of failure of ossification of lumbar and cervical spines, sacrum, and ischial and pubic bones. (Courtesy of Dr. R. Lachman, Harbor-UCLA Medical Center, and Dr. D. Rimoin, Cedars-Sinai Medical Center, Los Angeles, Calif.)

FIBROCHONDROGENESIS

Lazzaroni-Fossati described a patient with this early lethal disorder in 1978. Subsequently, seven additional patients have been reported. A distinctive fibrosis of the growth-plate cartilage led to the designation fibrochondrogenesis.

ABNORMALITIES
Growth. Short stature.

Craniofacies. Widely patent anterior fontanel, coronal and sagittal sutures. Protuberant eyes with large corneae. Hypoplastic nose with flat nasal bridge and anteverted nares. Long philtrum. Cleft palate. Short neck. Low-set, malformed ears.

Trunk. Flattened vertebrae with posterior vertebral hypoplasia and a sagittal midline cleft. Short, thin ribs with anterior and posterior cupping. Long, thin clavicles. Small chest.

Limbs. Rhizomelic shortening. Small hands and feet. Camptodactyly. Fifth finger clinodactyly. Hypoplastic finger and toenails. Short, dumbbell-shaped long bones with broad, irregular metaphyses. Prominent metaphyseal spurs adjacent to growth plates. Short fibulae.

Pelvis. Hypoplastic with ovoid ilia, irregular flattened acetabula with medial spikes and narrow sacrosciatic notches. Broad, hypoplastic ischii.

Other. Omphalocele. Hydrops.

NATURAL HISTORY. All affected individuals have been stillborn or have died in the neonatal period.

ETIOLOGY. Probably autosomal recessive.

COMMENT. Microscopic examination of long bones demonstrates gross disorganization of growth plate cartilage, fibrous appearance of the matrix, and normal metaphyseal and diaphyseal bone formation.

References

Lazzaroni-Fossati, F., et al.: La fibrochondrogenese. Arch. Fr. Pediatr., *35*:1096, 1978.

Eteson, D. J., et al.: Fibrochondrogenesis: Radiologic and histologic studies. Am. J. Med. Genet., *19*:277, 1984.

Whitely, C. B., et al.: Fibrochondrogenesis: Lethal, autosomal recessive chondrodysplasia with distinctive cartilage histopathology. Am. J. Med. Genet., *19*:265, 1984.

Bankier, A., et al.: Fibrochondrogenesis in male twins at 24 weeks gestation. Am. J. Med. Genet., *38*:95, 1991.

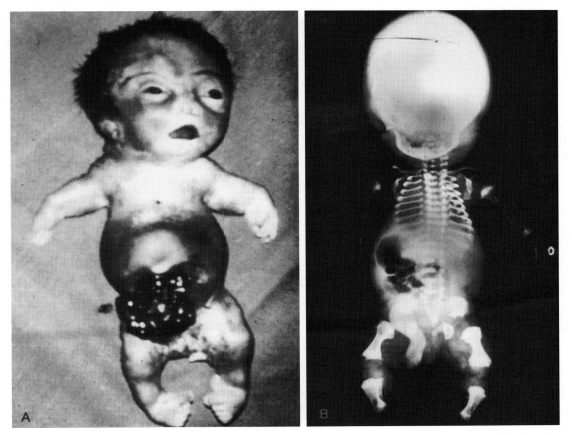

FIGURE 1. *A*, Stillborn infant with fibrochondrogenesis. Note the flat, wide nasal bridge, anteverted nares, short limbs, and equinovarus position of the feet. *B*, The radiograph reveals long, thin clavicles; short, thin ribs; flattened acetabula; narrow sacrosciatic notches; metaphyseal widening of the tibia and fibula; and dumbbell-shaped femora. (From Eteson, D. J., et al.: Am. J. Med. Genet., *19*:277, 1984, with permission.)

ATELOSTEOGENESIS, TYPE I

(Giant Cell Chondrodysplasia)

This early lethal short-limb dwarfing condition was set forth by Maroteaux et al. and Sillence et al. Atelosteogenesis derives from the Greek word for incomplete and relates to the marked lack of complete ossification of certain bones.

ABNORMALITIES
Growth. Short stature with proximal shortness of limbs.
Radiographs. Short humeri with proximal rounding and distal tapering. Absent fibula. Short femora with rounded proximal ends but square and tapered distal ends. Abnormally segmented and fused cervical vertebrae; thoracic platyspondyly with multiple coronal clefts throughout. Eleven pairs of ribs. Narrow thoracic cage. Markedly delayed ossification of proximal phalanges and middle phalanges with well-ossified distal phalanges.
Other. Polyhydramnios. Depressed nasal bridge.

OCCASIONAL ABNORMALITIES. Cleft palate. Laryngeal stenosis. Joint dislocations. Talipes equinovarus.

NATURAL HISTORY. All affected infants have been stillborn or have died immediately after birth.

ETIOLOGY. Unknown. All cases have been sporadic.

COMMENT. It has been suggested that atelosteogenesis is heterogeneous with three types (I, II, and III) differentiated on the basis of distinct radiologic and histologic features. Radiologic features specific for type I include 11 pairs of short ribs and dysharmonic ossification of metacarpals and phalanges; features specific for type II include a large gap between the first and second digits, a horizontal sacrum, and relatively large second and/or third metacarpals; features specific for type III include an "S"-shape curve of the cervical spine, evenly ossified metacarpals and phalanges with characteristic phalanges (large and wide with squared-off proximal ends).

References

Sillence, D. O., et al.: Spondylohumerofemoral hypoplasia (giant cell chondrodysplasia): A neonatally lethal short-limb skeletal dysplasia. Am. J. Med. Genet., *13*:7, 1982.
Maroteaux, P., et al.: Atelosteogenesis. Am. J. Med. Genet., *13*:15, 1982.
Sillence, D. O., et al.: Atelosteogenesis: Evidence for heterogeneity. Pediatr. Radiol., *17*:112, 1987.
Stern, H. J., et al.: Atelosteogenesis type III: A distinct skeletal dysplasia with features overlapping atelosteogenesis and oto-palatal-digital syndrome type II. Am. J. Med. Genet., *36*:183, 1990.
Temple, K., et al.: A case of atelosteogenesis. J. Med. Genet., *27*:194, 1990.

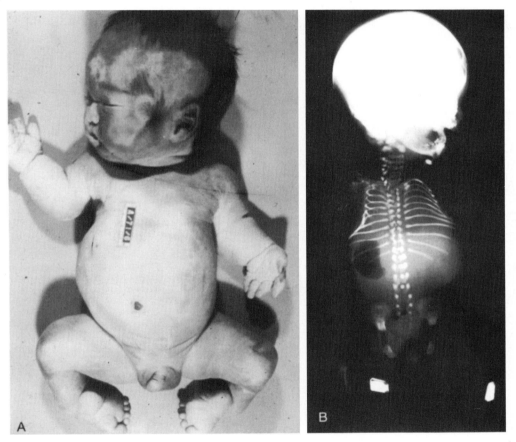

FIGURE 1. *A*, Stillborn with atelosteogenesis. Note the depressed nasal bridge, flexion contractures at knees, and equinovarus position of feet. *B*, The radiograph reveals lack of calcification of humerus and hypoplasia of much of the skeleton. (Courtesy of Dr. R. Lachman, Harbor-UCLA Medical Center, and Dr. D. Rimoin, Cedars-Sinai Medical Center, Los Angeles, Calif.)

SHORT RIB–POLYDACTYLY SYNDROME, TYPE I (Saldino-Noonan Type)

This disorder was originally described by Saldino and Noonan in 1972. Naumoff et al. and Yang et al. have published cases suggesting that short rib–polydactyly syndrome (SRP) type I represents two separate disorders, referred to as SRP type I and SRP type III. However, clinical, radiographic, and morphologic studies suggest that only one disorder exists, with wide variability in expression. This issue remains to be completely resolved.

ABNORMALITIES
Growth. Short stature.
Limbs. Short. Postaxial polydactyly of hands and/or feet. Syndactyly. Metaphyseal irregularities of long bones, with spurs extending longitudinally from medial and lateral segments. Underossified phalanges.
Trunk. Short, horizontal ribs. Notch-like ossification defects around periphery of vertebral bodies.
Pelvis. Small iliac bones with horizontal acetabular roof. Triangular ossification defect above lateral aspect of acetabulum.
Other. Cardiac defects, including transposition of great vessels, double-outlet left ventricle, double-outlet right ventricle, endocardial cushion defect, and hypoplastic right heart. Polycystic kidneys. Hypoplasia of penis. Defects of cloacal development. Imperforate anus.

OCCASIONAL ABNORMALITIES. Natal teeth. Preaxial polydactyly. Sex-reversal (phenotypic females with a 46XY karyotype).

NATURAL HISTORY. Death from respiratory insufficiency secondary to pulmonary hypoplasia has occurred in all infants within the first few hours after birth.

ETIOLOGY. Autosomal recessive.

References

Saldino, R. M., and Noonan, C. D.: Severe thoracic dystrophy with striking micromelia, abnormal osseous development, including the spine, and multiple visceral anomalies. Am. J. Roentgenol., *114:* 257, 1972.

Spranger, J., et al.: Short rib-polydactyly (SRP) syndromes, types Majewski and Saldino-Noonan. Z. Kinderheilkd., 116:73, 1974.

Naumoff, P., et al.: Short rib-polydactyly syndrome type 3. Radiology, 122:443, 1977.

Sillence, D. O.: Invited editorial comment: Non-Majewski short rib–polydactyly syndrome. Am. J. Med. Genet., 7:223, 1980.

Yang, S. S., et al.: Short rib-polydactyly syndrome, type 3 with chondrocytic inclusions: Report of a case and review of the literature. Am. J. Med. Genet., 7:205, 1980.

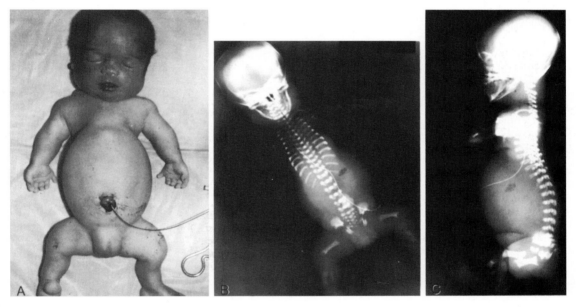

FIGURE 1. Short rib–polydactyly syndrome, Saldino-Noonan type. *A*, Stillborn male infant. Note the narrow thorax, short limbs, postaxial polydactyly, and hypoplastic penis. *B* and *C*, Radiographs show short, horizontal ribs; metaphyseal irregularities of long bones, with spurs extending from medial and lateral segments; and triangular ossification defects above lateral aspect of acetabulum.

SHORT RIB–POLYDACTYLY SYNDROME, TYPE II (Majewski Type)

In 1971, Majewski et al. described four infants with this early lethal form of short-limb dwarfism. Spranger et al. differentiated it from other forms of short rib–polydactyly in 1974, and subsequently a number of additional cases have been described.

ABNORMALITIES

Growth. Short stature with disproportionately short limbs.

Craniofacies. Midline cleft lip. Cleft palate. Short flat nose. Low-set, small, malformed ears.

Limbs. Both preaxial and postaxial polysyndactyly of hands and/or feet. Brachydactyly. Disproportionately short, oval-shaped tibiae. Short, rounded metacarpals and metatarsals. Premature ossification of proximal epiphyses of humeri, femora, and lateral cuboids. Underossified phalanges.

Trunk. Narrow thorax. Short, horizontal ribs. High clavicles.

Other. Ambiguous genitalia. Hypoplasia of epiglottis and larynx. Multiple glomerular cysts and focal dilatation of distal tubules of kidney.

OCCASIONAL ABNORMALITIES. Microglossia. Lobulated tongue. Absent gallbladder. Brain anomalies, including pachygyria, a small vermis, and absence of olfactory bulbs. Persisting left superior vena cava. Hydrops. Polyhydramnios.

NATURAL HISTORY. Respiratory insufficiency secondary to pulmonary hypoplasia has led to death soon after birth in all cases.

ETIOLOGY. Autosomal recessive.

COMMENT. It has been suggested that this disorder and oro-facial-digital syndrome type II may represent severe and mild ends of the spectrum of the same disorder.

References

Majewski, F., et al.: Polysyndaktylie, verkürzte Gliedmassen und Genitalfehlbildungen: Kennzeichen eines selbaständigen Syndroms? Z. Kinderheilkd., *111*:118, 1971.

Spranger, J., et al.: Short rib-polydactyly (SRP) syndromes, types Majewski and Saldino-Noonan. Z. Kinderheilkd., *116*:73, 1974.

Motegi, T., et al.: Short rib-polydactyly syndrome, Majewski type, in two males. Hum. Genet., *49*:269, 1979.

Chen, H., et al.: Short rib-polydactyly syndrome, Majewski type. Am. J. Med. Genet., *7*:215, 1980.

Silengo, M. C., et al.: Oro-facial-digital syndrome II. Transition types between the Mohr and Majewski syndromes: Report of 2 new cases. Clin. Genet., *31*:331, 1987.

Prudlo, J., et al.: Central nervous system alterations in a case of short-rib polydactyly syndrome, Majewski type. Devel. Med. Child. Neurol., *35*:158, 1993.

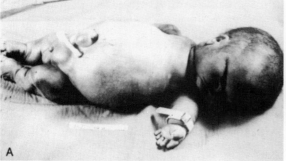

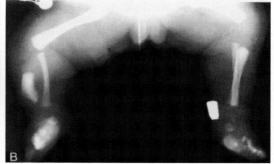

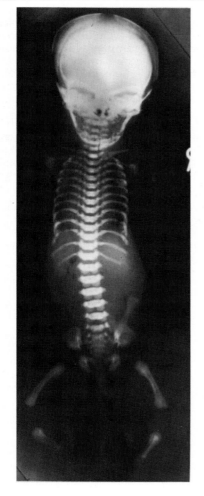

FIGURE 1. *A* to *C,* Neonate with short rib–polydactyly syndrome, Majewski type. Note the disproportionately short limbs, postaxial polydactyly, and, on the radiographs, the narrow thorax with short ribs and disproportionately short, abnormally shaped tibia. (Courtesy of Dr. R. Lachman, Harbor-UCLA Medical Center and Dr. D. Rimoin, Cedars-Sinai Medical Center, Los Angeles, Calif.)

THANATOPHORIC DYSPLASIA

Short Limbs, Flat Vertebrae, Large Cranium With Low Nasal Bridge

Maroteaux et al. set forth this disorder in 1967 and utilized the Greek term *thanatophoric* (death-bringing) to emphasize that such patients usually die shortly after birth. Langer et al. have separated this condition into two types. Type 1 (TD I) is most common and is characterized by curved long bones (most obviously the femora), and very flat vertebral bodies (35 per cent or less of the adjacent disk space in the lumbar region). Type 2 (TD II) is characterized by straight femora and taller vertebral bodies. Almost all cases of thanatophoric dysplasia with a severe cloverleaf skull (the kleeblattschädel anomaly) are TD II.

ABNORMALITIES

Central Nervous System. Severe abnormalities, the most common of which is temporal lobe dysplasia. Other defects include megalencephaly, hydrocephalus, brain stem hypoplasia, maldevelopment of inferior olivary and cerebellar dentate nuclei. Hypotonia, severe developmental delay in the few survivors.

Growth. Severe growth deficiency; 36 to 46 cm tall, with an average of 40 cm.

Craniofacial. Large cranium and fontanel; 36 to 47 cm, average of 37 cm. Small foramen magnum and short base of skull, with full forehead, low nasal bridge, bulging eyes, and small facies. Cloverleaf skull.

Limbs. Short, with small sausage-like fingers, bowed long bones with cupped spur-like irregular flaring of metaphyses, and lack of ossification in secondary centers at knee. Fibulae are shorter than tibiae. Disorganized chondrocytes and bony trabeculae, especially in central epiphyseal-metaphyseal region.

Thorax. Narrow with short ribs.

Spine. Short, flattened vertebrae with relatively wide intervertebral disk space. Lack of caudal widening of spinal canal.

Scapulae. Small and squarish.

Pelvis. Squarish and short, with small sciatic notch and medial spurs.

OCCASIONAL ABNORMALITIES.

Patent ductus arteriosus, auricular septal defect, horseshoe kidney, hydronephrosis, imperforate anus, radioulnar synostosis.

NATURAL HISTORY.

Feeble fetal activity and/or polyhydramnios is frequent in this disorder. These patients usually die shortly after birth, at least partially owing to the small thoracic cage and respiratory insufficiency. Although survival beyond the neonatal period is rare, two affected children, one who died at 5 years of age and the other still living at $3^6/_{12}$ years, have been reported. Both had profound developmental delay and severe growth deficiency. The author recommends offering no medical intervention toward survival for patients with this disorder.

ETIOLOGY.

Autosomal dominant. All cases represent fresh gene mutations. Greater than 50 per cent of patients with type I thanatophoric dysplasia (TD I) and 100 per cent of those tested with type II have mutations in the fibroblast growth factor receptor 3 (FGFR3) gene. Whereas individuals with achondroplasia have mutations in the transmembrane domain of FGFR3, TD I is associated with mutations in the extracellular domain of FGFR3 and TD II with mutations within the intracellular tyrosine kinase domain.

COMMENT.

Cloverleaf skull occurs only rarely in patients with TD I. In those cases, the cranial defect is mild. All cases of severe cloverleaf skull have occurred in patients with TD II.

References

Maroteaux, P., Lamy, M., and Robert, J. M.: Le nanisme thanatophore. Presse Med., *75*:2519, 1967.

Giedion, A.: Thanatophoric dwarfism. Helv. Paediatr. Acta, *23*:175, 1968.

Goutières, F., Aicardi, J., and Farkas-Bargeton, E.: Une malformation cérébrale particulière associée au nanisme thanatophore. Presse Med., *79*:960, 1971.

Thompson, B. H., and Parmley, T. H.: Obstetric features of thanatophoric dwarfism. Am. J. Obstet. Gynecol., *109*:396, 1971.

Horton, W. A., Harris, D. J., and Collins, D. L.: Discordance for the kleeblattschädel anomaly in monozygotic twins with thanatophoric dysplasia. Am. J. Med. Genet., *15*:97, 1983.

Langer, L. O., et al.: Thanatophoric dysplasia and cloverleaf skull. Am. J. Med. Genet. Suppl., *3*:167, 1987.

Knisely, A. S., and Amber, M. W.: Temporal lobe abnormalities in thanatophoric dysplasia. Pediatr. Neurosci., *14*:169, 1988.

Martinez-Frias, M. L., et al.: Thanatophoric dysplasia. An autosomal dominant condition? Am. J. Med. Genet., *31*:815, 1988.

MacDonald, I. M., et al.: Growth and development in thanatophoric dysplasia. Am. J. Med. Genet., *33*:508, 1989.

Tavorima, P. L., et al.: Thanatophoric dysplasia (types I and II) caused by distinct mutations in fibroblast growth factor receptor 3. Nat. Genet., *9*:321, 1995.

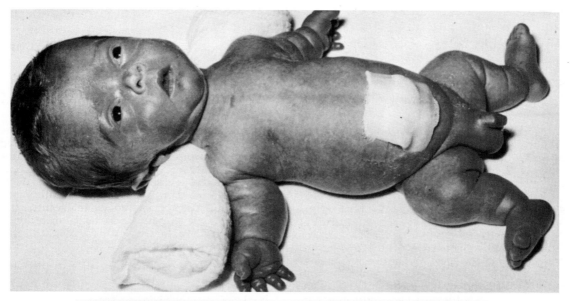

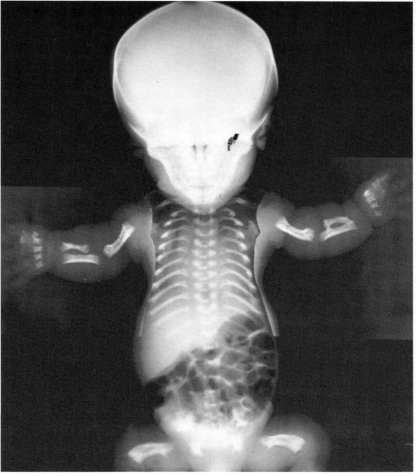

FIGURE 1. Thanatophoric dysplasia type I. Neonate. (From Giedion, A.: Helv. Paediatr. Acta, 23:175, 1968, with permission.)

JEUNE THORACIC DYSTROPHY

(Asphyxiating Thoracic Dystrophy)

Small Thorax, Short Limbs, Hypoplastic Iliac Wings

First described by Jeune et al. in 1955, over 100 cases have now been reported.

ABNORMALITIES

Growth. Short stature.

Skeletal. Infancy: Short horizontal ribs with irregular costochondral junctions and small thoracic cage. Hypoplastic iliac wings. Horizontal acetabular roofs with spur-like projections at lower margins of sciatic notches. Early ossification of capital femoral epiphysis. Childhood: Irregular epiphyses and metaphyses with relatively short limbs, especially the hands. Ulnae and fibulae relatively short. Cone-shaped epiphyses and early fusion between epiphyses and metaphyses of distal and middle phalanges.

Respiratory. Lung hypoplasia, presumably secondary to the small thoracic cage, is the major cause of death in early infancy.

Renal. Cystic tubular dysplasia and/or glomerular sclerosis.

Hepatic. Biliary dysgenesis with portal fibrosis and bile duct proliferation.

OCCASIONAL ABNORMALITIES.

Polydactyly, usually of hands and feet, notching of distal end of metacarpal and metatarsal bones; lacunar skull; direct hyperbilirubinemia with prolonged jaundice, pancreatic defects including fibrosis and cysts; retinal degeneration with predominantly cone-type cells remaining. Situs inversus. Mental retardation.

NATURAL HISTORY.

Early death, usually the consequence of asphyxia with or without pneumonia, occurs frequently. Expansion of the thoracic cage diameter with methyl methacrylate prosthesis has been used successfully in some patients. However, those who survive usually have progressive improvement in the relative growth of the thoracic cage and may have only slight to moderate shortness of stature. Chronic nephritis leading to renal failure is a serious potential feature of this disorder. Renal insufficiency may be evident by 2 years of age. Although infrequent, progressive hepatic dysfunction also occurs and may contribute to the relatively poor long-term prognosis for individuals with this disorder. Survival to the fourth decade has occurred.

ETIOLOGY.

Autosomal recessive. Prenatal diagnosis utilizing ultrasonography has been accomplished successfully at 18 weeks' gestation.

References

Jeune, M., Beraud, C., and Carron, R.: Dystrophie thoracique asphyxiante de caractère familial. Arch. Fr. Pediatr., 12:886, 1955.

Pirnar, T., and Neuhauser, E. B. D.: Asphyxiating thoracic dystrophy of the newborn. Am. J. Roentgenol. Radium Ther. Nucl. Med., 98:358, 1966.

Herdman, R. C., and Langer, L. O.: The thoracic asphyxiant dystrophy and renal disease. Am. J. Dis. Child., 116:192, 1968.

Langer, L. O.: Thoracic-pelvic-phalangeal dystrophy. Radiology, 91:447, 1968.

Friedman, J. M., Kaplan, H. G., and Hall, J. G.: The Jeune syndrome in an adult. Am. J. Med., 59:857, 1975.

Okerklaid, F., et al.: Asphyxiating thoracic dystrophy. Arch. Dis., Child., 52:758, 1977.

Allen, A. W., et al.: Ocular findings in thoracic-pelvic-phalangeal dystrophy. Arch. Ophthalmol., 97:489, 1979.

Shah, K. J.: Renal lesions in Jeune's syndrome. Br. J. Radiol., 53:432, 1980.

Elejalde, B. R., Mercedes de Elejalde, M., and Pansch, D.: Prenatal diagnosis of Jeune syndrome. Am. J. Med. Genet., 21:433, 1985.

Hudgins, L., et al.: Early cirrhosis in survivors with Jeune thoracic dystrophy. J. Pediatr., 120:754, 1992.

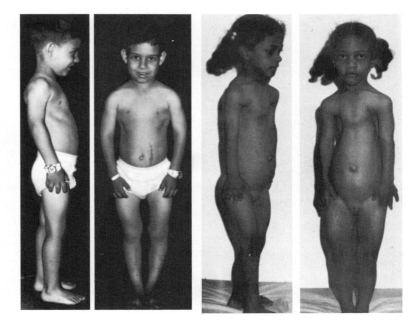

FIGURE 1. Affected children with Jeune thoracic dystrophy. Note the small thoracic cage, short hands, and mild bowing of legs. (Courtesy of Dr. Jaime Frias, University of South Florida, Tampa, Fla.)

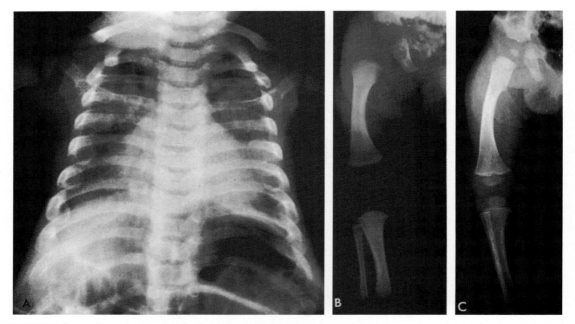

FIGURE 2. Jeune thoracic dystrophy. *A,* A 4-month-old. Note short ribs, high position of clavicles. *B* and *C,* Right lower extremity at 1 month and 10 months of age showing improvement in long bones and pelvis though fibula remains relatively short. (From Hanissian, A. S., et al.: J. Pediatr., *71:*855, 1967, with permission.)

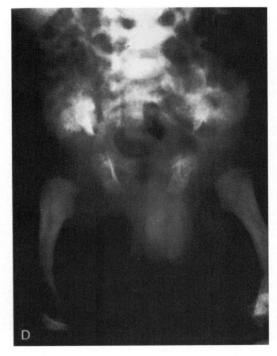

FIGURE 2. *Continued. D,* Horizontal acetablar roofs
with spur-like projections at lower margins of sciatic
notches.

CAMPOMELIC DYSPLASIA

Bowed Tibiae, Hypoplastic Scapulae, Flat Facies

Though reports of this condition appeared in the 1950s by Bound et al. and Bain and Barrett, it was not until the 1970s that the syndrome became more broadly recognized by Spranger et al. and Maroteaux et al., who utilized the term "camptomelique," meaning bent limb, to epitomize the disorder.

ABNORMALITIES
Growth. Prenatal onset growth deficiency with retarded osseous maturation and large head. Birth length, 35 to 49 cm. Average occipitofrontal circumference is 37 cm.

Central Nervous System. Tendency toward having large brain with gross cellular disorganization, most evident in cerebral cortex, thalamus, and caudate nucleus. Absence or hypoplasia of olfactory tract or bulbs. Hydrocephalus.

Facies. Flat-appearing small face with high forehead, anterior frontal upsweep, large anterior fontanel, low nasal bridge, micrognathia, cleft palate, short palpebral fissures, and malformed and/or low-set ears.

Limbs. Anterior bowing of tibiae with skin dimpling over convex area, short fibulae, mild bowing of femurs, and talipes equinovarus.

Radiographic. Short and somewhat flat vertebrae, particularly cervical. Hypoplastic scapulae, small thoracic cage with slender and/or decreased number of ribs, kyphoscoliosis, small iliac wings with relatively wide pelvic outlet. Absent mineralization of sternum. Lack of ossification of proximal tibial and distal femoral epiphysis and talus.

Tracheobronchial. Incomplete cartilaginous development with tracheobronchiomalacia.

Genitalia. Some of the affected XY individuals fail to develop masculine characteristics and have XY gonadal dysgenesis with ovarian, müllerian duct, and vaginal development.

OCCASIONAL ABNORMALITIES. Cardiac defects. Hydronephrosis. Polyhydramnios. Hypoplastic cochlea and semicircular canals. Anomalies in incus and stapes. Hearing loss.

NATURAL HISTORY. The great majority of patients die in the neonatal period from respiratory insufficiency, and those surviving into early infancy have feeding problems, failure to thrive, and evidence of serious central nervous system deficiency, including apneic spells. The oldest survivors include a 7-month-old, a 19-month-old, and a 17-year-old boy with an I.Q. of 45.

ETIOLOGY. Mutations in SOX9, a sex-determining region Y (SRY)–related gene located at 17q24 have been shown to cause both campomelic dysplasia and sex reversal. Previously, this disorder has been assumed to be recessively inherited based on seven families in which affected siblings have been born to unaffected parents. However, in none of the cases studied thus far have mutations in both SRY-related alleles been detected, indicating that the vast majority of cases of this disorder are due to an autosomal dominant gene that is usually lethal.

References

Bound, J. P., Finlay, H. V. L., and Rose, F. C.: Congenital anterior angulation of the tibia. Arch. Dis. Child., 27:179, 1952.

Bain, A. D., and Barrett, H. S.: Congenital bowing of the long bones: Report of a case. Arch. Dis. Child., 34:516, 1959.

Spranger, J., Langer, L. O., and Maroteaux, P.: Increasing frequency of a syndrome of multiple osseous defects? Lancet, 2:716, 1970.

Maroteaux, P., et al.: Le syndrome camptomélique. Maroteaux, P., et al.: Le syndrome camptomélique. Presse Med., 79:1157, 1971.

Hoefnagel, D., et al.: Camptomelic dwarfism. Lancet, 1:1068, 1972.

Schmickel, R. D., Heidelberger, K. P., and Poznanski, A. K.: The camptomelique syndrome. J. Pediatr., 82:299, 1973.

Hall, B. D., and Spranger, J. W.: Camptomelic dysplasia. Am. J. Dis. Child., 134:285, 1980.

Houston, C. S., et al.: The camptomelic syndrome: Review, report of 17 cases, and follow-up on the currently 17 year old boy first reported by Maroteaux et al. in 1971. Am. J. Med. Genet., 15:3, 1983.

Normann, E. K., et al.: Campomelic dysplasia—an underdiagnosed condition? Eur. J. Pediatr., 152:331, 1993.

Foster, J. W., et al.: Campomelic dysplasia and autosomal sex reversal caused by mutations in an SRY-related gene. Nature, 372:525, 1994.

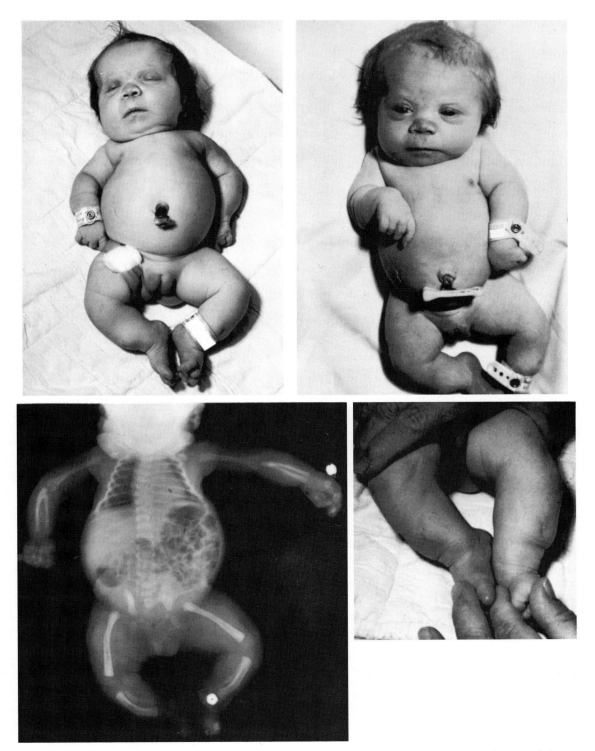

FIGURE 1. Campomelic dysplasia. Two newborn babies, showing low nasal bridge, micrognathia, small thorax, aberrant hand positioning, and bowed tibiae with dimples at the maximal point of bowing. Roentgenogram shows the slim, poorly developed bones and osseous immaturity (knee and foot). (From Hoefnagel, D., et al.: Lancet, *1*:1068, 1972, with permission. Copyrighted by The Lancet Ltd., 1972.)

ACHONDROPLASIA

Short Limbs, Low Nasal Bridge,
Caudal Narrowing of Spinal Canal

The most common chondrodysplasia, true achondroplasia, occurs with a frequency of about 1 in 15,000.

ABNORMALITIES

Growth. Small stature. Mean adult height in males is 131 ± 5.6 cm and in females is 124 ± 5.9 cm.

Craniofacial. Megalocephaly, small foramen magnum. Short cranial base with early spheno-occipital closure. Low nasal bridge with prominent forehead. Mild midfacial hypoplasia with narrow nasal passages.

Skeletal. Small cuboid-shaped vertebral bodies with short pedicles and progressive narrowing of lumbar interpedicular distance. Lumbar lordosis, mild thoracolumbar kyphosis with anterior beaking of first and/or second lumbar vertebra. Small iliac wings with narrow greater sciatic notch. Short tubular bones, especially humeri; metaphyseal flare with ball-and-socket arrangement of epiphysis to metaphysis. Short trident hand, fingers being similar in length, with short proximal and midphalanges. Short femoral neck; incomplete extension of elbow.

Other. Mild hypotonia. Early motor progress is often slow, although eventual intelligence is usually normal. Relative glucose intolerance evident with an oral glucose tolerance test.

OCCASIONAL ABNORMALITIES. Hydrocephalus secondary to a narrow foramen magnum may occur. Spinal cord and/or root compression can happen as a consequence of kyphosis, stenosis of the spinal canal, or disk lesions. About 46 per cent of patients have spinal complications, and therefore a cautious orthopedic-neurologic follow-up is merited.

NATURAL HISTORY. Macrocephaly may represent mild hydrocephaly relating to a small foramen magnum. Therefore, ultrasound studies of the brain should be seriously considered if the fontanel size is particularly large, the occipito-frontal circumference increases too rapidly, or any symptoms of hydrocephalus develop. Respiratory problems secondary to a small chest, upper airway obstruction, and sleep-disordered breathing are common. Although a relatively small foramen magnum is seen in all children with achondroplasia, symptoms related to cord compression at the cervicomedullary junction occur only rarely. For example, sudden death probably due to brain stem or upper cervical cord compression, a threat particularly during the first year of life, occurs in less than 3 per cent. Significant controversy exists as to when and if decompressive neurosurgery should be performed. It is important to recognize that evaluation of affected children with symptoms relating to cervical cord compression should be performed by individuals experienced with and aware of the natural history of achondroplasia. CT dimensions for the foramen magnum of children with achondroplasia have been established by Hecht et al. The physician should be alert to detect any neurologic complications due to bone or disk compression. Osteoarthritis is not a usual feature in the adult. Osteotomies for severe bowlegs are usually deferred until full growth has occurred. By discouraging the sitting position or other positions that cause the trunk to curve anteriorly until an age when good trunk strength has developed, a permanent gibbus or kyphosis which is due to anterior wedging of the first two lumbar vertebrae can be prevented as well as obviating many of the problems with spinal stenosis and spinal cord compression that are so debilitating to adults with this condition. Exercises may also be utilized in an attempt to flatten the lumbosacral curve. Relative overgrowth of the fibula may accentuate bowing and require early stapling. Short eustachian tubes may lead to middle ear infection and conductive hearing loss. Tympanic membrane tubes may be indicated. Verbal comprehension is frequently impaired. The mandibular teeth may become crowded, possibly requiring removal of one or more. Todorov et al. have developed a screening test that establishes normal milestones for children with achondroplasia up to 2 years of age. There is a tendency toward late childhood obesity, and females are more prone to have menorrhagia, fibroids, and large breasts.

ETIOLOGY. Autosomal dominant, about 90 per cent of the cases represent a fresh gene mutation. Older paternal age has been a contributing factor in these cases. Mutations in the gene encoding fibroblast growth factor receptor 3 (FGFR3) located at 4p16.3 have been documented in all cases reported to date. Interestingly, virtually all cases demonstrate the same single base pair substitution, possibly accounting for the consistency of the phenotype seen in this disorder.

COMMENT. Histologic evaluation at the epiphyseal line discloses shorter cartilage columns that lack the usual linear arrangement, and some cartilage cells appear to be undergoing a mucinoid degeneration.

References

Maroteaux, P., and Lamy, M.: Achondroplasia in man and animals. Clin. Orthop., 33:91, 1964.

Caffey, J.: Pediatric X-Ray Diagnosis, 5th ed. Chicago, Year Book Medical Publishers, 1967, p. 819.

Cohen, M. E., Rosenthal, A. D., and Matson, D. D.: Neurological abnormalities in achondroplastic children. J. Pediatr., 71:367, 1967.

Nelson, M. A.: Spinal stenosis in achondroplasia. Proc. R. Soc. Med., 65:1028, 1972.

Horton, W. A., et al.: Standard growth curves for achondroplasia. J. Pediatr., 93:435, 1978.

Oberklaid, F., et al.: Achondroplasia and hypochondroplasia. J. Med. Genet., 16:140, 1979.

Todorov, A. B., et al.: Developmental screening tests in achondroplastic children. Am. J. Med. Genet., 9:19, 1981.

Hall, J. G., et al.: Letter to the editor: Head growth in achondroplasia: Use of ultrasound studies. Am. J. Med. Genet., 13:105, 1982.

Stokes, D. C., et al.: Respiratory complications of achondroplasia. J. Pediatr., 102:534, 1983.

Hecht, J. T., et al.: Computerized tomography of the foramen magnum: Achondroplastic values compared to normal standards. Am. J. Med. Genet., 20:355, 1985.

Reid, C. S., et al.: Cervicomedullary compression in young patients with achondroplasia: Value of comprehensive neurologic and respiratory evaluation. J. Pediatr., 110:522, 1987.

Hall, J. G.: Kyphosis in achondroplasia: Probably preventable. J. Pediatr., 112:166, 1988.

Brinkman, G., et al.: Cognitive skills in achondroplasia. Am. J. Med. Genet., 47:800, 1993.

Shiang, R., et al.: Mutations in the transmembrane domain of FGFR3 causes the most common genetic form of dwarfism, achondroplasia. Cell, 78:335, 1994.

Committee on Genetics: Health supervision for children with achondroplasia. Pediatrics, 95:443, 1995.

Pauli, R. M., et al.: Prospective assessment of risk for cervico-medullary junction compression in infants with achondroplasia. Am. J. Hum. Genet., 56:732, 1995.

Rimoin, D. L.: Invited editorial: Cervicomedullary junction compression in infants with achondroplasia: When to perform neurosurgical decompression. Am. J. Hum. Genet., 56:824, 1995.

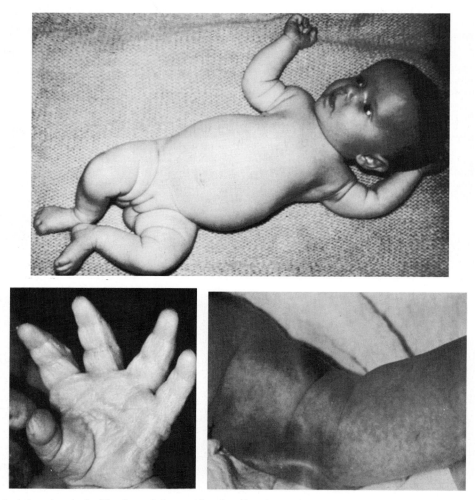

FIGURE 1. Achondroplasia. Newborn infant with achondroplasia, showing hypotonia, macrocephaly, low nasal bridge, relatively small thoracic cage, shortness of humeri and femurs (rhizomelia), "trident" position of the open, small hand, and inability to extend fully at the elbow.

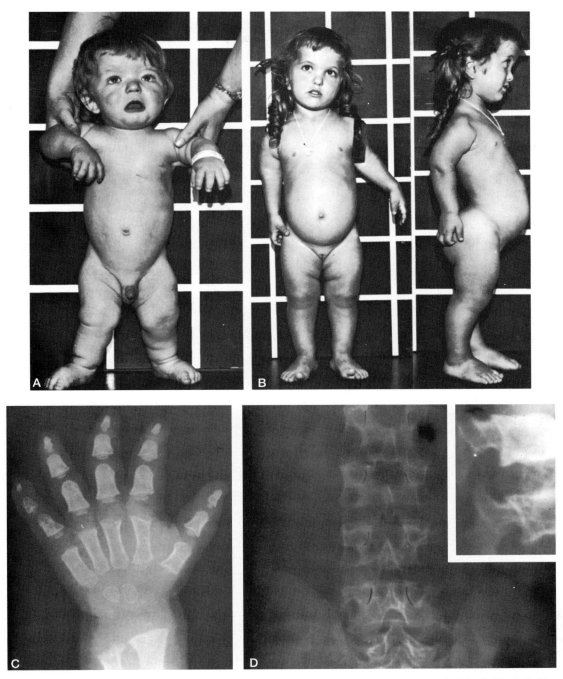

FIGURE 2. *Above*, Achondroplasia. *A*, A 1-year-old with height age of 4 months. (From Smith, D. W.: J. Pediatr., 70:504, 1967, with permission.) *B*, A 4-year-old with height age of 20 months. *Below*, *C*, Short "trident" hand with short metacarpals and phalanges. *D*, Caudal narrowing of spinal canal (pedicles marked) with short pedicles (*upper right*).

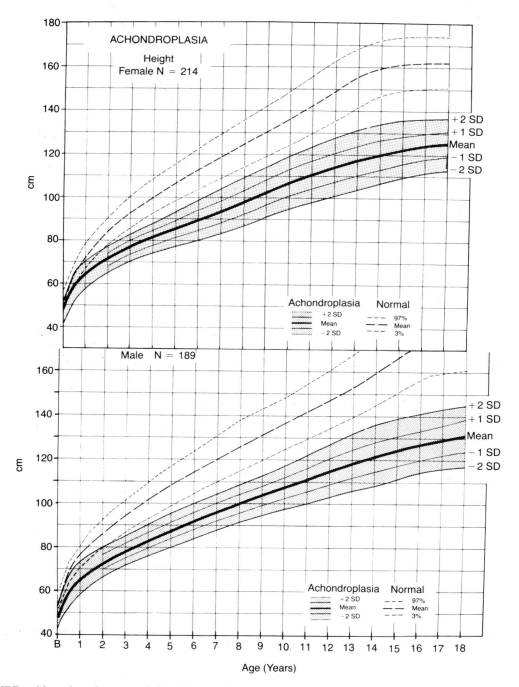

FIGURE 3. Note that about one half of the newborn babies with achondroplasia are within normal limits for length at birth, but there is a progressive deceleration of growth rate beginning in infancy. (From Horton, W. A., et al.: J. Pediatr., *93*:435, 1978, with permission.)

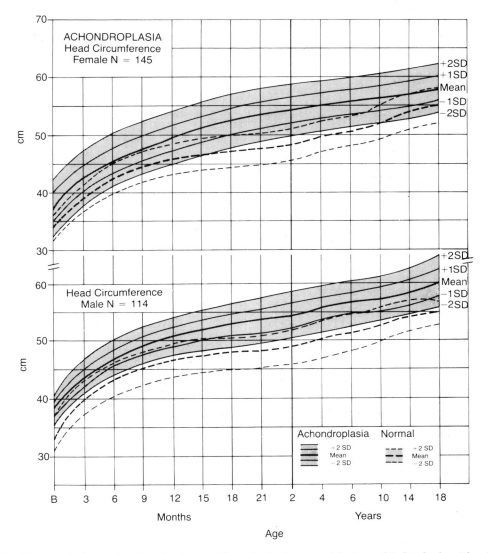

FIGURE 4. Macrocephaly, predominantly due to a large brain, is a usual feature of individuals with achondroplasia. (From Horton, W. A., et al.: J. Pediatr., *93*:435, 1978, with permission.)

HYPOCHONDROPLASIA

Short Limbs, Caudal Narrowing of Spine, Near-Normal Craniofacies

Though the features of this disorder were described by Ravenna in 1913, and its designation as hypochondroplasia and mode of inheritance were set forth in 1924, the majority of cases have been misdiagnosed as achondroplasia until recent times.

Hypochondroplasia has an incidence of about one twelfth that of achondroplasia and can be distinguished from it by the relative lack of craniofacial involvement and milder features in the hands and spine.

ABNORMALITIES

Growth. Small stature, usually of postnatal onset. Mean birth length, 47.7 cm; mean birth weight, 2.9 kg. Macrocephaly.

Limbs. Relatively short without rhizomelic, mesomelic, or acromelic predominance. Short tubular bones with mild metaphyseal flare. Short, broad femoral necks. Long distal fibulae, short distal ulnae, and long ulnar styloids. Brachydactyly. Bowing of legs. Stubby hands and feet. Mild limitation in elbow extension and supination.

Spine. Anteroposterior shortening of lumbar pedicles on lateral view. Spinal canal narrowing or unchanged caudally, with or without lumbar lordosis.

Pelvis. Squared and short ilia.

OCCASIONAL ABNORMALITIES. Mental deficiency, brachycephaly with short base of skull, mild frontal bossing, esotropia, cataract, ptosis, postaxial polydactyly of feet, high vertebrae, flat vertebrae.

NATURAL HISTORY. Slow growth, if not evident by birth, is usually obvious by 3 years of age. Final height attainment in adults ranged from 46.5 to 60 inches. Outward bowing of the lower limbs and genu varum may become pronounced with weight-bearing. Though this may improve in childhood, the condition may merit surgical straightening. The relatively long fibulae can result in inversion of the feet. Exercise may provoke mild aching in the knees, ankles, and/or elbows during childhood, and such discomfort is usually worse and may include the low back in the adult. Cesarean section is often required for delivery in pregnant women with this disorder. Mental deficiency, a rare feature in achondroplasia, was noted in 4 of the 13 cases reported by Walker et al., with I.Q.s ranging from 50 to 80, and in 9 per cent of the patients reported by Hall and Spranger.

ETIOLOGY. Autosomal dominant. Older paternal age has been documented in presumed fresh mutation cases. The altered gene for hypochondroplasia has been mapped to 4p16.3, the same locus as achondroplasia. This suggests that the two disorders may result from different mutations within the same gene.

References

Ravenna, F.: Achondroplasie et chondrohypoplasie: Contribution clinique. N. Iconog. Salpêtrière, *26*:157, 1913.

Léri, A., and Linossier (Mlle.): Hypochondroplasia héréditaire. Bull. Mem. Soc. Med. Hop. (Paris), *48*: 1780, 1924.

Beals, R. K.: Hypochondroplasia. A report of five kindred. J. Bone Joint Surg. [Am.], *51*:728, 1969.

Walker, B. A., et al.: Hypochondroplasia. Am. J. Dis. Child., *122*:95, 1971.

Hall, B. D., and Spranger, J.: Hypochondroplasia: Clinical and radiological aspects in 39 cases. Radiology, *133*:95, 1979.

Le Merrer, M., et al.: A gene for achondroplasia-hypochondroplasia maps to chromosome 4p. Nat. Genet., *6*:318, 1994.

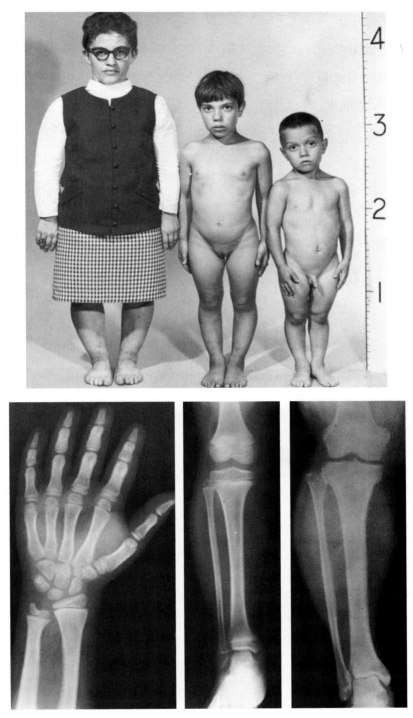

FIGURE 1. Hypochondroplasia. *Above,* Affected mother and children (7 and 6 years), showing short stature, most striking in the bowed lower limbs. *Lower left,* Note slight ulnar shortening, metaphyseal flaring with bulbous radial enlargement, and elongation of the styloid process (from a 10-year-old). *Lower middle,* A 7-year-old, showing elongation of distal fibula and slight "squaring off" of the proximal tibial epiphysis. *Lower right,* Adult, showing more striking squaring of proximal tibial epiphysis, with sharp flare of metaphysis and elongation of distal fibula with varus deformity of ankle mortise. (From Beals, R. K.: J. Bone Joint Surg. [Am.], *51*:728, 1969, with permission.)

353

PSEUDOACHONDROPLASIA
(Pseudoachondroplastic Spondyloepiphyseal Dysplasia)

Small Irregular Epiphyses, Irregular Mushroomed Metaphyses, Flattening and/or Anterior Beaking of Vertebrae, With Normal Craniofacial Appearance

Maroteaux and Lamy described three individuals with this pattern of altered bone morphogenesis in 1959. Numerous cases have been published.

ABNORMALITIES
Growth. Postnatal onset of short-limbed growth deficiency that becomes obvious between 18 months and 2 years. Adult stature, 82 to 130 cm.

Craniofacies. Normal head size and face.

Limbs. Disproportionately short. Hypermobility of major joints except elbows leading to genu varum, valgum, and recurvatum. Ulnar deviation of hands. Short fingers that are hypermobile.

Radiographs. Short long bones with wide metaphyses. Epiphyses are small, irregular, or "fragmented," especially the capital femoral epiphyses. Vertebral abnormalities consist of variable degrees of flattening with biconvex end plates and a central anterior boney protrusion from the anterior surface of the body. There is normal widening of the interpedicular distance from upper to lower lumbar spine. Odontoid aplasia or hypoplasia. Short sacral notches. Ribs tend to be spatulate. Terminal phalanges small.

Other. Lumbar lordosis, kyphosis, scoliosis.

NATURAL HISTORY. The patients have been described as "normal" at birth, with small size, short arms, and waddling gait becoming evident between 6 months and 4 years of age. Bowed lower extremities with waddling gait and scoliosis are the principal orthopedic problems, and there may be some limitation in joint motility. Intelligence is normal. Odontoid hypoplasia in association with hypermobility can result in increased motion of C1 on C2 leading to cord damage. Although the vertebral changes resolve with age, the epiphyseal changes of the long bones become more severe leading to progressive degeneration and severe osteoarthritis. A mild and severe form have been described.

ETIOLOGY. Autosomal dominant. The gene has been mapped to the pericentromeric region of chromosome 19. Mutations in the cartilage oligomeric matrix protein gene (COMP), which has been localized to chromosome 19p13.1, appear to lead to both the mild and severe forms of this disorder. Most of the cases have been sporadic and presumably represent fresh mutations. Rare cases of affected siblings born to unaffected parents are most likely the result of gonadal mosaicism. Based on what may well be an increased risk of gonadal mosaicism in this disorder, it has been estimated that unaffected parents who have had one affected child have a recurrence risk in the range of 4 per cent.

COMMENT. A mutation in the COMP gene also has been identified in multiple epiphyseal dysplasia, Fairbank type, suggesting that some forms of multiple epiphyseal dysplasia are allelic with pseudoachondroplasia.

References

Maroteaux, P., and Lamy, M.: Les formes pseudoachondroplastiques des dysplasies spondyloépiphysaires. Presse Med., *67*:383, 1959.

Ford, N., Silverman, F. N., and Kozlowski, K.: Spondyloepiphyseal dysplasia (pseudoachondroplastic type). Am. J. Roentgenol. Radium Ther. Nucl. Med., *86*:462, 1961.

Hall, J. G., et al.: Gonadal mosaicism in pseudoachondroplasia. Am. J. Med. Genet., *28*:143, 1987.

Briggs, M. D., et al.: Genetic linkage of mild pseudoachondroplasia (PSACH) to markers in the pericentromeric region of chromosome 19. Genomics, *18*:656, 1993.

Hecht, J. T., et al.: Linkage of typical pseudoachondroplasia to chromosome 19. Genomics, *18*:661, 1993.

Langer, L. O., et al.: Patient with double heterozygosity for achondroplasia and pseudoachondroplasia, with comments on these conditions and the relationship between pseudoachondroplasia and multiple epiphyseal dysplasia, Fairbank type. Am. J. Med. Genet., *47*:772, 1993.

Hecht, J. L., et al.: Mutations in exon 17B of cartilage oligomeric matrix protein (COMP) cause pseudoachondroplasia. Nat. Genet., *10*:325, 1995.

Briggs, M. D., et al.: Pseudoachondroplasia and multiple epiphyseal dysplasia due to mutations in the cartilage oligomeric matrix protein gene. Nat. Genet., *10*:330, 1995.

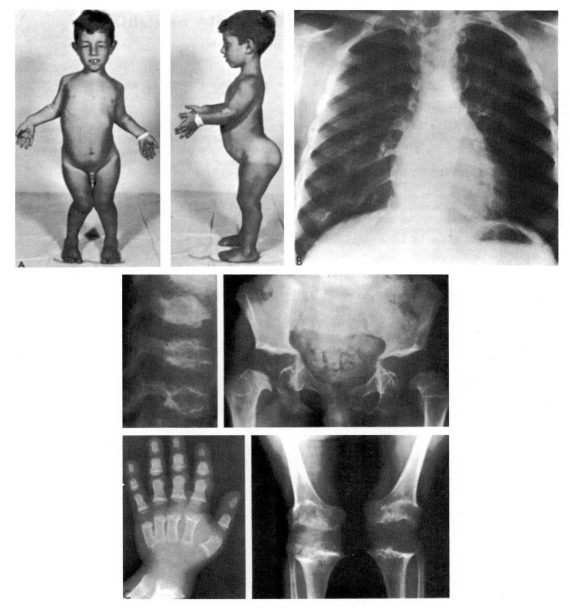

FIGURE 1. Pseudoachondroplastic spondyloepiphyseal dysplasia. *A*, An 8-year-old with height age of 3 years. *B*, Mildly spatulate ribs; scoliosis. *C*, Flattened irregular vertebral bodies, hypoplastic abnormal iliac wings, and short tubular bones with irregular "ball-in-socket" epiphyses in relation to metaphyses. (From Lindseth, R. E., et al.: Am. J. Dis. Child., *113*:721, 1967, with permission.)

ACROMESOMELIC DYSPLASIA

(Acromesomelic Dwarfism)

Short Distal Limbs, Frontal Prominence, Low Thoracic Kyphosis

Maroteaux et al. recognized this disorder in 1971, and Langer et al. summarized the manifestations in 19 patients in 1977. Approximately 30 cases have been reported.

ABNORMALITIES

Craniofacial. Disproportionately large head with relative frontal prominence, with or without relatively short nose.

Limbs. Short limbs with short hands and feet. Bowed forearms that are relatively shorter than upper arms. Limited elbow extension. Short fingers and toes with short but not dysplastic nails. Redundant skin develops over fingers in childhood.

Spine. Development of lower thoracic kyphosis.

Radiographs. Metacarpals and phalanges become increasingly shorter during the first year. Middle and proximal phalanges are broad. Cone-shaped epiphyses develop. Shortening of humerus, radius, and ulna progresses during first year. Bowed radius. Vertebral bodies are oval shaped in infancy, but with advancing age the posterior aspect of the bodies becomes shorter than the anterior. By 24 months, a central protrusion of bone develops anteriorly. Superiorly curved clavicles that appear located high. Flared metaphyses of long tubular bones. Hypoplasia of basilar portion of ilia and irregular ossification of lateral superior acetabular region in childhood.

OCCASIONAL ABNORMALITIES. Relatively large great toe. Corneal clouding. Hydrocephalus. Mild mental retardation.

NATURAL HISTORY. Birth weight may be normal, and the linear growth deficiency becomes more evident during the first year. Lower thoracic kyphosis, increased lumbar lordosis, and prominent buttocks are common. Most joints tend to be relatively lax. There may be some lag in gross motor performance because of the relatively large head and short limbs but intelligence is normal. Final height in nine adults ranged from 38 to 49 inches.

ETIOLOGY. Autosomal recessive.

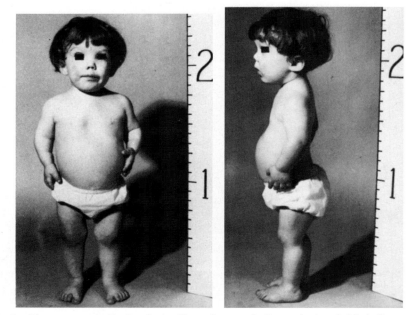

FIGURE 1. Infant with acromesomelic dysplasia. (From Langer, L. O., et al.: Am. J. Med. Genet., *1*:87, 1977, with permission.)

References

Maroteaux, P., Martinelli, B., and Campailla, E.: Le nanisme acromesomelique. Presse Med., 79:1838, 1971.

Langer, L. O., et al.: Acromesomelic dwarfism: Manifestations in childhood. Am. J. Med. Genet., 1:87, 1977.

Langer, L. O., and Garrett, R. T.: Acromesomelic dysplasia. Radiology, 137:349, 1980.

Fernandez del Moral, R., et al.: Report of a case: Acromesomelic dysplasia: Radiologic, clinical and pathological study. Am. J. Med. Genet., 33:415, 1989.

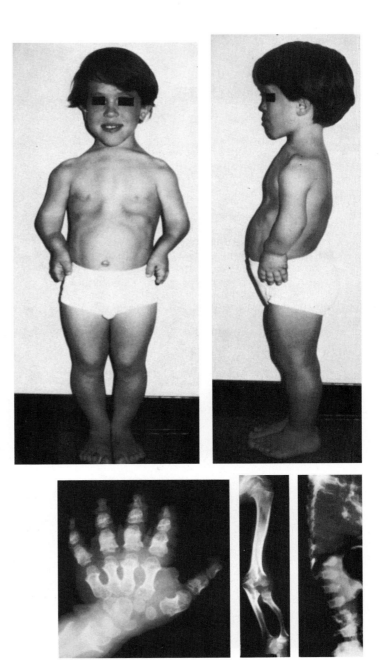

FIGURE 2. Child with acromesomelic dysplasia and roentgenographic findings. (From Langer, L. O., et al.: Am. J. Med. Genet., 1:87, 1977, with permission.)

SPONDYLOEPIPHYSEAL DYSPLASIA CONGENITA

Short Trunk, Lag in Epiphyseal Mineralization, Myopia

Spranger and Wiedemann established this disorder in 1966 when they reported six new cases and summarized 14 from the past literature. Numerous additional cases have been reported subsequently.

ABNORMALITIES. Onset at birth.

Growth. Prenatal onset growth deficiency; final height, 37 to 52 inches.

Facies. Variable flat facies, malar hypoplasia, cleft palate.

Eyes. Myopia, retinal detachment (50 per cent).

Spine. Short, including neck with ovoid flattened vertebrae with narrow intervertebral disk spaces, odontoid hypoplasia, kyphoscoliosis, lumbar lordosis.

Chest. Barrel chest with pectus carinatum.

Limbs. Lag in mineralization of epiphyses, which tend to be flat, with no os pubis, talus, calcaneus, or knee centers mineralized at birth. Coxa vara. Diminished joint mobility at elbows, knees, and hips.

Muscles. Weakness, easy fatigability, hypoplasia of abdominal muscles.

OCCASIONAL ABNORMALITIES. Talipes equinovarus, dislocation of hip.

NATURAL HISTORY. The hypotonic weakness and orthopedic situation contribute to a late on-set of walking, usually with a waddling gait. Myopia should be suspected, and frequent ophthalmologic evaluation is merited to guard against retinal detachment. Morning stiffness may be a feature, but there is usually no undue joint pain.

ETIOLOGY. Autosomal dominant. A variety of alterations in the COL2A1 gene, which codes for type II collagen including deletions, duplications, and single base substitutions, lead to spondyloepiphyseal dysplasia congenita. Instances of affected siblings born to unaffected parents is most likely due to germinal mosaicism.

References

Spranger, J., and Wiedemann, H. R.: Dysplasia spondyloepiphysaria congenita. Helv. Paediatr. Acta, *21*: 598, 1966.

Spranger, J., and Langer, L. O.: Spondyloepiphyseal dysplasia congenita. Radiology, *94*:313, 1970.

Harrod, M. J. E., et al.: Genetic heterogeneity in spondyloepiphyseal dysplasia congenita. Am. J. Med. Genet., *18*:311, 1984.

Spranger, J., et al.: The type II collagenopathies: A spectrum of chondrodysplasias. Eur. J. Pediatr., *153*: 56, 1994.

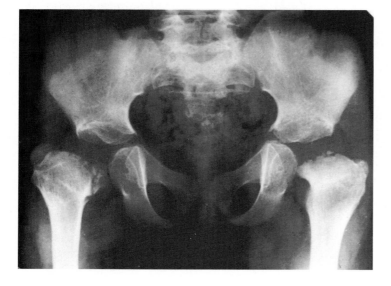

FIGURE 1. Spondyloepiphyseal dysplasia congenita. Pelvis at 7 years, showing horizontal acetabula and lack of ossification of femoral heads and femoral necks, which are in severe varus position. (Courtesy of Dr. Jurgen Spranger, Mainz, Germany.)

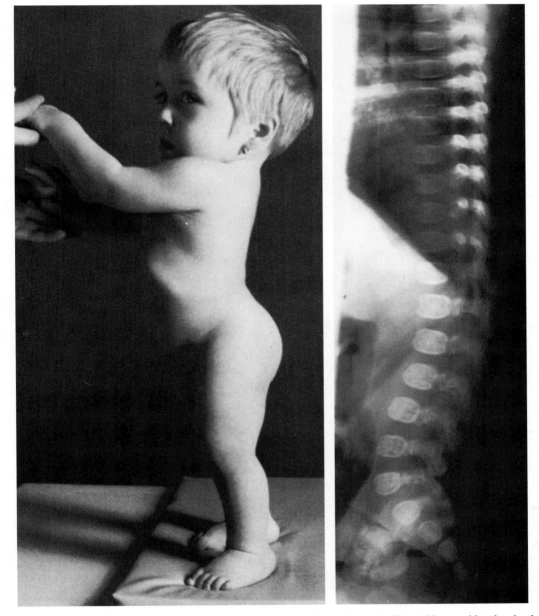

FIGURE 2. Spondyloepiphyseal dysplasia congenita. A 4-year-old boy. Note the flat midface and lumbar lordosis. Roentgenogram of spine at 9 months, showing mild dorsal flattening and minimal beaking at L2–L3. (Courtesy of Dr. Jurgen Spranger, Mainz, Germany.)

KNIEST DYSPLASIA

Flat Facies, Thick Joints, Platyspondyly

Though Kniest described this disorder in 1952, it has been more generally recognized only in recent years.

ABNORMALITIES

Growth. Disproportionate short stature with short, barrel-shaped chest.

Craniofacies. Flat facies with prominent eyes, low nasal bridge, myopia that may progress to retinal detachment, vitreoretinal degeneration, cleft palate with frequent ear infections. The head, which is of normal size, is relatively large.

Limbs. Enlarged joints with limited joint mobility and variable pain and stiffness. Short limbs, often with bowing. Some irregularity of epiphyses with late ossification of femoral heads. Flexion contractures in hips. Inability to form fist secondary to bony enlargements and soft tissue swelling at interphalangeal joints.

Other. Lumbar kyphoscoliosis. Inguinal and umbilical hernias, small pelvis, short clavicles. Hearing loss. Tracheomalacia. Cataracts. Lens dislocation.

Radiographs. Dumbbell-shaped femurs, hypoplastic pelvic bones, platyspondyly, and vertical clefts of vertebrae in newborn period. By age 3, pelvis becomes "dessert-cup shaped," ends of bones reveal irregular epiphyses, diffuse osteoporosis, and cloud-like radiodensities on both sides of epiphyseal plates. Thereafter, platyspondyly remains, intervertebral disk space is narrow, odontoid is large and wide. Flared metaphyses. Large epiphyses.

NATURAL HISTORY. Short extremities with stiff joints in neonatal period. Respiratory distress associated with tracheomalacia sometimes occurs in infancy. Marked lumbar lordosis and kyphoscoliosis lead to disproportionate shortening of trunk in childhood. Late walking because of orthopedic disability with contracted hips. Limitation of joint motion with pain, stiffness, and flexion contractures of major joints develops. Chronic otitis media related to cleft palate. Normal intelligence despite delayed motor milestones and speech. Final height, 106 to 145 cm. Frequent ophthalmologic evaluations are indicated in order to prevent retinal detachment.

ETIOLOGY. Autosomal dominant. Most cases represent a fresh gene mutation. This disorder represents one of a spectrum of chondrodysplasias due to defects in the gene for type II collagen, COL2A1. Others include type II achondrogenesis-hypochondrogenesis, spondyloepiphyseal dysplasia congenita, and Stickler syndrome.

References

Kniest, W.: Zur Abgrenzung der Dysostosis enchondralis von der Chondrodystrophie. Z. Kinderheilkd., 70:633, 1952.

Kim, H. J., et al.: Kniest syndrome with dominant inheritance and mucopolysacchariduria. Am. J. Hum. Genet., 77:755, 1975.

Rimoin, D. L., et al.: Metatropic dwarfism, the Kniest syndrome and the pseudoachondroplastic dysplasias. Clin. Orthop., 114:70, 1976.

Maumenee, I. H., and Traboulsi, E. I.: The ocular findings in Kniest dysplasia. Am. J. Ophthalmol., 100:155, 1985.

Spranger, J., et al.: The type II collagenopathies: A spectrum of chondrodysplasias. Eur. J. Pediatr., 153:56, 1994.

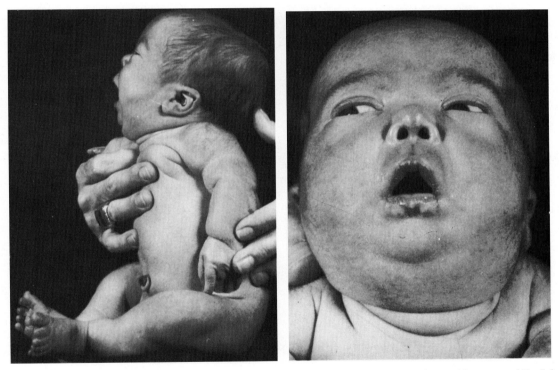

FIGURE 1. Infant with Kniest dysplasia, showing malproportionment and unusual facies. (Courtesy of Dr. John Graham, Cedars-Sinai Medical Center, Los Angeles, Calif.)

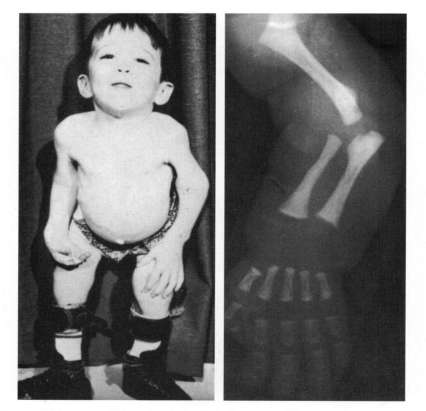

FIGURE 2. A 3-year-old boy with Kniest dysplasia. (*Left*, Courtesy of Dr. D. L. Rimoin, Cedars-Sinai Medical Center, Los Angeles, Calif. and *Right*, Courtesy of Dr. J. H. Graham, Cedars-Sinai Medical Center, Los Angeles, Calif.)

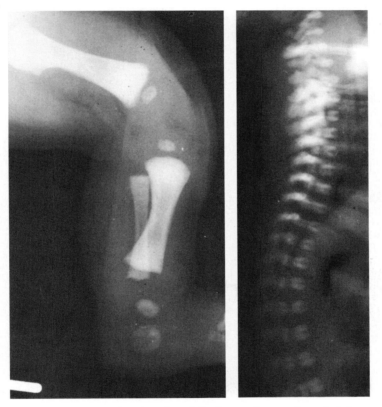

FIGURE 2. *Continued.* Roentgenograms showing altered limb morphogenesis and platyspondyly with coronal clefting. (Courtesy of Dr. J. H. Graham, Cedars-Sinai Medical Center, Los Angeles, Calif.)

DYGGVE-MELCHIOR-CLAUSEN SYNDROME

Initially described in 1962 by Dyggve et al., the clinical and radiographic features were set forth more completely in 1975 by Spranger et al. Approximately 50 cases have been reported.

ABNORMALITIES

Growth. Deficiency of postnatal onset, with short trunk dwarfism becoming evident before 18 months.

Performance. Mental deficiency.

Craniofacies. Microcephaly. Coarse facies. Prognathism. Facial bones large for cranium.

Spine. Flattened vertebrae with anterior pointing of the bodies and notch-like ossification defects of the superior and inferior end plates. Short neck. Odontoid hypoplasia. Scoliosis. Kyphosis. Lordosis.

Thorax. Sternal protrusion. Barrel chest.

Pelvis. Small ilia with irregularly calcified (lace-like) iliac crests in childhood developing into a marginal irregularity in adulthood. Lateral displacement of capital femoral epiphyses. Sloping, dysplastic acetabulae. Pubic ramus is wide.

Limbs. Restricted joint mobility. Waddling gait. Dislocated hips. Genu valga and vera. Rhizomelic limb shortening with irregular metaphyses and epiphyses. Malformed olecranons and radial heads. Broad hands and feet. Short metacarpals, particularly the first, and short notched phalanges. Cone-shaped epiphyses. Small carpals.

NATURAL HISTORY. Manifestations become evident between 1 and 18 months. Feeding problems frequently occur during infancy. Restriction of joint mobility primarily affects the elbows, hips, and knees. Spinal cord compression due to atlantoaxial instability is a preventable complication. The degree of mental retardation has varied from moderate to severe. Three known adults measured 128 cm, 127 cm, and 119 cm, respectively.

ETIOLOGY. Autosomal recessive.

COMMENT. Both sporadic and familial cases have been described with identical skeletal changes who have normal intelligence, suggesting that this disorder is heterogeneous.

References

Dyggve, H. V., Melchior, J. C., and Clausen, J.: Morquio-Ullrich's disease. An inborn error of metabolism? Arch. Dis. Child., 37:525, 1962.

Spranger, J., Maroteaux, P., Der Kaloustian, V. M.: The Dyggve-Melchior-Clausen syndrome. Radiology, 114:415, 1975.

Naffah, J.: The Dyggve-Melchior-Clausen syndrome. Am. J. Hum. Genet., 28:607, 1976.

Spranger, J., Bierbaum, B., and Herrmann, J.: Heterogeneity of Dyggve-Melchior-Clausen dwarfism. Hum. Genet., 33:279, 1976.

Bonafede, R. P., and Beighton, P.: The Dyggve-Melchior-Clausen syndrome in adult siblings. Clin. Genet., 14:24, 1978.

Beighton, P.: Dyggve-Melchior-Clausen syndrome. J. Med. Genet., 27:512, 1990.

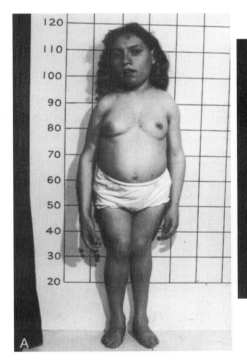

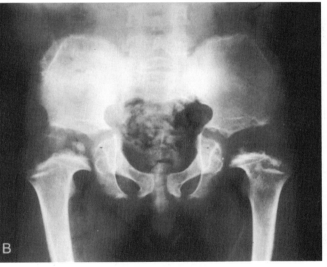

FIGURE 1. *A* and *B*, Adolescent with Dyggve-Melchior-Clausen syndrome. Note the irregularly calcified iliac crests. (Courtesy of Dr. R. Lachman, Harbor-UCLA Medical Center, and Dr. D. Rimoin, Cedars-Sinai Medical Center, Los Angeles, Calif.)

KOZLOWSKI SPONDYLOMETAPHYSEAL DYSPLASIA

(Kozlowski Spondylometaphyseal Chondrodysplasia)

Early Childhood Onset Short Spine, Irregular Metaphyses, Pectus Carinatum

Kozlowski et al. established this disorder in 1967, and several additional cases have been recognized. Spondylometaphyseal dysplasia comprises a group of disorders in which the spine and metaphyses of the tubular bones are affected. At least seven types have been classified based on minor radiographic differences and mode of transmission. The Kozlowski type is the most well known and the most common.

ABNORMALITIES

Growth. Growth deficiency, especially of trunk, from 1 to 4 years of age. Adult height, 4 feet 3 inches to 5 feet.

Spine. Short neck and trunk with dorsal kyphosis. Generalized platyspondyly with anterior narrowing in thoracolumbar region on lateral roentgenograms. On anteroposterior view, vertebral bodies extend more laterally to pedicles, producing an "open-staircase" appearance. Odontoid hypoplasia.

Thorax. Pectus carinatum.

Pelvis. Squarish, short iliac wings; flat, irregular acetabula.

Limbs. Irregular rachitic-like metaphyses, especially the proximal femur with very short femoral necks. Hypoplastic carpal bones with late ossification.

NATURAL HISTORY. Affected patients are usually normal at birth. A noticeably waddling gait with limitation of joint mobility becomes apparent at 15 to 20 months and is often the first sign of the disorder. Degenerative joint changes leading to discomfort occur at a relatively early age.

ETIOLOGY. Autosomal dominant, with most cases representing fresh mutation.

References

Kozlowski, K., Maroteaux, P., and Spranger, J.: La dysostose spondylo-métaphysaire. Presse Med., *75*: 2769, 1967.

Riggs, W., Jr., and Summitt, R. L.: Spondylometaphyseal dysplasia (Kozlowski). Report of affected mother and son. Radiology, *101*:375, 1971.

Le Quesne, G. W., and Kozlowski, K.: Spondylometaphyseal dysplasia. Br. J. Radiol., *46*:685, 1973.

Kozlowski, K., et al.: Spondylo-metaphyseal dysplasia. (Report of 7 cases and essay of classification). *In* Papadatos, C. J., and Bartsocas, C. S. (eds.): Skeletal Dysplasias. New York, Alan R. Liss, 1982, pp. 89–101.

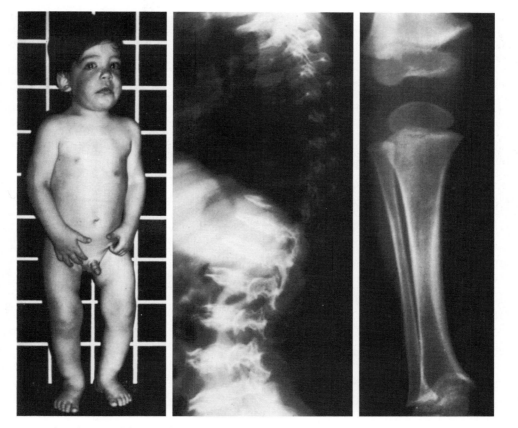

FIGURE 1. Kozlowski spondylometaphyseal dysplasia. Young boy. Note bowed legs, flattened vertebrae, and metaphyseal flare. (From Riggs, W., Jr., and Summitt, R. L.: Radiology, *101*:375, 1971, with permission.)

METATROPIC DYSPLASIA

(Metatropic Dwarfism Syndrome)

Small Thorax, Thoracic Kyphoscoliosis, Metaphyseal Flaring

Maroteaux et al. set forth this entity with five cases of their own and 12 unrecognized cases from the literature. The striking early findings, shown on the following three pages, include huge epiphyses. Over 50 cases have been reported.

ABNORMALITIES

Growth. Birth weight normal. Birth length greater than 97th percentile. Trunk, initially long relative to the limbs, becomes progressively short with the development of kyphoscoliosis, leading to short-trunk dwarfism.

Skeletal. Early platyspondyly with progressive kyphosis and scoliosis in infancy to early childhood. Odontoid hypoplasia. C1–C2 subluxation. Narrow thorax with short ribs. Short limbs with metaphyseal flaring and epiphyseal irregularity with hyperplastic trochanters. Prominent joints with restricted mobility at knee and hip but increased extensibility of finger joints. Hypoplasia of basilar pelvis with horizontal acetabula, short deep sacroiliac notch, and squared iliac wings.

OCCASIONAL ABNORMALITIES. Macrocephaly. Enlarged ventricles. Small foramen magnum. Clinical evidence of cord compression.

NATURAL HISTORY. Often evident at birth, the vertebral changes become severe during infancy. The trunk, originally long, becomes extremely short secondary to rapidly progressing kyphoscoliosis. Odontoid hypoplasia with C1–C2 subluxation can lead to cord compression, quadriplegia, and sometimes death. Cervical (C1–C2) fusion should be considered in all such cases. Measurements of the foramen magnum are indicated. Pelvic outlet constriction has led to colonic obstruction in at least one case.

ETIOLOGY. Genetic heterogeneity suggested by three different presentations: A nonlethal autosomal recessive form, a nonlethal autosomal dominant form with less severe spinal and pelvic changes, and a lethal autosomal recessive form with severe mushrooming and shortening of tubular bones and severe underossification of vertebral bodies.

References

Fleury, J., et al.: Un cas singulier de dystrophie osteochondrale congenitale (nanisme metatrophique de Maroteaux). Ann. Pediatr. (Paris), *13*:453, 1966.

Maroteaux, P., Spranger, I., and Wiedemann, H. R.: Der metatropische Zwergwucks. Arch. Kinderheilkd., *173*:211, 1966.

Larose, J. H., and Gay, B. G.: Metatropic dwarfism. Am. J. Roetgenol. Radium Ther. Nucl. Med., *106*:156, 1969.

Beck, M., et al.: Heterogeneity of metatropic dysplasia. Eur. J. Pediatr., *140*:231, 1983.

Shohat, M., et al.: Odontoid hypoplasia with vertebral cervical subluxation and ventriculomegaly in metatropic dysplasia. J. Pediatr., *114*:239, 1989.

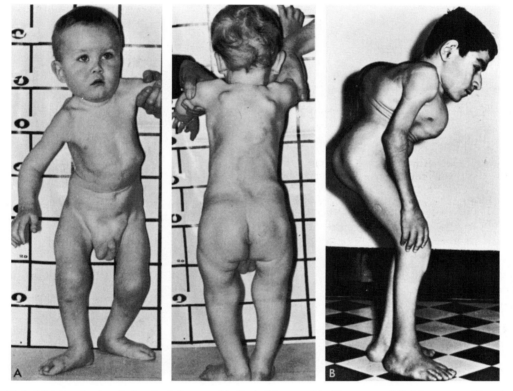

FIGURE 1. Metatropic dysplasia. *A*, A 2-year-old. *B*, A 16-year-old. (Courtesy of P. Maroteaux, Hospital des Enfants-Malades, Paris.)

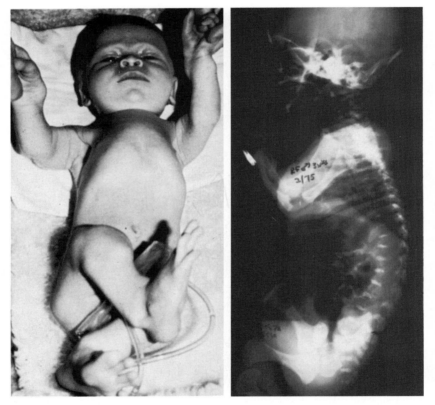

FIGURE 2. A 1-week-old with metatropic dwarfism and the platyspondyly at 3 weeks.

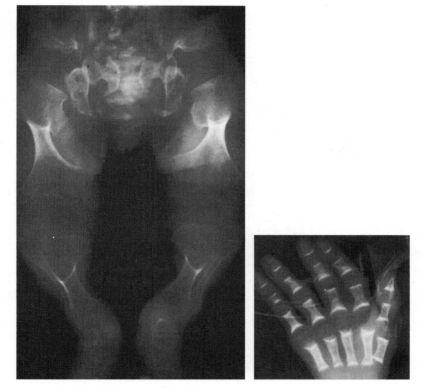

FIGURE 2. *Continued*. The grossly distorted metaphyses at 6 months and the hand at 2 months. (Courtesy of Dr. Paul S. Bergeson, Good Samaritan Hospital, Phoenix, Ariz.)

GELEOPHYSIC DYSPLASIA

Initially described by Spranger et al. in 1971, a total of 12 cases have now been reported. The term "geleophysic" (*geleos*, meaning happy; and *physis*, meaning nature) refers to the happy-natured facial appearance typical of this disorder.

ABNORMALITIES

Growth. Short stature predominantly of postnatal onset with normal upper/lower segment ratio. Span is decreased due to shortening of hands. Decreased birth length has been noted in one third of cases in which it was reported.

Craniofacies. Round, full face. Short nose with anteverted nares. Up-slanting palpebral fissures; long, smooth philtrum with thin, inverted vermilion and wide mouth. Thickened helix of normally formed ear. "Pleasant, happy-natured" appearance. Gradual coarsening occurs postnatally.

Limbs. Short hands and feet with markedly short tubular bones and relatively normal epiphyses. Wide shafts of first and fifth metacarpals and proximal and middle phalanges. Progressive contractures of multiple joints, particularly fingers and wrists. Small, irregular capital femoral epiphyses (after 4 years), but other epiphyses, metaphyses, and diaphyses are normal. J-shaped sella turcica.

Cardiac. Progressive thickening of heart valves, with incompetence.

Other. Hepatomegaly. Thickened, tight skin.

OCCASIONAL ABNORMALITIES. Narrowing of trachea and mainstem bronchi. Pectus excavatum. Paralysis of upward gaze due to abnormality of superior oblique muscle. Developmental delay. Seizures.

NATURAL HISTORY. Recognizable at birth because of typical face and small hands and feet, growth deficiency and the characteristic facies become more obvious with time. With respect to prognosis, two children have died secondary to tracheal stenosis at 3 and 4 years of age, respectively, and three died of heart failure secondary to progressive valvular disease at 5 months, 1 year, and 5 years of age, respectively. All the survivors have had cardiac involvement, although mild and asymptomatic in some. Two are now young adults.

ETIOLOGY. Autosomal recessive. Although the basic biochemical defect is unknown, lysosomal storage vacuoles have been found in skin epithelial cells, tracheal mucosa, liver, cartilage, and heart valves.

References

Spranger, J. W., et al.: Geleophysic dwarfism—a "focal" mucopolysaccharidosis? Lancet, 2:97, 1971.

Koiffmann, C. P., et al.: Brief clinical report: Familial recurrence of geleophysic dysplasia. Am. J. Med. Genet., *19*:483, 1984.

Spranger, J., et al.: Geleophysic dysplasia. Am. J. Med. Genet., *19*:487, 1984.

Wraith, J. E., et al.: Geleophysic dysplasia. Am. J. Med. Genet., *35*:153, 1990.

Shohat, M., et al.: Geleophysic dysplasia: A storage disorder affecting the skin, bone, liver, heart and trachea. J. Pediatr., *117*:227, 1990.

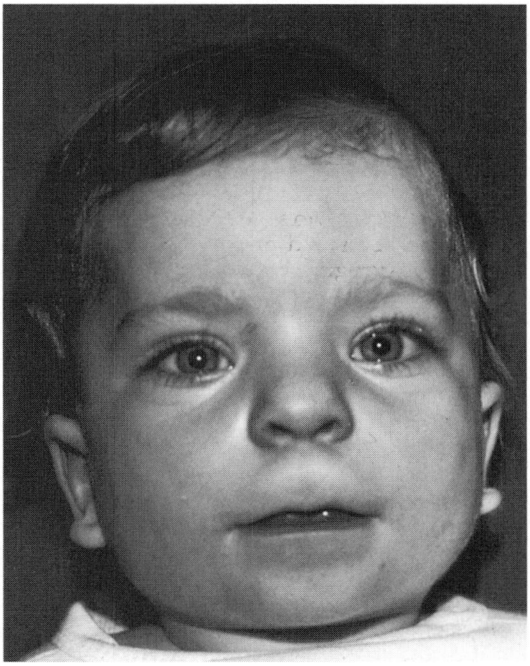

FIGURE 1. Geleophysic dysplasia. A 2-year-old boy. (From Spranger, J. W., et al.: Lancet, 2:97, 1971, with permission.)

CHONDROECTODERMAL DYSPLASIA

(Ellis-van Creveld Syndrome)

Short Distal Extremities,
Polydactyly, Nail Hypoplasia

Ellis and van Creveld set forth this entity in 1940. About 40 cases were reported by 1964 when McKusick et al. added 52 cases from an inbred Amish population. Well over 200 cases have now been reported.

ABNORMALITIES

Growth. Small stature of prenatal onset.

Skeletal. Disproportionate, irregularly short extremities. Polydactyly of fingers, occasionally of toes. Short, broad middle phalanges and hypoplastic distal phalanges. Malformed carpals, fusion of capitate and hamate, and extra carpal bones. Narrow thorax with short, poorly developed ribs. Hypoplasia of upper lateral tibia, with knock-knee. Pelvic dysplasia with low iliac wings and spur-like, downward projections at the medial and lateral aspects of the acetabula.

Nails. Hypoplastic.

Teeth. Neonatal teeth, partial anodontia, small teeth, and/or delayed eruption.

Mouth. Short upper lip bound by frenula to alveolar ridge; defects in alveolar ridge with accessory frenula.

Cardiac. About one half of the patients have a cardiac defect, most commonly an atrial septal defect; often with a single atrium.

OCCASIONAL ABNORMALITIES. Mental retardation, Dandy-Walker malformation, heterotopic masses of gray matter, scant or fine hair, cryptorchidism, epispadias, talipes equinovarus, renal agenesis.

NATURAL HISTORY. About one half of the patients die in early infancy as a consequence of cardiorespiratory problems. The majority of survivors are of normal intelligence. Eventual stature is in the range of 43 to 60 inches. There is usually some limitation in hand function, such as inability to form a clenched fist. Dental problems are frequent.

ETIOLOGY. Autosomal recessive.

References

Ellis, R. W. B., and van Creveld, S.: A syndrome characterized by ectodermal dysplasia, polydactyly, chondro-dysplasia and congenital morbus cordis. Report of three cases. Arch. Dis. Child., *15*:65, 1940.

McKusick, V. A., et al.: Dwarfism in the Amish. The Ellis-van Creveld syndrome. Bull. Hopkins Hosp., *115*:306, 1964.

Feingold, M., et al.: Ellis-van Creveld syndrome. Clin. Pediatr. (Phila.), *5*:431, 1966.

Rosemberg, S., et al.: Brief clinical report: Chondroectodermal dysplasia (Ellis-van Creveld) with anomalies of CNS and urinary tract. Am. J. Med. Genet., *15*:291, 1983.

Taylor, G. A., et al.: Polycarpaly and other abnormalities of the wrist in chondroectodermal dysplasia: The Ellis-van Creveld syndrome. Radiology, *151*: 393, 1984.

Quereshi, F., et al.: Skeletal histopathology in fetus with chondroectodermal dysplasia (Ellis-van Creveld syndrome). Am. J. Med. Genet., *45*:471, 1993.

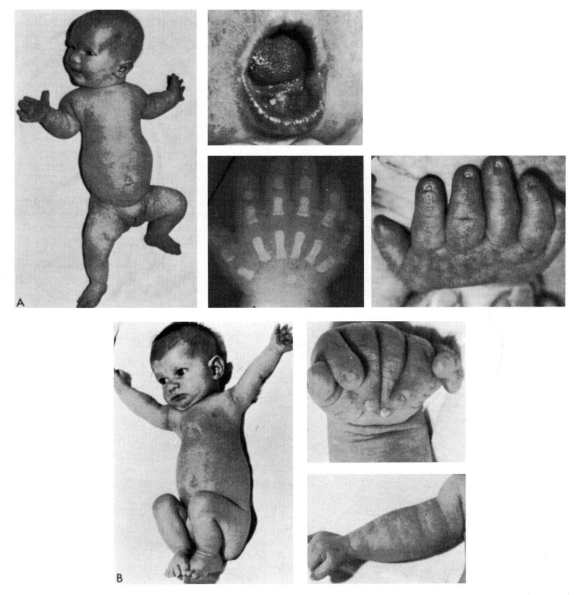

FIGURE 1. Chondroectodermal dysplasia. *A,* A 6-week-old. Note the hypoplasia of the alveolar ridge, with frenula and an aberrant tooth. The patient is now doing well at several years of age. *B,* A 5-month-old. Note the small thorax. The patient expired as a consequence of a congenital heart defect plus the small thorax. (*B* Courtesy of Professor H. Willi, Kantonsspital, Zurich.)

DIASTROPHIC* DYSPLASIA

(Diastrophic Nanism Syndrome)

Short Tubular Bones (Especially First Metacarpal), Joint Limitation With Talipes, Hypertrophied Auricular Cartilage

The 1960 report of Lamy and Maroteaux concerning three cases of their own and 11 similar cases from the literature established this pattern of malformation as a distinct entity. It is now recognized with frequency.

ABNORMALITIES

Growth. Disproportionate short stature of prenatal onset. Mean birth length, 42 cm.

Limbs. Talipes equinovarus plus limitation of flexion at proximal phalangeal joints and of extension at elbow, with or without dislocation of hip or knee with weight-bearing. Short and thick tubular bones with development of broad metaphyses and flattened irregular epiphyses that are late in mineralizing. Carpal bones may be accelerated in ossification in contrast with the remainder of the hand. First metacarpal unduly small. Abduction of thumbs (hitchhiker thumbs) and great toes. Variable symphalangism of proximal interphalangeal joints. Variable webbing at joints.

Spine. Scoliosis (49 per cent in females; 22 per cent in males). Spina bifida occulta from C3–C4 to upper thoracic vertebrae (73 per cent in females; 59 per cent in males). Hypoplasia of cervical vertebral bodies (29 per cent) with kyphosis and subluxation. Interpedicular narrowing from L1–L5.

Pinnae. Soft cystic masses in auricle develop into hypertrophic cartilage in early infancy in 84 per cent of patients.

OCCASIONAL ABNORMALITIES. Thick pectinate strands at root of iris, cleft palate (25 per cent), micrognathia, lateral displacement of patellae, subluxation of cervical vertebrae, elbow dislocation, hyperelasticity of skin, cryptorchidism. Early mineralization of ribs, intracranial calcification. Deafness secondary to fusion or lack of ossicles, stenosis of the external auditory canal. Laryngotracheal stenosis. Midfacial capillary hemangiomata.

NATURAL HISTORY. Two affected infants with cleft palate and micrognathia, similar in this respect to those with the Robin sequence,

died of respiratory obstruction. The mortality rate related to respiratory obstruction, including laryngeal stenosis, can be as high as 25 per cent in early infancy. For the survivors, general health is usually good, and the patients have normal intelligence, although there exists a risk for development of neurologic complications due to cervical spine anomalies. The possibility of atlantoaxial instability must always be considered. Unfortunately, the talipes equinovarus and the scoliosis that develop have been rather resistant to corrective orthopedic measures, and the functional problem is aggravated by the limitation in joint motility. Spinal cord compression may occur as a consequence of severe kyphoscoliosis. When present, the unusual defect of hypertrophied auricular cartilage may eventually give way to ossification. Linear growth is persistently slow; adult stature varies from 100 to 140 cm, with a mean of 125 cm.

ETIOLOGY. Autosomal recessive. The gene, which encodes a novel sulfate transporter, maps to the distal long arm of chromosome 5. It is likely that impaired function of its product leads to the production of undersulfated proteoglycans in cartilage matrix, the presumed basis for the clinical phenotype in this disorder.

References

Lamy, M., and Maroteaux, P.: Le nanisme diastrophique. Presse Med., 68:1977, 1960.

Langer, L. O.: Diastrophic dwarfism in early infancy. Am. J. Roentgenol. Radium Ther. Nucl. Med., 93: 399, 1965.

Walker, B. A., et al.: Diastrophic dwarfism. Medicine, 51:41, 1972.

Horton, W. A., et al.: The phenotypic variability of diastrophic dysplasia. J. Pediatr., 93:608, 1978.

Hastbacka, J., et al.: Diastrophic dysplasia gene maps to the distal long arm of chromosome 5. Proc. Natl. Acad. Sci. U. S. A., 87:8056, 1990.

Poussa, M., et al.: The spine in diastrophic dysplasia. Spine, 16:881, 1990.

Hastbacka, J., et al.: The diastrophic dysplasia gene encodes a novel sulfate transporter: Positional cloning by fine-structure linkage disequilibrium mapping. Cell, 78:1073, 1994.

---

*Diastrophic = crooked.

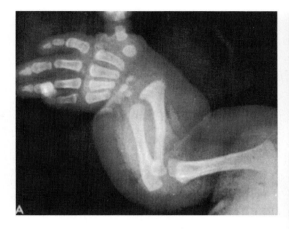

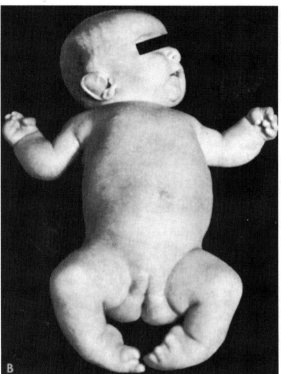

FIGURE 1. *A*, Diastrophic dwarfism in a 4-month-old. Note small first metacarpal. *B*, A 1-month-old. Note cystic swelling of ear. (From Langer, L. O.: Am. J. Roentgenol. Radium Ther. Nucl. Med., *93*: 399, 1965, with permission.) *C*, A 21-month-old. Note hypertrophy of ear and position of thumbs. (From Smith, D. W.: J. Pediatr., *70*:502, 1967, with permission.)

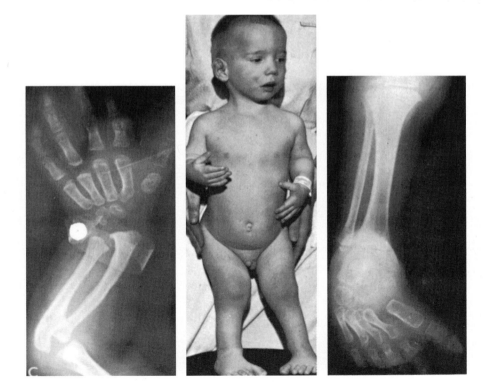

SPONDYLOEPIPHYSEAL DYSPLASIA TARDA

(X-Linked Spondyloepiphyseal Dysplasia)

Flattened Vertebrae of Midchildhood, Small Iliac Wings, Short Femoral Neck

This disorder was recognized in 1939 by Jacobsen.

ABNORMALITIES. Onset between 5 and 10 years of age.

Growth. Short stature; final height, 52 to 62 inches with an average of 55 inches. Trunk is disproportionately short.

Spine. Flattened vertebrae with hump-shaped mound of bone in central and posterior portions of vertebral end plates. Narrowing of disc spaces usually posteriorly. Lumbar spine is primarily affected. Kyphosis, mild scoliosis, short neck.

Pelvis. Small iliac wings.

Limbs. Short femoral neck. Mild epiphyseal irregularity with flattening of femoral head.

Joints. Eventual pain and stiffness in hips, shoulders, cervical and lumbar spine.

OCCASIONAL ABNORMALITIES. Corneal opacities.

NATURAL HISTORY. Symptoms are rare before 12 years. Vague back pain in adolescence is frequently the initial symptom. Back, knee, and especially hip pain due to osteoarthritis by 40 years of age; often disabling by 60 years. Total hip arthroplasty is commonly needed prior to 40 years of age.

ETIOLOGY. X-linked recessive in the vast majority of cases. It has been suggested that the locus for this disorder may be in the Xp2 region. In addition, both autosomal dominant and autosomal recessive late-onset spondyloepiphyseal dysplasia, clinically indistinguishable from the X-linked type, have been reported.

References

Jacobsen, A. W.: Hereditary ostochondrodystrophia deformans. A family with twenty members affected in five generations. J.A.M.A., *113*:121, 1939.

Maroteaux, P., Lamy, M., and Bernard, J.: La dysplasie spondyloepiphysaire tardive. Description clinique et radiologique. Presse Med., *65*:1205, 1957.

Langer, L. O.: Spondyloepiphyseal dysplasia tarda. Hereditary chondrodysplasia with characteristic vertebral configuration in the adult. Radiology, *82*:833, 1964.

Bannerman, R. M., Ingall, G. B., and Mohn, J. F.: X-linked spondyloepiphyseal dysplasia tarda. J. Med. Genet., *8*:291, 1971.

Szpiro-Tapia, S., et al.: Spondyloepiphyseal dysplasia tarda: Linkage with genetic markers from the distal short arm of the X chromosome. Hum. Genet., *81*:61, 1988.

Wells, J. A., et al.: Corneal opacities in spondyloepiphyseal dysplasia tarda. Cornea, *13*:280, 1994.

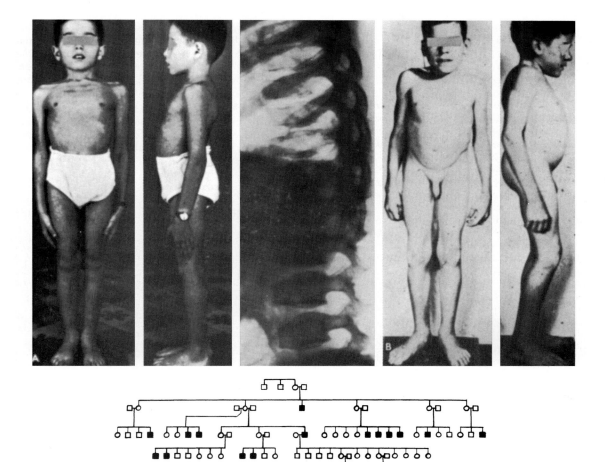

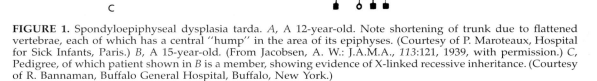

FIGURE 1. Spondyloepiphyseal dysplasia tarda. *A*, A 12-year-old. Note shortening of trunk due to flattened vertebrae, each of which has a central "hump" in the area of its epiphyses. (Courtesy of P. Maroteaux, Hospital for Sick Infants, Paris.) *B*, A 15-year-old. (From Jacobsen, A. W.: J.A.M.A., *113*:121, 1939, with permission.) *C*, Pedigree, of which patient shown in *B* is a member, showing evidence of X-linked recessive inheritance. (Courtesy of R. Bannaman, Buffalo General Hospital, Buffalo, New York.)

MULTIPLE EPIPHYSEAL DYSPLASIA

Small Irregular Epiphyses, Pain and Stiffness in Hips, Short Stature

This condition was described by Ribbing in 1937 and by Fairbank in 1947. It is frequently misdiagnosed as bilateral Legg-Perthes disease.

ABNORMALITIES

Growth. Slight to moderate shortness of stature. Adult stature, 145 to 170 cm.

Limbs. Late ossifying, small, irregular, mottled epiphyses with eventual osteoarthritis due to loss of articular cartilage in many large joints, especially in hips and knees. Short femoral neck. Mild metaphyseal flare. Shortness of metacarpals and phalanges leading to short stubby fingers. Approximately one third have symmetrical shoulder problems. Double-layered patellae that often dislocate laterally.

Spine. Although vertebral bodies are usually spared, they can be blunted, slightly ovoid, sometimes flattened.

NATURAL HISTORY. Evident from 2 to 10 years because of waddling gait and slow growth. Back pain is common. Slowly progressive pain and stiffness in joints, particularly in the hips, may be a complaint as early as 5 years, but usually not until 30 to 35 years. Joint replacement is often required.

ETIOLOGY. Autosomal dominant with wide variability in expression. More severely affected individuals are generally referred to as having the Fairbank type, whereas the Ribbing type is used to designate more mildly affected individuals. The two types do not overlap within families. Thus, in familial cases, the natural history can be predicted by taking into account the outcome in affected relatives. Two different genetic loci have been identified, one at 1p32 in the region containing the gene (COL9A2) that encodes the α_2 chain of type IX collagen and the other at 19p13.1. Regarding the latter, a mutation in the cartilage oligomeric matrix protein (COMP) gene, which has been localized to chromosome 19p13.1, has been identified in the Fairbank type. This indicates that the clinical phenotype of multiple epiphyseal dysplasia is genetically heterogeneous.

COMMENT. Mutations in the COMP gene also have been identified in pseudoachondroplasia demonstrating that some forms of multiple epiphyseal dysplasia are allelic with pseudoachondroplasia.

References

Ribbings, S.: Studien über hereditäre multiple ëpiphysenstörungen. Acta Radiol. [Suppl.], 34, 1937.

Fairbank, T.: Dysplasia epiphysealis multiplex. Br. J. Surg., 34:225, 1947.

Maudsley, R. H.: Dysplasia epiphysialis multiplex. A report of fourteen cases in three families. J. Bone Joint Surg., 37B:228, 1955.

Hoefnagel, D., et al.: Hereditary multiple epiphyseal dysplasia. Ann. Hum. Genet., 30:201, 1967.

Spranger, J.: The epiphyseal dysplasias. Clin. Orthop. Rel. Res., 114:46, 1976.

Ingram, R. R.: The shoulder in multiple epiphyseal dysplasia. J. Bone Joint Surg., 73B:277, 1991.

Oehlmann, R., et al.: Genetic linkage mapping of multiple epiphyseal dysplasia to the pericentromeric region of chromosome 19. Am. J. Hum. Genet., 54:3, 1994.

Briggs, M. D., et al.: Genetic mapping of a locus for multiple epiphyseal dysplasia (EDM2) to a region of chromosome 1 containing a type IX collagen gene. Am. J. Hum. Genet., 55:678, 1994.

Briggs, M. D., et al.: Pseudoachondroplasia and multiple epiphyseal dysplasia due to mutations in the cartilage oligomeric matrix protein gene. Nat. Genet., 10:330, 1995.

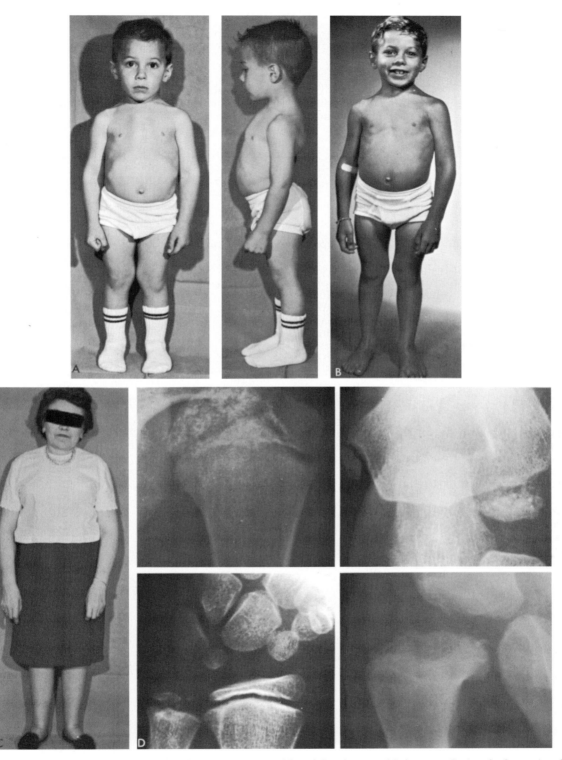

FIGURE 1. Multiple epiphyseal dysplasia. *A,* A 5-year-old with height age of 2⁶/₁₂ years. Patient had occasional aching in legs. *B,* Same patient at 8⁶/₁₂ years; height age, 4⁶/₁₂ years. He now has ankle and hip discomfort. *C,* Affected mother of patient shown in *A* and *B.* She is short of stature and has hip discomfort. *D,* Late and irregular mineralization of epiphyses, which may be small or aberrant in shape, or both.

METAPHYSEAL DYSPLASIA, SCHMID TYPE

Since the initial description by Schmid in 1949, several large pedigrees of affected individuals have been reported.

ABNORMALITIES

Growth. Mild to moderate shortness of stature. Adult height, 130 to 160 cm.

Skeletal. Relatively short tubular bones. Tibial bowing, especially at ankle. Waddling gait with coxa vara and genu varum. Flare to lower rib cage.

Radiographic. Enlarged capital femoral epiphyses before 10 years of age. Coxa vara beginning at 3 years. Femoral bowing. Metaphyseal abnormalities of distal and proximal femurs, proximal tibias, proximal fibulas, distal radius and ulna. Anterior cupping, splaying, and sclerosis of ribs. Metacarpals and phalanges as well as spine are normal. There is mild irregularity of acetabular roof.

NATURAL HISTORY. Bowed legs with waddling gait, the usual presenting sign, is usually evident in second year. Height, usually less than the fifth percentile, is rarely less than 7 SD below the mean. Pain in legs during childhood. Symptomatic and radiographic improvement beginning as early as 3 years of age, with orthopedic measures indicated only for unusual degrees of deformity and usually not until growth is complete. Since the epiphyses are not affected, there are usually no osteoarthritic symptoms. Intelligence and life expectancy are not affected.

ETIOLOGY. Autosomal dominant with variable expression. Mutations of the type X collagen (COL10A1) gene, which has been mapped to 6q22.3, are responsible for this pattern of malformation. Type X collagen expression is restricted to hypertrophic chondrocytes in areas undergoing endochondral ossification, such as growth plates.

References

Schmid, F.: Beitrag zur Dysostosis Enchondralis Metaphysaria. Monatsschr. Kinderheilkd., 97:393, 1949.

Stickler, G. B., et al.: Familial bone disease resembling rickets (hereditary metaphysial dysostosis). Pediatrics, 29:996, 1962.

Rosenbloom, A. L., and Smith, D. W.: The natural history of metaphyseal dysostosis. J. Pediatr., 66:857, 1965.

Lachman, R. S., et al.: Metaphyseal chondrodysplasia. Schmid type. Clinical and radiographic delineation with review of the literature. Pediatr. Radiol., 18:93, 1988.

Warman, M. L., et al.: A type X collagen mutation causes Schmid metaphyseal chondrodysplasia. Nat. Genet., 5:79, 1993.

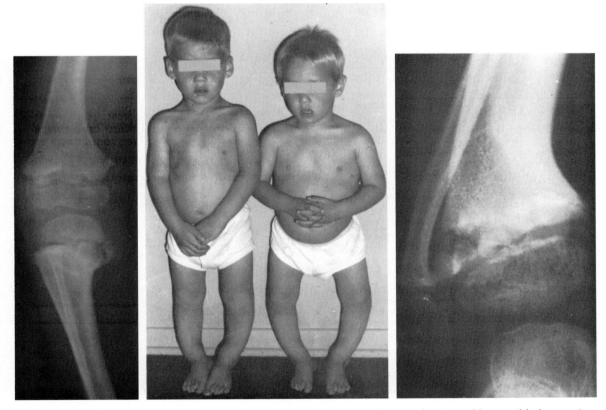

FIGURE 1. Metaphyseal dysplasia, Schmid type. Affected brothers showing bowing of legs, mild changes in thorax, and metaphyseal alterations. (From Rosenbloom, A. L., and Smith, D. W.: J. Pediatr., *66*:857, 1965, with permission.)

METAPHYSEAL DYSPLASIA, McKUSICK TYPE

(Cartilage-Hair Hypoplasia Syndrome)

Mild Bowing of Legs, Wide Irregular Metaphyses, Fine Sparse Hair

Discovered by McKusick et al. among an inbred Amish population, this condition has subsequently been detected in non-Amish individuals, particularly in the Finnish population.

ABNORMALITIES

Growth. Prenatal onset, short limb, long trunk, short stature evident neonatally in 76 per cent of cases and in 98 per cent by 1 year. Adult height, 104 to 149 cm. Decreased or absent pubertal growth spurt. Obesity in adults.

Hair. Fine, sparse, light, relatively fragile. Eyebrows, eyelashes, and body hair are also affected.

Skeletal. Relatively short limbs, mild bowing of legs. Prominent heel. Flat feet. Short hands, fingernails, toenails. Loose-jointed "limp" hands and feet. Incomplete extension of elbow. Mild flaring of lower rib cage with prominent sternum. Lumbar lordosis, scoliosis, small pelvic inlet.

Radiographic. Flared, scalloped, irregularly sclerotic metaphyses noted before closing of epiphyses primarily in knees and ankles, less frequently in hips. Epiphyses only minimally affected. Short tibia in relation to fibula.

Other. Diminished cellular immune response manifest by lymphopenia, decreased delayed hypersensitivity, and impaired in vitro responsiveness of lymphocytes to PHA. Mild macrocytic anemia. Neutropenia.

OCCASIONAL ABNORMALITIES. Brachycephaly. Malignancies (6 to 10 per cent). Esophageal atresia. Hirschsprung disease. Intestinal malabsorption in infancy. Altered T-cell responses. Congenital hypoplastic anemia.

NATURAL HISTORY. The early history is often indicative of an intestinal malabsorption problem, which tends to improve with time. The diminished cellular immunity often leads to severe or fatal response to varicella as well as other infections. The rare congenital hypoplastic anemia can occasionally be fatal. However, in most cases spontaneous recovery occurs before adulthood. The presence of anemia correlates with severity of the immunodeficiency and growth failure and to the neutropenia.

ETIOLOGY. Autosomal recessive. The gene for this disorder has been assigned to the proximal part of 9p using linkage analysis.

References

McKusick, V. A., et al.: Dwarfism in the Amish. II. Cartilage-hair hypoplasia. Bull. Hopkins Hosp., *116*: 285, 1965.

Lux, S. E., et al.: Chronic neutropenia and abnormal cellular immunity in cartilage-hair hypoplasia. N. Engl. J. Med., *282*:231, 1970.

Van der Burgt, I., et al.: Cartilage hair hypoplasia, metaphyseal chondrodysplasia type McKusick: Description of seven patients and review of the literature. Am. J. Med. Genet., *41*:371, 1991.

Makitie, O., and Kaitila, I.: Cartilage-hair hypoplasia–clinical manifestations in 108 Finnish patients. Eur. J. Pediatr., *152*:211, 1993.

Sulisalo, T., et al.: Cartilage-hair hypoplasia gene assigned to chromosome 9 by linkage analysis. Nat. Genet., *3*:338, 1993.

Makitie, O., et al.: Cartilage-hair hypoplasia. J. Med. Genet., *32*:39, 1995.

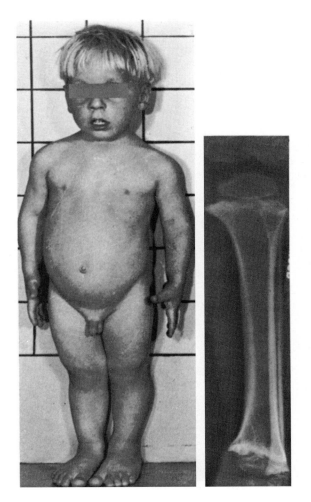

FIGURE 1. Metaphyseal dysplasia, McKusick type. A 5⁶/₁₂-year-old; height age, 18 months. (From McKusick, V. A., et al.: Bull. Hopkins Hosp., *116*:285, 1965, with permission.)

METAPHYSEAL DYSPLASIA, JANSEN TYPE

(Metaphyseal Dysostosis, Jansen Type)

Wide Irregular Metaphyses, Flexion Joint Deformity, Small Thorax

Since Jansen described this severe type of metaphyseal dysostosis, at least 14 cases have been reported.

ABNORMALITIES

Growth. Severe short stature of postnatal onset. Adult stature about 125 cm.

Facies. Small, immature in appearance, with prominent eyes. Mild supraorbital and frontonasal hyperplasia in the adult. Micrognathia.

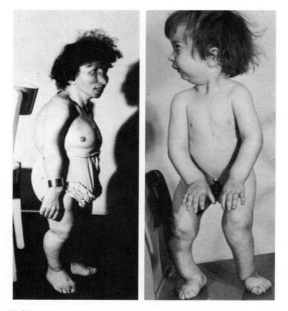

FIGURE 1. Metaphyseal dysplasia, Jansen type. Affected mother and daughter. (Courtesy of W. Lenz, Münster, Germany.)

Skeletal and Joint. Gross irregular cyst-like areas due to lack of metaphyseal ossification. Pelvis similarly affected. Small thoracic cage. Flexion deformities of joints, especially at knee and hip, yielding a squatting stance with symmetric para-articular widening.

Other. Waddling gait. Clinodactyly. Short clubbed fingers. Hyperostosis of calvarium with thick dense base of skull. Hypercalcemia. Variable deafness.

NATURAL HISTORY. Skeletal changes have been noted at birth or in early infancy. The defective growth and joint dysfunction are severe.

ETIOLOGY. Autosomal dominant, with most cases being fresh mutations.

COMMENT. Radiographic features change with age. At birth, diffuse radiolucency and irregularity of metaphyses of long bones. Wide growth plates of tubular bones. In childhood, cupping of metaphyses with a wide zone of irregular calcification. In adult, the large calcified masses in the metaphyses turn into bone, resulting in bulbous deformities at the ends of short, bowed long bones.

References

Jansen, M.: Über atypische Chondrodystrophie (Achondroplasia) und über eine noch nicht beschriebene angeborene Wachstummsstörung des Knochensystems: Metaphysäre Dysostosis. 2. Orthop. Chir., *61*:253, 1934.

Charrow, J., and Poznanski, A. K.: The Jansen type of metaphyseal chondrodysplasia: Confirmation of dominant inheritance and review of radiographic manifestations in the newborn and adult. Am. J. Med. Genet., *18*:321, 1984.

SHWACHMAN SYNDROME

(Metaphyseal Dysplasia With
Pancreatic Insufficiency and Neutropenia)

*Metaphyseal Chondrodysplasia,
Neutropenia, Exocrine Pancreatic Insufficiency*

In 1963, Shwachman et al. described five children with evidence of pancreatic insufficiency and leukopenia, none of whom had cystic fibrosis of the pancreas. Burke et al. subsequently documented the association of metaphyseal chondrodysplasia with this syndrome. Numerous cases have been documented.

ABNORMALITIES

Growth. Short stature of prenatal onset. Failure to thrive. Short-limb dwarfism.

Performance. I.Q. significantly lower than siblings. Mild mental retardation in one third.

Pancreas. Lack of exocrine pancreas, which is replaced by adipose tissue. Pancreatic trypsin, lipase, and amylase are absent.

Radiographic. Skeletal changes, including short ribs with widely flared costochondral junctions, ovoid vertebral bodies, widening and irregularity of metaphyses of long bones, which are short, and focal lack of mineralization in epiphyses. Narrow sacroiliac notch.

OCCASIONAL ABNORMALITIES. Anemia, thrombocytopenia, leukopenia, neutropenia, eczema, defective neutrophil chemotaxis, immunoglobulin deficiency, leukemia. Nephrocalcinosis. Intermittent and variable glycosuria. Generalized aminoaciduria. Type I renal tubular acidosis.

NATURAL HISTORY. Failure to thrive with diarrhea is the most common presenting situation at 2 to 10 months of age. Of interest is the observation that there is no steatorrhea; presumably the intestinal lipases are adequate in the absence of pancreatic lipase. The viscosity of duodenal secretions is also normal in contrast with cystic fibrosis of the pancreas, which can be readily excluded by sweat electrolyte studies.

The diarrhea tends to improve with age even without pancreatic enzyme replacement therapy. The therapy is followed by dramatic response in some patients but not in others. The leukopenia can occur intermittently and may be accompanied by a high frequency of bacterial infections.

ETIOLOGY. Autosomal recessive.

COMMENT. The exocrine pancreas is replaced by adipose tissue, whereas the islet cells of Langerhans are intact. Both are derived from a common endodermal outpouching from the foregut, and therefore, it is assumed that the exocrine pancreatic cells are lost early in life and replaced by fat. One possibility is a defect in the integrity of the lysozymes in these cells, allowing the cells to be destroyed by the very enzymes they produce.

References

Shwachman, H., et al.: Pancreatic insufficiency and bone marrow dysfunction. A new clinical entity. J. Pediatr., *63*:835, 1963.

Burke, V., et al.: Association of pancreatic insufficiency and chronic neutropenia in childhood. Arch. Dis. Child., *42*:147, 1967.

McLennan, T. W., and Steinbach, H. L.: Schwachman's syndrome: The broad spectrum of bone abnormalities. Radiology, *112*:167, 1974.

Danks, D. M., et al.: Metaphyseal chondrodysplasia, neutropenia, and pancreatic insufficiency presenting with respiratory distress in the neonatal period. Arch. Dis. Child., *51*:697, 1976.

Woods, W. G., et al.: The occurrence of leukemia in patients with the Shwachman syndrome. J. Pediatr., *99*:425, 1981.

Kent, A., et al.: Psychological characteristics of children with Shwachman syndrome. Arch. Dis. Child., *65*:1349, 1990.

CHONDRODYSPLASIA PUNCTATA, X-LINKED DOMINANT TYPE

(Conradi-Hünermann Syndrome)

Asymmetric Limb Shortness, Early Punctate Mineralization, Large Skin Pores

Initially described by Conradi and later by Hünermann, this disorder was clearly distinguished from the autosomal recessive type of chondrodysplasia punctata by Spranger et al.

ABNORMALITIES
Growth. Mild to moderate growth deficiency.
Facies. Variable low nasal bridge with flat facies; hypoplasia of malar eminences with downslanting palpebral fissures. Cataracts.
Limbs. Asymmetric shortening related to areas of punctate mineralization in epiphyses. Variable joint contractures.
Spine. Frequent scoliosis, even in infancy, related to areas of punctate mineralization.
Skin. Erythema and thick adherent scales in newborn period. In older children, variable follicular atrophoderma with large pores resembling "orange peel" and ichthyosis predominate. Sparse hair that tends to be coarse, and patchy areas of alopecia.

OCCASIONAL ABNORMALITIES. Dysplastic auricles. Minor nail anomalies. Nystagmus. Hazy cornea. Microphthalmus. Glaucoma. Atrophy of retina and optic nerve; short neck; hydramnios; hydrops; mild to moderate mental deficiency. Tracheal calcifications with associated tracheal stenosis; cardiac defects. Dislocated patella. Hexadactyly. Vertebral anomalies including clefting, wedging, and/or absence.

NATURAL HISTORY. Failure to thrive and/or infection may occur in early infancy. If the patient survives the first few months, the prognosis for survival is good. Stippling of the epiphyses of the long bones frequently resolves by 9 months. Orthopedic problems including scoliosis are frequent, and there is an enhanced risk of cataract formation.

ETIOLOGY. X-linked dominant.

COMMENT. In addition to this disorder and the autosomal recessive chondrodysplasia punctata, an X-linked recessive type exists. That condition is characterized by skeletal manifestation of chondrodysplasia punctata, ichthyosis due to steroid sulfatase deficiency, short stature, microcephaly, developmental delay, cataracts, and hearing loss. In addition, some affected males have anosmia and hypogonadism (Kallmann syndrome). The majority of patients have documented deletions and translocations of Xp22.3. Point mutations in the gene encoding arylsulfatase E (ARSE), which maps to Xp22.3, have been identified in a number of patients with this disorder, suggesting that the skeletal abnormalities are the result of altered ARSE activity.

References

Conradi, E.: Vorzeitiges Auftreten von Knochen und eigenartigen Verkalkungskernen bei Chondrodystrophia foetalis hypoplastica. Jahrb. Kinderheilkd., *80*:86, 1914.

Hünermann, C.: Chondrodystrophia calcificans congenita als abortive Form der Chondrodystrophie. Z. Kinderheilkd., *51*:1, 1931.

Spranger, J., Opitz, J. M., and Bidder, U.: Heterogeneity of chondrodysplasia punctate. Humangenetik, *11*:190, 1971.

Happle, R.: X-linked dominant chondrodysplasia punctata. Review of literature and report of a case. Hum. Genet., *53*:65, 1979.

Curry, C. J. R., et al.: Inherited chondrodysplasia punctata due to a deletion of the terminal short arm of an X chromosome. N. Engl. J. Med., *311*:1010, 1984.

Ballabio, A., and Andria, G.: Deletions and translocations involving the distal short arm of the human X chromosome: Review and hypothesis. Hum. Mol. Genet., *1*:221, 1992.

Wulfsberg, E. A., et al.: Chondrodysplasia punctata: A boy with X-linked recessive chondrodysplasia punctata due to an inherited X-Y translocation with a current classification of these disorders. Am. J. Med. Genet., *43*:823, 1992.

Franco, B., et al.: A cluster of sulfatase genes on Xp22.3: Mutations in chondrodysplasia punctata (CDPX) and implications for warfarin embryopathy. Cell, *81*:15, 1995.

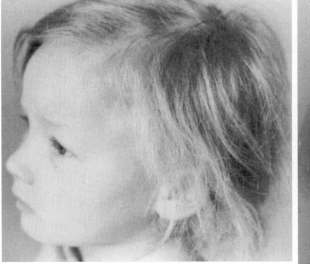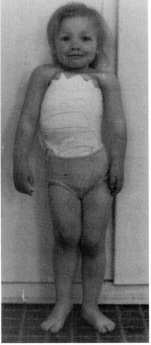

FIGURE 1. Chondrodysplasia punctata, X-linked dominant type. A 4⁶/₁₂-year-old girl, showing asymmetry (note shorter right leg), relatively short neck, scoliosis (casted), and coarse and somewhat sparse hair. She had large skin pores, most notably on the lower arms. Intelligence is normal. (Courtesy of P. MacLeod, Kingston, Ontario.)

AUTOSOMAL RECESSIVE CHONDRODYSPLASIA PUNCTATA
(Chondrodysplasia Punctata, Rhizomelic Type)

Short Humeri and Femora, Coronal Cleft in Vertebrae, Punctate Epiphyseal Mineralization

Spranger et al. clearly distinguished the rhizomelic (short proximal limb) type of chondrodysplasia punctata as a separate entity from the Conradi-Hünermann or X-linked dominant type of chondrodysplasia punctata. Besides the nine personal cases, Spranger et al. were able to find 33 additional cases from the literature.

ABNORMALITIES
Growth. Slow.
Central Nervous System. Mental deficiency, with or without spasticity, microcephaly.
Craniofacies. Low nasal bridge and flat facies with or without upward slanting palpebral fissures. Cataracts (72 per cent).
Limbs. Symmetric proximal shortening of humeri and femora. Metaphyseal splaying and cupping, especially at the knee, with sparse and irregular trabeculae. Epiphyseal and extraepiphyseal foci of calcification in early infancy with later epiphyseal irregularity. Multiple joint contractures.
Spine. Coronal cleft noted on lateral roentgenogram with dysplasia and irregularity of vertebrae.
Pelvis. Trapeziform dysplasia of upper ilium.

OCCASIONAL ABNORMALITIES. Ichthyosiform skin dysplasia (28 per cent).

NATURAL HISTORY. These patients usually have a severe problem in growth and mental development and die prior to 1 to 2 years of age. The majority die in the neonatal period of respiratory insufficiency. Only one patient is known to have survived to the age of 10 years. Effective management of the disorder has not been determined. Punctate epiphyseal and nonepiphyseal mineralization, which is not specific to this disorder, may not be found in all cases, especially when the diagnosis is not made in early infancy.

ETIOLOGY. Autosomal recessive. This condition is associated with a loss of specific peroxisomal functions. Peroxisomes are subcellular organelles that play an important role in several metabolic processes. Deficiencies in the two peroxisomal enzymes involved in phospholipid synthesis (dihydroxyacetone-phosphate-acyltransferase and alkyl dihydroxyacetone phosphate synthetase) have been found, and there is an impairment of phytanic acid oxidation.

References

Spranger, J. W., Opitz, J. M., and Bidder, U.: Heterogeneity of chondrodysplasia punctata. Humangenetik, *11*:190, 1970.

Spranger, J. W., Bidder, U., and Voelz, C.: Chondrodysplasia punctata (Chondrodystrophia calcifans). II. Der rhizomele Type. Fortschr. Geb. Roentgenstr. Nuklearmed., *114*:327, 1971.

Gilbert, E. F., et al.: Chondrodysplasia punctata: Rhizomelic form. Eur. J. Pediatr., *123*:89, 1976.

Heselson, N. G., Cremin, B. J., and Beighton, P.: Lethal chondrodysplasia punctata. Clin. Radiol., *29*:679, 1978.

Schutgens, R. B. H., et al.: Peroxisomal disorders: A newly recognized group of genetic diseases. Eur. J. Pediatr., *144*:430, 1986.

Schutgens, R. B. H., et al.: Prenatal and perinatal diagnosis of peroxisomal disorders. J. Inherit. Metab. Dis., *12*(Suppl. 1):118, 1989.

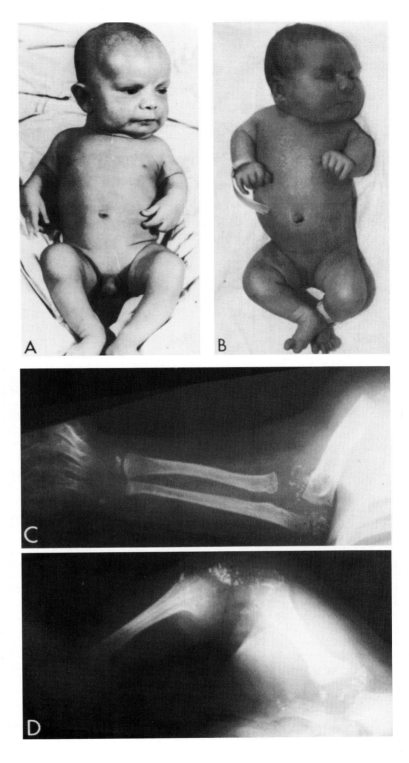

FIGURE 1. Autosomal recessive chondrodysplasia punctata syndrome. *A*, A 7-week-old male. (From Ford, G. D., et al.: Pediatrics, *8*:380, 1951, with permission.) *B*, Young infant. Note the short upper arms. (Courtesy of J. M. Opitz, Helena, Mont., and J. Spranger, Mainz, Germany.) *C* and *D*, Roentgenograms of the arm and leg of an infant, showing proximal shortening with aberrant form and punctate mineralization. (Courtesy of R. A. Hadley and G. Gibbs, University of Nebraska, Omaha, Neb.)

HYPOPHOSPHATASIA

(Perinatal Lethal Hypophosphatasia)

Poorly Mineralized Cranium, Short Ribs, Hypoplastic Fragile Bones

Rathbun recognized this disease in 1948, and numerous cases of this autosomal recessive, invariably lethal condition have been documented subsequently.

ABNORMALITIES
Growth. Short limb dwarfism.
Radiographic. Generalized lack of ossification. Poorly mineralized globular cranium. Poorly formed teeth. Hypoplastic fragile bone of varying density with irregular lack of metaphyseal mineralization, bowed lower extremities, characteristic "spurs" in midshaft of ulna and fibula sometimes protruding through skin, and short ribs with rachitic rosary and fractures. Small thoracic cage. Vertebral bodies, frequently unossified, but sometimes dense, rectangular/round, flattened, sagitally clefted, or butterfly shaped. Posterior elements are poorly ossified. Clavicles are least affected bones.

OCCASIONAL ABNORMALITIES. Polyhydramnios. Blue sclera.

NATURAL HISTORY. Death secondary to respiratory insufficiency during early infancy is usual. Of those who survive, early failure to thrive, hypotonia, irritability and occasionally seizures, anemia and/or hypercalcemia, and nephrocalcinosis are common.

ETIOLOGY. Autosomal recessive with marked radiographic variability. Affected infants have a severe deficiency of tissue and serum alkaline phosphatase and an excessive urinary excretion of phosphoethanolamine. Carriers may have a low value for serum alkaline phosphatase and mildly elevated phosphoethanolamine excretion. The gene for hypophosphatasia has been mapped to chromosome 1p36.1-p34 based upon linkage analysis in Canadian Mennonites. Prenatal diagnosis has been accomplished successfully with midtrimester ultrasonography and measurement of the liver/bone/kidney isoenzyme of alkaline phosphatase in chorionic villus sample taken between 10 and 12 weeks of gestation.

COMMENT. Based on age of onset and major clinical findings, four forms of hypophosphatasia have been characterized: A perinatal lethal form described above; an infantile form that presents within the first 6 months with growth deficiency, rachitic-like skeletal defects resulting in recurrent respiratory infection, increased intracranial pressure, and death in about 50 per cent of cases; a milder childhood type that presents after 6 months and is associated with premature loss of deciduous teeth, rachitic-appearing skeletal findings, and craniosynostosis; and an adult type that presents later in life with premature loss of adult teeth, recurrent fractures, and pseudofractures. Decreased activity of bone/liver/kidney serum alkaline phosphatase isoenzyme is a feature of all four types.

Based upon sibling recurrences, autosomal recessive inheritance has been implicated for both the perinatal lethal and infantile forms despite the fact that consanguinity is uncommon. Molecular analysis of the tissue nonspecific alkaline phosphatase gene locus on 1p has documented that most affected infants are compound heterozygotes (different mutations in each allele of the gene) for a number of different mutations likely accounting for the clinical variability. Compound heterozygosity has also been demonstrated in a few instances of the childhood and adult form of this disorder; since it appears that a variety of different mutations may account for the clinical findings, prediction of natural history needs to be based on the expression of the disorder in an individual family.

References

Rathbun, J. D.: "Hypophosphatasia." A new developmental anomaly. Am. J. Dis. Child., 75:822, 1948.

Rathbun, J. C., et al.: Hypophosphatasia: A genetic study. Arch. Dis. Child., 36:540, 1961.

Kellsey, D. C.: Hypophosphatasia and congenital bowing of the long bones. J. A. M. A., 179:187, 1962.

MacPherson, R. I., Kroeker, M., and Houston, C. S.: Hypophosphatasia. J. Can. Assoc. Radiol., 23:16, 1972.

Greenberg, C. R., et al.: Infantile hypophosphatasia: Localization within chromosome region 1p36.1-34 and prenatal diagnosis using linked DNA markers. Am. J. Hum. Genet., 46:286, 1990.

Brock, D. J. H., and Barron, L.: First-trimester diagnosis of hypophosphatasia: Experience with 16 cases. Prenat. Diagn., 11:387, 1991.

Shohat, M., et al.: Perinatal lethal hypophosphatasia: Clinical, radiologic and morphologic findings. Pediatr. Radiol., 21:421, 1991.

Henthorn, P. S., et al.: Different missense mutations at the tissue-nonspecific alkaline phosphatase gene locus in autosomal recessively inherited forms of mild and severe hypophosphatasia. Proc. Natl. Acad. Sci. U.S.A., 89:9924, 1992.

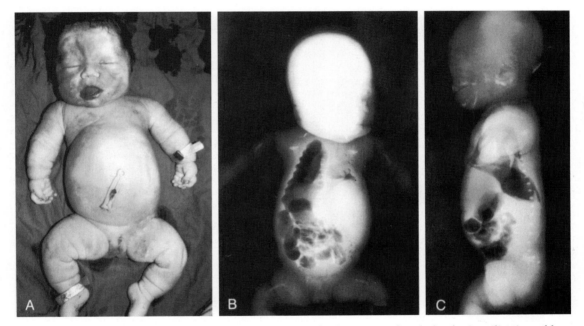

FIGURE 1. Hypophosphatasia. *A* to *C*, Stillborn infant with almost complete lack of mineralization of bony skeleton. Serum alkaline phosphatase was low, and there was an increased urinary phosphoethanolamine.

HAJDU-CHENEY SYNDROME

(Cheney Syndrome, Acro-osteolysis
Syndrome, Arthro-Dento-Osteo Dysplasia)

Early Loss of Teeth, Acro-osteolysis, Lax Joints

Originally described by Hajdu and Kauntze in 1948, and more extensively reported by Cheney, the features of this disorder in 13 patients were summarized by Herrmann et al. The basic defect appears to be one of connective tissue, most strikingly affecting the development and persistence of skeletal tissues. There are several other osteolytic disorders that are not set forth in this text.

ABNORMALITIES

Growth. Small stature, aggravated by osseous compression.

Cranium. Wormian bones, failure of ossification of sutures, thickened skull vault, absence of frontal sinus, elongated sella turcica; progressive basilar impression with foramen magnum impaction, hydrocephalus, and bathrocephaly.

Facies. Thick straight hair with prominent eyebrows and eyelashes. Down-slanting palpebral fissures. Low-set ears with prominent lobes. Broad nose with anteverted nares and long philtrum. Small mandible with diminished ramus.

Dentition. Resorption of alveolar process with early loss of teeth.

Spine. Biconcave vertebrae. Lumbar vertebral bodies are tall and disk spaces are narrow. Osteopenia can lead to collapse. Kyphoscoliosis. Cervical instability due to cervical osteolysis has rarely occurred. Short neck.

Limbs. Short distal digits and nails with acro-osteolysis and pseudoclubbing. Fingers are more severely affected than toes. Crowded carpal bones. Joint laxity. Discrepancy in lengths of paired long bones leading to valgus at knees and dislocation of radial heads. Fibulas are long and bowed. Osteopenia with fractures are common.

NATURAL HISTORY. Though the diagnosis is seldom made in childhood, the onset of the disorder usually occurs during that time, as indicated by the hand changes. Pain is a frequent manifestation, especially in the hands. The patients are often weak, and pathologic fractures are liable to occur. Osseous compression may actually result in a decrease in stature, and the basilar compression can be life threatening.

ETIOLOGY. Autosomal dominant, with sporadic cases presumably representing fresh gene mutation.

References

Hajdu, N., and Kauntze, R.: Cranio-skeletal dysplasia. Br. J. Radiol., *21*:42, 1948.

Cheney, W. D.: Acro-osteolysis. Am. J. Roentgenol. Radium Ther. Nucl. Med., *94*:595, 1965.

Herrmann, J., et al.: Arthro-dento-osteo-dysplasia (Hajdu-Cheney syndrome). Review of a genetic "acro-osteolysis" syndrome. Z. Kinderheilkd., *114*:93, 1973.

O'Reilly, M. A. R., and Shaw, D. G.: Hajdu-Cheney syndrome. Ann. Rheum. Dis., *53*:276, 1994.

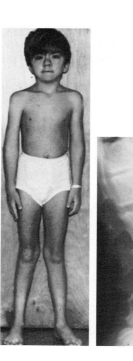

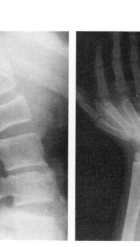

FIGURE 1. Hajdu-Cheney syndrome. Note the knock-knees, biconcave vertebra, diminished distal phalanges, crowded carpal bones, and relative lack of metaphyseal flare in the long bones. (From Herrmann, J., et al.: Z. Kinderheilkd., *114*:93, 1973, with permission.)

CRANIOMETAPHYSEAL DYSPLASIA

Bony Wedge Over Bridge of Nose,
Mild Splaying of Metaphyses

Often confused with the Pyle metaphyseal dysplasia syndrome, this disorder has more profound craniofacial hyperostosis and less metaphyseal broadening than in Pyle disease.

ABNORMALITIES

Craniofacial. Thick calvarium with dense base of cranial vault, facial bones, and mandible. Macrocephaly. Variable absence of pneumatization. Unusual thick bony wedge over bridge of nose and supraorbital area with hypertelorism and relatively small nose. Variable proptosis of eyes. Compression of foramina with cranial nerve deficits, headache, and narrow nasal passages with rhinitis.

Limbs. Mild to moderate metaphyseal broadening with diaphyseal sclerosis.

NATURAL HISTORY. The disease is evident from infancy, and these individuals may have serious problems from compression of the brain and cranial nerves, particularly the seventh, eighth, and optic nerves and from deafness. Hydrocephalus has occurred perhaps due to venous outlet obstruction. They are of normal intelligence. The autosomal recessive type is more severe and may result in facial paralysis and loss of vision.

ETIOLOGY. Both an autosomal dominant type and a presumed autosomal recessive type have been delineated, the latter being more severe in degree. The problem in bone morphogenesis is thought to be one of osteoclasis, with defective reabsorption and remodeling of secondary substantia spongiosa.

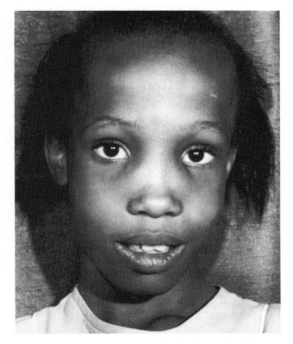

FIGURE 1. Craniometaphyseal dysplasia. An 11-year-old with the autosomal dominant type. The hyperostosis is already causing the fullness noted in the area of the nasal bridge. Hearing loss began at age 9 years. (Courtesy of D. L. Rimoin, Cedars-Sinai Medical Center, Los Angeles, Calif.)

References

Spranger, J., Paulsen, K., and Lehmann, W.: Die kraniometaphysare Dysplasia. Z. Kinderheilkd., *93*:64, 1965.

Millard, D. R., Jr., et al.: Craniofacial surgery in craniometaphyseal dysplasia. Am. J. Surg., *113*:615, 1967.

Gorlin, R. J., Spranger, J., and Koszalka, M.: Genetic craniotubular bone dysplasias and hyperostoses. A critical analysis. Birth Defects, *5*:79, 1969.

Penchaszadeh, V. B., Gutierrez, E. R., and Figuero, P.: Autosomal recessive craniometaphyseal dysplasia. Am. J. Med. Genet., *5*:43, 1980.

Hudgins, R. J., and Edwards, M. S. B.: Craniometaphyseal dysplasia associated with hydrocephalus: Case report. Neurosurgery, *20*:617, 1987.

Cole, D. E. C., and Cohen, M. M.: A new look at craniometaphyseal dysplasia. J. Pediatr., *112*:577, 1988.

FRONTOMETAPHYSEAL DYSPLASIA

Prominent Supraorbital Ridges,
Joint Limitations, Splayed Metaphyses

More than 20 cases of this disorder have been recognized since Gorlin and Cohen's initial report in 1969.

ABNORMALITIES

Craniofacial. Coarse facies with wide nasal bridge and prominent supraorbital ridges. Incomplete sinus development. Partial anodontia, delayed eruption, and retained deciduous teeth. High palate. Small mandible with decreased angle and prominent antigonial notch.

Limbs. Flexion contracture of fingers, wrists, elbows, knees, and ankles. Arachnodactyly with disproportionately wide and elongated phalanges. Increased density in diaphyseal region with lack of modeling in metaphyseal region, giving Erlenmeyer-flask appearance to femur and tibia. Partial fusion of carpal and of tarsal bones.

Other Skeletal. Wide foramen magnum with various cervical vertebral anomalies and wide interpedicular distance of vertebrae. Flared pelvis with constriction of supraacetabular area; chest cage deformities; winged scapulae; scoliosis.

Other. Mixed conductive and sensorineural hearing loss, which progresses. Wasting of muscles of arms and legs, especially hypothenar and interosseous muscles of hands.

OCCASIONAL ABNORMALITIES. Mental retardation. Ocular hypertelorism with downslanting palpebral fissures. Obstructive uropathy. Cardiac murmur, cause unknown. Subglottic tracheal narrowing.

NATURAL HISTORY. Affected individuals are usually asymptomatic at birth. The restriction of joint mobility and development of contractures are progressive. Respiratory difficulties including subglottic stenosis can lead to significant morbidity and even death. Anesthesia can be a significant problem. All patients should be evaluated to rule out urologic abnormalities.

ETIOLOGY. X-linked with severe manifestations in males and variable but more mildly affected females.

References

Gorlin, R. J., and Cohen, M. M.: Frontometaphyseal dysplasia: A new syndrome. Am. J. Dis. Child., *118*: 487, 1969.

Danks, D. M., et al.: Fronto-metaphyseal dysplasia. A progressive disease of bone and connective tissue. Am. J. Dis. Child., *123*:254, 1972.

Gorlin, R. J., and Winder, R. B.: Frontometaphyseal dysplasia—evidence for X-linked inheritance. Am. J. Med. Genet., *5*:81, 1980.

Fitzsimmons, J. S., et al.: Frontometaphyseal dysplasia. Further delineation of the clinical syndrome. Clin. Genet., *22*:195, 1982.

Mehta, Y., and Shou, H.: The anaesthetic management of an infant with frontometaphyseal dysplasia (Gorlin-Cohen syndrome). Acta Anaesthesiol. Scand., *32*:505, 1988.

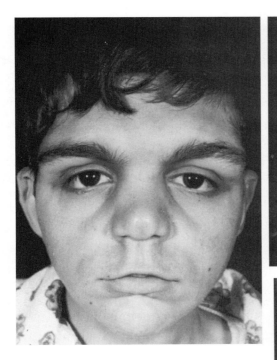

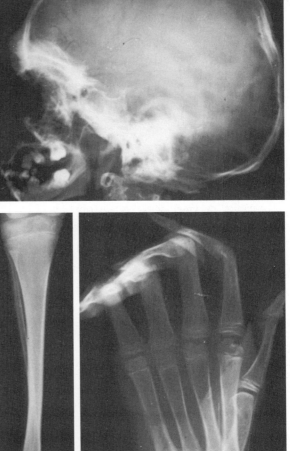

FIGURE 1. Frontometaphyseal dysplasia. An 11-year-old. Note broad, prominent nasal bridge and thickened tissue with prominent philtrum. The skull shows supraorbital bossing with small paranasal sinuses. Note the bowing of the fibula and metaphyseal flaring of tibia; long, poorly modeled tubular bones of hands; and partial lysis of carpal bones. (From Danks, D. M., et al.: Am. J. Dis. Child., *123*:254, 1972, with permission.)

PYLE METAPHYSEAL DYSPLASIA

(Pyle Disease)

*Marked Splaying Metaphyses, Mild
Supraorbital Hyperplasia, Genu Valgum*

Described in 1931 by Pyle, this disorder was more fully characterized and distinguished from craniometaphyseal dysplasia by Gorlin et al. in 1970. More than 20 cases have been recognized.

ABNORMALITIES

Craniofacial. Mild supraorbital hyperplasia and thickening of calvarium.

Limbs. Marked Erlenmeyer-flask–like flare of distal femur and proximal tibia, with cortical thinning and osteoporosis. Similar but less striking changes in other distal long bones plus distal metacarpals and proximal phalanges. Genu valgum. Limited elbow extension.

Other Skeletal. Thickening of sternal ends of ribs, pubic and ischial bones, and medial ends of clavicle.

OCCASIONAL ABNORMALITIES. Muscle weakness, joint pain, scoliosis, platyspondyly, fractures, carious and misplaced teeth, prognathism, elongated big toe.

NATURAL HISTORY. Affected individuals are often asymptomatic. Genu valgum, problems related to fractures, and misplaced teeth sometimes require management.

ETIOLOGY. Autosomal recessive.

References

Pyle, E.: A case of unusual bone development. J. Bone Joint Surg. [Am.], *13*:874, 1931.

Gorlin, R. J., Koszalka, M. F., and Spranger, J.: Pyle's disease (familial metaphyseal dysplasia). J. Bone Joint Surg. [Am.], *52*:347, 1970.

Heselson, N. G., et al.: The radiological manifestations of metaphyseal dysplasia (Pyle disease). Br. J. Radiol., *52*:431, 1979.

Beighton, P.: Pyle disease (metaphyseal dysplasia) J. Med. Genet., *24*:321, 1987.

K

K. OSTEOCHONDRODYSPLASIA WITH OSTEOPETROSIS

OSTEOPETROSIS: AUTOSOMAL RECESSIVE—LETHAL

(Severe Osteopetrosis)

Dense, Thick, Fragile Bone; Secondary Pancytopenia; Cranial Nerve Compression

More than 100 cases of this lethal disorder have been reported since its initial description.

ABNORMALITIES
Skeletal. Thick, dense, fragile bone with modeling alterations such as obtuse mandibular angle, partial aplasia of distal phalanges, straight femora, blocky "bone within a bone" metacarpals, and macrocephaly with frontal bossing. Marrow compression leads to pancytopenia, and compression of cranial foramina may lead to deafness, blindness, vestibular nerve dysfunction, extraocular muscle paralysis, other cranial nerve palsies, blindness, and/or hydrocephalus. Primary molars and permanent dentition tend to be distorted and teeth fail to erupt. Periodontal attachment is poor, allowing for exfoliation. Early decay. Fractures are common.
Metabolic. Serum calcium level may be low and serum phosphorus level elevated. Increased alkaline phosphatase.
Other. Hepatosplenomegaly. Mental retardation.

NATURAL HISTORY. Often evident at birth, with subsequent severe complications and death from anemia, bleeding, or overwhelming infection in infancy or childhood. Ocular involvement, occurring at a median age of 2 months, is the most common presenting sign followed by seizures from hypocalcemia. The natural course of the disease results in survival of 30 per cent of patients at 6 years of age. No affected person has survived adolescence. Problems of dentition and dental infection may become serious.

ETIOLOGY. Autosomal recessive. There appears to be defective reabsorption of immature bone. Two less severe forms of osteopetrosis exist. A rare autosomal recessive disorder that usu-

ally presents in the second year of life with fractures and is associated with renal tubular acidosis, cerebral calcifications, and low levels of carbonic anhydrase II; and a relatively common mild form of osteopetrosis with delayed manifestations and autosomal dominant inheritance. In this latter form, diagnosis is often made by chance when radiographs are taken for other reasons. Bone pain occurs in 25 per cent of cases. Facial palsy and deafness, as well as involvement of the optic and trigeminal nerves, occur infrequently. Osteomyelitis, particularly of the mandible, occurs frequently. Mild skeletal changes become apparent in childhood. Life span is normal.

COMMENT. Allogeneic bone marrow transplantation is the only potentially curative approach for this disorder. Some success has been reported using this treatment.

References

Albers-Schönberg, H.: Eine bisher nicht beschriebene Allgemeinekrankung des Skelettes im Röntgenbilde. Fortschr. Geb. Roentgenstrahlen Nuklearmed., 11:261, 1907.

Tips, R. L., and Lynch, H. T.: Malignant congenital osteopetrosis resulting from a consanguineous marriage. Acta Paediatr. Scand., 51:585, 1962.

Beighton, P., Horan, F., and Hamersma, H.: A review of the osteopetroses. Postgrad. Med. J., 53:507, 1977.

Shapiro, F.: Osteopetrosis: Current clinical considerations. Clin. Orthop., 294:34, 1993.

Gerritsen, E. J. A., et al.: Autosomal recessive osteopetrosis: Variability of findings at diagnosis and during the natural course. Pediatrics, 93:247, 1994.

Gerritsen, E. J. A., et al.: Bone marrow transplantation for autosomal recessive osteopetrosis. J. Pediatr., 125:896, 1994.

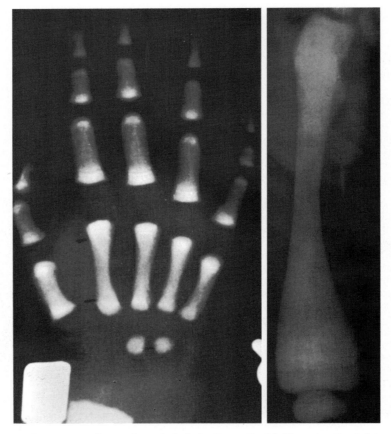

FIGURE 1. Osteopetrosis: autosomal recessive—lethal. An 8-month-old. The sclerotic skeleton shows the ''bone within a bone'' (endobone) appearance, vertical striations at the metaphyseal-diaphyseal juncture, and broad metaphyses.

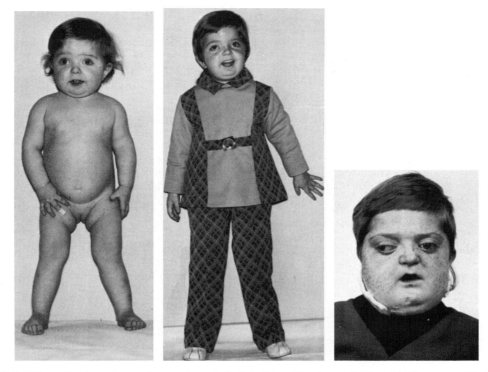

FIGURE 2. Osteopetrosis: autosomal recessive—lethal. *Left* to *right*, Same child at (*A*) 2 years, with length at third percentile and beginning genu valgum; at (*B*)$3^{9}/_{12}$ years, who lost vision, despite attempted decompression of optic nerve; and at (*C*) $10^{6}/_{12}$ years, with proptosis and mandibular osteitis. Her death at 11 years resulted from carotid artery compression. (Courtesy of Dr. Dag Aarskog, Bergen, Norway.)

SCLEROSTEOSIS

Syndactyly, Thickening and Overgrowth of Bone

Hansen described the disorder in 1967, and Beighton et al. set forth the findings in 25 individuals in 1976. Greater than 60 cases of this disorder have now been reported.

ABNORMALITIES. Progressive thickening and overgrowth of bone.

Growth. Overgrowth leading to mild or moderate gigantism becomes evident in midchildhood.

Craniofacies. Development of prominent, sometimes asymmetric mandible by 5 years of age. Cranial hyperostosis leads to occlusion of cranial foramina resulting in deafness and facial palsy in later childhood. Proptosis of eyes occurs in adulthood, and blindness may be a consequence.

Limbs. Syndactyly of second to third fingers (not 100 per cent), deviation of terminal phalanges, nail dysplasia, thickening of bones.

NATURAL HISTORY. The progression of the dense thickening of bone leads to severe distortion of the face, dental malocclusion, proptosis, and relative midfacial hypoplasia, as well as occlusion of multiple cranial foramina and increased intracranial pressure. The latter may cause headaches, intellectual impairment, deterioration of vision, and may even be fatal. Sudden death from impaction of medulla oblongata in the foramen magnum has occurred. Most patients require prophylactic craniectomy in early adulthood. Hearing aids may be helpful. Orthodontia is always indicated.

ETIOLOGY. Autosomal recessive. The majority of cases have occurred in the Afrikaner population of South Africa. Similar clinical and radiographic manifestations have led Beighton et al. to suggest that a fundamental link exists between sclerosteosis and Van Buchem disease. The only significant difference between the two is greater severity and syndactyly in the majority of patients with sclerosteosis.

References

Hansen, H. G.: Sklerosteose. *In* Opitz, J., and Schmid, F. (eds.): Handbuch der Kinderheilkunde, Vol. 6. New York, Berlin, 1967, pp. 351–355.

Beighton, P., Durr, L., and Hamersma, H.: The clinical features of sclerosteosis. Ann. Intern. Med., *84*:393, 1976.

Beighton, P., et al.: The syndrome status of sclerosteosis and Van Buchem disease. Clin. Genet., *25*:175, 1984.

Beighton, P.: Sclerosteosis. J. Med. Genet., *25*:200, 1988.

du Plessis, J. J.: Sclerosteosis: Neurosurgical experience with 14 cases. J. Neurosurg., *78*:388, 1993.

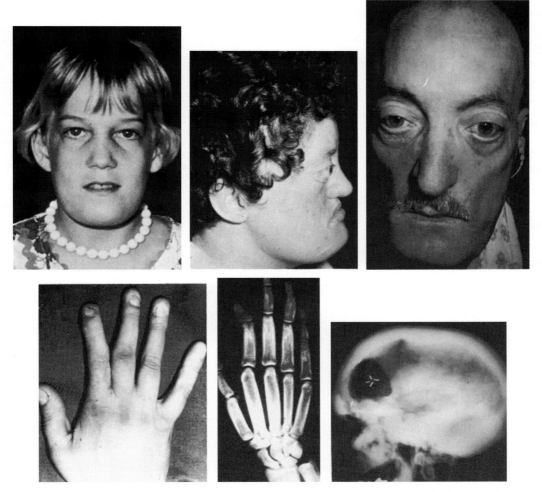

FIGURE 1. Sclerosteosis. Facies showing mandibular overgrowth, asymmetry, and proptosis; hand showing nail hypoplasia, irregular fingers, diaphyseal thickening with dense bone; and skull showing dense thickening. A piece of calvarium was removed to reduce the increased intracranial pressure. (From Beighton, P., et al.: Ann. Intern. Med., *84*:393, 1976, with permission.)

LENZ-MAJEWSKI HYPEROSTOSIS SYNDROME

Dense, Thick Bone; Symphalangism; Hypotrophic Skin

Since 1974, when Lenz and Majewski first proposed this condition as a distinct syndrome, only five patient reports have appeared in the literature. However, at least three other isolated cases have been published as "unknown" multiple malformation syndromes. The features in infancy differ greatly from those in older childhood, producing difficulties in early diagnosis.

ABNORMALITIES

Growth. Early failure to thrive, postnatal short stature. Eventual severe emaciation.

Performance. Moderate to severe mental deficiency.

Craniofacial. Disproportionately large cranium with broad and prominent forehead late closure of large fontanels. Hypertelorism with protuberant eyes. Frequent choanal stenosis or atresia, nasolacrimal duct stenosis.

Skin. Cutis laxa in infancy. Later, skin becomes hypotrophic and thin with prominent, subcutaneous veins, especially over the scalp. Cutaneous syndactyly of the digits. Absence of elastic fibers on skin biopsy.

Hair. Sparse in infancy.

Teeth. Dysplastic enamel.

Skeletal. Proximal symphalangism, delayed ossification of ulnar rays, short or absent middle phalanges, and dorsiflexion of fingers. Broad, thick ribs and calvicles. Widespread cortical sclerosis and thickening of bone in diaphyses, calvarium, and skull base. Shallow and distorted orbits. Long, flared, and radiolucent metaphyses, osteopenic epiphyses. Delayed bone age.

Genitalia. Cryptorchidism and inguinal hernia in boys.

OCCASIONAL ABNORMALITIES. Large,

floppy ears, small tongue, micrognathia, cerebral atrophy, flexion-contractures at elbows and knees, hypospadias/chordee, dislocated hips (one case), early death.

NATURAL HISTORY. At birth, cutis laxa, large fontanels, and syndactyly are the most prominent features. Progressive hyperostosis becomes evident only after the first 6 months of life, often leading to erroneous diagnosis in infancy. Choanal stenosis may cause respiratory insufficiency and repeated episodes of pneumonia. Later, this problem may be aggravated by relative thoracic immobility due to rib widening. Poor weight gain and slow statural growth persist even after resolution of infantile feeding difficulties. No affected patient has yet survived to adulthood.

ETIOLOGY. Unknown. All cases have been sporadic. New mutation for a dominant gene has been suggested because of a tendency toward increased parental age.

References

Kaye, C. I., Fischer, D. E., and Esterly, B. E.: Cutis laxa, skeletal anomalies and ambiguous genitalia. Am. J. Dis. Child., 127:115, 1974.

Lenz, W. D., and Majewski, F. A.: A generalized disorder of the connective tissues with progeria, choanal atresia, symphalangism, hypoplasia of dentine and craniodiaphyseal hyperostosis. Birth Defects, X(12):133, 1974.

Robinow, M., Johanson, A. J., and Smith, T. H.: The Lenz-Majewski hyperostotic dwarfism: A syndrome of multiple congenital anomalies, mental retardation and progressive skeletal sclerosis. J. Pediatr., 91:417, 1977.

Gorlin, R. J., and Whitley, C. B.: Lenz-Majewski syndrome. Radiology, 149:129, 1983.

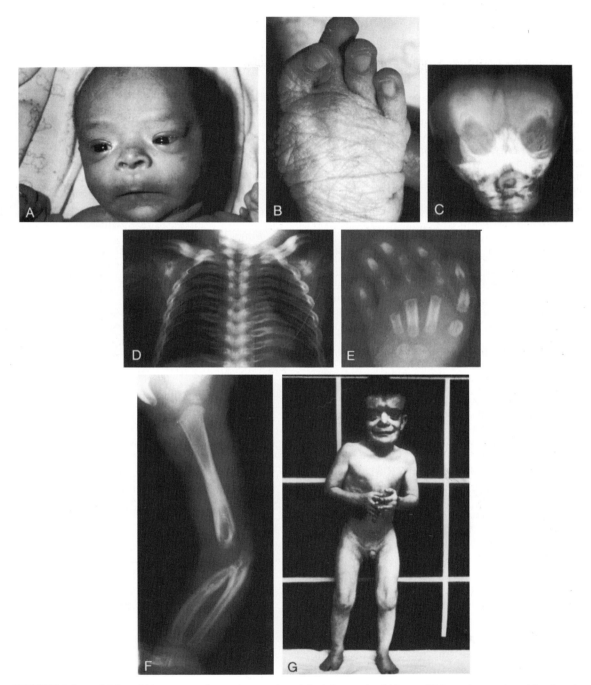

FIGURE 1. Lenz-Majewski hyperostosis syndrome. *A* and *B*, A 2-month-old boy with broad, prominent forehead, ocular hypertelorism, cutaneous syndactyly with dorsiflexed fingers, and cutis laxa. Radiographs of the same patient at 1 year reveal sclerosis of skull base (*C*), broad ribs and clavicles (*D*), symphalangism and hypoplasia of middle phalanges (*E*), and diaphyseal undermodeling and cortical thickening with radiolucent metaphyses and epiphyses (*F*). (*A* to *F* Courtesy of Dr. Jon Aase, University of New Mexico, Albuquerque, N. M.) *G*, The changing phenotype is demonstrated by a boy, 4$7/12$ years old, who has a square forehead with bifrontal bossing, ocular hypertelorism, and flexion contractures at elbows and knees. (*G* Courtesy of Dr. Meinhard Robinow, Children's Medical Center, Dayton, Ohio.)

PYKNODYSOSTOSIS

*Osteosclerosis, Short Distal
Phalanges, Delayed Closure of Fontanels*

Though cleidocranial dysostosis associated with osteosclerosis and bone fragility had been recognized prior to 1962, this condition was not well clarified until Maroteaux and Lamy described it as pyknodysostosis (*pyknos* meaning dense).

ABNORMALITIES

Growth. Small stature with adult height of less than 150 cm.

Skeletal. Osteosclerosis with tendency toward transverse fracture.

Craniofacial. Frontal and occipital prominence, delayed closure of sutures, persistence of anterior fontanel, wormian bones, lack of frontal sinus. Facial hypoplasia with prominent nose and narrow grooved palate. Obtuse angle to mandible, which may be small.

Dentition. Irregular permanent teeth with or without partial anodontia, delayed eruption, caries.

Clavicle. Dysplasia to loss of acromion end.

Digits. Acro-osteolytic dysplasia of distal phalanges, especially of index finger. Wrinkled skin over dorsa of distal fingers. Flattened and grooved nails.

OCCASIONAL ABNORMALITIES. Mental retardation (6 of 32). Scoliosis. Vertebral arch defects in the interarticular parts or pedicles, most frequently at L5.

NATURAL HISTORY. About two thirds of the patients have had fractures, most commonly the mandible, clavicle, and lower extremities, including the metatarsals. There may be a progressive degeneration of the distal phalanges and outer calvicle and persistent open fontanels, especially posteriorly. Special dental care is often indicated.

ETIOLOGY. Consanguinity in 7 of 32 families and sibship occurrence from unaffected parents are indicative of an autosomal recessive determination. However, Shuler discovered the syndrome in a maternal uncle of an affected male and therefore raised the question of X-linked recessive inheritance in that family.

COMMENT. The artist Toulouse-Lautrec is considered to have had pyknodysostosis.

References

Thomsen, G., and Guttadauro, M.: Cleidocranial dysostosis associated with osteosclerosis and bone fragility. Acta Radiol., 37:559, 1952.

Maroteaux, P., and Lamy, M.: La pycnodysostose. Presse Med., 70:999, 1962.

Shuler, S. E.: Pycnodysostosis. Arch. Dis. Child., 38: 620, 1963.

Elmore, S. M.: Pycnodysostosis: A review. J. Bone Joint Surg. [Am.], 49A:153, 1967.

Mills, K. L. G., and Johnson, A. W.: Pyknodysostosis. J. Med. Genet., 25:550, 1988.

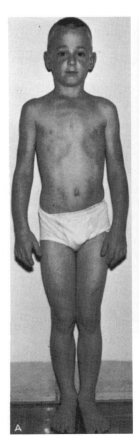

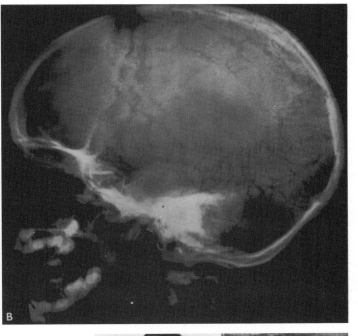

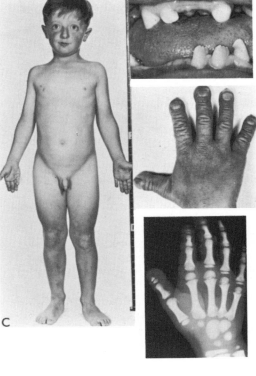

FIGURE 1. Pyknodysostosis. *A*, A 10-year-old with height age of 8⁶/₁₂ years. *B*, Patient shown in *A*. Note the open fontanel and lamboid suture, absence of frontal sinus or mastoid air cells, obtuse angle of mandible, and delay in eruption of permanent dentition. *C*, A 7⁶/₁₂-year-old with height age of 4⁶/₁₂ years. Note the generally dense bone and partial loss of several distal phalanges. (*C* From Shuler, S. E.: Arch. Dis. Child., *38*:620, 1963, with permission.)

CLEIDOCRANIAL DYSOSTOSIS

*Defect of Clavicle, Late Ossification of
Cranial Sutures, Delayed Eruption of Teeth*

A possible example of this rather generalized dysplasia of osseous and dental tissues was detected in the skull of a Neanderthal man. The more obvious features of the defect in the clavicle and cranium prompted Marie and Sainton to utilize the term cleidocranial dysostosis for this condition. However, the more generalized dysplasia of bone and teeth has been emphasized, and the term cleidocranial dysostosis depicts only a portion of the abnormal development. Well over 500 cases have been reported.

ABNORMALITIES. The following are frequent but not constant features:

Growth. Slight to moderate shortness of stature.

Craniofacial. Brachycephaly with bossing of frontal, parietal, and occipital bones; late closure of fontanels and mineralization of sutures; late or incomplete development of accessory sinuses and mastoid air cells; wormian bones; small sphenoid bones. Calvarial thickening. Midfacial hypoplasia with low nasal bridge, narrow high-arched palate. Hypertelorism.

Dentition. Late eruption, especially the permanent teeth, which are often abnormal with aplasia, malformed roots, retention cysts, enamel hypoplasia, enhanced caries, supernumerary teeth.

Clavicle and Chest. Partial to complete aplasia of clavicle with associated muscle defects, small thorax with short oblique ribs.

Hands. Hand anomalies including asymmetric length of fingers with long second metacarpal, short middle phalanges of second and fifth fingers, short and tapering distal phalanges with or without down-curving nails, cone-shaped phalangeal epiphyses in childhood, accessory proximal metacarpal epiphyses that fuse in childhood, and slow rate of carpal ossification.

Other Skeletal. Delayed mineralization of pubic bone, with wide symphysis pubis, narrow pelvis, broad femoral head with short femoral neck, with or without coxa vara. Lateral notching of proximal femoral ossification centers. Spondylolysis. Spondylolisthesis.

OCCASIONAL ABNORMALITIES. Cervical rib, small scapulae, syringomyelia, scoliosis, kyphosis, flat acetabula, osteosclerosis, increased bone fragility, deafness, cleft palate, micrognathia.

NATURAL HISTORY. Though stature is often reduced, mentality is usually normal. Hearing should be assessed, and dental problems should be anticipated. Removal of deciduous teeth does not seem to hasten the eruption of permanent teeth, and the permanent teeth may be difficult to extract because of malformed roots. A narrow pelvis may necessitate cesarean section in the pregnant female with this condition. A narrow thorax may lead to respiratory distress in early infancy.

ETIOLOGY. Autosomal dominant with wide variability in expression, but usually showing penetrance. About one third of the cases represent fresh mutations. A gene for this disorder has been mapped to chromosome 6p21. A rare autosomal recessive form of this disorder has been described in three individuals from two consanguineous families.

COMMENT. The degree of variance in expression includes a lack of defective clavicular development. Many of the radiologic signs, such as metacarpal pseudoepiphyses and late mineralization of the pubic ramus, depend on the age of the patient.

References

Marie, P., and Sainton, P.: Observation d'hydrocephalie héréditaire (père et fils) par vice de développement du crane et du cerveau. Bull. Mem. Soc. Med. Hop. (Paris), 14:706, 1897.

Grieg, D. M.: Neanderthal skull presenting features of cleidocranial dysostosis and other peculiarities. Edinburgh Med. J., 40:407, 1933.

Lasker, G. W.: The inheritance of cleidocranial dysostosis. Hum. Biol., 18:103, 1946.

Jackson, W. P. U.: Osteo-dental dysplasia (cleidocranial dysostosis). The "Arnold head." Acta Med. Scand., 139:292, 1951.

Forland, M.: Cleidocranial dysostosis. A review of the syndrome and report of a sporadic case, with hereditary transmission. Am. J. Med., 33:792, 1962.

Fauré, C., and Maroteaux, P.: Cleidocranial dysplasia. In Kaufman, H. J. (ed.): Progress in Pediatric Radiology, Vol. 4. Basel, Karger, 1973, pp. 211–238.

Jarvis, J. L., and Keats, T. E.: Cleidocranial dysostosis. A review of 40 new cases. Am. J. Roentgenol., 121: 5, 1974.

Goodman, R. M., et al.: Evidence for an autosomal recessive form of cleidocranial dysostosis. Clin. Genet., 8:20, 1975.

Mundlos, S., et al.: Genetic mapping of cleidocranial dysplasia and evidence of a microdeletion in one family. Hum. Mol. Genet., 4:71, 1995.

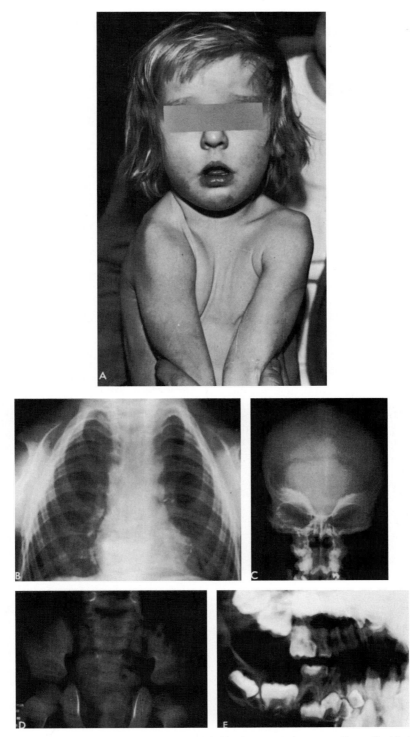

FIGURE 1. Cleidocranial dysostosis. *A*, A 3⁶/₁₂-year-old; height age, 2⁶/₁₂ years. (From Smith, D. W.: J. Pediatr., *70*:500, 1967, with permission.) *B*, Absent clavicles. *C*, Poorly mineralized cranial sutures. *D*, Hypoplasia of ilia, widespread pubic rami. *E*, Mandible showing delay in eruption of permanent teeth in a 7-year-old. (*C* and *E* Courtesy of R. Scherz, General Hospital, Tacoma, Wash.)

YUNIS-VARON SYNDROME

Yunis and Varon reported five patients from three families with this disorder in 1980. An additional eight affected children have been described subsequently.

ABNORMALITIES. (Based on 13 patients.)

Performance. Severe developmental delay in two out of three children who survived the neonatal period.

Growth. Prenatal growth deficiency (approximately 50 per cent of patients); severe failure to thrive postnatally.

Craniofacial. Microcephaly; sparse scalp hair, eyebrows, and eyelashes; wide calvarial sutures and enlarged fontanels; short upslanting palpebral fissures; anteverted nares; labiogingival retraction; short philtrum; thin lips; low-set/dysplastic ears with hypoplastic lobes; loose nuchal skin; broad secondary alveolar ridge; micrognathia.

Limbs. Agenesis/hypoplasia of thumbs and great toes; short tapering fingers and toes with nail hypoplasia; agenesis/hypoplasia of distal phalanges of fingers and toes, middle phalanges of fingers and first metatarsals; simian crease.

Other Skeletal. Absence or hypoplasia of one or both clavicles; absent sternal ossification; pelvic dysplasia; hip dislocation; abnormal scapula.

OCCASIONAL ABNORMALITIES. Absent nipples, external genital anomalies; sclerocornea; cataracts; mild ocular hypertelorism; premature loss of deciduous teeth; cystic dental follicles; glossoptosis; CNS malformations including arhinencephaly, agenesis of the corpus callosum, abnormality of cerebellar vermis; tetralogy of Fallot; cardiomyopathy; syndactyly of fingers and toes.

NATURAL HISTORY. Death in the neonatal period has occurred in 8 of 11 live-born infants. Although intellectual performance was normal in one mildly affected 3-year-old boy, the other two children who survived the neonatal period had severe developmental delay at 1 and 4 years of age, respectively.

ETIOLOGY. Autosomal recessive.

References

Yunis, E., and Varon, H.: Cleidocranial dysostosis, severe micrognathism, bilateral absence of thumbs and first metatarsal bones, and distal aphlangia: A new genetic syndrome. Am. J. Dis. Child., *134*:649, 1980.

Hughes, H. E., and Partington, M. W.: Brief clinical report: The syndrome of Yunis and Varon—report of a further case. Am. J. Med. Genet., *14*:539, 1983.

Garrett, G., et al.: Yunis-Varon syndrome with osteodysplasia. J. Med. Genet., *27*:114, 1990.

Ades, L. D., et al.: Congenital heart malformation in Yunis-Varon syndrome. J. Med. Genet., *30*:788, 1993.

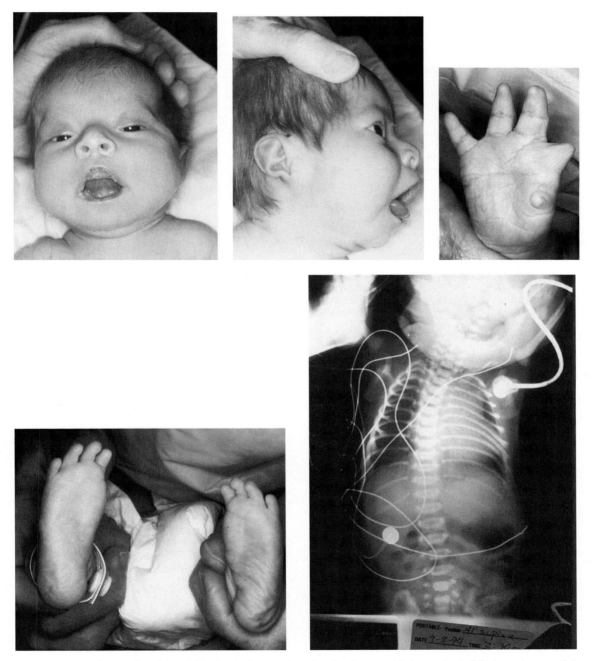

FIGURE 1. Newborn infant. Note labiogingival retraction, dysplastic ears with hypoplastic lobules, micrognathia, typical limb anomalies, and hypoplasia of clavicles.

L

L. CRANIOSYNOSTOSIS SYNDROMES

SAETHRE-CHOTZEN SYNDROME

Brachycephaly With Maxillary Hypoplasia, Prominent Ear Crus, Syndactyly

Originally described by Saethre and by Chotzen in the early 1930s, this disorder was more recently appreciated as a distinct entity. In the experience of the author, this has been the most common heritable disorder in which coronal craniostenosis may be an associated feature.

ABNORMALITIES. Variability of almost all features.

Craniofacial. Disturbance of cranial development including craniosynostosis of coronal, lambdoid, and/or metopic sutures; late closing fontanels, parietal foramina; and both ossification defects and hyperostosis of the calvarium. Brachycephaly with high flat forehead. Low frontal hairline. Maxillary hypoplasia with narrow palate. Facial asymmetry with deviation of nasal septum. Shallow orbits. Hypertelorism. Ptosis of eyelid. Lacrimal duct abnormalities. Prominent ear crus extending from the root of the helix across the concha. Small ears.

Limbs. Cutaneous syndactyly, usually partial, most commonly of second and third fingers and/or third and fourth toes. Mild to moderate brachydactyly with small distal phalanges and clinodactyly of fifth finger. Single upper palmar crease. Short angulated or flattened thumbs. Broad great toes with valgus deformity. Finger-like thumbs. Limited elbow extension.

Other. Short clavicles with distal hypoplasia.

OCCASIONAL ABNORMALITIES. Craniosynostosis to the point of increased intracranial pressure. Mental deficiency, small stature, cleft palate, deafness, strabismus, radioulnar synostosis, vertebral anomalies, short fourth metacarpals, hallucal reduplication, notched terminal phalanges of great toe, presumed cardiac anomaly (murmur), cryptorchidism, renal anomaly.

NATURAL HISTORY. Though most patients are apparently of normal intelligence, mental deficiency of mild to moderate degree has been a feature. Whether this is secondary to craniosynostosis remains to be clarified. Facial appearance tends to improve during childhood.

ETIOLOGY. Autosomal dominant. The gene has been mapped to 7p21-p22. A rather wide variance in expression exists. The author has evaluated one family in which the child had coronal craniostenosis requiring early surgical intervention but did not have limb defects. The father, who had no craniosynostosis, had syndactyly of the hands and feet and broad thumbs and toes. Combining the findings in the father and son yielded most of the variable features of Saethre-Chotzen syndrome.

References

Saethre, H.: Ein Beitrag zum Turmschaedelproblem (Pathogenese, Erblichkeit und Symptomatologie). Z. Nervenheilkd., *117*:533, 1931.

Chotzen, F.: Eine eigenartige familiare Entwicklungsstörung. (Akrocephalosyndaktylie, Dysostosis craniofacialis und Hypertelorismus). Monatsschr. Kinderheilkd., *55*:97, 1932.

Aase, J. M., and Smith, D. W.: Facial asymmetry and abnormalities of palms and ears: A dominantly inherited developmental syndrome. J. Pediatr., *76*:928, 1970.

Pantke, O. A., et al.: The Saethre-Chotzen syndrome. Birth Defects, *XI*(2):190, 1975.

Friedman, J. M., et al.: Saethre-Chotzen syndrome: A broad and variable pattern of skeletal malformations. J. Pediatr., *91*:929, 1977.

Brueton, L. A., et al.: The mapping of a gene for craniosynostosis: Evidence for linkage of the Saethre-Chotzen syndrome to distal chromosome 7p. J. Med. Genet., *29*:681, 1992.

Reardon, W., and Winter, R. M.: Saethre-Chotzen syndrome. J. Med. Genet., *31*:393, 1994.

Rose, C. S. P., et al.: Localization of the genetic locus for Saethre-Chotzen syndrome to a 6 cM region of chromosome 7 using four cases with apparently balanced translocations at 7p21.2. Hum. Molec. Genet., *3*:1405, 1994.

FIGURE 1. Saethre-Chotzen syndrome. Five affected family members. Note the variable ptosis, facial asymmetry, and strabismus. The hand of the girl shows a simian crease, clinodactyly, and mild webbing between the second and third fingers (the only individual with syndactyly *noted* in this family). The ear of the boy shows the unusually prominent crus across the concha, found in all affected individuals in this family. (From Aase, J. M., and Smith, D. W.: J. Pediatr., 76:928, 1970, with permission.)

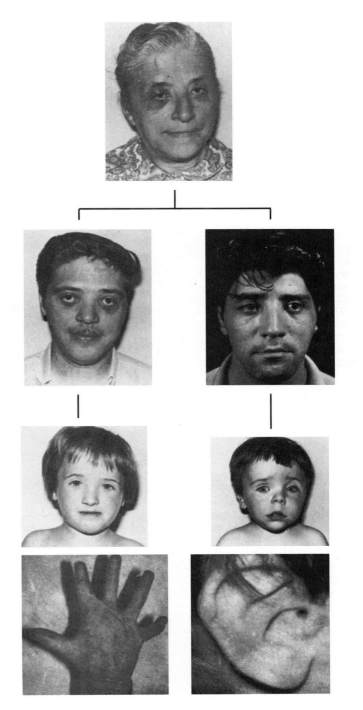

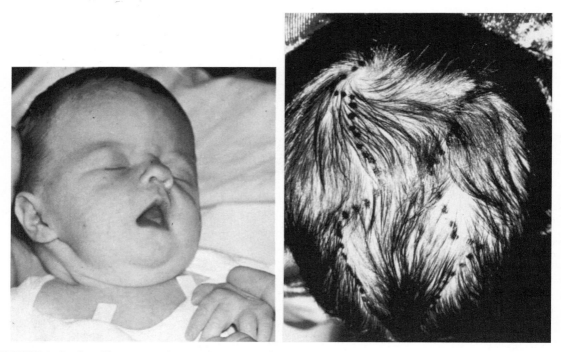

FIGURE 2. Saethre-Chotzen syndrome. *Left*, Infant with bilateral craniosynostosis and third and fourth finger syndactyly. *Right*, Infant with huge anterior and posterior fontanels (outlined). (Courtesy of Dr. J. M. Friedman, University of British Columbia, Vancouver, British Columbia.)

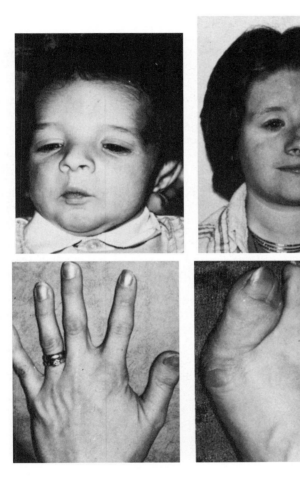

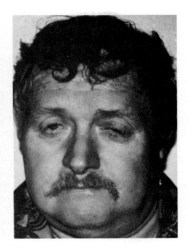

FIGURE 3. Saethre-Chotzen syndrome. Three affected family members. *Above*, Variable ptosis, facial asymmetry, and down-slanting palpebral fissures. *Left*, Partial syndactyly of second and third fingers and broad thumb and great toe, the latter in valgus position. (From Friedman, J. M., et al.: J. Pediatr., *91:*929, 1977, with permission.)

PFEIFFER SYNDROME
(Pfeiffer-type Acrocephalosyndactyly)

Brachycephaly, Mild Syndactyly, Broad Thumbs and Toes

Since this disorder was reported by Pfeiffer in 1964, more than 30 cases have been published.

ABNORMALITIES
Craniofacial. Brachycephaly with craniosynostosis of coronal, with or without sagittal sutures with full high forehead, ocular hypertelorism, small nose with low nasal bridge, narrow maxilla.

Hands and Feet. Broad distal phalanges of thumb and big toe, proximal phalanx of thumb and great toe is frequently a delta phalanx, small middle phalanges of fingers, partial syndactyly of second and third fingers and second, third, and fourth toes.

OCCASIONAL ABNORMALITIES.
Choanal atresia. Cartilaginous trachea. Laryngo-, tracheo-, and bronchomalacia. Kleeblattschädel anomaly (cloverleaf skull). Radiohumeral synostosis of elbow. Symphalangism of index finger. Fused vertebrae. Mental retardation. Hydrocephalus. Arnold-Chiari malformation. Seizures. Fifth finger clinodactyly. Imperforate anus.

NATURAL HISTORY AND COMMENT.
Three clinical subtypes have been delineated by Cohen that are significant with respect to prognosis. Patients with type 1 have the "classic" phenotype with craniosynostosis, broad thumbs and great toes, variable degrees of syndactyly, and normal to near normal intelligence. This type is compatible with life. Type 2 is associated with cloverleaf skull, severe ocular proptosis, severe CNS involvement, elbow ankylosis/synostosis, broad thumbs and great toes, and a variety of low-frequency visceral anomalies. Affected individuals do poorly, with early death. Type 3 Pfeiffer syndrome is associated with craniosynostosis, severe ocular proptosis in the absence of cloverleaf skull, shallow orbits, shortness of the anterior cranial base, elbow ankylosis, and various visceral anomalies. Neurologic compromise is common. Affected patients die early.

ETIOLOGY.
Autosomal dominant inheritance as well as sporadic cases presumably due to fresh gene mutation have been seen in type 1. All cases of types 2 and 3 Pfeiffer syndrome reported to date have been sporadic. Muenke et al. provided evidence that some cases of Pfeiffer syndrome are due to mutations in the fibroblast growth factor receptor 1 (FGFR1) gene, which maps to chromosome 8p11.22-p12. However, Rutland et al. reported mutations in the fibroblast growth factor receptor 2 (FGFR2) gene, which maps to chromosome 10q25-q26, indicating that Pfeiffer syndrome is genetically heterogeneous. It is presently unclear what relationship if any exists between the clinical subclassification of Pfeiffer syndrome set forth by Cohen and the molecular genetics. The value of the subclassification relates primarily to providing the family with a realistic prognosis.

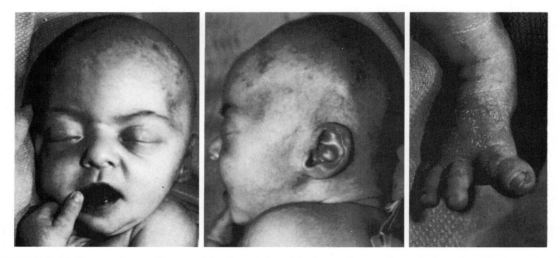

FIGURE 1. Pfeiffer syndrome. Presumed fresh mutational instance of coronal craniostenosis with aberrant and mildly broad toe and questionable mildly altered thumbs.

References

Pfeiffer, R. A.: Dominant erbliche Akrocephalosyndactylie. Z. Kinderheilkd., *90*:301, 1964.

Martsolf, J. T., et al.: Pfeiffer syndrome. An unusual type of acrocephalosyndactyly with broad thumbs and great toes. Am. J. Dis. Child., *121*:257, 1971.

Cohen, M. C.: Pfeiffer syndrome update, clinical subtypes, and guidelines for differential diagnosis. Am. J. Med. Genet., *45*:300, 1993.

Muenke, M., et al.: A common mutation in the fibroblast growth factor receptor 1 gene in Pfeiffer syndrome. Nat. Genet., *8*:268, 1994.

Rutland, P., et al.: Identical mutations in the FGFR2 gene cause both Pfeiffer and Crouzon syndrome phenotypes. Nat. Genet., *9*:173, 1995.

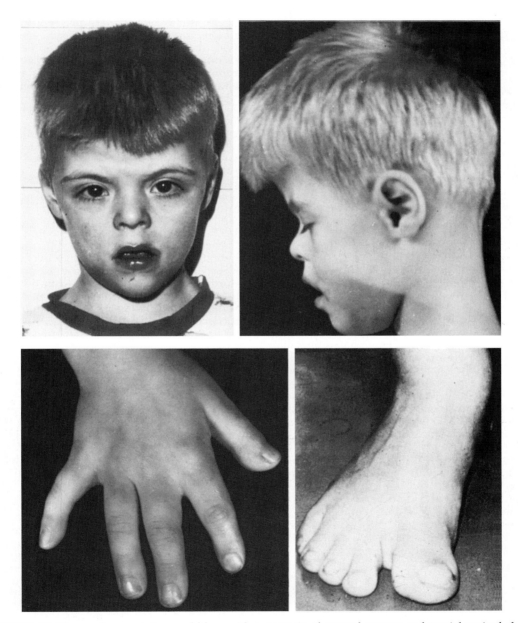

FIGURE 2. Pfeiffer syndrome. A 4-year-old boy with synostosis of coronal sutures and partial sagittal closure, broad thumbs and great toes, and partial syndactyly between second and third fingers and second through fourth toes. (From Martsolf, J. T., et al.: Am. J. Dis. Child., *121*:257, 1971, with permission.)

APERT SYNDROME

(Acrocephalosyndactyly)

Irregular Craniosynostosis, Midfacial Hypoplasia,
Syndactyly, Broad Distal Phalanx of Thumb and Big Toe

The condition was reported by Wheaton in 1894. In 1906, Apert summarized nine cases, and in 1920, Park and Powers published an exceptional essay on this entity. Numerous cases have been reported.

ABNORMALITIES

Growth. Mean birth length and weight above the 50th percentile. In childhood deceleration of linear growth occurs such that most values are between the 5th and 50th percentiles. Deceleration becomes more pronounced after adolescence.

Performance. Mental deficiency is present in a significant number of patients. In two separate studies mean I.Q. was 74 with a range from 52 to 89, and 61 with a range from 44 to 90, respectively. In a third study, 52 per cent had an I.Q. less than 70.

Central Nervous System. Although their incidence is unknown, the following defects occur: Agenesis of corpus callosum, nonprogressive ventriculomegaly, progressive hydrocephalus, absent or defective septum pallucidum, gyral abnormalities, hippocampal abnormalities, and megalencephaly.

Craniofacial. Short anteroposterior diameter with high, full forehead and flat occiput. Irregular craniosynostosis, especially of coronal suture. Fontanels may be large and late in closure. Flat facies, supraorbital horizontal groove, shallow orbits, hypertelorism, strabismus, down-slanting of palpebral fissures, small nose, maxillary hypoplasia. Narrow palate with median groove, with or without cleft palate or bifid uvula. Dental anomalies include delayed and/or ectopic eruption and shovel-shaped incisors. Malocclusion.

Limbs. Osseous and/or cutaneous syndactyly, varying from total fusion to partial fusion, most commonly with complete fusion of second, third, and fourth fingers. Distal phalanges of the thumbs are often broad and in valgus position. Fingers may be short. Cutaneous syndactyly of all toes with or without osseous syndactyly. Distal hallux may be broad and malformed.

Skin. Moderate to severe acne, including the forearms, at adolescence.

Other. Fusion of cervical vertebrae usually at C5–C6.

OCCASIONAL ABNORMALITIES.
Short humerus, synostosis of radius and humerus, limitation of joint mobility, genu valga. Gastrointestinal anomalies in 1.5 per cent including pyloric stenosis, esophageal atresia, and ectopic anus. Respiratory anomalies in 1.5 per cent including pulmonary aplasia and anomalous tracheal cartilage. Cardiac defects in 10 per cent including pulmonic stenosis, overriding aorta, ventricular septal defect, and endocardial fibroelastosis. Genitourinary anomalies in 10 per cent including polycystic kidney, hydronephrosis, bicornuate uterus, vaginal atresia, and cryptorchidism.

NATURAL HISTORY. Early surgery for craniosynostosis is indicated when there is evidence of increased intracranial pressure. However, early neurosurgical treatment does not prevent mental retardation, which is most likely related to malformations of the CNS. Upper airway compromise due to a combination of reduction in size of the nasopharynx and reduction in patency of the choanae as well as lower airway compromise due to anomalies of the tracheal cartilage may be responsible for early death. There should be vigorous early management of the syndrome. When the thumb is immobilized, early surgery to allow for a pincer grasp is indicated, with later attempts at further improvement of hand function. Hearing loss secondary to chronic otitis media and/or congenital fixation of the stapedial footplate is not uncommon. Newer techniques allow for vastly improved facial cosmetic reconstruction.

ETIOLOGY. Autosomal dominant. The vast majority of cases are sporadic and have been associated with older paternal age. Mutations in the fibroblast growth factor receptor 2 gene (FGFR2), which maps to chromosome 10q25-10q26, cause Apert syndrome. Different mutations in the same gene cause Crouzon syndrome as well as Pfeiffer syndrome. The recurrence risk for the unaffected parents of a child with Apert syndrome is negligible, whereas the recurrence risk for the affected individual is 50 per cent.

COMMENT. The osseous developmental pathology appears to be irregular bridging between the early islands of mesenchymal blastema that will become bone, especially in the distal extremities and cranium. Indications of hypoplasia and abnormal shape of bone are also evident, and the mutant gene may adversely affect the organization of other tissues. This is evident in the occurrence of mental deficiency and the greater than expected concurrence of a number of nonskeletal malformations. Therefore, every neonate suspected of having Apert syndrome deserves a complete evaluation for other malformations.

References

Wheaton, S. W.: Two specimens of congenital cranial deformity in infants associated with fusion of the fingers and toes. Trans. Pathol. Soc. Lond., 45:238, 1894.

Apart, E.: De l'Acrocephalosyndactylie. Bull. Soc. Med., 23:1310, 1906.

Park, E. A., and Powers, G. F.: Acrocephaly and scaphocephaly with symmetrically distributed malformations of the extremities. A study of the so-called "acrocephalosyndactylism." Am. J. Dis. Child., 20:235, 1920.

Blank, C. E.: Apert's syndrome (a type of acrocephalosyndactyly). Observations on British series of thirty-nine cases. Ann. Hum. Genet., 24:151, 1960.

Cohen, M. M., and Kreiborg, S.: The central nervous system in the Apert syndrome. Am. J. Med. Genet., 35:36, 1990.

Cohen, M. M., et al.: An updated pediatric perspective on the Apert syndrome. Am. J. Dis. Child., 147:989, 1993.

Wilkie, A. O. M., et al.: Apert syndrome results from localized mutations of FGFR2 and is allelic with Crouzon syndrome. Nat. Genet., 9:165, 1995.

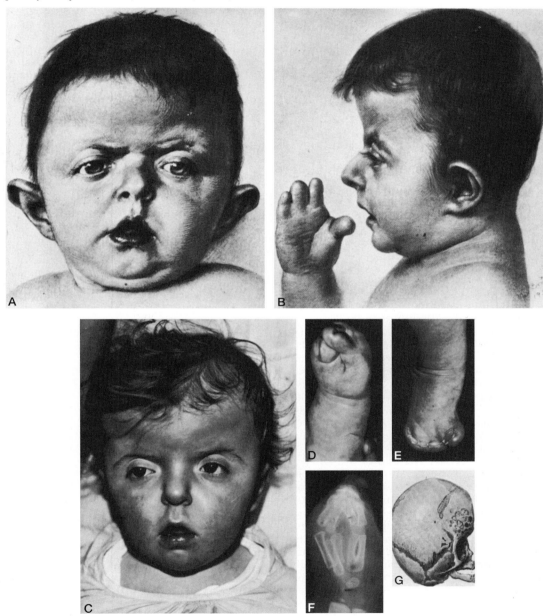

FIGURE 1. Apert syndrome. *A* and *B*, A girl, drawn by the late M. Brödel. *C*, A 2-year-old girl, her hand (*D*), foot (*E*), and x-ray film of the hand (*F*). *G*, The cranium of an infant with Apert syndrome, showing the irregular synostosis of the coronal suture and the aberrant development in the frontal bone. (*A*, *B*, and *G* from Park, E. A., and Powers, G. F.: Am. J. Dis. Child., 20:235, 1920, with permission.)

CROUZON SYNDROME

(Craniofacial Dysostosis)

*Shallow Orbits, Premature
Craniosynostosis, Maxillary Hypoplasia*

Originally described in 1912 by Crouzon in a mother and her daughter, this condition usually has an adverse effect on craniofacial development alone. With complete examination, including the hands and feet, many of the patients who have been diagnosed as having Crouzon syndrome in the past have been recognized as having Saethre-Chotzen syndrome. Furthermore, others represent the coronal stenosis sequence due to fetal head constraint in utero, a nongenetic type of disorder.

ABNORMALITIES

Craniofacial. Ocular proptosis due to shallow orbits with or without divergent strabismus, hypertelorism. Frontal bossing. Exposure conjunctivitis or keratitis. Unexplained poor visual acuity. Optic atrophy. Nystagmus. Hypoplasia of maxilla with or without curved parrot-like nose, inverted V shape to palate. Conductive hearing loss. Craniosynostosis, especially of coronal, lambdoid, and sagittal sutures with palpable ridging. Short anteroposterior and wide lateral dimensions of the cranium may occur.

OCCASIONAL ABNORMALITIES. Mental retardation. Hydrocephalus. Seizures. Agenesis of corpus callosum. Keratoconus. Iris coloboma. Atresia of auditory meatus. Cleft lip with or without cleft palate. Bifid uvula. Subluxation of radial heads. Acanthosis nigricans involving eyelids, perioral, perialar, and neck skin predominantly.

NATURAL HISTORY. The degree of craniosynostosis, as well as the age of onset, is variable. One infant is described who showed no roentgenographic evidence of craniosynostosis at 4 months but complete sutural closure by 11 months of age. Surgical morcellation procedures to allow for more normal brain development are indicated when there is increased intracranial pressure. Otherwise, the indications are usually cosmetic, and the decision toward surgery is usually mitigated by the severity of the aberrant shape plus the competency of the surgeon who will perform the procedure. Newer techniques allow for cosmetic reconstruction of the facial bones. Obstruction of the upper airway frequently results in obligatory mouth breathing but rarely leads to acute respiratory distress.

ETIOLOGY. Autosomal dominant with variable expression, shallow orbits being the most consistent feature. About one quarter of the reported cases have had a negative family history and presumably represent fresh mutations. Mutations in the fibroblast growth factor receptor 2 gene (FGFR2), which maps to chromosome 10q25-q26, cause Crouzon syndrome. Some cases of Pfeiffer syndrome are caused by an identical mutation in the same gene. Different mutations in the same gene cause Apert syndrome as well as Jackson-Weiss syndrome, a disorder associated with craniosynostosis and broad great toes with medial deviation and tarsal-metatarsal coalescence.

References

Crouzon, O.: Dysostose cranio-faciale héréditaire. Bull. Mem. Soc. Med. Hop. (Paris), *33*:545, 1912.

Bertelsen, T. I.: The premature synostosis of the cranial sutures. Acta Ophthalmol. [Suppl. 51] (Kbh.), *1*:176, 1958.

Dodge, H. W., Jr., Wood, M. W., and Kennedy, R. L. J.: Craniofacial dysostosis: Crouzon's disease. Pediatrics, *23*:98, 1959.

Kreiborg, S.: Crouzon syndrome: A clinical and roentgencephalometric study. Scand. J. Plast. Reconstr. Surg., Suppl. 18, 1981.

Perlman, J. M., and Zaidman, G. W.: Bilateral keratoconus in Crouzon's syndrome. Cornea, *13*:80, 1994.

Reardon, W., et al.: Mutations in the fibroblast growth factor receptor 2 gene cause Crouzon syndrome. Nat. Genet., *8*:98, 1994.

Jabs, E. W., et al.: Jackson-Weiss and Crouzon syndromes are allelic with mutations in fibroblast growth factor receptor 2. Nat. Genet., *8*:275, 1994.

Rutland, P., et al.: Identical mutations in the FGFR2 gene cause both Pfeiffer and Crouzon syndrome phenotypes. Nat. Genet., *9*:173, 1995.

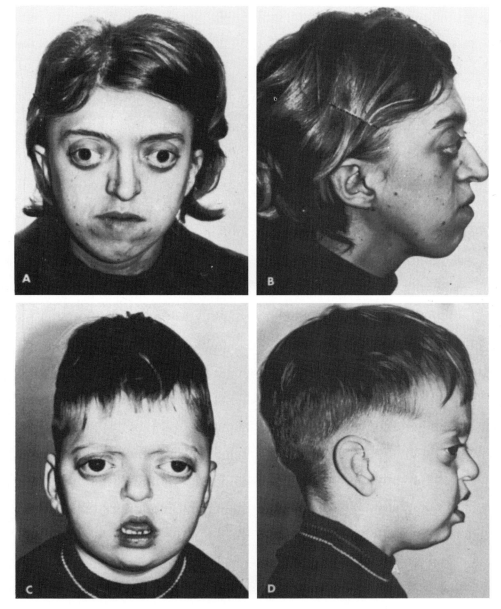

FIGURE 1. Mother (*A* and *B*) and son (*C* and *D*) with Crouzon syndrome. (Courtesy of Dr. Michael Cohen, Dalhousie University, Halifax, Nova Scotia.)

CRANIOFRONTONASAL DYSPLASIA

The name craniofrontonasal dysplasia was introduced by Cohen in 1979 to designate this condition. Through analysis of 58 families and 8 males from 18 families, Grutzner and Gorlin have set forth the differences in the clinical phenotype between males and females with this disorder. This is one of the few conditions in which females are more severely affected than males.

ABNORMALITIES

Cranial. Females—craniosynostosis, brachycephaly, and frontal bossing. Males—increased bony interorbital distance. Craniosynostosis has never been seen.

Facial. Females and males—hypertelorism, facial asymmetry, broad nasal root, bifid nasal tip.

Limbs. Females and males—longitudinal splitting of nails, syndactyly of toes, broad first toe, clinodactyly. Females—syndactyly of fingers.

OCCASIONAL ABNORMALITIES. Females—telecanthus, exotropia, nystagmus, strabismus, and Sprengel deformity. Females and males—cleft lip/palate, webbed neck, and mental retardation. Males—short stature, pectus excavatum, pseudoarthrosis of clavicles, brachydactyly, pre-axial and postaxial polydactyly, deviated distal phalanges of fingers and toes, wide space between first and second toes, hypospadias, shawl scrotum, and diaphragmatic hernia.

ETIOLOGY. Probably X-linked dominant. However, the far milder manifestation of the disorder in males is unusual and not adequately explained.

COMMENT. This condition is primarily diagnosed in females. All reported males have been identified based on a confirmed diagnosis in a female relative.

References

Slover, R., and Sujanski, E.: Frontonasal dysplasia with coronal craniosynostosis in three sibs. Birth Defects, *XV(5B)*:75, 1979.

Cohen, M. M.: Craniofrontonasal dysplasia. Birth Defects, *XV(5B)*:85, 1979.

Young, I. D.: Craniofrontonasal dysplasia. J. Med. Genet., *24*:193, 1987.

Grutzner, E., and Gorlin, R. J.: Craniofrontonasal dysplasia: Phenotypic expression in females and males and genetic considerations. Oral Surg. Oral Med. Oral Pathol., *65*:436, 1988.

FIGURE 1. A 2-month-old female with ocular hypertelorism, facial asymmetry, and right coronal craniosynostosis. (Courtesy of Dr. Marilyn C. Jones, Children's Hospital, San Diego, Calif.)

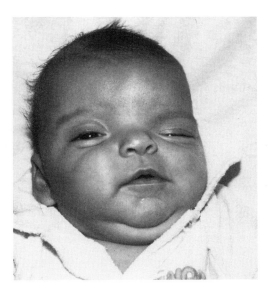

CARPENTER SYNDROME

*Acrocephaly, Polydactyly and
Syndactyly of Feet, Lateral Displacement of Inner Canthi*

Although Carpenter described this condition in 1901, it was not firmly established as an entity until Temtamy's report in 1966. Approximately 40 cases have been reported.

ABNORMALITIES

Growth. Postnatal growth less than 25th percentile. Obesity.

Performance. Variable delay in intellectual performance. I.Q.s have ranged from 52 to 104.

Craniofacial. Brachycephaly with variable synostosis of coronal, sagittal, and lambdoid sutures. Shallow supraorbital ridges. Flat nasal bridge. Lateral displacement of the inner canthi with or without inner canthal folds. Corneal opacity, maldeveloped or microcornea, optic atrophy and/or blurring of disk margins. Low-set and malformed ears. Hypoplastic mandible and/or maxilla. Narrow, highly arched palate.

Limbs. Brachydactyly of hands with clinodactyly, partial syndactyly, and camptodactyly. Single flexion crease. Subluxation at distal interphalangeal joints. Angulation deformities at knees. Preaxial polydactyly of the feet with partial syndactyly. Short or missing middle phalanges of fingers and toes.

Cardiovascular. Defects in 50 per cent including ventricular septal defect, atrial septal defect, patent ductus arteriosus, pulmonic stenosis, tetralogy of Fallot, and transposition of great vessels.

Other. Hypogenitalism. Cryptorchidism. Umbilical hernia. Omphalocele.

OCCASIONAL ABNORMALITIES.

Postaxial polydactyly, preauricular pits, short muscular neck, delayed loss of deciduous teeth, partial anodontia, duplication of second phalanx of thumb, metatarsus varus, flat acetabulum, flare to pelvis, coxa valga, genu valgum, lateral displacement of patellae, pilonidal dimple, accessory spleen. Hydronephrosis with or without hydroureter. Precocious puberty. Conductive and neurosensory hearing loss.

NATURAL HISTORY. Recent reports indicate that mental retardation is not an obligate feature of this condition and probably does not relate to the timing of craniofacial surgery. Fine motor dysfunction secondary to the digital anomalies is a continuing problem. Articulation errors attributed to inability to perform rapidly alternating movements of the lips and tongue can lead to speech problems. Eustachian tube dysfunction is secondary to the short cranial base.

ETIOLOGY. Autosomal recessive.

References

Carpenter, G.: Two sisters showing malformations of the skull and other congenital abnormalities. Rep. Soc. Study Dis. Child. Lond., *1*:110, 1901.

Temtamy, S. A.: Carpenter's syndrome: Acrocephalopolysyndactyly, an autosomal recessive syndrome. J. Pediatr., *69*:111, 1966.

Frias, J. L., et al.: Normal intelligence in two children with Carpenter syndrome. Am. J. Med. Genet., *2*: 191, 1978.

Robinson, L. K., et al.: Carpenter syndrome: Natural history and clinical spectrum. Am. J. Med. Genet., *20*:461, 1985.

Cohen, D. M., et al.: Acrocephalopolysyndactyly type II—Carpenter syndrome: Clinical spectrum and an attempt at unification with Goodman and Summit syndromes. Am. J. Med. Genet., *28*:311, 1987.

Richieri-Costa, A., et al.: Carpenter syndrome with normal intelligence: Brazilian girl born to consanguineous parents. Am. J. Med. Genet., *47*:281, 1993.

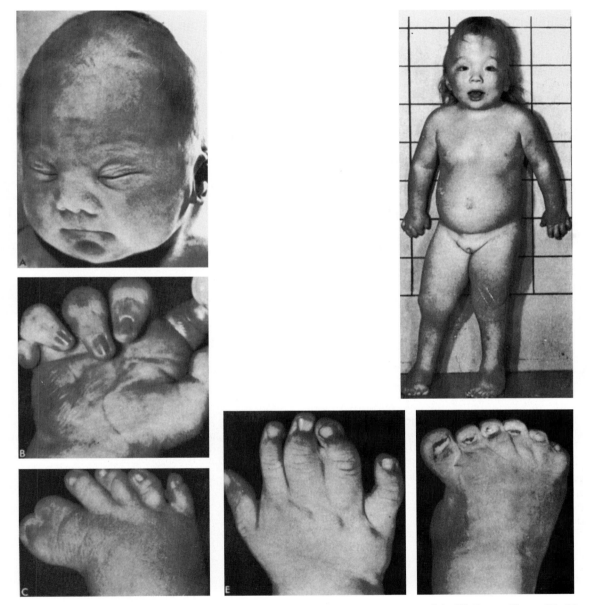

FIGURE 1. Carpenter syndrome. *A* to *C*, Neonate, necropsy photos. (Courtesy of A. W. Bauer, Group Health Cooperative, Seattle, Wash.) *D* and *E*, A 3-year-old. (From Temtamy, S. A.: J. Pediatr., *69*:111, 1966, with permission.)

GREIG CEPHALOPOLYSYNDACTYLY SYNDROME

Preaxial and Postaxial Polydactyly, Syndactyly, Frontal Bossing

Initially described by Greig in 1926, additional cases were reported by Temtamy and McKusick, Marshall and Smith, and Hootnick and Holmes. Subsequently, more than 50 cases have been published.

ABNORMALITIES
Craniofacies. High forehead (70 per cent). Frontal bossing (58 per cent). Macrocephaly (52 per cent). Apparent hypertelorism. Broad nasal root (79 per cent).

Hands. Postaxial polydactyly (78 per cent). Broad thumbs (90 per cent). Syndactyly, primarily fingers 3 and 4 (82 per cent).

Feet. Preaxial polydactyly (81 per cent). Broad halluces (89 per cent). Syndactyly, primarily toes 1 to 3 (90 per cent).

OCCASIONAL ABNORMALITIES. Broad, late-closing cranial sutures. Advanced bone age. Down-slanting palpebral fissures. Mild mental deficiency. Agenesis of corpus callosum (one patient). Mild degrees of hydrocephaly. Craniosynostosis. Camptodactyly. Radiographic evidence of preaxial polydactyly of hands and postaxial polydactyly of feet. Osseous syndactyly.

ETIOLOGY. The majority of cases are familial with an autosomal dominant mode of inheritance. Three families with dominantly inherited Greig syndrome segregating with balanced translocations involving 7p13 have been reported. In addition, a few sporadic cases have been described with an interstitial deletion involving 7p with breakpoints at the same location confirming the localization of this disorder to 7p13.

References

Greig, D. M.: Oxycephaly. Edinburgh Med. J., *33*:189, 1926.

Temtamy, S., and McKusick, V. A.: Synopsis of hand malformation with particular emphasis on genetic factors. Birth Defects, *V(3)*:125, 1969.

Marshal, R. E., and Smith, D. W.: Frontodigital syndrome: A dominant inherited disorder with normal intelligence. J. Pediatr., *77*:129, 1970.

Hootnick, D., and Holmes, L. B.: Family polysyndactyly and craniofacial anomalies. Clin. Genet., *3*:128, 1972.

Tommerup, N., and Nielsen, F.: A familial translocation t(3;7) (p21.1;p13) associated with the Greig polysyndactyly-craniofacial anomalies syndrome. Am. J. Med. Genet., *16*:313, 1983.

Gollop, T. R., and Fontes, L. R.: The Greig cephalopolysyndactyly syndrome: Report of a family and review of the literature. Am. J. Med. Genet., *22*:59, 1985.

Pettigrew, A. L., et al.: Greig syndrome associated with an interstitial deletion of 7p: Confirmation of the localization of Greig syndrome to 7p13. Hum. Genet., *87*:452, 1991.

Ausems, M. G. E. M., et al.: Greig cephalopolysyndactyly syndrome in a large family. A comparison of the clinical signs with those described in the literature. Clin. Dysmorphol., *3*:21, 1994.

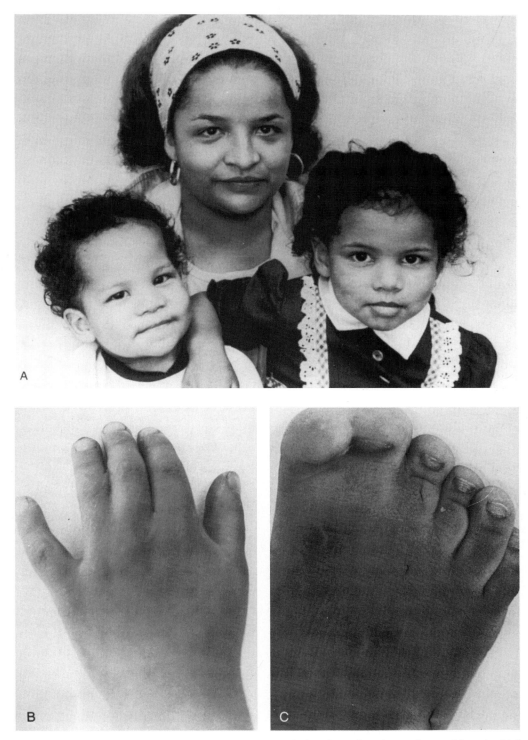

FIGURE 1. *A* to *C,* Mother and her children with Greig cephalopolysyndactyly syndrome. Note the high forehead, syndactyly of fingers 3 and 4, and preaxial polydactyly of foot. (From Duncan, P. A., et al.: Am. J. Dis. Child., *133:*818, 1979, with permission.)

ANTLEY-BIXLER SYNDROME

(Multisynostotic Osteodysgenesis,
Trapezoidcephaly/Multiple Synostosis)

Craniosynostosis, Choanal Atresia, Radiohumeral Synostosis

First described by Antley and Bixler in 1975, subsequent cases have been reported by De-Lozier et al. and Robinson et al. Schinzel et al. documented the first instance of affected siblings.

ABNORMALITIES

Craniofacial. Brachycephaly (100 per cent). Frontal bossing (100 per cent). Large anterior fontanel (90 per cent). Craniosynostosis (70 per cent). Midfacial hypoplasia (100 per cent). Depressed nasal bridge (100 per cent). Proptosis (100 per cent). Choanal stenosis and/or atresia (80 per cent). Dysplastic ears (100 per cent). Stenotic external auditory canals (50 per cent).

Limbs. Radiohumeral synostosis (100 per cent). Joint contractures, including inability to extend fingers and decreased range of motion at wrists, hips, knees, and ankles (100 per cent). Arachnodactyly associated with enlarged interphalangeal joints, increased numbers of flexion creases, and distal tapering with narrow nails (70 per cent). Femoral bowing (100 per cent). Femoral fractures (50 per cent) Rocker-bottom feet (60 per cent).

OCCASIONAL ABNORMALITIES.
Hydrocephalus. Preauricular tags. Vaginal atresia. Hypoplastic labia majora. Fused labia minora. Clitoromegaly. Atrial septal defects. Renal defect. Multiple hemangiomata. Partial cutaneous syndactyly. Narrow chest and pelvis.

NATURAL HISTORY.
Respiratory compromise secondary to upper airway obstruction has varied from severe nasal congestion to multiple apneic episodes leading to death in the first few months of life in 80 per cent of cases. Survivors frequently require tracheostomy, and the placement of a gastrostomy tube is often necessary. Although gross and fine motor function have been difficult to assess because of joint contractures, prognosis may be reasonably good once the difficult perinatal period has passed. Joint contractures have improved with age and passive range-of-motion exercises. There has been no propensity to fracture postnatally. Resection of the radiohumeral synostosis was attempted in one child at 6 months of age. However, recurrence of the bone fusion recurred within 3 months. That same child, now 10 years of age, functions intellectually and socially as a normal fifth grader.

ETIOLOGY.
Probable autosomal recessive inheritance based on one example of affected sisters born to unaffected parents.

References

Antley, R. M., and Bixler, D.: Trapezoidcephaly, midface hypoplasia, and cartilage abnormalities with multiple synostoses and skeletal fractures. Birth Defects, *XI(2)*:397, 1975.

DeLozier, C. D., et al.: The syndrome of multisynostotic osteodysgenesis with long-bone fractures. Am. J. Med. Genet., *7*:391, 1980.

Robinson, L. K., et al.: The Antley-Bixler syndrome. J. Pediatr., *101*:201, 1982.

Schinzel, A., et al.: Antley-Bixler syndrome in sisters: A term newborn and a prenatally diagnosed fetus. Am. J. Med. Genet., *14*:139, 1983.

Escobar, L. F., et al.: Antley-Bixler syndrome from a prognostic perspective: Report of a case and review of the literature. Am. J. Med. Genet., *29*:829, 1988.

DeLozier, C. D.: Antley-Bixler syndrome from a prognostic perspective. Am. J. Med. Genet., *32*:262, 1989.

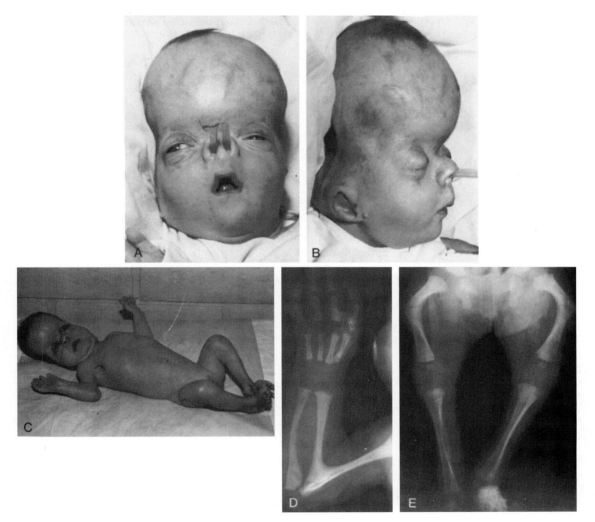

FIGURE 1. Antley-Bixler syndrome. *A* to *E*, Newborn female infant with severe maxillary hypoplasia, depressed nasal bridge, proptosis, and dysplastic ears. Note the multiple joint contractures, radiohumeral synostosis, and femoral bowing. (From Robinson, L. K., et al.: J. Pediatr., *101*:201, 1982, with permission.)

BALLER-GEROLD SYNDROME

(Craniosynostosis–Radial Aplasia Syndrome)

Baller described a 26-year-old woman in 1950, and Gerold subsequently reported affected siblings. Over 20 cases have been reported.

ABNORMALITIES

Performance. Fifty per cent of those followed beyond infancy have been mentally deficient.

Growth. Prenatal and postnatal growth deficiencies.

Craniofacies. Craniosynostosis involving any or all sutures (100 per cent). Low-set and posteriorly rotated ears (64 per cent). Micrognathia (50 per cent). Prominent nasal bridge (32 per cent). Down-slanting palpebral fissures (32 per cent). Microstomia (32 per cent). Epicanthal folds (27 per cent). Flattened forehead (27 per cent).

Limbs. Radial aplasia/hypoplasia (77 per cent). Short, curved ulna (68 per cent). Missing carpals, metacarpals, and phalanges. Fused carpals. Absent or hypoplastic thumbs (100 per cent).

Anal. Anomalies in 40 per cent including imperforate anus and/or anteriorly placed anus.

Urogenital. Anomalies in 35 per cent including ectopic, hypoplastic, dysplastic, and/or absent kidney, and persistence of the cloaca.

OCCASIONAL ABNORMALITIES.
Epicanthal folds. Bifid uvula. Cleft palate. Choanal stenosis. Strabismus. Optic atrophy. Myopia. Seizures. Polymicrogyria. Hydrocephalus. Absent corpus callosum. Conductive hearing loss. Capillary hemangiomata over nose and philtrum. Hypoplastic ala nasi. Vertebral defects. Rib fusions. Scoliosis. Hypoplastic humerus. Decreased range of motion at shoulders, elbows, and knees. Hypoplastic patellae. Coxa valga. Spina bifida occulta. Cardiac defects (25 per cent) include subaortic valvular hypertrophy, ventricular septal defect, and tetralogy of Fallot.

NATURAL HISTORY. Twenty per cent of the live-borns died unexpectedly during the first year of life. For the remainder, postnatal growth deficiency is common. Of the 13 affected individuals for whom developmental performance was mentioned, 6 were mentally retarded; 2, both of whom were less than 2 years of age, had moderate motor delay; and 5 were normal.

ETIOLOGY. Autosomal recessive inheritance

References

Baller, F.: Radiusaplasie und Inzucht. Z. Menschl. Vererb.-Konstit.-Lehre, *29*:782, 1950.

Gerold, M.: Frakturheilung bei einem seltenen Fall kongenitaler Anomalie der oberen Gliedmassen. Zentralbl. Chir., *84*:831, 1959.

Greitzer, L. J., et al.: Craniosynostosis–radial aplasia syndrome. J. Pediatr., *84*:723, 1974.

Lin, A. E., et al.: Further delineation of the Baller-Gerold syndrome. Am. J. Med. Genet., *45*:519, 1993.

Ramos Fuentes, F. J., et al.: Phenotypic variability in the Baller-Gerold syndrome: Report of a mildly affected patient and review of the literature. Eur. J. Pediatr., *153*:483, 1994.

FIGURE 1. Baller-Gerold syndrome. *A* and *B*, Newborn infant with metopic craniosynostosis, mildly dysplastic ears, and radial dysplasia with absent thumbs. (From Greitzer, L. J.: J. Pediatr., *84*:723, 1974, with permission.)

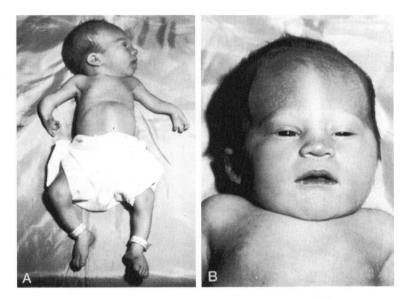

M

M. OTHER SKELETAL DYSPLASIAS

MULTIPLE SYNOSTOSIS SYNDROME
(Symphalangism Syndrome)

Symphalangism, Hypoplasia of Alae Nasi

In the past, this disorder was generally termed symphalangism (synostosis of finger joints), a nonspecific anomaly. The multiple synostosis character of the disorder herein set forth was emphasized by Maroteaux et al.

ABNORMALITIES

Facies. Narrow, with hypoplasia of alae nasi, hypoplastic nasal septum, fusion of the nasal bone and the frontal process of the maxilla, short philtrum, thin vermilion of upper lip, occasional strabismus.

Limbs. Multiple fusion of midphalangeal joints, elbows, and carpal and tarsal bones (especially navicular to talus). Variable clinodactyly, brachydactyly, and distal bone hypoplasia or aplasia in phalanges. Aplasia/hypoplasia of fingernails/toenails. Cutaneous syndactyly. Limited forearm pronation/supination, rotation of hips, and abduction of shoulders. Short feet and hallux.

Spine. Vertebral anomalies.

Middle Ear. Variable fusion of middle ear ossicles, with conductive deafness, most commonly fusion of stapes to the round window.

Other. Pectus excavatum. Prominent costochondral junction.

OCCASIONAL ABNORMALITIES. Moderate mental deficiency. Klippel-Feil anomaly. Short sternum. Good muscle development. Short arms and legs.

ETIOLOGY. Autosomal dominant with appreciable variance in expression.

COMMENT. Potential for significant partial or complete restoration of hearing by otologic surgery is excellent. Symphalangism is progressive and is not always present in childhood.

References

Vesell, E. S.: Symphalangism, strabismus and hearing loss in mother and daughter. N. Engl. M. Med., *263:* 839, 1960.

Fuhrmann, W., et al.: Dominant erbliche Brachydaktylie mit Gelenksaplasien. Humangenetik, *1:*337, 1965.

Strasburger, A. K., et al.: Symphalangism: Genetic and clinical aspects. Bull. Johns Hopkins Hosp., *117:*108, 1965.

Elkington, S. G., and Huntsman, R. G.: The Talbot fingers. A study in symphalangism. Br. Med. J., *1:*407, 1967.

Maroteaux, P., Bouvet, J. P., and Briard, M. L.: La maladie des synostoses multiples. Nouv. Presse Med., *1:*3041, 1972.

Herrmann, J.: Symphalangism and brachydactyly syndrome. Birth Defects, *X(5):*23, 1974.

de-Silva, E. O., Filho, S. M., and de Albuquerque, S. C.: Multiple synostosis syndrome: Study of a large Brazilian kindred. Am. J. Med. Genet., *18:*237, 1984.

Hurvitz, S. A., et al.: The facio-audio-symphalangism syndrome: Report of a case and review of the literature. Clin. Genet., *28:*61, 1985.

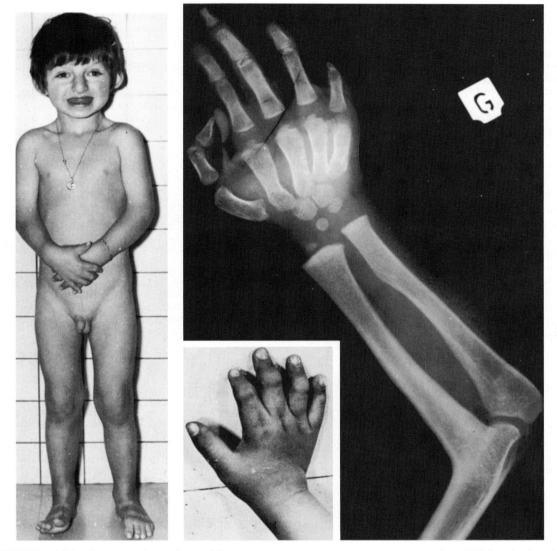

FIGURE 1. Multiple synostosis syndrome. Note narrow nose; prominent external ear; and variable brachydactyly, aplasia of distal phalanges, and synostoses. (From Maroteaux, P., et al.: Nouv. Presse Med., *1*:3041, 1972, with permission.)

SPONDYLOCARPOTARSAL SYNOSTOSIS SYNDROME

Disproportionate Short Stature, Block Vertebrae, Carpal Synostosis

This disorder was delineated in 1994 by Langer et al., who described six affected individuals and reviewed an additional six from the literature.

ABNORMALITIES

Growth. Disproportionate short stature with short trunk.

Thorax. Failure of normal spinal segmentation which when symmetric leads to block vertebrae, and when asymmetric leads to mild scoliosis and lordosis. The presence of a unilateral unsegmented bar results in severe scoliosis and lordosis.

Hands and Feet. Carpal synostosis most commonly capitate-hamate and lunate-triquetrum. Tarsal synostosis. Pes planus.

OCCASIONAL ABNORMALITIES. Cleft palate. Sensorineural or mixed hearing loss. Preauricular skin tag. Round broad face with ocular hypertelorism, and short nose with anteverted nares and broad, square nasal tip. Enamel hypoplasia. Decreased range of motion at elbows. Postaxial polydactyly. Renal cyst. Odontoid hypoplasia.

NATURAL HISTORY. Progressive scoliosis and lordosis are the major complications and are sometimes associated with restrictive impairment of total lung capacity. Cervical vertebral instability has been described. The unsegmented bar is difficult to identify radiographically in early life because it is cartilaginous. Serial follow-up x-rays are indicated. Tomography is often helpful.

ETIOLOGY. Autosomal recessive inheritance.

References

Langer, L. O., and Moe, J. M.: A recessive form of congenital scoliosis different from spondylothoracic dysplasia. Birth Defects, *11(6)*:83, 1975.

Wiles, C. R., et al.: Congenital synspondylism. Am. J. Med. Genet., *42*:288, 1992.

Langer, L. O., et al.: Spondylocarpotarsal synostosis syndrome (with or without unilateral unsegmented bar). Am. J. Med. Genet., *51*:1, 1994.

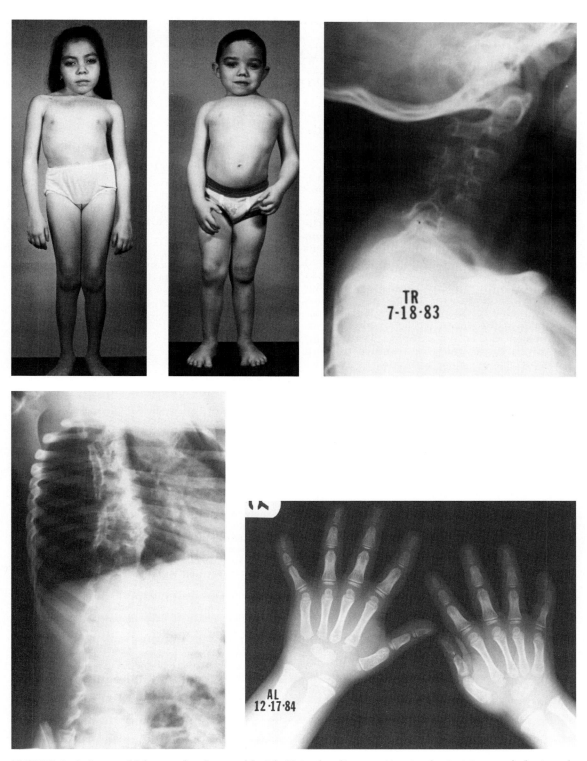

FIGURE 1. A 5-year-old boy and a 9-year-old girl. Note the disproportionate short stature and short neck, synostosis of the cervical vertebrae, the unilateral unsegmented bar and the carpal synostosis. (From Langer, L. L., et al.: Am. J. Med. Genet., *51*:1, 1994, with permission of Wiley-Liss, a division of John Wiley & Sons.)

435

MULTIPLE EXOSTOSES SYNDROME

(Diaphyseal Aclasis, External Chondromatosis Syndrome)

Diaphyseal Outgrowths Leading to Limb
Deformity, With or Without Short Metacarpals

More than 1000 cases have been reported.

ABNORMALITIES

Skeletal. Diaphyseal juxtaepiphyseal out-growths develop, capped by hyaline carti-lage, and tend to grow away from the joint, leading to deformity. Though often present at birth, they are usually not appreciated until early childhood. There is a slowing in their growth at adolescence, and no further growth occurs in the adult. They are most prominent at the ends of long bones, espe-cially at the knees, with variable involve-ment of the pelvis, scapulae, and ribs. In-volved bone may be relatively short, especially the ulna, with consequent bow-ing of the forearm. Shortness of stature with a mean male adult height of 170 cm with a range of 155 to 190.5 cm and a mean female adult height of 155 cm with a range of 127 to 173 cm. Thirty-seven per cent of male and 44 per cent of female heights less than the fifth percentile.

OCCASIONAL ABNORMALITIES. Enchon-dromata. Short metacarpal (fourth and fifth) bones.

NATURAL HISTORY. New outgrowths and en-largement of old exostoses may occur through adolescence. Thereafter, no further growth takes place, although there is a 3 per cent incidence of sarcoma from such lesions, with an age at iden-tification ranging from 11 to 64 years. In a ret-rospective review of 43 affected individuals and 137 of their affected relatives, Luckert-Wicklund et al. documented the following: Approximately two thirds of patients have surgery for removal of at least one exostosis; for those patients 21 years or older the mean number of exostosis re-moved was 3.5; compression of peripheral nerves occurred in 22.6 per cent, of blood vessels in 11.3 per cent, and of the spinal cord in one patient; arthritis with age of onset of 36 years occurred in 14 per cent; and during pregnancy changes in the exostosis occurred in 10.5 per cent.

ETIOLOGY. Autosomal dominant. Linkage studies have identified three chromosomal lo-cations for multiple exostosis genes at 8q24.1, the pericentric region of 11, and 19p. It has been suggested that these are most likely tumor-sup-pressor genes.

References

Solomon, L.: Hereditary multiple exostosis. Am. J. Hum. Genet., *16*:351, 1964.

Shapiro, F., Simon, S., and Glimcher, M. J.: Hereditary multiple exostosis. J. Bone Joint Surg., *61A*:815, 1979.

Cook, A., et al.: Genetic heterogeneity in families of hereditary multiple exostoses. Am. J. Hum. Genet., *53*:71, 1993.

Wu, Y.-Q., et al.: Assignment of a second locus for multiple exostoses to the pericentric region of chro-mosome 11. Hum. Mol. Genet., *3*:167, 1994.

Le Merrer, M., et al.: A gene for hereditary multiple exostoses maps to chromosome 19p. Hum. Mol. Ge-net., *3*:717, 1994.

Ahn, J., et al.: Cloning of the putative tumour sup-pressor gene for hereditary multiple exostosis (EXT 1) Nature Genetics, *11*:137, 1995.

Luckert-Wicklund, C., et al.: Natural history study of hereditary multiple exostoses. Am. J. Med. Genet., *55*:43, 1995.

Hecht, J. T., et al.: Hereditary multiple exostoses and chondrosarcoma: Linkage to chromosome 11 and loss of heterozygosity for EXT-linked markers on chromosome 11 and 8. Am. J. Hum. Genet., *56*:1125, 1995.

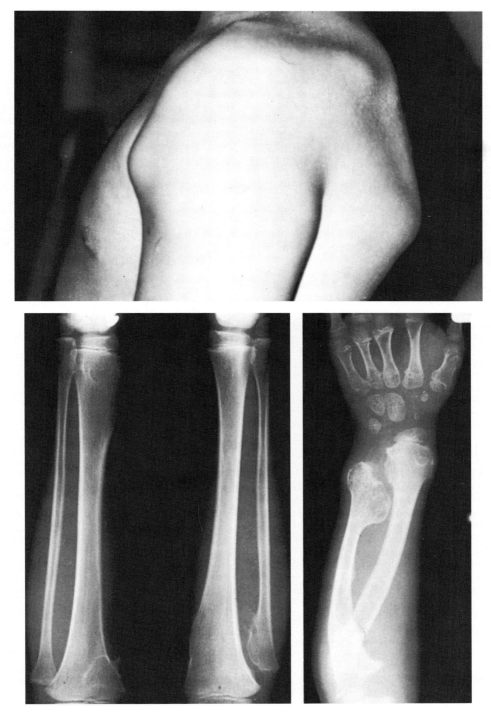

FIGURE 1. Multiple exostoses syndrome. *Upper*, Grossly evident exostoses in upper humerus and in scapula. *Lower*, Metaphyseal distribution of exostoses, which may be deforming, as seen in the wrist in this example.

NAIL-PATELLA SYNDROME
(Hereditary Osteo-onychodysplasia)

Nail Dysplasia, Patella Hypoplasia, Iliac Spurs

Little's report in 1897, limited to a presentation of the patellar defect, is usually credited as the initial description of this syndrome, whereas this pattern includes multiple other dysplasias of osseous as well as nonosseous mesenchymal tissues. Well over 400 cases have been reported.

ABNORMALITIES
Nails. Hypoplasia, splitting, most commonly of thumbnail; discoloration, longitudinal ridging, poorly formed lunulae and triangular lunulae (98 per cent).
Knees. Hypoplastic to absent patella, hypoplasia of lateral femoral condyle and small head of fibula (92 per cent).
Elbows. Incomplete extension. Hypoplastic capitellum, small head of radius (90 per cent).
Ilia. Spur in midposterior ilium, 71 per cent palpable (81 per cent).
Scapulae. Hypoplasia, convex thick outer border (44 per cent).
Irides. Dark, "cloverleaf" pigmentation at inner margin (46 per cent).
Renal. Proteinuria with or without hematuria, casts, renal insufficiency (48 per cent).
Other Frequent Features. Absence of distal phalangeal joints. Delayed ossification of secondary centers of ossification. Valgus deformity of femoral neck. Talipes. Madelung deformity.

OCCASIONAL ABNORMALITIES
Skeletal. Prominent outer clavicle, hypoplasia of first ribs, malformed sternum, spina bifida, scoliosis, enlarged ulnar styloid process, clinodactyly of fifth finger, dislocation of head of radius, antecubital pterygium, polyarteritis-like vasculitis.
Eyes. Keratoconus, microcornea, microphakia, cataract, ptosis.
Muscles. Aplasia of pectoralis minor, biceps, triceps, quadriceps.
Central Nervous System. Occasional mental deficiency, psychosis.
Other. Cleft lip/palate. Sensorineural hearing loss.

NATURAL HISTORY. Patients may have problems due to limitation of joint mobility, dislocation, or both, especially at the elbows and knee, where osteoarthritis may eventually limit function. Children should be closely followed for scoliosis. Albuminuria is the most common early indication of a renal problem. Studies show thickening of the glomerular basement membrane and presence of fibrillar, collagen-like material within it and fusion of epithelial foot processes, cause unknown. Renal failure, which develops in approximately 30 per cent of patients with nephropathy, sometimes occurs in teenage years, but is rare prior to the fourth decade. It has been suggested that the 3.9 per cent of affected patients with antecubital pterygia all develop severe renal problems.

ETIOLOGY. Autosomal dominant, always showing some expression. The gene has been mapped to 9q34.1 with close linkage to the gene loci for the ABO blood group.

References

Little, E. M.: Congenital absence or delayed development of the patella. Lancet, 2:781, 1897.

Carbonara, P., and Alpert, M.: Hereditary osteoonychodysplasia (Hood). Am. J. Med. Sci., 248:139, 1964.

Lucas, G. L., and Opitz, J. M.: The nail-patella syndrome. Clinical and genetic aspects of 5 kindreds with 38 affected family members. J. Pediatr., 68:273, 1966.

Darlington, D., and Hawkins, C. F.: Nail-patella syndrome with iliac horns and hereditary nephropathy. Necropsy report and anatomical dissection. J. Bone Joint Surg. [Br.], 49-B:164, 1967.

Beals, R. K., and Eckardt, A. L.: Hereditary onychoosteodysplasia. A report of nine kindreds. J. Bone Joint Surg. [Am.], 51:505, 1969.

Daniel, C. R., Osment, L. S., and Noojin, R. O.: Triangular lunulae. Arch. Dermatol., 116:448, 1980.

Looij, B. J., et al.: Genetic counseling in hereditary osteo-onychodysplasia (HOOD, nail-patella syndrome) with nephropathy. J. Med. Genet., 25:682, 1988.

Rizzo, R., et al.: Familial bilateral pterygia with severe renal involvement in nail-patella syndrome. Clin. Genet., 44:1, 1993.

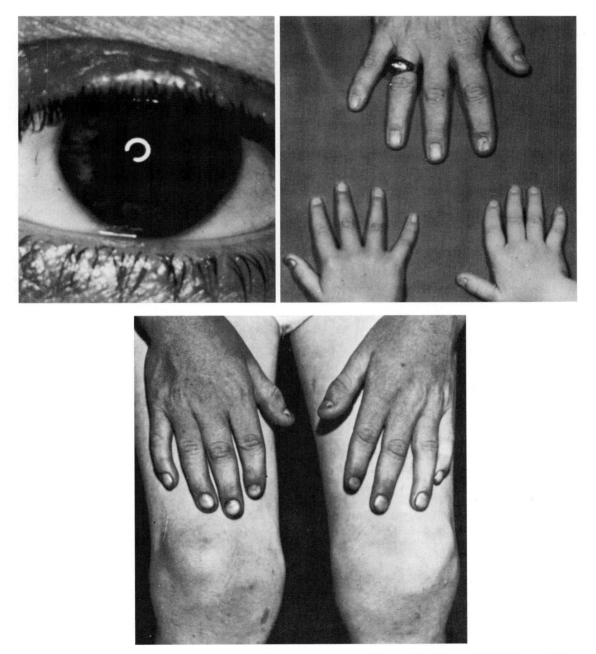

FIGURE 1. Nail-patella syndrome. *Upper left*, Aberrant patterning of inner iris. *Upper right*, Father and two affected offspring showing nail hypoplasia, most striking for the thumbnails. *Below*, Adolescent showing nail hypoplasia, especially of thumbs, and displacement of small patellae. (Bottom photo courtesy of J. Opitz, Helena, Mont.)

LERI-WEILL DYSCHONDROSTEOSIS

*Short Forearms With Madelung
Deformity, With or Without Short Lower Leg*

Leri and Weill described this condition in 1929. Most patients previously categorized as having Madelung deformity have Leri-Weill dyschondrosteosis.

ABNORMALITIES

Growth. Variable small stature, adult height from 135 cm to normal.

Extremities. Short forearm with bowing of radius and distal hypoplasia of the dorsally dislocated ulna leading to a widened gap between radius and ulna, and altered osseous alignment at wrist (Madelung deformity). May have partial dislocation of ulna at wrist, elbow, or both, with limitation of movement. Short lower leg.

OCCASIONAL ABNORMALITIES.

Short hands and feet with metaphyseal flaring in metacarpal and metatarsal bones, short fourth metacarpal and/or metatarsal bones, curvature of tibia, exostoses from proximal tibia and/or fibula, abnormal femoral neck, coxa valga, abnormal tuberosity of humerus.

NATURAL HISTORY.

Associated paramyotonia has been noted in affected individuals in one family; whether this is a frequent feature remains to be determined. Otherwise, the only problems are moderate shortness of stature and limitation of joint mobility at the wrist, elbow, or both.

ETIOLOGY. Autosomal dominant, with an excess of affected females in the recorded cases.

References

Leri, A., and Weill, J.: Une affection congenitale et symétrique du développement osseus: la dyschondrosteose. Bull. Mem. Soc. Med. Hop. (Paris), *45:* 1491, 1929.

Langer, L. O.: Dyschondrosteosis, a hereditary bone dysplasia with characteristic roentgenographic features. Am. J. Roentgenol. Radium Ther. Nucl. Med., *45:*178, 1965.

Herdman, R. C., Langer, L. O., and Good, R. A.: Dyschondrosteosis. The most common cause of Madelung's deformity. J. Pediatr., *68:*432, 1966.

Felman, A. H., and Kirkpatrick, J. A.: Dyschondrosteose. Am. J. Dis. Child., *120:*329, 1970.

Beals, R. K.: Dyschondrosteosis and Madelung's deformity: Report of three kindreds and review of the literature. Clin. Orthoped., *116:*24, 1976.

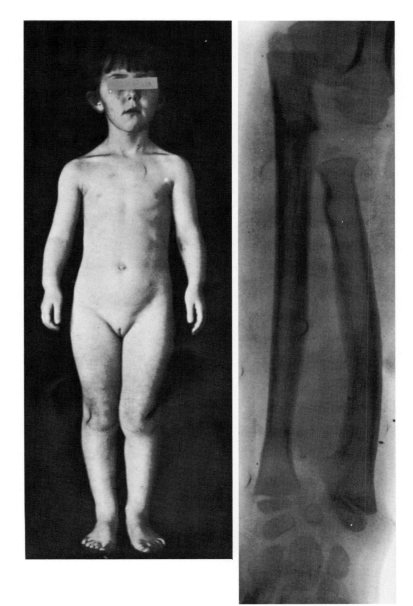

FIGURE 1. Leri-Weill dyschondrosteosis. Age, 7⁵/₁₂
years; height age, 5⁶/₁₂ years.
(From Lamy and Maroteaux:
Les chondrodystrophies géno-
typiques. Paris, L'expansion
Scientifique Française, 1960,
with permission.)

LANGER MESOMELIC DYSPLASIA
(Homozygous Leri-Weill Dyschondrosteosis Syndrome)

Mesomelic Dwarfism, Rudimentary Fibula, Micrognathia

Langer summarized this disorder as a distinctive entity in 1967, citing numerous cases from past literature. The original report was presented by Brailsford.

ABNORMALITIES
Facies. Small mandible.

Limbs. Short, especially forearms and lower legs (mesomelia). The fibula is rudimentary, the tibia is short with proximal hypoplasia, the ulna is reduced distally, and the radius is dorsolaterally bowed and short.

NATURAL HISTORY. One adult male was 130 cm tall. Normal intelligence with surprisingly good function.

ETIOLOGY. The homozygous state of the autosomal dominant gene for Leri-Weill dyschondrosteosis syndrome. Heterozygote individuals with the latter disorder have mild to moderate shortness of stature and relatively short forearms with the Madelung deformity. The homozygous state is associated with a much more severe shortness of stature with striking smallness of the forearms and lower legs (mesomelia) plus the additional feature of micrognathia.

References

Brailsford, J. F.: Dystrophies of the skeleton. Br. J. Radiol., *8*:533, 1935.

Blockey, N. J., and Lawrie, J. H.: An unusual symmetrical distal limb deformity in siblings. J. Bone Joint Surg. [Br.], *45*:745, 1963.

Langer, L. O.: Mesomelic dwarfism of the hypoplastic ulna, fibula, mandible type. Radiology, *89*:654, 1967.

Espiritu, C., Chen, H., and Woolley, P. V., Jr.: Probable homozygosity for the dyschondrosteosis genes. Am. J. Dis Child., *129*:375, 1975.

Kunze, J., and Klemm, T.: Mesomelic dysplasia, type Langer—a homozygous state for dyschondrosteosis. Eur. J. Pediatr., *134*:269, 1980.

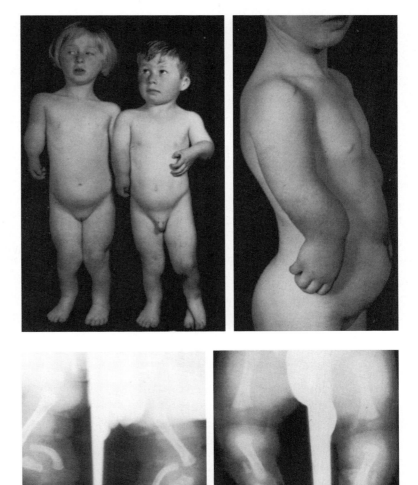

FIGURE 1. Langer mesomelic dysplasia. Siblings with unusual shortness of stature with disproportionate smallness of forearms and lower legs, especially the ulnae and fibulae. (From Blockley, N. J., and Lawrie, J. H.: J. Bone Joint Surg. [Br.], *45*:745, 1963, with permission.)

ACRODYSOSTOSIS

*Short Hands With Peripheral
Dysostosis, Small Nose, Mental Deficiency*

Maroteaux and Malamut first described this disorder in three patients in 1968, and there are now over 40 published cases.

ABNORMALITIES

Growth. Mild to moderate prenatal onset growth deficiency. Short stature (55 per cent).

Performance. Mental deficiency in 77 per cent. Average I.Q. of 61 with a range from 24 to 85. Hearing deficit (67 per cent).

Craniofacial. Brachycephaly, low nasal bridge, broad and small upturned nose (97 per cent), tendency to hold mouth open, hypoplastic maxilla (100 per cent) with prognathism. Increased mandibular angle (68 per cent).

Limbs. Short, especially distally, with progressive deformity in distal humerus, radius, and ulna, and cone-shaped epiphyses that fuse prematurely in hands and feet. Hands appear short and broad, with wrinkling of dorsal skin. Large great toe.

Other. Vertebral defects including loss of normal caudal widening of the lumbar interpedicular distance (75 per cent), small vertebrae that may collapse, spinal canal stenosis, and scoliosis. Advanced bone age. Epiphyseal stippling noted in neonatal period principally involving the lumbosacral and cervical vertebral bodies, the carpus, tarsus, proximal humerus, terminal phalanges, knees, and hips. Stippling regresses by 4 months and is almost always gone by 8 months of age.

OCCASIONAL ABNORMALITIES. Epicanthal

folds (39 per cent), hypertelorism (35 per cent), optic atrophy, dimpled nasal tip, malocclusion of teeth, delayed tooth eruption (23 per cent), hypodontia (3 per cent), calvarial hyperostosis, hydrocephalus, pigmented nevi, hypoplastic genitalia (29 per cent), cryptorchidism (29 per cent), irregular menses (18 per cent), hypogonadism, dislocated radial heads, renal anomalies (3 per cent).

NATURAL HISTORY. Most patients do relatively well except for the problems of mental deficiency and arthritic complaints. Progressive restriction of movement of the hands, elbows, and spine may occur.

ETIOLOGY. Autosomal dominant.

COMMENT. It has been suggested that individuals felt to have this disorder in fact have Albright hereditary osteodystrophy. Complete resolution of this issue awaits further study.

References

Maroteaux, P., and Malamut, G. L.: L'acrodysostose. Presse Med., *76*:2189, 1968.

Robinow, M., et al.: Acrodysostosis. A syndrome of peripheral dysostosis, nasal hypoplasia, and mental retardation. Am. J. Dis. Child., *121*:195, 1971.

Butler, M. G., et al.: Acrodysostosis: report of a 13 year old boy with review of literature and metacarpophalangeal pattern profile analysis. Am. J. Med. Genet., *30*:971, 1988.

Viljoen, D., and Beighton, P.: Epiphyseal stippling in acrodysostosis. Am. J. Med. Genet., *38*:43, 1991.

Steiner, R. D., and Pagon, R. A.: Autosomal dominant transmission of acrodysostosis. Clin. Dysmorphol., *1*:201, 1992.

Davies, S. J., and Hughes, H. E.: Familial acrodysostosis: Can it be distinguished from Albright's hereditary osteodystrophy. Clin. Dysmorphol., *1*:207, 1992.

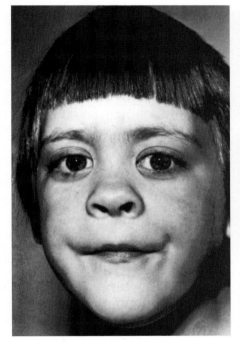

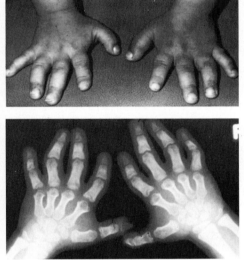

FIGURE 1. Acrodysostosis. A 5-year-old female. Note the low nasal bridge, epicanthal folds, prominent mandible, short, broad fingers with skin wrinkling, and the broad and short metacarpals and phalanges with cone-shaped epiphyses.

ALBRIGHT HEREDITARY OSTEODYSTROPHY

(Pseudohypoparathyroidism,
Pseudopseudohypoparathyroidism)

parathyroid →
↑ Ca absorption

↑♀

Short Metacarpals, Rounded Facies, With or Without Hypocalcemia and/or Vicarious Mineralization

Albright described this condition in 1942 and referred to it as pseudohypoparathyroidism because of hypocalcemia and hyperphosphatemia that were unresponsive to parathormone. Subsequently, patients were detected with a comparable phenotype but with normocalcemia, even in the same family as a patient with hypocalcemia. The term pseudopseudohypoparathyroidism was utilized to designate such instances. Because it is now obvious that hypocalcemia is a variable expression in this heritable disease, the term Albright hereditary osteodystrophy seems preferable. Both phenotypes appear to result from decreased activity of the alpha subunit of the trimeric G_s regulatory protein, the function of which is to couple membrane receptors to adenyl cyclase, an action that stimulates cyclic adenosine monophosphate.

ABNORMALITIES

Growth. Small stature; final height, 54 to 60 inches; occasionally normal. Moderate obesity. Span decreased for height.

Performance. Mental deficiency, I.Q.s of 20 to 99, mean I.Q. of approximately 60; occasionally normal.

Face and Neck. Rounded, low nasal bridge. Short neck. Cataracts.

Dentition. Delayed dental eruption, aplasia, and/or enamel hypoplasia.

Limbs. Short metacarpals and metatarsals, especially the fourth and fifth. Short distal phalanx of thumb. Cone-shaped epiphyses. Osteoporosis.

Extraskeletal Calcification. Areas of mineralization in subcutaneous tissues, basal ganglia.

Calcium and Phosphorus. Variable hypocalcemia and hyperphosphatemia.

OCCASIONAL ABNORMALITIES. Hypothyroidism, hypogonadism with or without gonadal dysgenesis, peripheral lenticular opacities, nystagmus, unequal size of pupils, blurring of disk margins, tortuosity of vessels, diplopia, microphthalmia, optic atrophy, macular degeneration, hypertelorism, thick calvarium, short ulna, short phalanges, genu valgum, fibrous dysplasia, exostosis, osteitis fibrosa cystica, epiphyseal dysplasia, advanced bone age, clavicular abnormalities, cervical vertebral anomalies with associated spinal cord compression, osteochondroma.

NATURAL HISTORY. The shortened metacarpal and/or phalangeal bones represent early epiphyseal fusion and may not be evident until several years of age. Hypocalcemia, when present, usually becomes evident in childhood, seizures being the most common presenting symptom. Hypocalcemia may become manifest during periods of increased calcium utilization, as in adolescence or in pregnancy. Cautious vitamin D therapy in a dosage of 25,000 to 100,000 units/day may be necessary; however, the therapy should be discontinued every few years to reassess the situation, because spontaneous amelioration of the hypocalcemia may occur with time.

ETIOLOGY. Autosomal dominant. A variety of different mutations in the gene encoding the α subunit of the membrane-bound G_s protein (GNAS1) that stimulates adenyl cyclase activity accounts for the cases studied to date. The gene is localized to chromosome 20q13.11. The 2:1 female-to-male sex ratio reported in the literature is currently not explained.

References

Albright, F., et al.: Pseudohypoparathyroidism—an example of "Seabright-bantam syndrome." Report of three cases. Endocrinology, 30:922, 1942.

Christiaen, L., et al.: Le pseudohypoparathyroidisme chronique. A propos de trois cas familiaux. Acta Paediatr. Belg., 21:5, 1967.

Spranger, J. W.: Skeletal dysplasia and the eye: Albright's hereditary osteodystrophy. Birth Defects, 5: 122, 1969.

Poznanski, A. K., Werder, E. A., and Giedion, A.: The patterning of shortening of the bones of the hand in PHP and PPHP. Pediatr. Radiol., 123:707, 1977.

Fitch, N.: Albright's hereditary osteodystrophy: A review. Am. J. Med. Genet., 11:11, 1982.

Levine, M. A., et al.: Genetic deficiency of the α subunit of the guanine nucleotide-binding protein G_s as the molecular basis for Albright hereditary osteodystrophy. Proc. Natl. Acad. Sci. U. S. A., 85:615, 1988.

Patten, J. L., et al.: Mutation in the gene encoding the stimulatory G protein of adenylate cyclase in Albright's hereditary osteodystrophy. N. Engl. J. Med., 322:1412, 1990.

Gejman, P. V., et al.: Genetic mapping of the G$_S$-α subunit gene (GNAS1) to the distal long arm of chromosome 20 using a polymorphism detected by denaturing gradient gel electrophoresis. Genomics, 9: 782, 1991.

Wilson, L. C., and Trembath, R. C.: Albright's hereditary osteodystrophy. J. Med. Genet., 31:779, 1994.

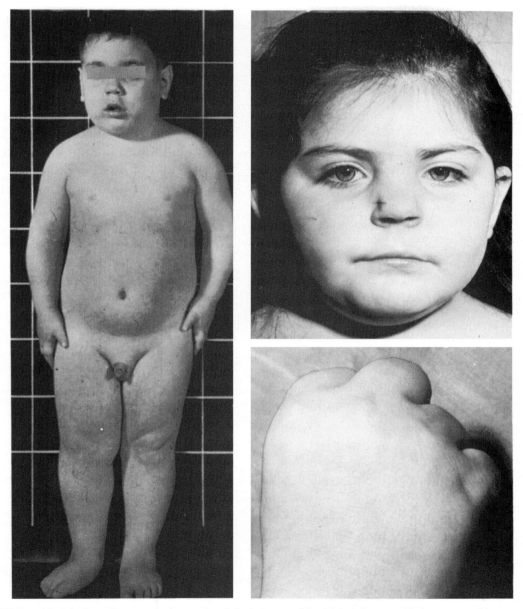

FIGURE 1. Albright hereditary osteodystrophy. *Left*, A 5-year-old with height age of 3⁶/₁₂ years and bone age of 5 years. Hypocalcemia and hyperphosphatemia were first detected at 1 year of age. *Right*, Moderately retarded girl showing rounded facies and indications of short fourth and fifth metacarpal bones in fisted hand.

WEILL-MARCHESANI SYNDROME

(Brachydactyly-Spherophakia Syndrome)

*Brachydactyly, Small
Spherical Lens, Short Stature*

More than 18 instances of this condition have been described since the initial recognition by Weill in 1932 and the broader description by Marchesani in 1939.

ABNORMALITIES

Growth. Small stature.

Craniofacial. Broad skull, small shallow orbits, mild maxillary hypoplasia with narrow palate.

Eyes. Small spherical lens, shallow anterior chamber, myopia with or without glaucoma, ectopia lentis in half of cases, blindness in one third.

Teeth. Malformed and malaligned.

Limbs. Brachydactyly with broad metacarpals and phalanges, with or without late ossification of epiphyses. Stiff joints, particularly of hands.

OCCASIONAL ABNORMALITY. Cardiac anomaly.

NATURAL HISTORY. The mean age of recognition of an ocular problem in this disorder is 7.5 years, the youngest recorded age being 9 months. Dilatation of the pupil is often necessary to appreciate the lens defect. Intelligence is usually not affected. There is the occasional development of carpal tunnel nerve compression at adolescence or later. Since glaucoma can be induced in affected individuals by provoking miosis, miotics are contraindicated.

ETIOLOGY. Autosomal recessive inheritance with partial expression in the heterozygote, manifested by short stature. Gorlin et al. reported a family in which a father and two of his three children were affected, suggesting genetic heterogeneity or the possibility of pseudodominance.*

References

Weill, G.: Ectopie du cristallin et malformations générales. Ann. Ocul. (Paris), *169:*21, 1932.

Marchesani, O.: Brachydaktylie und angeborene Kugellinse als Systemerkrankung. Klin. Monatsbl. Augenheilkd., *103:*392, 1939.

Zabriskie, J., and Reisman, M.: Marchesani syndrome. J. Pediatr., *52:*158, 1958.

Feinberg, S. B.: Congenital mesodermal dysmorphodystrophy (brachymorphic type). Radiology, *74:*218, 1960.

Gorlin, R. J., L'Heureux, P. R., and Shapiro, I.: Weill-Marchesani syndrome in two generations: Genetic heterogeneity or pseudodominance. J. Pediatr. Ophthalmol., *11:*139, 1974.

Wright, K. W., and Chrousos, G. A.: Weill-Marchesani syndrome with bilateral angle-closure glaucoma. J. Pediatr. Ophthalmol. Strabismus, *22:*129, 1985.

---

*Transmission of a recessive gene from parent to child due to the mating of a homozygous affected individual with a heterozygote for the same disorder or with an individual who is deleted at the gene locus on one homologue.

FIGURE 1. Weill-Marchesani syndrome. A 9-year-old with height age of 5⁶/₁₂ years. Small lens and myopia. (From Zabriskie, J., and Reisman, M.: J. Pediatr., 52:158, 1958, with permission.)

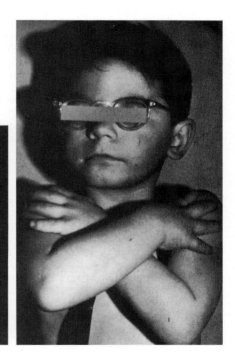

N

N. STORAGE DISORDERS

GENERALIZED GANGLIOSIDOSIS SYNDROME, TYPE I (SEVERE INFANTILE TYPE)

(Caffey Pseudo-Hurler Syndrome,
Familial Neurovisceral Lipidosis)

Coarse Facies, Joint Limitation, Kyphosis in Early Infancy

In 1951, Caffey described two neonates who had many of the features of Hurler syndrome, but of prenatal onset. Landing et al. reported pathologic studies in similar cases showing foamy histiocytes in the liver and spleen, swollen neurons, and vacuoles in the glomerular epithelium. They interpreted the storage material as a glycolipid and set forth the name "familial neurovisceral lipidosis," which was changed to "generalized gangliosidosis" by Okada and O'Brien on the basis of finding elevated levels of ganglioside GM_1 in the liver, spleen, and brain tissue from a patient. The molecular defect has been shown to be a deficiency of ganglioside GM_1 β-galactosidase.

ABNORMALITIES

Growth. Deficiency, with relatively low birth weight and severe postnatal growth deficit.

Performance. Severe early defect in developmental performance with hypotonia, poor coordination, and later, spasticity.

Orofacial. Coarse features with low nasal bridge, broad nose, flaring alae nasi, frontal bossing, long philtrum, hypertrophied alveolar ridges with prominent maxilla and mild macroglossia. Hirsutism.

Eyes. Cherry-red macular spot in about one half of the patients.

Skeletal. Moderate joint limitation with thick wrists, contractures at the elbows and knees, and development of clawhand. Early roentgenograms show poorly mineralized, coarsely trabeculated long bones with medullary midshaft broadening and a "cloak" of subperiosteal new bone formation, especially evident in the humerus. Some metaphyseal cupping and epiphyseal irregularity are usually present. With time, the bones appear more like those of the Hurler syndrome, including kyphosis with anterior bullet wedging of vertebrae. Ribs are thick, legs may be bowed, and talipes may be present. Short broad hands. Kyphoscoliosis.

Viscera. Variable hepatosplenomegaly with some foamy histiocytes. Vacuolation in glomerular epithelial cells containing swollen lysosomes.

Leukocytes. Vacuolation within cytoplasm of leukocytes and foam cells in marrow.

Urinary Excretion. Mucopolysaccharides occasionally may be increased with the excretion of keratan sulfate–like materials.

Other. Facial and peripheral edema in early infancy. Inguinal hernia. Angiokeratoma corporis diffusum (telangiectases or warty growths, in groups, together with thickening of the epidermis).

NATURAL HISTORY. Severe developmental lag with hypotonia, feeding problems with failure to thrive, and frequent infections usually culminate in death during early infancy. Deterioration of cerebral function is rapid if the patient survives the first year, leading to a decerebrate status with seizures and death prior to 2 years of age. The mean age of survival for 17 patients was 13.5 months, with a range from 3.5 to 25 months. No form of therapy other than life-supportive tube feeding and antibiotic management of infections has been effective. Considering the natural history of this disorder, the author favors discussion with the parents followed by the withholding of life-supportive medical treatment, if this course of management is acceptable to the parents.

ETIOLOGY. Autosomal recessive. The human β-galactosidase gene has been assigned to chromosome 3p21.33. Okada and O'Brien detected a deficit (one twentieth of normal) of the lysosomal enzyme β-galactosidase in the liver from these patients. The presumed developmental pathology of the disease is as follows: (1) inability to cleave the terminal galactose from ganglioside and mucopolysaccharide, (2) accumulation of these products within lysosomes where they would normally be degraded, and (3) the storage disease.

The diagnosis can be confirmed by the assay of β-galactosidase in the peripheral leukocytes or in cultured skin fibroblasts. Prenatal diagnosis has been established on the basis of cultured amniotic fluid cells.

COMMENT. In patients with GM, gangliosidosis, and Morquio syndrome, type B, there is a deficiency of β-galactosidase. Different mutations in the β-GAL gene result in both disorders.

References

Caffey, J.: Gargoylism (Hunter-Hurler disease, dysostosis multiplex, lipochondrodystrophy); prenatal and neonatal bone lesions and their early postnatal evolution. Bull. Hosp. Joint Dis., *12*: 38, 1951.

Landing, B. H., et al.: Familial neurovisceral lipidosis. An analysis of eight cases of a syndrome previously reported as "Hurler-variant," "Pseudo-Hurler disease," and "Tay-Sachs disease with visceral involvement." Am. J. Dis. Child., *108*:503, 1964.

Okada, S., and O'Brien, J. S.: Generalized gangliosidosis: Beta-galactosidase deficiency. Science, *160*: 1002, 1968.

Kaback, M. M., et al.: Gangliosidosis type I: In-utero detection and fetal manifestations. J. Pediatr., *82*: 1037, 1973.

Takano, T., and Yamanouchi, Y.: Assignment of human β-galactosidase-A gene to 3p21.33 by fluorescence in situ hybridization. Hum. Genet., *92*:403, 1993.

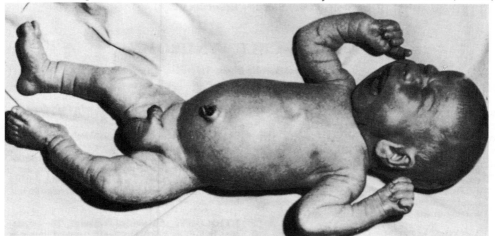

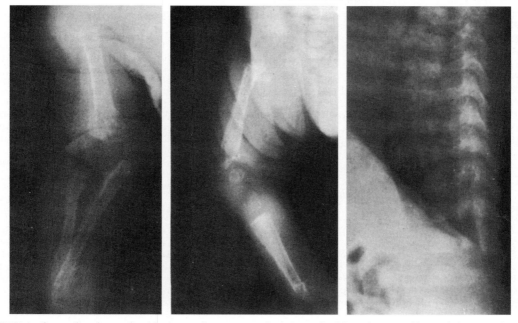

FIGURE 1. Generalized gangliosidosis syndrome, type I. A 2-week-old with x-ray films of the arm, leg, and thoracolumbar vertebrae. Note the coarse facies, hypertrophied alveolar ridges, broad wrists, periosteal cloaking with thin cortices, altered shape of head of humerus and femur, and hypoplastic vertebrae. (From Scott, C. R., et al.: J. Pediatr., *71*:357, 1967, with permission.)

LEROY I-CELL SYNDROME

(Mucolipidosis II)

Early Alveolar Ridge Hypertrophy, Joint Limitation, Thick Tight Skin in Early Infancy

This disorder was recognized by Leroy and DeMars when they noted unusual cytoplasmic inclusions in the cultured fibroblasts of a girl who had been considered to have the Hurler syndrome despite the fact that she did not have cloudy corneas or excessive acid mucopolysaccharide in the urine.

ABNORMALITIES

Growth. Birth weight less than $5\frac{1}{2}$ pounds. Marked growth deficiency with lack of linear growth after infancy.

Performance. Slow progress from early infancy, reaching a plateau at approximately 18 months with no apparent deterioration subsequently.

Craniofacial. High, narrow forehead. Thin eyebrows, puffy eyelids, inner epicanthal folds, clear or faintly hazy corneas. Low nasal bridge, anteverted nostrils. Long philtrum.

Mouth. Progressive hypertrophy of alveolar ridges.

Skeletal and Joints. Moderate joint limitation in flexion, especially of hips. Dorsolumbar kyphosis. Broadening of wrists and fingers. Roentgenographic findings in the later phases similar to those seen in children with the Hurler syndrome. In early infancy, periosteal new bone formation leading to a "cloaking" of the long tubular bones is best seen in femora and humeri.

Skin. Thick, relatively tight skin during early infancy that becomes less tight as the patients become older. Cavernous hemangiomata.

Other. Minimal hepatomegaly. Diastasis recti. Inguinal hernia (one case). Systolic murmurs after 1 year of age.

Note. No metachromatic granules noted in leukocytes. Urinary mucopolysaccharides normal to mildly increased.

NATURAL HISTORY. By 18 months of age, most patients can sit with support, and some stand with support. However, severe progressive retardation of growth and development occur. Recurrent bouts of bronchitis, pneumonia, and otitis media have been frequent during early childhood. Death, which usually occurs by 5 years of age, is often associated with congestive heart failure.

ETIOLOGY. Autosomal recessive. The consistent finding is a deficiency of lysosomal enzymes within cultured skin fibroblasts and an increase in lysosomal enzymes in plasma, cerebrospinal fluid, and urine. This defective processing of lysosomal enzymes is the result of a deficiency of phospho-N-acetylglucosamine transferase seen in this disorder as well as in pseudo-Hurler polydystrophy (mucolipidosis III). A marked increase in serum activity of beta-hexosaminidase, iduronate sulfatase, and arylsulfatase A is seen in both disorders.

Heterozygotes cannot be detected. Prenatal diagnosis can be established on the basis of cultured amniotic fluid cells.

References

Leroy, J. G., and DeMars, R. I.: Mutant enzymatic and cytological phenotypes in cultured human fibroblasts. Science, *157*:804, 1967.

Matalon, R., et al.: Lipid abnormalities in a variant of the Hurler syndrome. Proc. Natl. Acad. Sci. U. S. A., *59*:1097, 1968.

Leroy, J. G., DeMars, R. I., and Opitz, J. M.: "I-cell" disease. *In* Bergsma, D. S. (ed.): The First Conference on the Clinical Delineation of Birth Defects, Part IV. Baltimore, Williams & Wilkins, 1969.

Leroy, J. G, et al.: I-cell disease, a clinical picture. J. Pediatr., *79*:360, 1971.

Hickman, S., and Neufeld, E. F.: A hypothesis for I-cell disease: Defective hydrolases that do not enter lysosomes. Biochem. Biophys. Res. Commun., *49*:992, 1972.

Kaplan, A., Achord, D. T., and Sly, W. S.: Phosphohexosyl components of a lysosomal enzyme are recognized by pinocytosis receptors on human fibroblasts. Proc. Natl. Acad. Sci. U. S. A., *74*:2026, 1977.

Neufeld, E. F.: Lysosomal storage diseases. Ann. Rev. Biochem. *60*:257, 1991.

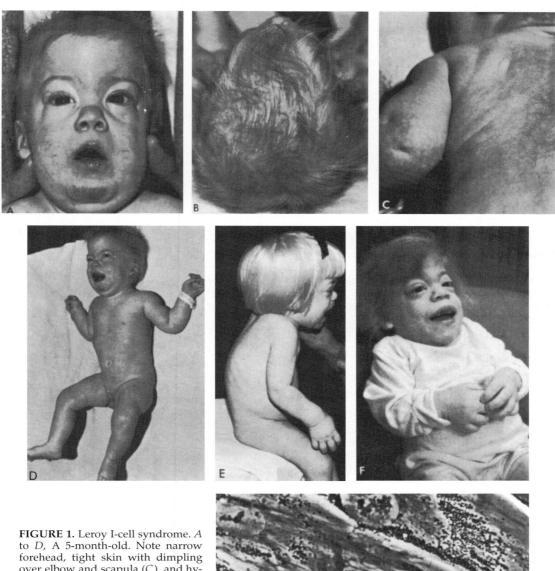

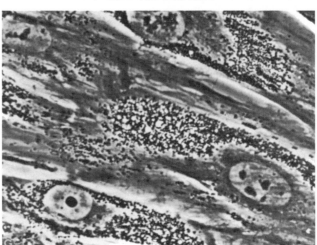

FIGURE 1. Leroy I-cell syndrome. *A to D*, A 5-month-old. Note narrow forehead, tight skin with dimpling over elbow and scapula (*C*), and hypertrophy of alveolar ridge (*D*). *E*, Same patient at 2⁶/₁₂ years; height age, 14 months. *F*, Same patient at 6 years; height age, 14 months. *G*, Phase contrast photo of cultured fibroblasts, showing cytoplasmic inclusions. Magnification about 700 ×. (*G* from Leroy, J. G., and DeMars, R. I.: Science, *157*:804, 1967, with permission. Copyright 1967 American Association for the Advancement of Science.)

PSEUDO-HURLER POLYDYSTROPHY SYNDROME

(Mucolipidosis III)

*Coarse Facies, Stiff Joints by
2 to 4 Years, No Mucopolysacchariduria*

This disorder was recognized by Maroteaux and Lamy in 1966. Clinically, the disorder is of milder degree than the Hurler syndrome and is similar to the Scheie syndrome, but the patients do not have hepatosplenomegaly, cloudy corneas, or mucopolysacchariduria.

ABNORMALITIES. Onset usually appreciated at 4 to 5 years.
Growth. Decreasing growth rate in early childhood.
Performance. Mild mental deficiency, I.Q.s of 64 to 85.
Facies. Development of mildly coarse facies by 6 years.
Eyes. Mild corneal opacities, evident by slit lamp, by 6 to 8 years.
Joints. Stiffness, especially in hands, elbows, shoulders, and knees.
Skeletal. Mild platyspondyly, flaring iliac wings, flattening of femoral epiphyses, changes in hands.
Cardiac. Aortic valve disease, often with regurgitation.
Other. Inguinal hernia. Acne.

NATURAL HISTORY. Stiffness of joints usually becomes evident by 4 to 5 years of age. Carpal tunnel compression is a potential complication. Mild to moderate deterioration of central nervous system function. Some patients have lived into their 20s.

ETIOLOGY. Autosomal recessive inheritance. Marrow plasma cells show vacuolated plasma cells with swollen lysosomes, but there is no mucopolysacchariduria. Lysosomal enzymes are elevated in the serum and decreased in cultured fibroblasts. The disorder is considered similar to I-cell disease, but is of a milder nature. As with mucolipidosis II, there is a marked increase in serum beta-hexosaminidase, iduronate sulfatase, and arylsulfatase A and a deficiency of phospho-N-acetylglucosamine transferase. These two disorders are best differentiated by their clinical courses.

References

Maroteaux, P., and Lamy, M.: La pseudopolydystrophie de Hurler. Presse Med., 74:2889, 1966.

Scott, C. I., Jr., and Grossman, M. S.: Pseudo-Hurler polydystrophy. Birth Defects, 4(5):349, 1969.

McKusick, V. A.: Heritable Disorders of Connective Tissue, 4th ed. St. Louis, C. V. Mosby Co., 1972, p. 652.

Melhem, R., et al.: Roentgen findings in mucolipidosis III (pseudo-Hurler polydystrophy). Radiology, 106: 153, 1973.

Thomas, G. H., et al.: Mucolipidosis III (pseudo-Hurler polydystrophy): Multiple lysosomal enzyme abnormalities in serum and cultured fibroblast cells. Pediatr. Res., 7:751, 1973.

Lang, L., et al.: Lysosomal enzyme phosphorylation in human fibroblasts: Kinetic parameters offer a biochemical rationale for two distinct defects in the uridine diphospho-N-acetylglucosamine: Lysosomal enzymic precursor N-acetylglucosamine-1-phosphotransferase. J. Clin. Invest., 76:2191, 1985.

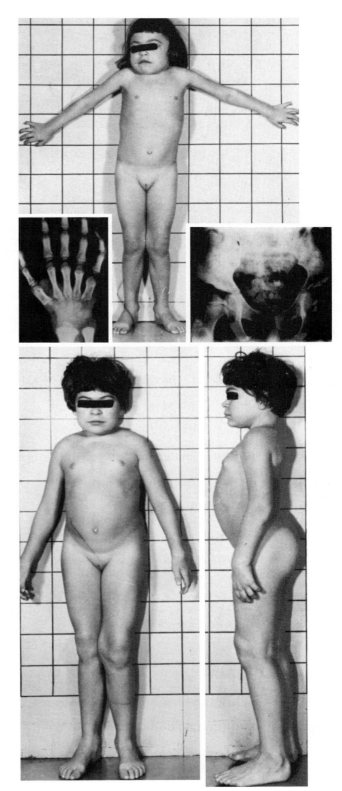

FIGURE 1. Pseudo-Hurler polydystrophy syndrome. *Above,* A 6-year-old girl with roentgenograms of hand and pelvis. *Below,* Early adolescent girl showing mild facial coarsening, joint contractures, and lumbar lordosis. (From Scott, C. I., Jr., and Grossman, M. S.: Birth Defects, 4:349, 1969, with permission.)

HURLER SYNDROME

(Mucopolysaccharidosis I H, MPS 1 H)

Coarse Facies, Stiff Joints, Mental Deficiency, Cloudy Corneas by 1 to 2 Years

Hurler set forth this entity in 1919, 2 years after the Hunter syndrome was described.

ABNORMALITIES
Growth. Deceleration of growth between 6 and 18 months; maximal stature, 110 cm.

Performance. Grossly retarded progress at 6 to 12 months, with failure of advancement by 2 to 5 years.

Craniofacial and Eyes. Scaphocephalic macrocephaly with frontal prominence, coarse facies with full lips, flared nostrils, low nasal bridge, and tendency toward hypertelorism. Inner epicanthal folds. Hazy corneas, retinal pigmentation.

Mouth. Hypertrophied alveolar ridge and gums with small malaligned teeth. Enlarged tongue.

Skeletal and Joints. Diaphyseal broadening of short misshapen bones and joint limitation result in the clawhand and other joint deformities, with more limitation of extension than flexion. Flaring of the rib cage. Kyphosis and thoracolumbar gibbus secondary to anterior vertebral wedging, short neck. Odontoid hypoplasia. J-shaped sella turcica. Widening of medial end of clavicle.

Cardiac. Murmurs; cardiac failure may be due to intimal thickening in the coronary vessels or the cardiac valves.

Other. Hirsutism, hepatosplenomegaly, inguinal hernia, umbilical hernia, dislocation of hip, mucoid rhinitis, deafness.

Urinary Excretion. Dermatan sulfate and heparan sulfate.

OCCASIONAL ABNORMALITIES.
Communicating hydrocephalus, presumably a result of thickened meninges. Arachnoid cysts. Retinal dysfunction. Open-angle glaucoma. Cardiomyopathy. Hydrocele. Nephrotic syndrome. Carpal tunnel syndrome. Hypoplasia of mandibular condyles.

NATURAL HISTORY.
Growth during the first year actually may be more rapid than usual, with subsequent deterioration. Subtle changes in the facies, macrocephaly, hernias, limited hip motility, noisy breathing, and frequent respiratory tract infections may be evident during the first 6 months.

Upper airway obstruction secondary to thickening of the epiglottis and tonsillar and adenoidal tissues as well as tracheal narrowing due to mucopolysaccharide accumulation can lead to sleep apnea and serious airway compromise. Because of the upper airway problems as well as odontoid hypoplasia with or without C1–C2 subluxation, anesthesia is a significant risk. Deceleration of developmental and mental progress is evident during the latter half of the first year. Hearing loss is almost always present. These patients are usually placid, easily manageable, and often lovable. Hypertension frequently occurs and is either centrally mediated or secondary to aortic coarctation. Death usually occurs in childhood secondary to respiratory tract or cardiac complications, and survival past 10 years of age is unusual.

ETIOLOGY.
Autosomal recessive. The primary defect is an absence of the lysosomal hydrolase α-L-iduronidase (IDUA) which is responsible for the degradation of the glycosaminoglycans, heparan sulfate and dermatan sulfate. The pathologic consequence is an accumulation of mucopolysaccharides in parenchymal and mesenchymal tissues and the storage of lipids within neuronal tissues. The IDUA gene has been mapped to chromosome 4p16.3. Diagnosis is confirmed by the physical appearance, the excretion of dermatan sulfate and heparan sulfate in the urine, and the absence of α-L-iduronidase in cultured fibroblasts. Heterozygote detection is available. Prenatal diagnosis is possible by measuring α-L-iduronidase in cultured amniotic fluid cells.

References

Hurler, G.: Ueber einen Typ multipler Abartungen, vorwiegend am Skelettsystem. Z. Kinderheilkd., *24*:220, 1919.

Leroy, J. G., and Crocker, A. C.: Clinical definition of the Hurler-Hunter phenotypes. A review of 50 patients. Am. J. Dis. Child., *112*:518, 1966.

Matalon, R., and Dorfman, A.: Hurler's syndrome, and α-L-iduronidase deficiency. Biochem. Biophys. Res. Commun., *47*:959, 1972.

Muenzer, J.: Mucopolysaccharidoses. Adv. Pediatr., *33*:269, 1989.

Adachi, K., and Chole, R. A.: Management of tracheal lesions in Hurler syndrome. Arch. Otolaryngol. Head Neck Surg., *116*:1205, 1990.

Scott, H. S., et al.: Chromosomal localization of the human α-L-Iduronidase gene (IDUA) to 4p16.3 Am. J. Hum. Genet., *47*:802, 1990.

Belani, K. G., et al.: Children with mucopolysaccharidosis: Perioperative care, morbidity, mortality and new findings. J. Pediatr. Surg., *28*:403, 1993.

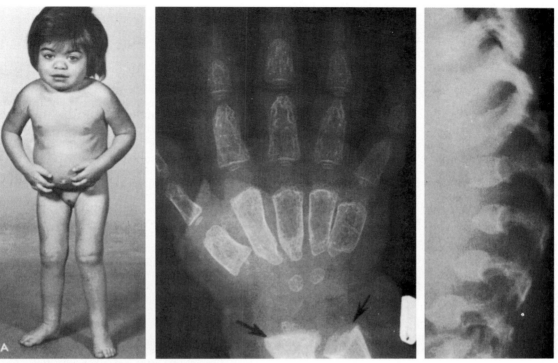

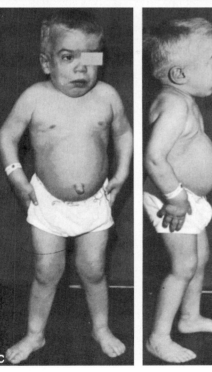

FIGURE 1. Hurler syndrome. *A*, A 2-year-old who sat at 1 year and walked at 21 months. Height age at 6 months was 10 months; at 1 year, 16 months; and at 2 years, 2 years. *B*, Broad, irregular bone, especially at metaphyses. Thoracic and lumbar vertebrae are short with anterior wedging. *C*, A 5-year-old with height age of 3 years.

SCHEIE SYNDROME

(Mucopolysaccharidosis I S, MPS I S)

Broad Mouth With Full Lips,
Early Corneal Opacity, Normal Mentality

This disorder was originally described by Scheie et al. in 1962.

ABNORMALITIES

General. Little, if any, impairment of intelligence.

Facies. Broad mouth with full lips by 5 to 8 years of age. Mandibular prognathism.

Corneas. Uniform clouding of cornea in early stage, becoming most dense in periphery.

Limbs. Joint limitation leading to clawhand, small carpal bones, femoral head dysplasia. Broad and short hands and feet.

Cardiac. Aortic valvular defect.

Other. Body hirsutism. Retinal pigmentation. Inguinal and umbilical hernias. Short neck.

Urinary Excretion. Proportionately more dermatan sulfate than usual.

OCCASIONAL ABNORMALITIES. Edema-like swelling of optic disk and macula. Carpal tunnel narrowing may cause median nerve compression. Psychosis and possible mental deterioration may occur. Mild impairment of growth. Hearing loss. Hepatomegaly. Macroglossia. Glaucoma, myopia. Sleep apnea. Progressive juxta-articular cystic lesions in hands and feet.

NATURAL HISTORY. Onset of symptoms usually occurs after 5 years of age. Diagnosis made in most cases between 10 and 20 years. Cardiac evaluation is suggested at regular intervals because of the increased incidence of aortic valvular disease. Visual impairment is the most significant handicap. Life span is relatively normal.

ETIOLOGY. Autosomal recessive, with excess urinary excretion of dermatan sulfate and absence of α-L-iduronidase in cultured fibroblasts. The α-L-iduronidase gene, different mutations of which lead to Hurler syndrome, Scheie syndrome, and Hurler-Scheie syndrome, is located at chromosome 4p16.3. Differentiation between these three disorders by biochemical measurements is difficult.

References

Scheie, H. G., Hambrick, G. W., Jr., and Barness, L. A.: A newly recognized forme fruste of Hurler's disease (gargoylism). Am. J. Ophthalmol., *53*:753, 1962.

Emerit, I., Maroteaux, P., and Vernant, P.: Deux observations de mucopolysaccharidose avec atteinte cardiovasculaire. Arch. Fr. Pediatr., 23:1075, 1966.

Scott, H. S., et al.: Identification of mutations in the α-L-iduronidase gene (IDUA) that cause Hurler and Scheie syndromes. Am. J. Hum. Genet., *53*:973, 1993.

Summers, C. G., et al.: Dense peripheral corneal clouding in Scheie syndrome. Cornea, *13*:277, 1994.

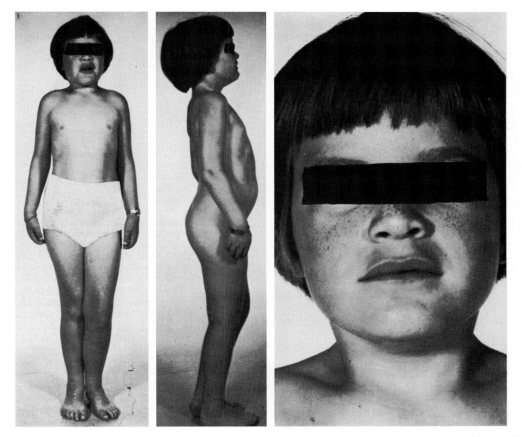

FIGURE 1. Scheie syndrome. Child, 9 9/12 years old, with height age of 9 years and I.Q. of 102. Mild to moderate limitation of shoulder, elbow, and hand movement. Mild corneal opacity. (Courtesy of R. Scott, University of Washington, Seattle, Wash.)

HURLER-SCHEIE SYNDROME

(Mucopolysaccharidosis I H/S, MPS I H/S)

Stevenson et al. set forth this disorder in 1976 and suggested that it represented a genetic compound of the Hurler syndrome and the Scheie syndrome. However, the birth of children with this disorder to consanguineous parents indicates that, like MPS I S and MPS I H some patients with MPS I H/S represent a different mutation of the α-L-iduronidase (IDUA) gene. The clinical phenotype is intermediate between the severe MPS I H and the mild MPS I S.

ABNORMALITIES

Performance. Mild mental deficiency to normal.

Growth. During the first year, growth may be accelerated; thereafter, it decelerates to growth deficiency.

Craniofacial. Development of scaphocephaly with macrocephaly, low nasal bridge, prominent lips, corneal clouding. Micrognathia.

Skin. Thickened, with fine hirsutism.

Skeletal. Moderate joint limitation. Mild to moderate dysostosis multiplex changes with broadening of bones but without gibbus.

Other. Chronic rhinorrhea, middle ear fluid, inguinal hernia with or without umbilical hernia, hepatosplenomegaly, with or without cardiac valvular changes. Deafness. Arachnoid cyst.

NATURAL HISTORY. The progression is intermediate between that of Hurler syndrome and that of Scheie syndrome. Onset of symptoms usually between 3 and 8 years with survival into the 20s common. Onset of corneal clouding, joint limitations, cardiac valvular abnormalities, and hearing impairment frequently develop by the early to mid teens. Anesthesia can be associated with significant complications.

ETIOLOGY. Autosomal recessive, with excess urinary excretion of dermatan sulfate and heparan sulfate and a deficiency of α-L-iduronidase (IDUA) in cultured fibroblasts. Different mutations in the IDUA gene located at chromosome 4p16.3 lead to MPSI H/S as well as MPS I H and MPS I S.

References

Stevenson, R. E., et al.: The iduronidase-deficient mucopolysaccharidoses; clinical and roentgenographic features. Pediatrics, 57:111, 1976.

Roubicek, M., et al.: The clinical spectrum of α-L-iduronidase deficiency. Am. J. Med. Genet., 20:471, 1985.

Schmidt, H., et al.: Radiological findings in patients with mucopolysaccharidosis I H/S (Hurler-Scheie syndrome). Pediatr. Radiol., 17:409, 1987.

Nicholson, S. C., et al.: Management of a difficult airway in a patient with Hurler-Scheie syndrome during cardiac surgery. Anesth. Analg., 75:830, 1992.

Scott, H. S., et al.: Identification of mutations in the α-L-iduronidase gene (IDUA) that cause Hurler and Scheie syndromes. Am. J. Hum. Genet., 53:973, 1993.

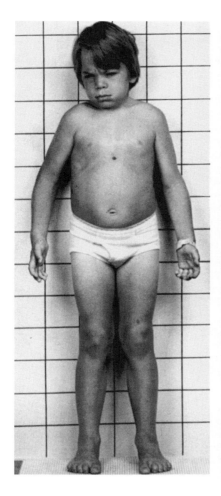

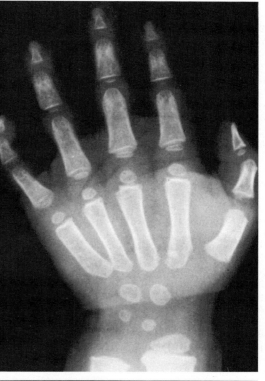

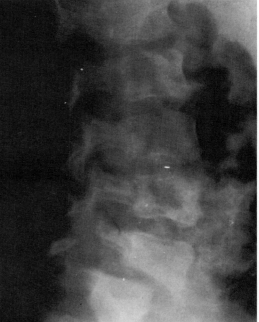

FIGURE 1. Hurler-Scheie syndrome. *Left*, Young boy showing mildly altered facies and joint limitations that are most evident at elbow and in the fingers. *Right*, Subtle dysostosis multiplex type of changes in hand and in lumbar spine. (From Stevenson, R. E., et al.: Pediatrics, *57*:111, 1976, with permission.)

HUNTER SYNDROME

(Mucopolysaccharidosis II)

*Coarse Facies, Growth Deficiency,
Stiff Joints by 2 to 4 Years, Clear Corneas*

Hunter described this condition found in two brothers in 1917. A mild and severe type have been delineated, based on the age of onset, degree of central nervous system involvement, and rapidity of deterioration. Both types have the same deficiency of iduronate sulfatase. The severe type is outlined below.

ABNORMALITIES. Onset at about 2 to 4 years.
Growth. Deficiency, onset at 1 to 4 years. Adult height, 120 to 150 cm.
Performance. Juvenile type: Mental and neurologic deterioration at approximately 2 to 5 years of age to the point of severe mental deficiency with aggressive hyperactive behavior and spasticity.
Craniofacial. Coarsening of facial features, full lips. Macrocephaly. Macroglossia.
Joints and Skeletal. Stiff partial contracture of joints, clawhand. Broadening of bones.
Other. Hepatosplenomegaly, hypertrichosis, inguinal hernias, mucoid nasal discharge, progressive deafness. Delayed tooth eruption. Dentigerous cysts. Hoarse voice.

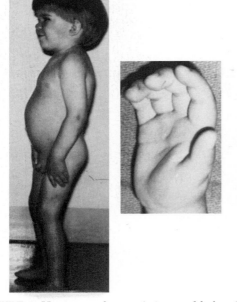

FIGURE 1. Hunter syndrome. A 4-year-old showing evidence of tight joints, especially fingers. Presumably the "mild type," as his intelligence seemed within normal limits at 4 years of age.

Urinary Excretion. Dermatan sulfate and heparan sulfate.

OCCASIONAL ABNORMALITIES. Diarrhea, nodular skin lesions over scapular area and on arms, kyphosis, pes cavus, osteoarthritis of head of femur, retinal pigmentation, chronic disk edema, ptosis, congestive heart failure, coronary occlusion. Hydrocephalus. Airway obstruction. Seizures. Neurogenic bladder secondary to a narrow cervical spinal canal with myelopathy.

IMPORTANT DIFFERENCES IN CONTRAST WITH THE HURLER SYNDROME. (1) Clear corneas, (2) less severe gibbus, (3) no affected females, and (4) more gradual onset of features.

NATURAL HISTORY. Gradual decline in growth rate from 2 to 6 years. Deafness frequently is evident by 2 to 3 years. Severe neurologic complications develop in the late stages. Cardiac complications resulting from valvular, myocardial, and ischemic factors as well as airway obstruction caused by macroglossia, a deformed pharynx, a short thick neck, and gradual deformation and collapse of the trachea not uncommonly lead to death prior to 15 years.

COMMENT. The mild type has been associated with maintenance of intelligence into adult life. Survival into the fifth and sixth decades is not unusual. Adult hearing loss is frequent. Carpal tunnel syndrome and joint contractures are common. Somatic involvement occurs in patients with the mild type but the rate of progression is much less rapid.

ETIOLOGY. The primary defect is a deficiency of iduronate sulfatase, which can be measured in peripheral white blood cells. Excess dermatan sulfate and heparan sulfate are found in urine. The gene for Hunter syndrome has been mapped to Xq27-q28. The broad variability of expression, which includes the severe and mild types, is due to different mutations in the same gene. Carrier females may be determined by assaying for iduronate sulfatase in peripheral white blood cells. However, results have been ambiguous in approximately 15 per cent of obligate carriers.

References

Hunter, C.: A rare disease in two brothers. Proc. R. Soc. Med., *10*:104, 1917.

Leroy, J. G., and Crocker, A. C.: Clinical definition of the Hurler-Hunter phenotypes. A review of 50 patients. Am. J. Dis. Child., *112*:518, 1966.

Upadhyaya, M., et al.: Localization of the gene for Hunter syndrome on the long arm of X chromosome. Hum. Genet., *74*:391, 1986.

Muenzer, J.: Mucopolysaccharidoses. Adv. Pediatr., *33*: 269, 1986.

Sasaki, C. T.: Hunter's syndrome: A study in airway obstruction. Laryngoscope, *97*:280, 1987.

Wilson, P. J.: Frequent deletions at Xq28 indicate genetic heterogeneity in Hunter syndrome. Hum. Genet., *86*:505, 1991.

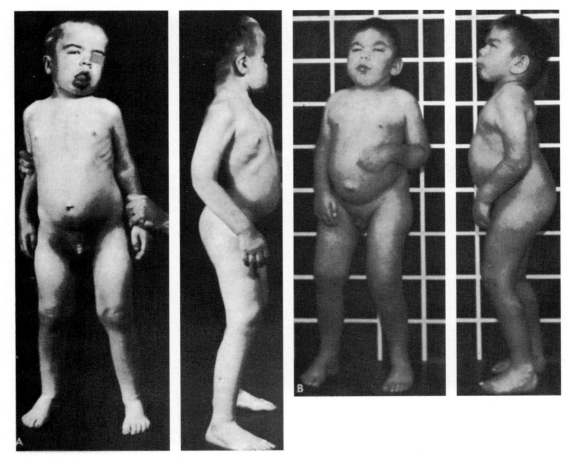

FIGURE 2. Hunter syndrome. *A*, A 9⁶/₁₂-year-old with height age of 7⁸/₁₂ years. (Courtesy of A. C. Crocker, Boston Children's Hospital, Boston, Mass.) *B*, A 13⁶/₁₂-year-old with height age of 7 years.

SANFILIPPO SYNDROME

(Mucopolysaccharidosis III, Types A, B, C, and D)

Mild Coarse Facies, Mild Stiff Joints, Mental Deficiency

This clinical disorder was recognized by Sanfilippo et al. in 1963 and appears to be the most common mucopolysaccharidosis disorder. The excess urinary excretion of mucopolysaccharide is heparan sulfate alone. These individuals usually have clear corneas.

ABNORMALITIES. Onset in early childhood.

Growth. Normal to accelerated growth for 1 to 3 years, followed by slow growth.

Performance. Slowing mental development by $1^{6}/_{12}$ to 3 years, followed by deterioration, including gait, speech, and behavior. Hyperactivity.

Craniofacies. Dense calvarium. Mildly coarse facies with synophrys.

Other. Variable hepatosplenomegaly. Obliteration of pulp chambers of teeth by irregular secondary dentin. Ovoid dysplasia of vertebrae. Mild cardiac involvement.

NATURAL HISTORY. Sleep disturbances and frequent upper respiratory tract infections may be early evidence of the disorder prior to the slowing of growth and mental deterioration. Unfortunately, the usual result is severe mental deficiency in a strong, often difficult to manage, individual. The syndrome may be compatible with long survival, but many die of pneumonia by 10 to 20 years.

ETIOLOGY. Autosomal recessive. Sanfilippo A is a defect of heparan N-sulfatase; Sanfilippo B, a deficiency of N-acetyl-α-D-glucosaminidase; Sanfilippo C, a deficiency of acetyl-CoA:α-glucosaminide-N-acetyltransferase; and Sanfilippo D, a deficiency of N-acetyl-α-D-glucosaminide-6-sulfatase. Excess heparan sulfate is excreted in the urine in all four types, and the clinical phenotype is identical in each. The gene for D-glucosaminide sulfatase has been localized to chromosome 12q14.

References

Sanfilippo, S. J., et al.: Mental retardation associated with acid mucopolysacchariduria (heparitin sulfate type). J. Pediatr., *63*:837, 1963.

Spranger, J., et al.: Die HS-Mucopolysaccharidose von Sanfilippo (Polydystrophe Oligophrenie). Bericht über 10 Patienten. Z. Kinderheilkd., *101*:71, 1967.

Kriel, R. L., et al.: Neuroanatomical and EEG correlations in Sanfilippo syndrome, type A. Arch. Neurol., *35*:838, 1978.

Andria, G., et al.: Sanfilippo B syndrome. Clin. Genet., *15*:500, 1979.

Nidiffer, F. D., and Kelly, T. E.: Developmental and degenerative patterns associated with cognitive, behavioral and motor difficulties in Sanfilippo syndrome. An epidemiology study. J. Ment. Defic. Res., *27*:185, 1983.

Van Schrojenstein-de Valk, H. M. J., et al.: Follow-up on seven adult patients with mid Sanfilippo B disease. Am. J. Med. Genet., *28*:125, 1987.

Robertson, D. A., et al.: Chromosomal localization of the gene for human glucosamine-6-sulfatase to 12q14. Hum. Genet., *79*:175, 1988.

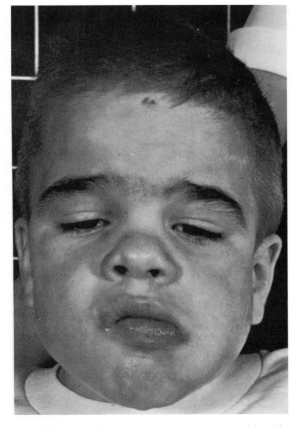

FIGURE 1. Sanfilippo syndrome. A 7-year-old with the height age of 5⁹/₁₂ years. His capabilities have been regressing, and his present I.Q. is about 50. A sibling is similarly affected. (Courtesy of R. Scott, University of Washington School of Medicine, Seattle, Wash.)

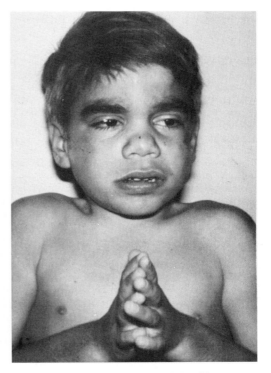

FIGURE 2. A 9-year-old boy with Sanfilippo syndrome, type B, whose I.Q. was about 20. (Courtesy of Dr. Robert Summitt, University of Tennessee College of Medicine, Memphis, Tenn.)

MORQUIO SYNDROME

(Mucopolysaccharidosis IV, Types A and B)

Onset at 1 to 3 Years of Age, Mild Coarse Facies, Severe Kyphosis and Knock-Knees, Cloudy Corneas

Mistakenly interpreted by Osler in 1898, this condition was described by Morquio in 1919; it was recognized as a mucopolysaccharidosis in 1963. Deficiencies of two different enzymes leading to a severe form, mucopolysaccharidosis IV A, and a mild form, mucopolysaccharidosis IV B, are now recognized. Within both forms, marked clinical heterogeneity has been documented that is most likely due to different mutations of the same gene.

ABNORMALITIES. Onset between 1 and 3 years.

Growth. Severe limitation with cessation by later childhood. Adult stature 82 to 115 cm.

Craniofacial. Mild coarsening of facial features, with broad mouth and short anteverted nose.

Eyes. Cloudy cornea evident by slit lamp examination, usually after 5 to 10 years of age.

Skeletal and Joints. Marked platyspondyly, with vertebrae changing to ovoid, ovoid with anterior projection, to flattened form with short neck and trunk plus kyphoscoliosis. Odontoid hypoplasia. Early flaring of rib cage progressing to bulging sternum. Short, curved long bones with irregular tubulation, widened metaphyses, abnormal femoral neck, flattening of femoral head, knock-knee with medial spur of tibial metaphysis, conical bases of widened metacarpals, irregular epiphyseal form, osteoporosis. Short, stubby hands. Joint laxity, most evident at wrists and small joints, and joint restriction in some of the larger joints, especially the hips.

Mouth. Widely spaced teeth with thin enamel that tends to become grayish in color.

Cardiac. Late onset of aortic regurgitation.

Other. Hearing loss. Inguinal hernia. Hepatomegaly.

Urinary Excretion. Keratan sulfate.

OCCASIONAL ABNORMALITIES. Macrocephaly, mental deficiency. Pigmentary retinal degeneration in older patients. Glaucoma. Hydrops fetalis.

NATURAL HISTORY. The earliest recognized indications of the disease have been flaring of the lower rib cage, prominent sternum, frequent upper respiratory tract infections (including otitis media), hernias, and growth deficiency, all becoming evident by 18 to 24 months of age. Severe defects of vertebrae may result in cord compression or respiratory insufficiency. These and cardiac complications may result in death prior to 20 years. In the milder form, longer survival is the rule, dental enamel is normal, and C2–C3 subluxation has been documented in addition to C1–C2 subluxation. Mentality is usually normal in both the severe and the mild forms.

ETIOLOGY. Autosomal recessive. The basic defect in type IVA is a deficiency of N-acetylgalactosamine-6-sulfatase, whereas in type IVB there is a deficiency of β-galactosidase. The gene for N-acetylgalactosamine-6-sulfatase has been isolated and mapped to 16q24.3. The gene for β-galactosidase, different mutations of which cause type IVB Morquio syndrome and generalized gangliosidosis syndrome, type I, has been mapped to 3p21.33. Confirmation of the diagnosis is dependent upon two-dimensional electrophoresis or thin-layer chromatography of isolated urinary glycosaminoglycans, since false-negative screening tests for urinary mucopolysaccharides occur and/or the deficiency of the enzyme in cultured skin fibroblasts or leukocytes. Heterozygote detection is possible. Prenatal diagnosis has been performed using both amniotic fluid cells and chorionic villi.

References

Osler, W.: Sporadic cretinism in America. Trans. Congr. Am. Phys., 4:169, 1898.

Morquio, L.: Sur une forme de dystrophie osseuse familiale. Arch. Med. Enf., 32:129, 1929.

Robins, M. M., Stevens, H. F., and Linker, A.: Morquio's disease: An abnormality of mucopolysaccharide metabolism. J. Pediatr., 62:881, 1963.

Langer, L. O., and Carey, L. S.: The roentgenographic features of the ks mucopolysaccharidosis of Morquio (Morquio-Brailsford's disease). Am. J. Roentgenol. Radium Ther. Nucl. Med., 97:1, 1966.

Linker, A., Evans, L. R., and Langer, L. O.: Morquio's disease and mucopolysaccharide excretion. J. Pediatr., 77:1039, 1970.

Matalon, R., et al.: Morquio's syndrome: Deficiency of a chondroitin sulfate N-acetylhexosamine sulfatase. Biochem. Biophys. Res. Commun., 61:759, 1974.

Muenzer, J.: Mucopolysaccharidoses. Adv. Pediatr., *33*: 269, 1986.

Applegarth, D. A., et al.: Morquio disease presenting as hydrops fetalis and enzyme analysis of chorionic villus tissue in a subsequent pregnancy. Pediatr. Pathol., 7:593, 1987.

Morris, C. P., et al.: Morquio A syndrome: Cloning, sequence and structure of the human *N*-acetylgalac-tosamine 6-sulfatase (GALNS) gene. Genomics, 22: 652, 1994.

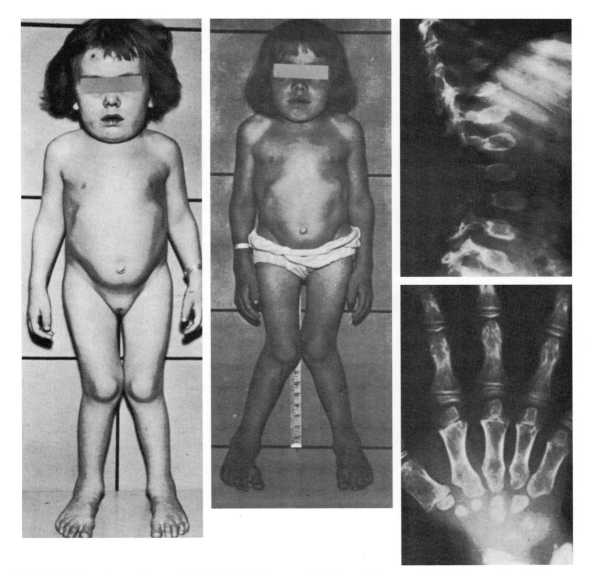

FIGURE 1. Morquio syndrome. *Left*, Patient at 3⁶/₁₂ years; height age, 2⁹/₁₂ years. *Center*, Same patient at 7 years; height age, 2⁹/₁₂ years. *Right*, X-ray films of patient at 7 years. (From Robins, M. M., et al.: J. Pediatr., *62*:881, 1963, with permission.)

MAROTEAUX-LAMY MUCOPOLYSACCHARIDOSIS SYNDROME (MILD, MODERATE, AND SEVERE TYPES)

(Mucopolysaccharidosis VI)

Coarse Facies, Stiff Joints, Cloudy Corneas in Infancy, No Mental Deterioration

Maroteaux et al. recognized this disorder as being distinct from Hurler syndrome in that mental deterioration did *not* occur during early childhood. Three clinical subtypes have been indicated, based on age of onset, rate of progression, and the extent of involvement of affected organs. Symptoms begin by 1 to 3 years in the severe type, by late childhood in the intermediate type, and after the second decade in the mild type.

ABNORMALITIES
Growth. Deficiency.
Craniofacial. Coarse facies with large nose and thick lips. Low nasal bridge.
Eyes. Fine corneal opacity. Cornea may be thick and/or large.
Skeletal and Joints. Mild stiffness of joints. Metaphyses, slightly broad and irregular. Epiphyseal irregularity, especially femoral epiphysis. Vertebrae flattened with anterior wedging of T12 and L1. Prominent sternum. Broad ribs. Elongated sella turcica. Odontoid hypoplasia. Lumbar kyphosis, genu valgum.
Other. Umbilical and inguinal hernias. Skin, thick and tight. Small, widely spaced teeth with late eruption. Hepatosplenomegaly. Varying degrees of deafness. Cytoplasmic granules in leukocytes.

OCCASIONAL ABNORMALITIES.
Macroglossia. Macrocephaly. Hydrocephalus. Involvement of heart valves. Glaucoma. Hearing impairment. Cervical myopathy due to thickening of the cervical dura mater.

NATURAL HISTORY.
Macrocephaly; frequent upper respiratory tract infections; diarrhea; hernias; and limitation of knee, hip, and elbow movement may be present in infancy. Thereafter, the three clinical subtypes diverge. Those with the severe type rapidly deteriorate physically and by 3 to 6 years have serious deformity. The longest survivor of the severe type is into the 20s. Most die from cardiopulmonary complications by the second or third decade. The age of onset of growth deficiency is usually a little later than in the Hurler syndrome; the extent of skeletal broadening, joint limitation, hepatosplenomegaly, and corneal opacification is generally less than with Hurler syndrome; and mental deficiency has not been noted during childhood. The data on prognosis for the mild and intermediate types are inadequate. Anesthesia, due to airway management, can pose a significant risk.

ETIOLOGY. Autosomal recessive. The molecular defect is a deficiency of N-acetylgalactosamine-4-sulfatase (arylsulfatase B). The enzyme is missing in all tissues, including cultured fibroblasts. The gene for N-acetylgalactosamine-4-sulfatase maps to chromosome 5q13-q14. There is an increased urinary excretion of mucopolysaccharides consisting predominantly of dermatan sulfate. Heterozygote detection and prenatal diagnosis may be feasible in selected laboratories.

References

Maroteaux, P., et al.: Une nouvelle dysostose avec élimination urinaire de chondroitine-sulfate B. Presse Med., 71:1849, 1963.

Maroteaux, P., and Lamy, M.: Hurler's disease, Morquio's disease, and related mucopolysaccharidoses. J. Pediatr., 67:312, 1965.

Fallis, N., Barnes, F. L., II, and di Ferrante, N.: A case of polydystrophic dwarfism with urinary excretion of dermatan sulfate and heparan sulfate. J. Clin. Endocrinol. Metab., 28:26, 1968.

O'Brien, J. F., Cantz, M., and Spranger, J.: Maroteaux-Lamy disease, subtype A: Deficiency of an N-acetylgalactosamine-4-sulfatase. Biochem. Biophys. Res. Commun., 60:1170, 1974.

Litgens, T., et al.: Chromosomal localization of ARSB, the gene for human N-acetylygalactosamine-4-sulfatase. Hum. Genet., 82:67, 1989.

Tan, C. T. T., et al.: Valvular heart disease in four patients with Maroteaux-Lamy syndrome. Circulation, 85:188, 1992.

Isbrandt, D., et al.: Mucopolysaccharidosis VI (Maroteaux-Lamy syndrome): Six unique arylsulfatase B gene alleles causing variable disease phenotypes. Am. J. Hum. Genet., 54:454, 1994.

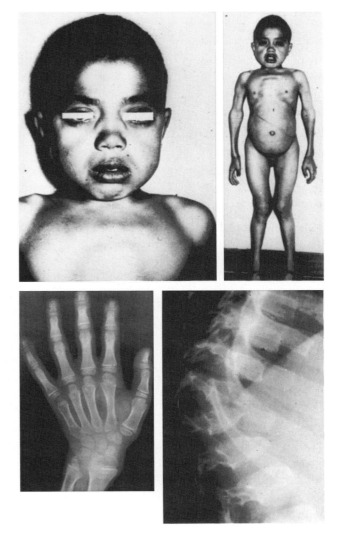

FIGURE 1. Maroteaux-Lamy mucopolysaccharidosis syndrome. Older boy, short of stature, with normal intelligence. (Courtesy of P. Maroteaux, Hôpital des Enfants-Malades, Paris.)

MUCOPOLYSACCHARIDOSIS VII

(Sly Syndrome, β-Glucuronidase Deficiency)

Initially described by Sly et al. in an infant with short stature, skeletal deformities, hepatosplenomegaly, and mental deficiency, approximately 32 cases have been reported subsequently. A widely variable clinical phenotype has been noted from severely affected infants to mildly affected adults.

ABNORMALITIES
Growth. Postnatal growth deficiency.
Performance. Moderately severe mental deficiency.
Craniofacies. Macrocephaly. Coarsened facies.
Eyes. Corneal clouding in the severe form.
Skeletal. Thoracolumbar gibbus. Metatarsus adductus. Flaring of lower ribs. Prominent sternum. J-shaped sella turcica. Acetabular dysplasia, narrow sciatic notches, and hypoplastic basilar portions of ilia. Widening of ribs. Pointed proximal metacarpals.
Other. Inguinal hernia. Hepatosplenomegaly.

OCCASIONAL ABNORMALITIES. Joint contractures. Hydrocephalus. Involvement of heart valves. Odontoid hypoplasia. Shortening and anterior irregularities of vertebral bodies, wedge deformities of lumbar vertebrae. Anterior, inferior beaking of lower thoracic and lumbar vertebrae. Hip dysplasia. Hydrops fetalis.

NATURAL HISTORY. Unlike the other known mucopolysaccharidoses, MPS VII is sometimes recognizable in the neonatal period, associated with hydrops fetalis and hepatosplenomegaly. For them, death occurs in the first few months. A more mild form, also presenting in the newborn period, is associated with developmental delay, much less rapid deterioration, and survival into adolescence.

ETIOLOGY. Autosomal recessive. The basic defect is a deficiency of β-glucuronidase, which can be documented in fibroblasts and leukocytes. The gene for β-glucuronidase has been mapped to the proximal long arm of chromosome 7 at 7q21.1-7q22.

COMMENT. The existence of multiple allelic forms of this disorder most likely explains the wide variability in the clinical phenotype. There exists at least one form of β-glucuronidase deficiency that presents during the second decade of life and is characterized by mild skeletal abnormalities and normal intelligence.

References

Sly, W. S., et al.: Beta glucuronidase deficiency. Report of clinical radiologic, and biochemical features of a new mucopolysaccharidosis. J. Pediatr., *82*:249, 1973.

Daves, B. S., and Degnan, M.: Different clinical and biochemical phenotype associated with beta glucuronidase deficiency. *In* Bergsma, D. (ed.): Skeletal Dysplasias. New York, National Foundation March of Dimes, 1974, p. 251.

Hoyme, H. E., et al.: Presentation of mucopolysaccharidosis VII (β-glucuronidase deficiency) in infancy. J. Med. Genet., *18*:237, 1981.

Allanson, J. E., et al.: Deletion mapping of the β-glucuronidase gene. Am. J. Med. Genet., *29*:517, 1988.

Wallace, S. P., et al.: Degeneration of speech, language, and hearing in a patient with mucopolysaccharidosis VII. Int. J. Pediatr. Otorhinolaryngol., *19*:97, 1990.

Wu, B. M., et al.: Overexpression rescues the mutant phenotype of L176F mutation causing β-glucuronidase deficiency mucopolysaccharidosis in two Mennonite siblings. J. Biol. Chem., *38*:23681, 1994.

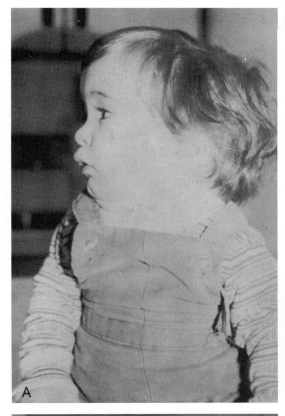

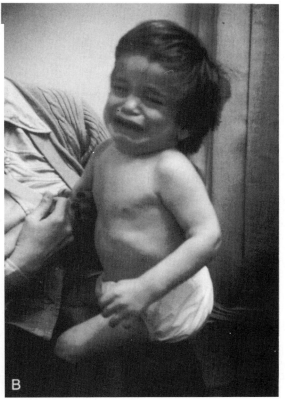

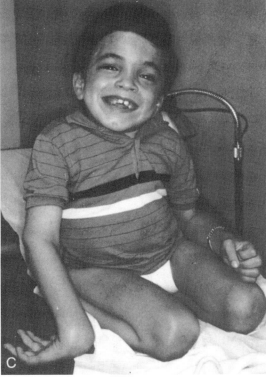

FIGURE 1. Mucopolysaccharidosis VII. Same child at 1 year (*A*), 2 years (*B*), and 8 years (*C*) of age. Note the coarse facies and joint contractures.

O

O. CONNECTIVE TISSUE DISORDERS

MARFAN SYNDROME

Arachnodactyly With Hyperextensibility, Lens Subluxation, Aortic Dilatation

Described as dolichostenomelia in the initial report by Marfan, this disorder has been extensively studied and recognized as a connective tissue disorder by McKusick.

ABNORMALITIES
Skeletal. Tendency toward tall stature with long slim limbs, little subcutaneous fat, and muscle hypotonia. Arachnodactyly. Pes planus. Decreased upper to lower segment ratio. Joint laxity with scoliosis (60 per cent) and kyphosis. Pectus excavatum or carinatum. Narrow facies with narrow plate.
Eyes. Lens subluxation, usually upward, with defect in suspensory ligament. Increased axial globe length. Myopia. Retinal detachment.
Cardiovascular. Dilatation with or without dissecting aneurysm of ascending aorta, less commonly of thoracic or abdominal aorta or pulmonary artery. Secondary aortic regurgitation. Mitral valve prolapse.
Other. Inguinal and/or femoral hernias. Dural distention leading in some cases to meningocele.

OCCASIONAL ABNORMALITIES. Large ears, cataracts, retinal detachment, glaucoma, strabismus, refractive errors including anisometropia and amblyopia, striae in pectoral or deltoid area, diaphragmatic hernia, pulmonary malformation contributing to spontaneous pneumothorax and/or emphysema with an increased susceptibility to respiratory tract infection. Hemivertebrae, colobomata of iris, cleft palate, incomplete rotation of colon. Ventricular dysrhythmias. Sleep apnea. Neuropsychologic impairment, including learning disability and attention deficit disorder, in 42 per cent of 19 individuals (5 to 18 years of age) despite normal I.Q. Schizophrenia.

NATURAL HISTORY. During childhood and adolescence, special care should be directed toward prevention of scoliosis. The serious vascular complications may develop at any time from fetal life through old age and are the chief cause of death. A significantly reduced rate of aortic dilatation and its associated complications has been documented in affected individuals treated with β-adrenergic blocking agents, leading Salim et al. to recommend that patients with Marfan syndrome be treated with β-adrenergic blockers as soon as the diagnosis is made. In addition, based on a follow-up study of 50 consecutive patients (age range, 9 to 52 years) who received a graft for the complete replacement of the ascending aortic aneurysm and aortic valve, Gott et al. recommend prophylactic repair for any patient with Marfan syndrome who has an ascending aorta with a diameter of 6 cm or more, regardless of symptoms or the presence of aortic regurgitation. Secondary glaucoma may occur, especially when the lens dislocates into the anterior chamber of the eye. The mean age of survival is 43 for men and 46 for women. These individuals are of normal intelligence.

ETIOLOGY. Autosomal dominant, with sufficiently wide variability in expression that the diagnosis is often tenuous in sporadic nonfamilial cases. The disorder can occur without ectopia lentis and without pronounced arachnodactyly. Mutations in the fibrillin (FBN1) gene located on chromosome 15q21.1 are responsible for the pattern of defects seen in Marfan syndrome. Fibrillin is a glycoprotein that is a major component of the suspensory ligament of the eye as well as being a substrate for elastin in the aorta and other elastic tissues. Although a defect in fibrillin metabolism occurs in Marfan syndrome, not all patients with alterations in fibrillin have Marfan syndrome. Since multiple FBN1 mutations have been identified, there is no screening test for a common mutation. Only in families in which there are multiple affected members can linkage analysis be used to identify probable carriers of the FBN1 gene.

COMMENT. A severe neonatal form of Marfan syndrome in children diagnosed in the first 3 months of life has been delineated. Serious cardiac defects including mitral valve prolapse, valvular regurgitation, and aortic root dilatation occur in about 80 per cent of cases, and congenital contractures are present in 64 per cent. A characteristic facies, dolichocephaly, a high arched palate, micrognathia, hyperextensible joints, arachnodactyly, pes planus, chest deformity, iridodenesis, megalocornea, and lens dislocation are also frequently present. Fourteen per cent of affected children die during the first year. A different mutation in the FBN1 gene causes the severe neonatal form.

References

Marfan, A. B.: Un cas de déformation congénitales des quatre membres plus prononcée aux extrémities charactérisée par l'allongement des os avec un certain degré d'amincissement. Bull. Mem. Soc. Med. Hop. (Paris), *13*:220, 1896.

Pyeritz, R. E., and McKusick, V. A.: The Marfan syndrome: Diagnosis and management. N. Engl. J. Med., *300*:772, 1979.

Hofman, K. J., Bernhardt, B. A., and Pyeritz, R. E.: Increased incidence of neuropsychologic impairment in the Marfan syndrome. Am. J. Hum. Genet., *37*:4A, 1985.

Gott, V. L., et al.: Surgical treatment of aneurysms of the ascending aorta in the Marfan syndrome. Results of composite-graft repair in 50 patients. N. Engl. J. Med., *314*:1070, 1986.

Morse, R. P. et al.: Diagnosis and management of infantile Marfan syndrome. Pediatrics, *86*:888, 1990.

Lee, B., et al.: Linkage of Marfan syndrome and a phenotypically related disorder to two different fibrillin genes. Nature, *352*:330, 1991.

Kainulainen, K., et al.: Mutations in the fibrillin gene responsible for dominant ectopic lentis and neonatal Marfan syndrome. Nat. Genet., *6*:64, 1994.

Salim, M. A., et al.: Effect of beta-adrenergic blockade on aortic root rate of dilatation in the Marfan syndrome. Am. J. Cardiol., *74*:629, 1994.

Shores, J., et al.: Progression of aortic dilitation and the benefit of long-term β-adrenergic blockade in Marfan's syndrome. N. Engl. J. Med., *330*:1335, 1994.

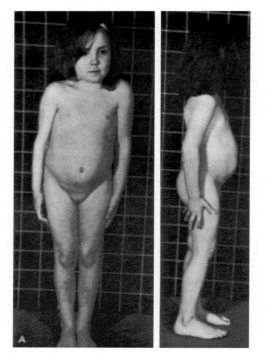

FIGURE 1. Marfan syndrome. *A*, A 3⁶/₁₂-year-old, with height age of 5 years, who has lens dislocation, mild arachnodactyly of the hands and feet, unusually soft skin, and narrow palate. The family history of the Marfan syndrome in the mother and grandfather tends to confirm the diagnosis in this case.

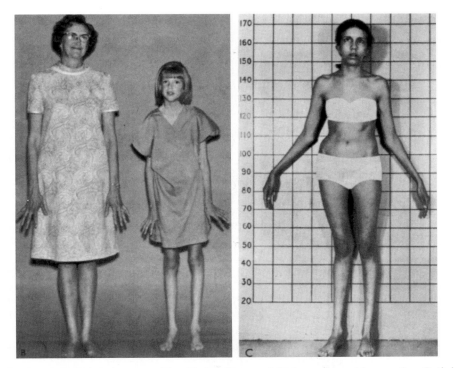

FIGURE 1. *Continued.* *B*, Girl, 9³/₁₂ years old, with height age of 12³/₁₂ years, and her mother. Both have arachnodactyly, but only the mother has dislocation of the lenses. *C*, A 16-year-old with arachnodactyly, hyperextensible hands and knees, limitation of extension at elbow, scoliosis, systolic and diastolic murmurs, superiorly dislocated lenses, glaucoma, and retinal detachments, despite numerous surgical procedures. She represents a fresh mutation in that no other family members are affected. (*C* courtesy of Dr. Victor McKusick, Johns Hopkins Hospital, Baltimore, Md., and Dr. Judith Hall, University of British Columbia, Vancouver, British Columbia.)

BEALS SYNDROME

(Beals Contractural Arachnodactyly Syndrome)

Joint Contractures, Arachnodactyly, "Crumpled" Ear

Beals and Hecht described this syndrome in 1971. They found 11 probable past reports of the same entity, including the original Marfan report.

ABNORMALITIES

Limbs. Long slim limbs (dolichostenomelia) with arachnodactyly (86 per cent). Camptodactyly (78 per cent). Ulnar deviation of fingers. Joint contractures, especially of knees (81 per cent), elbows (86 per cent), and hips (26 per cent).

Other Skeletal. Kyphoscoliosis (46 per cent), relatively short neck. Metatarsus varus. Mild talipes equinovarus (32 per cent). Hypoplasia of calf muscles (65 per cent).

Ears. "Crumpled" appearance with poorly defined conchas and prominent crura from the root of the helix (75 per cent).

Other. Mitral valve prolapse with regurgitation.

OCCASIONAL ABNORMALITIES.
Micrognathia (26 per cent). Cranial abnormalities including scaphocephaly, brachycephaly, dolichocephaly, and frontal bossing (29 per cent). Iris coloboma. Ectopia lentis. Keratoconus. Myopia. Subluxation of patella. Atrial septal defect, ventricular septal defect, hypoplasia of aorta. Sternal defects.

NATURAL HISTORY.
There tends to be gradual improvement in the joint limitations, but the scoliosis may be progressive.

ETIOLOGY.
Autosomal dominant inheritance. Linkage of Beals syndrome families to a fibrillin locus on chromosome 5q23-31 (FBN2) has been documented. Mutations in the FBN2 gene have been demonstrated in two patients.

References

Beals, R. K., and Hecht, F.: Delineation of another heritable disorder of connective tissue. J. Bone Joint Surg. [Am.], *53*:987, 1971.

Hecht, F., and Beals, R. K.: "New" syndrome of congenital contractural arachnodactyly originally described by Marfan in 1896. Pediatrics, *49*:574, 1972.

Anderson, R. A., Koch, S., and Camerini-Otero, R. D.: Cardiovascular findings in congenital contractural arachnodactyly: Report of an affected kindred. Am. J. Med. Genet., *18*:265, 1984.

Ramos Arroyo, M. A., Weaver, D. D., and Beals, R. K.: Congenital contractural arachnodactyly. Report of four additional families and review of literature. Clin. Genet., *25*:570, 1985.

Lee, B., et al.: Linkage of Marfan syndrome and a phenotypically related disorder to two different fibrillin genes. Nature, *352*:330, 1991.

Viljoen, D.: Congenital contractural arachnodactyly (Beals syndrome). J. Med. Genet., *31*:640, 1994.

Putnam, E. A., et al.: Fibrillin-2 (FBN2) mutations result in the Marfan-like disorder, congenital contractural arachnodactyly. Nat. Genet., *11*, 456: 1995.

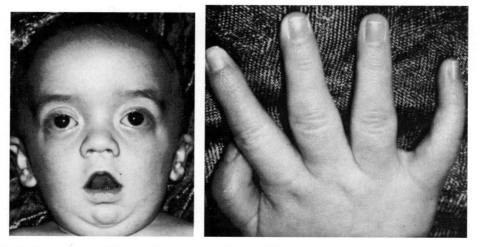

FIGURE 1. Beals syndrome. Young infant showing facies, folded helixes of ears, and relative arachnodactyly with minor camptodactyly. He developed severe scoliosis by 2 years of age.

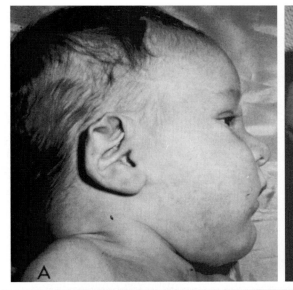
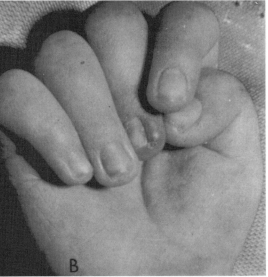
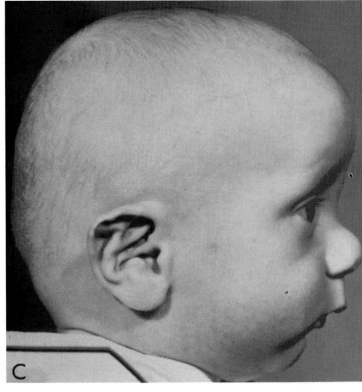
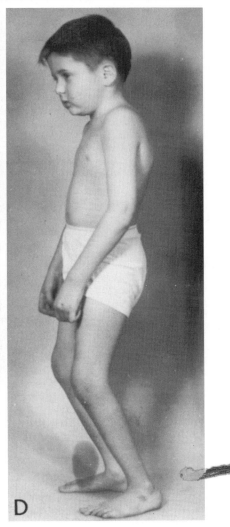

FIGURE 2. Beals syndrome. *A* and *B*, Infant showing "crumpled" ear and aberrant position of contracted fingers. *C*, Note similar appearance of ear to that in *A*. *D*, A 6-year-old sibling of infant in *C*. (*C* and *D* from Beals, R. K., and Hecht, F.: J. Bone Joint Surg. [Am.], 53:987, 1971, with permission.)

HOMOCYSTINURIA SYNDROME

Subluxation of Lens, Malar Flush, Osteoporosis

Urinary amino acid screening of mentally defective patients resulted in the independent discovery of this entity by Carson et al. and Gerritsen and Waisman in 1963. Finkelstein et al. found a lack of cystathionine synthetase activity in the liver of affected individuals, and this enzyme defect apparently leads to the accumulation of homocystine and methionine with a deficiency of cystathionine and cystine. Vitamin B_6–responsive and vitamin B_6–nonresponsive forms of this disorder have been delineated.

ABNORMALITIES
General. Mental defect in 58 per cent of 38 patients.
Eye. Subluxation, usually downward, of the lens by the age of 10 years, the earliest instance noted being 2 years. Myopia.
Skeletal. Slim skeletal build, arachnodactyly, pectus excavatum or carinatum, genu valgum, pes cavus, everted feet with or without kyphoscoliosis. Osteoporosis.
Vasculature. Medial degeneration of aorta and elastic arteries with intimal hyperplasia and fibrosis leading to pads and ridges within the vessels. Both arterial and venous thromboses are frequent.
Skin. Malar flush with tendency toward patchy erythematous blotches elsewhere.
Hair. Tends to be fine, sparse, dry, and light in color.

OCCASIONAL ABNORMALITIES.
Cataracts, glaucoma, optic atrophy, cystic retinal degeneration or detachment, irregular crowded teeth, high arched palate, hernias, hepatomegaly with fatty liver.

NATURAL HISTORY.
Seizures, with onset from 6 months to 5 years of age, have been noted, and the EEG pattern is usually abnormal. Excessive nervousness may be a feature, occasionally with schizophrenic behavior. Neurologic defect, especially spasticity, may be present and is often asymmetric—presumably the consequence of vascular thrombosis that can be arterial or venous and not infrequently involves the coronary artery. Venipuncture or surgical procedures may be followed by excessive vascular thrombosis and should be avoided when possible. Thromboembolic phenomena constitute the most life-threatening feature of this disease. Another problem, osteoporosis, frequently leads to partial collapse of vertebrae, and there is an increased likelihood of fractures.

Failure to thrive has been a feature of some cases, with severe mental defect. However, normal to tall stature is the more usual growth pattern.

A long-term follow-up evaluation of 629 affected patients has been reported. Lens dislocation at 10 years of age, initial clinically detected thromboembolic events at 15 years, spinal osteoporosis at 15 years, and mortality at age 30 occurred less frequently in untreated vitamin B_6–responsive patients than in untreated vitamin B_6–nonresponsive patients. Thromboembolic events and hypoglycemia can complicate anesthesia.

ETIOLOGY. Autosomal recessive. Decreased cystathionine synthetase activity has been found in the liver of the parents of homocystinuric individuals, supporting the contention that they are heterozygotes. Interference with collagen cross-linking by sulfhydryl groups of homocystine causes ectopia lentis and skeletal changes. Sulfation factor–like effects contribute to the disruption of vascular endothelium, leading to platelet thrombosis and then to arterial and venous occlusions. Pyridoxine therapy may be beneficial in some cases when begun in infancy.

COMMENT. The urinary cyanide nitroprusside test may not always yield a positive result in patients with homocystinuria, and specific amino acid studies therefore constitute the most important diagnostic measure. A completely successful mode of therapy has not yet been demonstrated. A low-methionine, high-cystine diet is beneficial in preventing mental retardation in vitamin B_6–nonresponsive patients if begun in the neonatal period.

References

Carson, N. A. J., et al.: Homocystinuria: A new inborn error of metabolism associated with mental deficiency. Arch. Dis. Child., *38*:425, 1963.

Finkelstein, J. D., et al.: Homocystinuria due to cystathionine synthetase deficiency: The mode of inheritance. Science, *146*:785, 1964.

Gerritsen, T., and Waisman, H. A.: Homocystinuria, an error in the metabolism of methionine. Pediatrics, *33*:413, 1964.

White, H. H., et al.: Homocystinuria. Trans. Am. Neurol. Assoc., *89*:24, 1964.

Grieco, H. J.: Homocystinuria; pathogenetic mechanisms. Am. J. Med. Sci., *273*:120, 1977.

Mudd, S. H., et al.: The natural history of homocystinuria cystathionine β-sulfatase deficiency. Am. J. Hum. Genet., *37*:1, 1985.

Lowe, S., et al.: Anesthetic implications of the child with homocystinuria. J. Clin. Anesth., *6*:142, 1994.

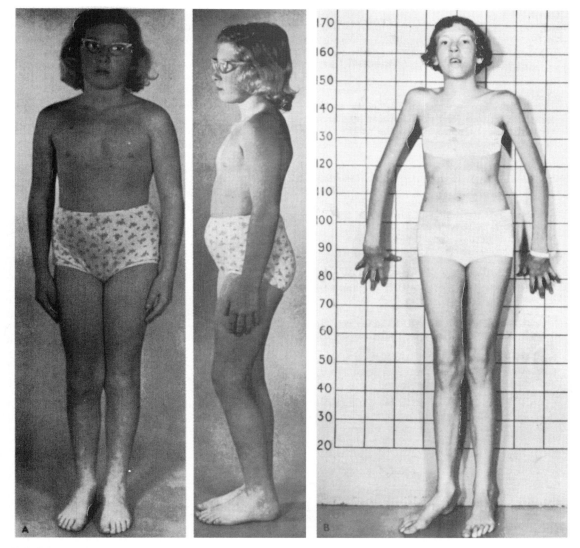

FIGURE 1. *A*, A 10-year-old girl with homocystinuria, who presented with lens subluxation that was first noted at 4 years of age. Her early developmental progress was within normal limits, but she has been receiving special schooling and her I.Q. is 67. *B*, A 12-year-old girl with arachnodactyly, "tight" joints, and inferiorly and nasally dislocated lenses. She is of low normal intelligence with a "schizoid personality" and has had two episodes of gastrointestinal bleeding, one documented as being secondary to a gastric infarct. (*B* courtesy of Dr. Victor McKusick, Johns Hopkins Hospital, Baltimore, Md., and Dr. Judith Hall, University of British Columbia, Vancouver, British Columbia.)

CAMURATI-ENGELMANN SYNDROME

(Progressive Diaphyseal Dysplasia)

Diaphyseal Dysplasia, Weakness, Leg Pain

Originally described by Cockayne in 1920, this disorder was further delineated by Camurati and then Engelmann in the 1920s. More than 80 cases have been reported.

ABNORMALITIES
Radiographic. Progressive diaphyseal broadening with thickened cortices and an abrupt transition toward more normal metaphyseal bone, most evident in femora and tibiae. There is thickening of the bone, irregular endosteal and periosteal apposition, and narrowing of the medullary canal. Erlenmeyer flask defects, sclerosis of skull base, and involvement of mandible in severe cases. Vertebral sclerosis confined to the posterior part of the vertebral bodies and arches on CT scan.
Muscles. Relative weakness, most severe around pelvic girdle. Muscle biopsy may show atrophic fibers with degeneration.
Function. Waddling gait, leg pains, weakness.

OCCASIONAL ABNORMALITIES.
Deafness, exophthalmos, headaches, scoliosis, late adolescence.

NATURAL HISTORY.
Severely affected patients may have feeding problems, waddling gait, and leg pains even in infancy and often have an asthenic "malnourished" appearance. Mild cases may only be evident by roentgenogram. Hyperostosis may progress to optic nerve compression, for which surgical intervention is merited. Although the progression of the disorder is difficult to predict, it probably starts early in life, reaches advanced stages in adolescence, and either remains stationary or advances slowly in adulthood.

ETIOLOGY. Autosomal dominant with wide variance in expression and variable penetrance.

References

Cockayne, E. A.: Case for diagnosis. Proc. R. Soc. Med., *13*:132, 1920.

Camurati, M.: Di un raro caso di osteite simmetrica erediatria degli arti inferiori. Chir. Organi. Mov., *6*: 662, 1922.

Engelmann, G.: Ein Fall von Osteopathic hyperostotica (sclerotans) multiplex infantilis. Fortschr. Roentgenstr., *39*:1101, 1929.

Sparkes, R. S., and Graham, C. B.: Camurati Engelmann disease. Genetics and clinical manifestations with a review of the literature. J. Med. Genet., *9*:73, 1972.

Yen, J. K., et al.: Camurati-Engelmann disease. J. Neurosurg., *48*:138, 1978.

Yoshioka, H., et al.: Muscular changes in Engelmann's disease. Arch. Dis. Child., *55*:716, 1980.

Kaftori, J. K., et al.: Progressive diaphyseal dysplasia (Camurati-Englemann): Radiographic follow-up and CT findings. Radiology, *164*:777, 1987.

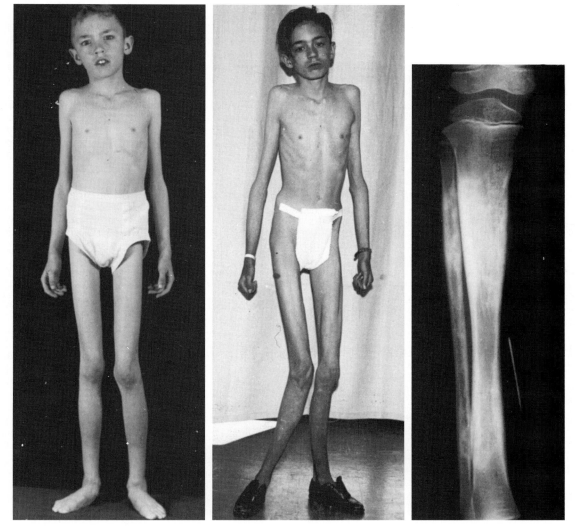

FIGURE 1. Camurati-Engelmann syndrome. A 10-year-old and an 18-year-old patient showing slim habitus, with bowing and angulation at the knees, and flat feet. Roentgenogram shows irregular cortical thickening with diaphyseal broadening. (From Clawson, D. K., and Loop, J. W.: J. Bone Joint Surg. [Am.], 46:143, 1964, with permission.)

EHLERS-DANLOS SYNDROME

Hyperextensibility of Joints, Hyperextensibility of Skin, Poor Wound Healing With Thin Scar

Originally described by Van Meekeren in 1682, this condition was further clarified by Ehlers in 1901 and Danlos in 1908. More than 100 cases have been described. The possibility has been raised that the celebrated violinist Paganini may have had Ehlers-Danlos syndrome, thus accounting for his unusual dexterity and reach.

Ten distinct forms of the Ehler-Danlos syndrome have now been delineated. Only type I has been set forth in detail in this text.

ABNORMALITIES. The most consistent features are set forth below.
Face. Narrow maxilla.
Auricles. Hypermobile, with tendency toward "lop ears."
Skin. Velvety, hyperextensible, and fragile, with poor wound healing leaving parchment-thin scars. Small, movable subcutaneous spherules contain either mucinous material or adipose.
Joints. Hyperextensibility with liability toward dislocation at hip, shoulder, elbow, knee, or clavicle. Pes planus.
Blood Vessels. Easy bruisability.
Cardiac. Mitral valve prolapse with or without tricuspid valve prolapse. Aortic root and/or sinus of Valsalva dilatation.

OCCASIONAL ABNORMALITIES
Eyes and Facies. Wide nasal bridge. Epicanthal folds, blue sclerae, myopia, microcornea, keratoconus, glaucoma, ectopia lentis, retinal detachment.
Skeletal. Small stature, kyphoscoliosis (27 per cent), long neck, slim skeletal build, downsloping ribs, talipes deformity, overlapping toes. Talipes equinovarus.
Dentition. Small; irregular placement; partial anodontia.
Cardiovascular. Dissecting aneurysm, intracranial aneurysm, hemorrhage. Atrial septal defect, abnormal aortic arch, other heart defects, mitral valve prolapse.
Gastrointestinal. Inguinal hernia, diaphragmatic hernia, ectasia of intestine, intestinal diverticuli.
Renal. Ureteropelvic anomaly, renal tubular acidosis.
Other. Mental deficiency. Autism.

NATURAL HISTORY. Barabas discovered that most patients with Ehlers-Danlos syndrome are born prematurely following premature rupture of the membranes, possibly the first obvious indication of relative friability of tissues in these individuals. The integrity of tissues is easily disturbed, as evidenced by the fragility of skin and blood vessels. Wound healing is delayed, with relatively inadequate scar tissue, and prolonged hemorrhage may occur following trauma. Both of these factors, plus the tendency of sutures to tear out, rule out unnecessary surgical procedures. These patients should be cautioned to avoid traumatic situations. Gastrointestinal hemorrhage or hemoptysis may be a problem. The poor integrity of vessels occasionally may lead to a dissecting aneurysm, and affected women are liable to have postpartum hemorrhage. Whether or not the tendency to have chilblains and acrocyanosis is secondary to vascular alterations is undetermined.

The peculiar fat- or mucinoid-containing subcutaneous spherules, most commonly found in areas of frequent mild trauma, may mineralize and thereby be evident on roentgenograms.

ETIOLOGY. Autosomal dominant with wide variance in expression.

COMMENT. Major features of types II through X are summarized here.
Type II. A similar but much milder clinical picture and autosomal dominant inheritance.
Type III. Striking joint hypermobility, frequent joint dislocation, soft but otherwise normal skin, and autosomal dominant inheritance. Osteoarthritis by 30 to 40 years of age.
Type IV. The vascular or ecchymotic type. Characteristic face with large eyes, a thin pinched nose and thin lips. The hands and feet appear prematurely aged. Thin or translucent skin with easily visible underlying veins, easy bruising, normal joint mobility with the exception of the small joints of the hands, bowel and/or arterial rupture leading to death, as well as uterine rupture during pregnancy, neurovascular manifestations including spontaneous carotid-cavernous fistulae, intracranial aneurysms, and carotid artery aneurysms, and autosomal dominant inheritance in the majority of cases. Mutations in the type III collagen gene COL3A1 lead to a defect in type III collagen that is responsible for the clinical phenotype. Death usually occurs before the fifth decade.
Type V. A clinical picture similar to that of type II but with X-linked recessive inheritance. The female carriers are asymptomatic.

Type VI. Soft, hyperextensible skin with moderate scarring and easy bruising, joint laxity, scoliosis, muscle hypotonia, ocular fragility, and keratoconus. Lysyl hydroxylase deficiency resulting in hydroxylysine-deficient collagen, and autosomal recessive inheritance. The gene for lysyl hydroxylase has been cloned and mapped to chromosome 1p36. Diagnosis can be confirmed by assay of lysyl hydroylase in skin fibroblasts.

Type VII. Hyperextensible and easily bruisable skin that is not usually fragile, marked joint hyperextensibility, congenital hip dislocation. Type VII has been subclassified into three types: EDS VII A due to a mutation in the COL1A1 gene; EDS VII B due to a mutation in the COL1A2 gene; and EDS VII C due to a deficiency in procollagen *N*-proteinase activity. Types A and B are autosomal dominant and type C is autosomal recessive.

Type VIII. Periodontitis, marked bruising, mild or no joint hypermobility, thin skin with hyperextensibility, poor wound healing, and autosomal dominant inheritance.

Type IX. Soft, mildly extensible skin, occipital horn-like exostosis, short humeri, short broad clavicles, chronic diarrhea, bladder diverticulae with a propensity to bladder rupture, and X-linked recessive inheritance. Abnormal copper utilization has been noted. Diagnosis is confirmed by decreased serum copper and ceruloplasmin.

Type X. Joint hypermobility and dislocation, mildly hyperextensible fragile skin with poor wound healing, a platelet aggregation defect that corrects with the addition of fibrinectin, and autosomal recessive inheritance.

References

Van Meekeren, J. A.: De dilatabiltate extraordinaria cutis. Chapter 32 in Observations Medicochirogicae. Amsterdam, 1682.

Ehlers, E.: Cutis laxa, Neigung zu Harmorrhagien in der Haut, Lockerung mehrer Artikulationen. Dermat. Ztschr., *8*:173, 1901.

Danlos, H.: Un cas de cutis laxa avec tumeurs par contusion chronique des coudes et des genoux (santhome juvenile pseudodiabetique de MM. Hallopeau et Mace de Lepinay). Bull. Soc. Fr., Dermat. Syph., *19*:70, 1908.

Wechsler, H. L., and Fisher, E. R.: Ehlers-Danlos syndrome. Pathologic, histochemical, and electron microscopic observations. Arch. Pathol., *77*:613, 1964.

Barabas, A. P.: Ehlers-Danlos syndrome: Associated with prematurity and premature rupture of foetal membranes; possible increase in incidence. Br. Med. J., *2*:682, 1966.

Leier, C. V., et al.: The spectrum of cardiac defects in Ehlers-Danlos syndrome, types I and III. Ann. Intern. Med., *92*:171, 1980.

Yeowell, H. N., and Pinnell, S. R.: The Ehlers-Danlos syndrome. Semin. Dermatol., *12*:229, 1993.

Schievink, W. I., et al.: Neurovascular manifestations of heritable disorders of connective tissue. Stroke, *25*:889, 1994.

Tilstra, D. J., and Byers, P. H.: Molecular basis of hereditary disorders of connective tissue. Annu. Rev. Med., *45*:149, 1994.

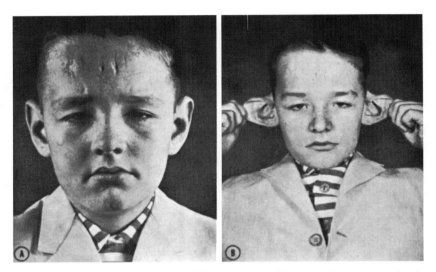

FIGURE 1. Ehlers-Danlos syndrome. A 12-year-old boy showing thin persisting scars on forehead (*A*), hyperelasticity of auricles and skin (*B* and *D*), and hyperextensibility of joints (*C*). (From Rees, T. D., et al.: Plast. Reconstr. Surg., 32:39, 1963, with permission.)

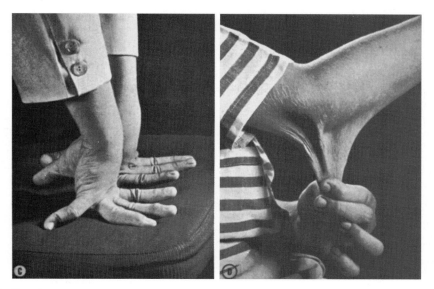

FIGURE 1. *Continued.*

OSTEOGENESIS IMPERFECTA SYNDROME, TYPE I

(Autosomal Dominant Osteogenesis Imperfecta, Lobstein Disease)

Fragile Bone, Blue Sclerae, Hyperextensibility, Presenile Deafness

At least four types of osteogenesis imperfecta exist. Only type I and type II are discussed in detail in this text.

ABNORMALITIES

Growth. Postnatal onset growth deficiency (50 per cent).

Dentition. Hypoplasia of dentin and pulp with translucency of teeth, which have a yellowish or bluish gray coloration, and susceptibility to caries, irregular placement, and late eruption.

Sclerae and Skin. The skin and sclerae tend to be thin and translucent; partial visualization of the choroid gives the sclerae a blue appearance. Easy bruising (75 per cent).

Skeletal. Postnatal onset of mild limb deformity, primarily anterior or lateral bowing of femora and anterior bowing of tibiae (20 per cent). Fractures (92 per cent). Scoliosis (mild to moderate in 17 per cent; severe in 3 per cent). Kyphosis (mild to moderate in 18 per cent; severe in 2 per cent). Hyperextensible joints (100 per cent). Wormian bones in cranial sutures.

Hearing. Impairment in 35 per cent, secondary to otosclerosis, and usually first noted in third decade.

Other. Macrocephaly (18 per cent). Triangular facial appearance (30 per cent). Inguinal and/or umbilical hernia.

OCCASIONAL ABNORMALITIES.
Prenatal growth deficiency (7 per cent), embryotoxon (opacity in the peripheral cornea), keratoconus, megalocornea. Syndactyly. Floppy mitral valve.

NATURAL HISTORY. Eight per cent of patients have first fracture noted at birth, 23 per cent in the first year, 45 per cent in preschool, and 17 per cent during school years. Bowing of the limbs is almost never noted in newborns. After adolescence, the likelihood of fracture diminishes, although inactivity, pregnancy, or lactation can apparently enhance the likelihood of fracture. Scoliosis, usually not diagnosed before the end of the first decade, progresses during puberty and in some cases can be severe in adulthood. Loss of stature secondary to progressive platyspondyly and kyphosis due to spinal osteoporosis occurs in adults. Hearing impairment is common in adults, who often require hearing aids or surgery for osteosclerosis. Virtually all patients are ambulatory.

ETIOLOGY. Autosomal dominant with marked variability in expression. From the molecular standpoint, osteogenesis imperfecta type I results from mutations that cause a quantitative defect in the production of type I collagen, the result (in most cases studied) of decreased synthesis of the pro-α-1(I) chain of type I procollagen.

COMMENT. Major features of types III and IV are summarized here.

Type III. Prenatal onset growth deficiency. Macrocephaly with a triangular facial appearance. Multiple fractures usually present at birth. Progressive bone deformities from birth through childhood and adolescence. The sclera, although bluish in infancy, are usually normal in adults. Dentinogenesis imperfecta and hearing loss often occur. Severe kyphoscoliosis sometimes leads to respiratory compromise. Autosomal dominant, in most cases the result of dominant mutations in one of the two genes, COL1A1 and COL1A2 that encode the pro-α-1(I) and pro-α-2(I) chains of type I collagen. A rare autosomal recessive variety has also been described that may be the most common form of osteogenesis imperfecta in South African blacks.

Type IV. An autosomal dominant disorder associated with normal to moderately short stature with significant bone deformity, normal sclera, femoral bowing in the newborn period that straightens with time, and often dentinogenesis imperfecta. Mutations at both COL1A1 and COL1A2 loci can lead to type IV.

References

Freda, V. J., Vosburgh, G. J., and Di Liberti, C.: Osteogenesis imperfecta congenita. A presentation of 16 cases and review of the literature. Obstet. Gynecol., *18*:535, 1961.

Sillence, D. O., Senn, A., and Danks, D. H.: Genetic heterogeneity in osteogenesis imperfecta. J. Med. Genet., *16*:101, 1979.

Byers, P. H., Bonadio, J. F., and Steinmann, B.: Invited editorial comment: Osteogenesis imperfecta: Update and perspective. Am. J. Med. Genet., *17*:429, 1984.

Sillence, D. O., et al.: Osteogenesis imperfecta type III. Delineation of the phenotype with reference to genetic heterogeneity. Am. J. Med. Genet., *23*:821, 1986.

Byers, P. H.: Osteogenesis imperfecta: An update. Growth Genet. Horm., *4*:1, 1988.

Willing, M. C., et al.: Osteogenesis type I is commonly due to a COL1A1 null allele of type I collagen. Am. J. Hum. Genet., *51*:508, 1992.

Molyneux, K., et al.: A single amino acid deletion in the α-2(I) chain of type I collagen produces osteogenesis imperfecta type III. Hum. Genet., *90*:621, 1993.

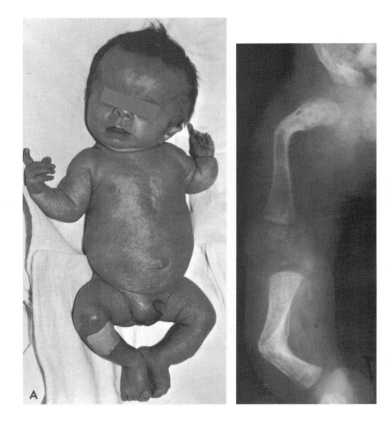

FIGURE 1. Osteogenesis imperfecta syndrome, type I. *A*, A 2-month-old. Length, 19 inches; blue sclerae, inguinal hernia, hepatosplenomegaly.

FIGURE 2. *B,* A 17-month-old with a third fracture that was healing well by 18 months. Note the thin cortices and the ground glass, "washed-out" appearance of the bone.

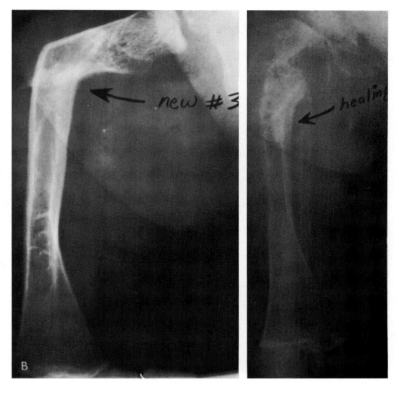

OSTEOGENESIS IMPERFECTA SYNDROME, TYPE II

(Osteogenesis Imperfecta Congenita, Vrolik Disease)

Short Broad Long Bones, Multiple Fractures, Blue Sclerae

A perinatally lethal variety of osteogenesis imperfecta, this disorder is characterized by short limbs, short, broad long bones, radiologic evidence of severe osseous fragility, and defective ossification. Based on subtle differences in radiographic features, Sillence et al. have subdivided this disorder into three groups. Type A is characterized by short, broad crumpled femora and continuously beaded ribs; type B by short, broad crumpled femora but normal ribs or ribs with incomplete beading; and type C by long, thin, inadequately modeled, rectangular long bones with multiple fractures and thin, beaded ribs.

ABNORMALITIES
Growth. Prenatal short-limbed growth deficiency.

Craniofacial. Poorly mineralized, soft calvarium with large fontanels and multiple wormian bones. Deep blue sclerae, shallow orbits, small nose, low nasal bridge.

Limbs. Short, thick, ribbon-like, poorly mineralized long bones with multiple fractures and callus formation, especially in lower limbs.

Other. Flattened vertebrae, hypotonia, inguinal hernias, variable hydrocephalus. Hydrops.

NATURAL HISTORY. These patients usually are stillborn or die in early infancy of respiratory failure.

ETIOLOGY. In virtually all cases, this disorder is due to a dominant mutation in one of the two type I collagen genes (COL1A1 or COL1A2). The majority of cases of type II osteogenesis imperfecta are the result of sporadic mutations of an autosomal dominant gene. For these cases, a recurrence rate of about 6 per cent has been observed and is felt to be the result of parental germ cell mutation. Autosomal recessive inheritance has been implicated for the rare osteogenesis imperfecta type II B and osteogenesis imperfecta type II C.

References

Sillence, D. O., et al.: Osteogenesis imperfecta, type II. Delineation of the phenotype with reference to genetic heterogeneity. Am. J. Med. Genet., 17:407, 1984.

Spranger, J.: Invited editorial comment: Osteogenesis imperfecta: A pasture for splitters and lumpers. Am. J. Med. Genet., 17:425, 1984.

Byers, P. H., Bonadio, J. F., and Steinmann, B.: Invited editorial comment: Osteogenesis imperfecta. Update and perspective. Am. J. Med. Genet., 17:429, 1984.

Horwitz, A. L., Lazda, V., and Byers, P. H.: Recurrent type II (lethal) osteogenesis imperfecta: Apparent dominant inheritance. Am. J. Hum. Genet., 37:A59, 1985.

Tsipouras, P., et al.: Osteogenesis imperfecta type II is usually due to new dominant gene. Am. J. Hum. Genet., 37:A79, 1985.

Byers, P. H., et al.: Perinatal lethal osteogenesis imperfecta (OI type II): A biochemically heterogeneous disorder usually due to new mutations in the gene for type I collagen. Am. J. Hum. Genet., 42:237, 1988.

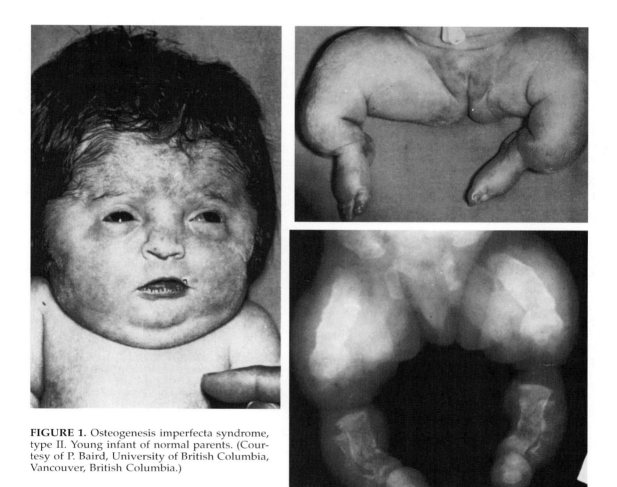

FIGURE 1. Osteogenesis imperfecta syndrome, type II. Young infant of normal parents. (Courtesy of P. Baird, University of British Columbia, Vancouver, British Columbia.)

FIBRODYSPLASIA OSSIFICANS PROGRESSIVA SYNDROME

Short Hallux, Fibrous Dysplasia Leading to Ossification in Muscles and Subcutaneous Tissues

This condition, described in a letter by Guy Patin in 1692, was extensively reviewed by Rosenstirn in 1918. More than 500 cases have been reported.

ABNORMALITIES

Digits. Short hallux, often with synostosis. Less frequently, short thumb.

Fibrous Tissues. Swellings, sometimes with pain and fever, in aponeuroses, fasciae, and tendons, leading to ossification in muscles and fibrous tissue; most prominent in neck, dorsal trunk, and proximal limbs, with sternocleidomastoid and masseters frequently involved.

Other. Progressive cervical vertebral spine fusion. Scoliosis.

OCCASIONAL ABNORMALITIES. Short phalanges other than hallux or thumb, clinodactyly of fifth finger, short femoral neck, flat broadened mandibular condyle, hip synovial osteochondromatosis, hernia. Widely spaced teeth. Hypogenitalism and/or delayed sexual development. Easy bruising. Hearing loss. Cardiac conduction abnormalities.

NATURAL HISTORY. The unusual fibrodysplasia leading to ossification may become evident during fetal life or as late as 25 years, with most patients experiencing onset at 5 years. Ossification is usually evident within 2 to 8 months of the time swelling occurs. Eighty per cent of patients develop some restrictive heterotopic ossification by 7 years, and by the age of 15 more than 95 per cent develop severely restricted mobility of their arms. The most common locations for the initial heterotopic ossification are the neck, spine, and shoulder. Areas with lower risk include the wrists, ankles, and jaw. Diaphragm, tongue, extraocular, facial, and cardiac muscles are usually spared. No effective treatment has been discovered, although symptomatic relief of pain may be achieved by salicylates or hydrocortisone analogue therapy. The natural history tends toward exacerbation and remission, and therefore, the results of therapy should be interpreted with caution. Another matter for caution is the interpretation of biopsies from affected tissues. The pathologic interpretation may be osteogenic sarcoma, although such a malignant growth is not a feature of this disease. Furthermore, any kind of trauma, including biopsy, surgery, and/or intramuscular injection, can be a focus for an area of ectopic ossification. Problems with anesthesia including difficulties with tracheal intubation, restrictive pulmonary disease, and abnormalities of cardiac conduction have occurred.

ETIOLOGY. Autosomal dominant with almost full penetrance for short hallux and varying expression for the fibrodysplasia. About 90 per cent of patients represent fresh mutations, for which older paternal age has been noted as a factor.

COMMENT. Although the fundamental defect in fibrous tissue is unknown, it is obvious that it allows for ossification to normal-appearing bone in tissues in which ossification normally would not occur.

References

Rosenstirn, J.: A contribution to the study of myositis ossificans progressiva. Ann. Surg., *68*:485, 1918.

Tünte, W., Becker, P. E., and v. Knorr, G.: Zur Genetik der Myositis ossificans progressiva. Humangenetik, *4*:320, 1967.

Rogers, I. G., and Geho, W. B.: Fibrodysplasia ossificans progressiva. J. Bone Joint Surg. [Am.], *61*:909, 1979.

Newton, M. C., et al.: Fibrodysplasia ossificans progressiva. B. J. Anaesth., *64*:246, 1990.

Cohen, R. B., et al.: The natural history of heterotopic ossification in patients who have fibrodysplasia ossificans progressiva. J. Bone Joint Surg. [Am.], *75*: 215, 1993.

Rocke, D. M., et al.: Age and joint-specific risk of initial heterotopic ossification in patients who have fibrodysplasia ossificans progressiva. Clin. Orthop., *301*:243, 1994.

Shah, P. B., et al.: Spinal deformity in patients who have fibrodysplasia ossificans progressiva. J. Bone Joint Surg. [Am.], *76*:1442, 1994.

FIGURE 1. Fibrodysplasia ossificans progressiva syndrome. A 13-year-old showing progressive ossification in back musculature and short valgus hallux.

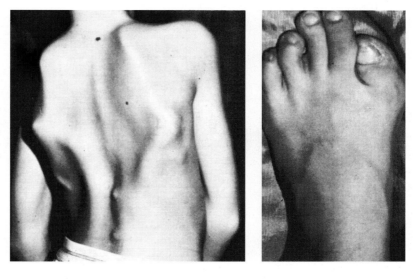

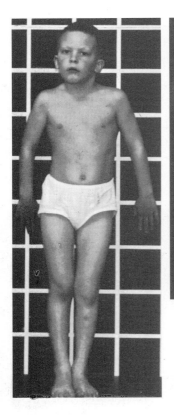

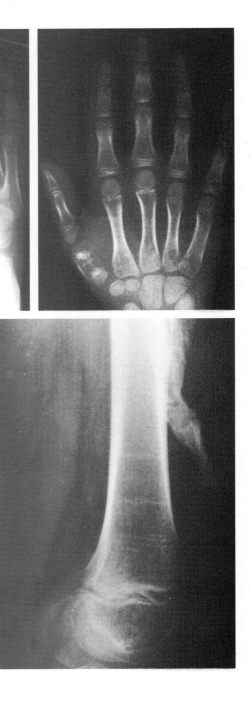

FIGURE 2. Fibrodysplasia ossificans progressiva syndrome. A 7-year-old with secondary torticollis, scoliosis, and partial contractures at elbow, hip, and knee joints. Note the short and deformed first metatarsal, hallux, and first metacarpal. Aberrant ossification is evident in the lower thigh. (From Herrmann, J., et al.: Birth Defects, 5(5): 1969. Courtesy of Dr. John M. Opitz, Helena, Mont.)

P

P. HAMARTOSES

STURGE-WEBER SEQUENCE

*Flat Facial Hemangiomata,
Meningeal Hemangiomata With Seizures*

The association and localization of aberrant vasculature in the facial skin, eyes, and meninges are compatible with a defect arising in a limited part of the cephalic neural crest, cells of which migrate to the supraocular dermis, choroid, and pia mater.

ABNORMALITIES

Facial. Pink to purplish red nonelevated cutaneous hemangiomata, most commonly in a trigeminal facial distribution, sometimes involving the choroid of the eye with secondary buphthalmos and/or glaucoma as well as the conjunctiva or episcleral region. Involvement usually unilateral, is sometimes bilateral.

Meninges and Central Nervous System. Hemangiomata of arachnoid and pia mater, especially in occipital and temporal areas with secondary cerebral cortical atrophy, sclerosis, and "double contour" convolutional calcification. Seizures, paresis, mental deficiency.

OCCASIONAL ABNORMALITIES. Hemangiomatosis in nonfacial areas, CNS, and other tissues. Klippel-Trenaunay-Weber syndrome. Macrocephaly. Cavernous hemangiomata. Colobomata of iris, retinal vasculature tortuosity, iris heterochromia, retinal detachment, and strabismus. Coarctation of aorta, abnormal external ears.

NATURAL HISTORY. The surface cutaneous hemangiomata are usually present at birth and seldom progress. Seizures most commonly begin between 2 and 7 months of age and are grand mal in type, often asymmetric. The degree of CNS involvement is variable, with 30 per cent having paresis and 56 per cent having seizures; 39 per cent have normal intelligence. Cerebral calcification is usually not evident by radiography until later infancy, the earliest occurring in a patient 13 months of age, first being noted in the occipital region.

Medical anticonvulsant treatment is of limited value, and occasionally, partial extirpation of affected meninges, brain tissue, or both may be merited in unilateral cases as a measure to control the seizures. The presence of seizure activity in the first year of life is associated with a very poor outcome with respect to intellectual performance and independent living. Glaucoma presents before 2 years of age if tissues destined to form the anterior chamber angle are affected. If conjunctival and episcleral vascular tissues are involved, glaucoma frequently does not occur until after 5 years of age.

ETIOLOGY. Unknown. Sporadic, with rare exceptions. Occasionally, other family members may have hemangiomata of a lesser degree.

COMMENT. Port-wine facial nevi occur frequently without eye or brain abnormalities. Only patients with lesions involving the opthalmic distribution of the trigeminal nerve are at risk for neuro-ocular complications.

References

Chaeo, D. H.-C.: Congenital neurocutaneous syndromes of childhood. III. Sturge-Weber disease. J. Pediatr., 55:635, 1959.

Butterworth, T., and Strean, L. P.: Clinical Genodermatology. Baltimore, Williams & Wilkins Co., 1962.

Enolras, O., Riche, M. C., and Merland, J. J.: Facial port-wine stains and Sturge-Weber syndrome. Pediatrics, 76:48, 1985.

Oakes, W. J.: The natural history of patients with the Sturge-Weber syndrome. Pediatr. Neurosurg., 18: 287, 1992.

Sullivan, T. J., et al.: The ocular manifestation of the Sturge-Weber syndrome. J. Pediatr. Ophthalmol. Strabismus, 29:349, 1992.

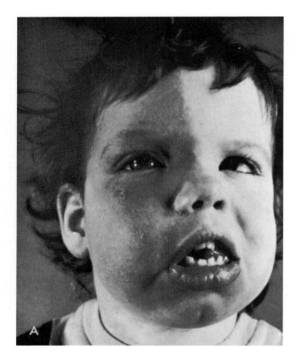

FIGURE 1. Sturge-Weber sequence. *A,* Affected child who has had grand mal seizures.

FIGURE 1. *Continued. B,* Note the fine mineralization (*left*), which tends to reflect the convolutional pattern of the brain.

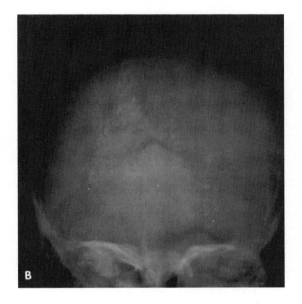

NEUROCUTANEOUS MELANOSIS SEQUENCE

Melanosis of Skin and Pia-arachnoid, Central Nervous System Deterioration

This melanocytic hamartomatosis of the skin and pia-arachnoid was first described in 1861. More than 100 cases have been reported.

ABNORMALITIES

Skin. Giant pigmented nevi (66 per cent) usually in a "bathing trunk" or lumbosacral distribution; less frequently in the occipital region or upper back. Numerous congenital nevi without a prominent large lesion (34 per cent). Associated small or medium-sized congenital melanocytic nevi on the scalp, face, or neck occur in association with the larger lesions.

Pia-arachnoid. Thick and pigmented with nests and sheets of melanotic cells, 88 per cent with cranial involvement and 88 per cent with spinal involvement. Leptomeningeal melanoma.

Central Nervous System. Liable to development of seizures and deterioration of CNS function. Hydrocephalus secondary to blockage of cisternal pathways or obliteration of arachnoid villi by the tumor. Involvement of spinal cord and its coverings. Cranial nerve palsies, particularly VI and VII.

OCCASIONAL ABNORMALITIES. Syringomyelia. Psychosis. Meckel diverticulum. Urinary tract anomalies including renal pelvis and ureteral malformations, unilateral renal cysts, rhabdomyosarcoma. Extracranial melanoma probably representing metastases from meningeal melanoma.

NATURAL HISTORY. The cutaneous melanosis is grossly evident at birth. Central nervous system function may be normal initially, but seizures and mental deterioration may begin before 1 year of age, apparently related to progression of the melanoblastic involvement of the pia-arachnoid, leading to increased intracranial pressure, spinal cord compression, and to diffuse or localized malignancy that occurs in greater than 50 per cent of patients.

The CNS consequences of the disorder often result in early demise. Three of the recognized patients were stillborn; the majority died before 2 years of age, and only 10 per cent of the patients are known to have survived past the age of 25 years. The interval between the age at initial presentation and death ranges from immediate to 21 years, with more than one half occurring within 3 years of initial diagnosis. Although the frequency of leptomeningeal involvement in children with giant hairy nevi is unknown, patients without nevi on the head or neck or the posterior midline rarely develop neurologic complications.

The risk of malignant melanoma degeneration of the cutaneous melanosis is said to be 10 to 13 per cent, with half becoming evident by 5 years of age. Thus, surgery to reduce the skin lesions is indicated in patients in whom careful evaluation has documented a lack of leptomeningeal involvement.

ETIOLOGY. Sporadic, cause unknown. Presumed to be an aberration in growth of early melanoblasts of neural crest origin, which contribute to the skin and pia-arachnoid. The sex incidence has been equal, and a family history of melanomata was noted in only one case.

References

Rokitansky, J.: Ein ausgezeichneter Fall von Pigment-mal mit ausgebreiteter Pigmentirung der inneren Hirn- und Rückenmarkshäute. Allg. Wien Med. Ztg., *6*:113, 1861.

Van Bogaert, L.: La Mélanose neurocutanée diffuse hérédofamiale. Bull. Acad. R. Med. Belg. (6th Series), *13*:397, 1948.

Fox, H., et al.: Neurocutaneous melanosis. Arch. Dis. Child., *39*:508, 1964.

Hoffman, H. J., and Freeman, A.: Primary malignant leptomeningeal melanoma in association with giant hairy nevus. J. Neurosurg., *26*:62, 1967.

Kadonaga, J. H., and Frieden, I. J.: Neurocutaneous melanosis: Definition and review of literature. J. Am. Acad. Dermatol., *24*:747, 1991.

Frieden, I. J., et al.: Giant congenital melanocytic nevi: Brain magnetic resonance findings in neurologically asymptomatic children. J. Am. Acad. Dermatol., *31*:423, 1994.

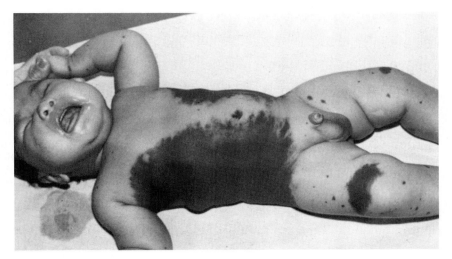

FIGURE 1. Neurocutaneous melanosis sequence. Infant who as yet shows no signs of CNS involvement. (Courtesy of S. Bintliff, Kauikeolani Children's Hospital, Honolulu, Hawaii.)

LINEAR SEBACEOUS NEVUS SEQUENCE
(Nevus Sebaceus of Jadassohn, Epidermal Nevus Syndrome)

Midfacial Nevus Sebaceus, Seizures, Mental Deficiency

Nevus sebaceous of Jadassohn is most commonly found in an otherwise normal individual. However, the association of this type of lesion in the midfacial area with seizures and mental deficiency has been reported in at least 100 cases.

ABNORMALITIES
Growth. Asymmetric overgrowth. Advanced bone age.

Skin. Nevus sebaceous with hyperpigmentation and hyperkeratosis. Lesions most commonly in the midfacial area, from the forehead down into the nasal area, tending to be linear in distribution. May also affect trunk and limbs.

Central Nervous System. Seizures of major motor, focal, or minor motor types. Mental deficiency.

OCCASIONAL ABNORMALITIES
Skeletal. Cranial asymmetry or hemimacrocephaly. Premature closure of sphenoid frontal sutures, sphenoid bone malformation, and abnormalities of sella turcica. Scoliosis, kyphosis, abnormalities of ulna, head of radius, humerus, and fibula. Polydactyly. Syndactyly. Vitamin D–resistant rickets.

Eyes. Esotropia, lipodermoid of conjunctiva, cloudy cornea, colobomata of eyelid, coloboma of iris disk and choroid, atrophy of optic nerve, subretinal neovascularization. Microphthalmia.

Central Nervous System. Micro- and/or macrocephaly. Cerebral and cerebellar hypoplasia, arachnoid cysts, hydrocephalus. Hemiparesis. Cranial nerve palsy. Cortical blindness. Hypertonia. Cerebral vascular changes. Intracerebral calcifications. Cerebral neoplasia/hamartoma.

Other. Short palpebral fissures. Pigmented nevi, spotty alopecia, coarctation of aorta, patent ductus arteriosus, hypoplastic left heart, ventricular septal defect, cardiac arrhythmias, hypoplasia of renal and/or pulmonary artery, cleft palate, hypoplastic teeth. Renal hamartomata, nephroblastoma. Double urinary collecting system. Horseshoe kidneys. Enlarged clitoris. Undescended testes. Cystic biliary adenoma of liver. Dental anomalies.

NATURAL HISTORY. The nevus sebaceous is usually present at birth as a slightly yellow to orange to tan waxy appearing lesion containing deficiencies and/or papillomatous excesses of epidermal elements, especially sebaceous glands and immature hair follicles. With time, the lesions tend to become verrucous and unsightly.

Early surgical removal should be considered, since there is a 15 to 20 per cent risk of tumor, especially basal cell epithelioma. Furthermore, there may be unpredictable periods of rapid growth of the lesions. In the cases with associated CNS features, the onset of seizures has been from 2 months to 2 years, and they are difficult to control. The mental deficiency has been moderate to severe, though an occasional patient may have normal intelligence. The vitamin D–resistant rickets that sometimes occurs is a variant of tumor-induced osteomalacia. The associated rickety lesions, muscle weakness, and bone pain, as well as the biochemical abnormalities (hypophosphatemia, a low renal tubular maximum for reabsorption of inorganic phosphate, a decreased circulating 1,25 dihydroxy vitamin D level, and a normal or elevated serum 25 hydroxy vitamin D concentration) reverse following surgical removal of the skin lesions. If that is impossible, successful treatment has been accomplished with the continued use of calcitriol and phosphorus.

ETIOLOGY. Unknown. Whether this constitutes a single etiologic entity remains to be determined. Bianchine noted seizures and/or mental deficiency without skin lesions in several first-degree relatives of one patient. Hence, a cautious family evaluation is indicated in cases of this clinical disorder.

References

Mehregan, A. H., and Pinkus, H.: Life history of organoid nevi. Special reference to nevus sebaceus of Jadassohn. Arch. Dermatol., 91:574, 1965.

Marden, P. M., and Venters, H. D.: A new neurocutaneous syndrome. Am. J. Dis. Child., 112:79, 1966.

Bianchine, J. W.: The nevus sebaceus of Jadassohn. A neurocutaneous syndrome and a potentially premalignant lesion. Am. J. Dis. Child., 120:223, 1970.

Lansky, L. L., et al.: Linear sebaceous nevus syndrome. Am. J. Dis. Child., 123:587, 1972.

Leonidas, J. C., et al.: Radiographic features of the linear sebaceous syndrome. Am. J. Roentgenol., 132: 277, 1979.

Carey, D. E., et al.: Hypophosphatemic rickets/osteomalacia in linear sebaceous nevus syndrome: A variant of tumor-induced osteomalacia. J. Pediatr., 109: 994, 1986.

Alfonso, I., et al.: Linear nevus sebaceous syndrome: A review. J. Clin. Neuroophthalmol., 7:170, 1987.

Grebe, T. A., et al.: Further delineation of the epidermal nevus syndrome: Two cases with new findings and literature review. Am. J. Med. Genet., 47:24, 1993.

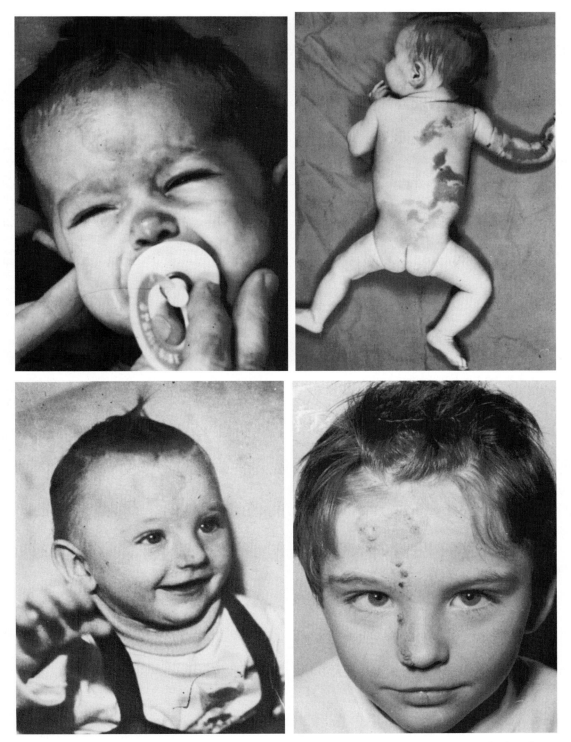

FIGURE 1. Linear sebaceous nevus sequence. *Above,* A 2-week-old with facial and extensive body sebaceous nevi. Intractable seizures began at 5 months, and the patient died at 9 months with pneumonia. Necropsy revealed renal nodular nephronoblastomatosis. (From Lansky, L. L., et al.: Am. J. Dis. Child., *123*:587, 1972, with permission.) *Below,* Verrucous change in sebaceous nevus from infancy to older childhood. (From Bianchine, J. W.: Am. J. Dis. Child., *120*:223, 1970, with permission.)

INCONTINENTIA PIGMENTI SYNDROME

(Bloch-Sulzberger Syndrome)

Irregular Pigmented Skin Lesions With or Without Dental Anomaly, Patchy Alopecia

Bardach originally described the condition in twin sisters in 1925, and soon thereafter Bloch set forth the term incontinentia pigmenti to depict the unusual skin lesions. A major review of 635 cases by Carney includes only 16 affected males.

ABNORMALITIES

Skin. Most consistent feature. Blisters, preceded by erythema, develop typically in a linear distribution along the limbs and around the trunk within the first few weeks. As the blisters begin to heal, hyperkeratotic lesions develop on the distal limbs and scalp and rarely on the trunk or face. Hyperpigmentation, most apparent on the trunk distributed along lines of Blaschko, occur in streaks and whorls, usually developing after the blisters have disappeared. Pale, hairless patches or streaks most evident on the lower legs develop usually at the time the hyperpigmentation disappears.

Dentition. Eighty per cent have hypodontia, delayed eruption, and/or conical form.

Hair. Fifty per cent have minor abnormalities. Atrophic patchy alopecia, especially on the posterior scalp at the vertex, is common. Lusterless, wiry, coarse hair as well as thin, sparse hair in early childhood.

Nails. Abnormalities in 40 per cent ranging from mild ridging or pitting to severe nail disruption.

Central Nervous System. About one third have mental deficiency, microcephaly, spasticity, and/or seizures.

Eyes. About 30 per cent have strabismus, often with refractive errors. Abnormalities of the retinal vessels and underlying pigment cells in 40 per cent leading to retinal ischemia, new vessel proliferation, bleeding, and fibrosis. Retinal detachment, ureitis, keratitis, cataract, microphthalmos, and optic atrophy occur infrequently.

Osseous. About 20 per cent have hemivertebrae, kyphoscoliosis, extra rib, syndactyly, hemiatrophy, and/or short arms and legs.

OCCASIONAL ABNORMALITIES. Nail dystrophy, breast hypoplasia, abnormalities in nipple pigmentation, supernumerary nipple, nipple hypoplasia, dacryostenosis, eczema, short stature, hydrocephalus. Subungual keratotic tumors.

NATURAL HISTORY. Bullous skin lesions are generally present in early infancy and tend to progress from inflammatory or vesicular to pigmented and may fade in childhood. General eosinophilia is often present in infancy and the vesicles contain eosinophils. Verrucous lichenoid lesions develop during infancy in about one third of cases, especially over the dorsum of the hands and feet. During the period when the blisters are present, the lesions should be kept dry and protected from trauma. The development of the irregular marble cake–like pigmentation may or may not coincide with the sites of bullous or verrucous lesions. The pigmented areas gradually fade in the second to third decades, and the adult may show only slightly atrophic depigmented "achromic stains," especially over the lower legs. Since the retinal vascular changes sometimes progress during the neonatal period, monthly ophthalmologic evaluations are recommended during the first 2 to 3 months of life. In approximately 10 per cent of cases, this process progresses to severe scarring with significant visual loss. About one half of the patients show other features, the most serious being the CNS abnormalities. Seizures in the neonatal period represent an ominous sign relative to future neurologic development. In their absence, prognosis is, in most cases, good.

ETIOLOGY. Family studies suggest X-linked dominance with lethality in affected males. The ratio of females to males in affected sibships is 2:1, with one half of the females affected. Several studies have confirmed linkage of familial incontinentia pigmenti to Xq28. The parents, especially the mother, should be closely examined for residual skin lesions, including achromatic spots, before genetic counseling is rendered.

References

Bardach, M.: Systematisierte Naevusbildungen bei einem cineiigen Zwillingspaar. Ein Beitrag zur Naevusätiologie. Z. Kinderheilkd., 39:542, 1925.

Bloch, B.: Eigentümliche bisher nicht beschriebene Pigmentaffektion (Incontinentia pigmenti). Schweiz. Med. Wochenschr., 56:404, 1926.

Carney, R. G.: Incontinentia pigmenti, a world statistical analysis. Arch. Dermatol., 112:535, 1976.

Sefiani, A., et al.: The gene for incontinentia pigmenti is assigned to Xq28. Genomics, 4:427, 1989.

Landy, S. J., and Donnai, D.: Incontinentia pigmenti (Bloch-Sulzberger syndrome). J. Med. Genet., 30:53, 1993.

Sybert, V. P.: Incontinentia pigmenti nomenclature. Am. J. Hum. Genet., 55:209, 1994.

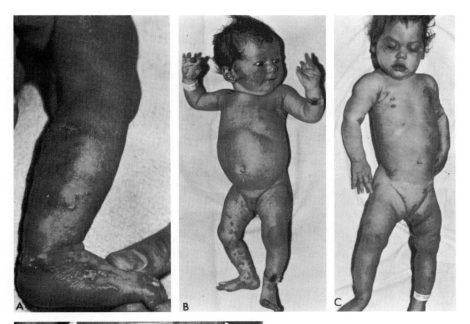

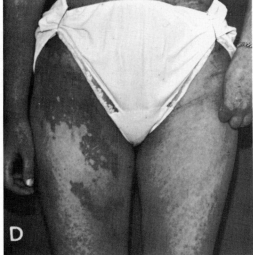

FIGURE 1. Incontinentia pigmenti syndromes. *A,* Early lesions in the young infant shown in *B. C,* Older mentally deficient infant with reticular pigmentation. *D,* Mentally deficient woman with spasticity and pseudogliomatous retinal detachment, showing advanced skin pigmentary change. *E,* Minor abnormalities of dentition in an affected girl. *F,* Reticular pigmentation in a 3-year-old mentally deficient girl. (*A* to *E* courtesy of J. M. Opitz, Helena, Mont.)

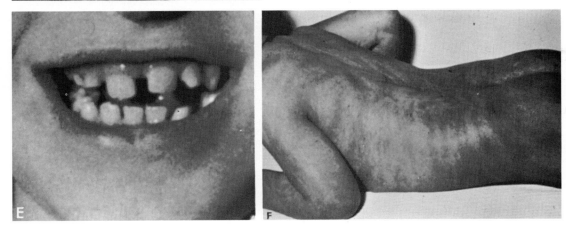

HYPOMELANOSIS OF ITO

(Incontinentia Pigmentosa Achromians)

Initially described by Ito in 1952, numerous affected individuals subsequently have been reported. The characteristic skin lesions involve streaked, whorled, or mottled areas of hypopigmentation on limbs and/or trunk usually evident in infancy. It is now clear that hypomelanosis of Ito is not a specific disorder, but is an etiologically heterogeneous physical finding that is frequently indicative of chromosomal or genetic mosaicism. Approximately 70 per cent of reported cases have associated anomalies. With the exception of mental retardation (67 per cent), seizures (35 per cent), and cerebral atrophy (16 per cent), all other associated abnormalities have occurred in less than 8 per cent.

ASSOCIATED ABNORMALITIES

Central Nervous System. Variable mental retardation, seizures, neurologic problems.

Craniofacies. Macrocephaly. Coarse facies. Hypertelorism. Epicanthal folds. Thick lips. Cleft lip/palate. Malformed auricles.

Eyes. Iridial heterochromia. Abnormal retinal pigmentation. Strabismus.

Hair, Teeth. Hypertrichosis. Diffuse alopecia. Dysplasia of teeth. Irregularly spaced teeth.

Limbs. Clinodactyly. Syndactyly. Ectrodactyly. Polydactyly. Triphalangeal thumb. Genu valga.

Skeletal. Kyphoscoliosis/lordosis. Short stature.

NATURAL HISTORY. The skin lesions, which are best appreciated by a Wood lamp examination, do not go through a prodrome phase as in incontinentia pigmenti. The prognosis depends on the type and extent of associated abnormalities.

ETIOLOGY. Hypomelanosis of Ito is etiologically heterogeneous. Karyotyping of characteristic skin findings to rule out chromosomal mosaicism when developmental delay or structural anomalies are also present is indicated. Recurrence risk is low except in those chromosomally abnormal individuals in which a balanced parental translocation is present. A single-gene basis for hypomelanosis of Ito probably does not exist.

References

Ito, M.: Studies on melanin XI. Incontinentia pigmenti; achromians. Tohoku J. Exp. Med., *55*(Suppl.):57, 1952.

Ritter, C. L., et al.: Chromosome mosaicism in hypomelanosis of Ito. Am. J. Med. Genet., *35*:14, 1990.

Flannery, D. B.: Pigmentary dysplasia: Hypomelanosis of Ito, and genetic mosaicism. Am. J. Med. Genet., *35*:18, 1990.

Sybert, V. P., et al.: Pigmentary abnormalities and mosaicism for chromosomal aberration: Association with clinical features similar to hypomelanosis of Ito. J. Pediatr., *116*:581, 1990.

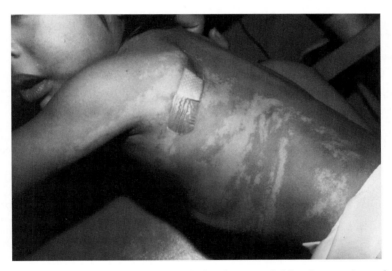

FIGURE 1. Hypomelanosis of Ito. A 14-month-old with developmental delay, hypotonia, and seizures. Note the irregular, streaky distribution of hypopigmentation. (Courtesy of Dr. Marilyn Jones, University of California, San Diego, Calif.)

TUBEROUS SCLEROSIS SYNDROME
(Adenoma Sebaceum)

*Hamartomatous Skin Nodules,
Seizures, Phakomata, Bone Lesions*

Von Recklinghausen is said to have described this disease, but Bourneville is usually given credit for its recognition in 1880. Hamartomatous lesions develop in many tissues, especially the skin and brain. Diagnostic criteria have been set forth by the National Tuberous Sclerosis Association.

ABNORMALITIES
Brain and Eyes. Glioma-angioma lesions in cortex and white matter, with seizures (93 per cent) and mental deficiency (62 per cent) as apparent consequences. Behavioral problems and autism. Roentgenographic evidence of intracranial mineralization (51 per cent), most commonly in basal ganglia or periventricular region. However, the periventricular lesions may be noted early in the clinical course by CT scan as one of the most consistent features. Hamartomas of retina or optic nerve in 53 per cent; in half of these, the hamartomas are bilateral.

Skin. Fibrous-angiomatous lesions (83 per cent), varying in color from flesh to pink to yellow to brown, develop in the nasolabial fold, cheeks, and elsewhere. White macules classified into three types: "Thumb-print" macules, "lance-ovate" macules (one end rounded, the other with a sharp tip) or ash leaf macule, and the confetti macules (tiny 1- to 3-mm macules). Café au lait spots. Fibromatous plaques and nodules.

Bone. Cyst-like areas in phalanges (66 per cent) and elsewhere, with areas of periosteal thickening yielding roentgenographic evidence of "sclerosis."

Renal. Angiomyolipomata in 45 to 81 per cent, usually multiple and benign. Tubular enlargement and cyst formation with hyperplasia of tubular cells.

Dentition. Pit-shaped enamel defects, most evident by close inspection of labial premolar surfaces.

OCCASIONAL ABNORMALITIES.
Other hamartomata: fibromata (especially gingival and subungual), lipomata, angiomata, nevi, shagreen patches (goose flesh–like). Rhabdomyomata and angiomata of heart, cystic changes in lung, hamartomata of liver and pancreas. Hamartomatous rectal polyps, hypothyroidism, thyroid adenomata. Sexual precocity. Astrocytoma.

NATURAL HISTORY. Hamartomata usually become evident in early childhood and may increase at adolescence. Facial nodular lesions are present in 50 per cent of children by 5 years, whereas white macules are present at birth or in early infancy in almost all patients, and are easily visualized with help of the Wood lamp. Malignant transformation may occur, and about 6 per cent of patients develop a brain tumor. However, malignant transformation of the periventricular nodules is rare. The seizures, which tend to develop in early childhood, may initially be myoclonic and later grand mal in type and are difficult to control. Electroencephalographic abnormality is found in 87 per cent of patients and may be of the grossly disorganized hypsarrhythmic pattern. The seizures and mental defect seem to be related to the extent of hamartomatous change in the brain. For those with mental deficiency, 100 per cent have seizures, 88 per cent by 5 years of age; whereas of those without serious mental deficiency, 69 per cent have seizures, 44 per cent by 5 years of age. Mental deterioration is unusual, except in relation to frequent seizures of status epilepticus.

An unknown percentage of patients die prior to 20 years of age as the consequence of status epilepticus, general debility, pneumonia, or tumor. It should be appreciated that there is wide variability in expression of the disease; all patients with skin lesions do not develop seizures, mental deficiency, or both, and the earlier noted pattern of abnormality is biased toward the more severe cases. One general survey showed a 69 per cent incidence of mental deficiency. However, of the nine patients diagnosed at a hospital for skin diseases, none were mentally deficient, whereas 93 per cent of those admitted to a children's hospital were mentally deficient.

ETIOLOGY. Autosomal dominant, with about 86 per cent representing fresh mutations from unaffected parents. Two genetic loci have been identified for tuberous sclerosis using linkage analysis: one on 9q34 and one on 16p13. There are no differences in the incidence of mental retardation, periungual fibromas, or facial angiofibromas among individuals in the different linkage groups. Affected individuals usually show some manifestations of the disorder by adulthood. A search for depigmented spots and/or hairs, enamel defects, and subungual hamartomas, as well as CT scan for periventricular lesions and renal ultrasound for angiomyolipomas should be considered in first-degree relatives of affected individuals prior to genetic counseling.

References

Bourneville, D.: Sclereuse tubereuse des circonvolutions cerebrales. Idiote et epilepsie hemiplegique. Arch. Neurol. (Paris), 1:81, 1880.

Lagos, J. C., and Gomez, M. R.: Tuberous sclerosis: Reappraisal of a clinical entity. Mayo Clin. Proc., 42: 26, 1967.

Bundey, S., and Evans, K.: Tuberous sclerosis: A genetic study. J. Neurol. Neurosurg. Psychiatry, 32:591, 1969.

Hoff, M., et al.: Enamel defects associated with tuberous sclerosis. Oral Surg., 40:261, 1976.

Kenishi, Y., et al.: Tuberous sclerosis. Early neurologic manifestations and CT features in 18 patients. Brain Dev., 1:31, 1979.

Shepherd, C. W., et al.: Causes of death in patients with tuberous sclerosis. Mayo Clin. Proc., 66:792, 1991.

Roach, E. S., et al.: Diagnostic criteria: Tuberous sclerosis complex. Report of the diagnostic criteria committee of the National Tuberous Sclerosis Association. J. Clin. Neurol., 7:221, 1992.

Janniger, C. K., and Schwartz, R. A.: Tuberous sclerosis: Recent advances for the clinician. Cutis, 51:167, 1993.

Povey, S., et al.: Two loci for tuberous sclerosis: One on 9q34 and one of 16p13. Ann. Hum. Genet., 58: 107, 1994.

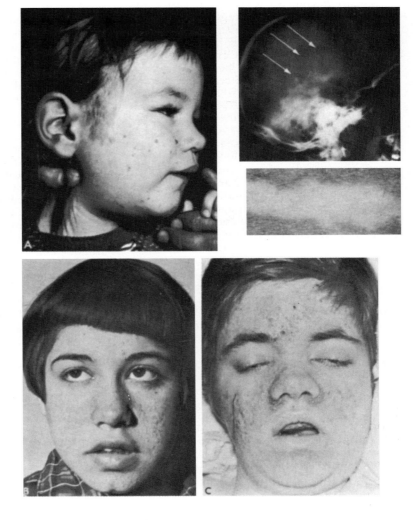

FIGURE 1. Tuberous sclerosis syndrome. *A*, A 2-year-old with early pink to red nodular and flat skin lesions and seizures. *B*, Girl with mental deficiency and seizures. *C*, Young woman with mental deficiency and seizures, on Dilantin (phenytoin) therapy. (*B* and *C* courtesy of L. Dobbs, Rainier State Training School, Buckley, Wash.) *Upper right*, Skull roentgenogram showing periventricular calcification and skin showing depigmented "ash leaf" lesions. (Courtesy of Michael M. Cohen, J., D.D.S., Dalhousie University, Halifax, Nova Scotia.)

NEUROFIBROMATOSIS SYNDROME

Multiple Neurofibromata, Café au Lait Spots, With or Without Bone Lesions

Von Recklinghausen described this disease in 1882. It is estimated to affect 1 in 3500 individuals.

ABNORMALITIES

Skin. Areas of hyper- or hypopigmentation with café au lait spots in 94 per cent. Roughly three fourths of affected individuals have six or more spots measuring 1.5 cm or greater in size, most commonly on trunk. Rarely present at birth, they occur in 80 per cent by 1 year of age and 100 per cent by 4 years. "Freckling" in axilla, inguinal folds, and perineum are common after 3 years of age.

Tumors. Benign tumors consisting of extracellular matrix, Schwann-like cells, fibroblasts, mast cells, endothelial cells, and perineural cells that arise from the peripheral nervous system. Cutaneous neurofibromas are usually small, raised, soft, pigmented nodules. Plexiform neurofibromas, which occur along nerve bundle tracts, can be large and appear at birth or in early childhood.

Other. Lisch nodules or pigmented iris hamartomata (95 per cent after 6 years; 100 per cent after 20 years). Macrocephaly of postnatal onset. Mild short stature.

OCCASIONAL ABNORMALITIES

Central Nervous System. Tumors, including optic gliomas (15 per cent) and other astrocytomas, neurilemmomas, meningiomas, and neurofibromas, occurring in 5 to 10 per cent. Seizures and/or EEG abnormalities in about 20 per cent. Mental deficiency in 2 to 5 per cent, with learning disability, hyperactivity, and/or speech problems in 50 per cent. Cerebral vascular compromise. Headaches.

Skeletal. Scoliosis. Hypoplastic bowing of lower legs, with pseudoarthrosis at birth. Osseous lesions with localized osteosclerosis, rib fusion, spina bifida, absence of patella, dislocation of radius and ulna, local overgrowth, and scalloping of vertebral bodies with deformed pedicles. Sphenoid wing dysplasia.

Hamartomata. Cutaneous nevi, lipomata, angiomata, neurofibroma in kidney, stomach, heart, tongue, and bladder.

Other. Syndactyly. Glaucoma. Ptosis. Corneal opacity. Potentially malignant melanoma of iris. Verrucous nevus. Pheochromocytoma. Pulmonic stenosis. Vascular hyperplasia of the intima and media. Pruritus.

NATURAL HISTORY. The majority of affected individuals have a benign course. Neurofibromas rarely develop in children less than 6 years of age. They may increase in size and number at puberty, during pregnancy, and between 50 and 70 years of age. The complications of neurofibromatosis can be divided into those that are structural (macrocephaly, segmental hypertrophy, scoliosis, pseudoarthrosis, cardiac defects), those that are functional (seizures, speech and learning disorders, hypertension, intellectual deficits), and those that relate to neoplasia. Screening for structural and functional complications can be done effectively through comprehensive physical evaluation every 6 months. The author believes that routine radiologic screening for CNS and visceral tumors is not warranted in the majority of cases. Rather, clinicians following affected individuals should maintain a high index of suspicion and evaluate specific signs and symptoms as they develop. Malignant change can occur in all types of neurofibromas. The overall risk of neurofibrosarcoma is about 5 per cent. Pain, increasing tumor size, and focal neurologic deficit should all raise concern relative to malignant transformation. Only about 5 per cent of patients become symptomatic from gliomas, no matter where in the optic nerve or chiasma it is located.

ETIOLOGY. Autosomal dominant with high penetrance but wide variability in expression. The neurofibromatosis type 1 (NF1) gene is located in the pericentromeric region of the long arm of chromosome 17. The extremely large size of the gene is consistent with the high spontaneous mutation rate of neurofibromatosis. About 50 per cent of patients have a fresh gene mutation. The NF1 gene encodes a protein designated neurofibromin, which may function as a tumor suppressor.

COMMENT. In addition to the classic form of neurofibromatosis, a second disorder exists, referred to as neurofibromatosis type 2 or acoustic neurofibromatosis. Also autosomal dominant, it is characterized by a later age of onset, the presence of bilateral acoustic neuromas, which generally develop over the second and third decades, as well as neurofibromas, meningiomas, gliomas, schwannomas, and/or juvenile posterior subcapsular cataracts. Usually only a few café au lait spots and cutaneous neurofibromas are present. NF2 is often more severe than NF1 in that multiple intracranial tumors can develop in childhood or early adulthood and schwannomas of the dorsal spinal roots occur. The NF2 gene is located on the long arm of chromosome 22 at 22q11.2. Finally, there exists a segmental form of neurofibromatosis characterized by café au lait spots, cutaneous neurofibromas, and intrathoracic and/or intra-abdominal neurofibromas limited to a circumscribed body segment. Unilateral Lisch nodules occur only when the involved segment includes one of the eyes. Because this disorder is most likely due to a somatic mutation, it has been suggested that recurrence risk is negligible. However, cases of genetic transmission have been reported.

References

Von Recklinghausen, F.: Ueber die multiplen Fibroma der Haut und ihre Beziehung zu den multiplen Neuromen. Berlin. A. Hirschwald, 1882.

Crowe, F. W., Schull, W. J., and Neel, J. V.: Multiple Neurofibromatosis. American Lecture Series No. 281. Springfield, Ill., Charles C Thomas, 1952.

Mena, E., et al.: Neurofibromatosis and renovascular hypertension in children. Am. J. Roentgenol. Radium Ther. Nucl. Med., 118:39, 1973.

Miller, R. M., and Sparkes, R. S.: Segmental neurofibromatosis. Arch. Dermatol., 113:837, 1977.

Eldridge, R.: Central neurofibromatosis with bilateral acoustic neuromas. Adv. Neurol., 29:57, 1981.

Riccardi, V. M.: Von Recklinghausen neurofibromatosis. N. Engl. J. Med., 305:1617, 1981.

Mackool, B. T., and Fitzpatrick, T. B.: Diagnosis of neurofibromatosis by cutaneous examination. Semin. Neurol., 12:358, 1992.

Ragge, N. K.: Clinical and genetic patterns of neurofibromatosis 1 and 2. Br. J. Ophthalmol, 77:662, 1993.

Vickochil, D., et al.: The neurofibromatosis type I gene. Annu. Rev. Neurosci., 15:183, 1993.

The Concensus Developmental Panel. National Institutes of Health Consensus Developmental Conference Statement on Acoustic Neuroma, December 11–13, 1991. Arch. Neurol., 51:210, 1994.

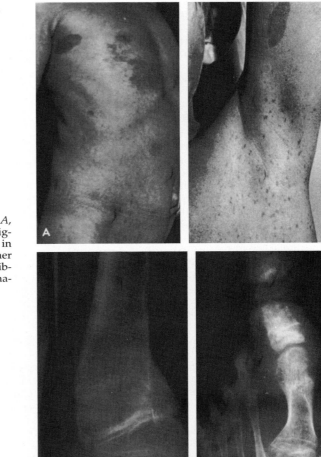

FIGURE 1. Neurofibromatosis syndrome. *A*, Café au lait, ovoid, irregular, and minute pigmentary spots on the trunk of one child and in the axilla—axillary "freckling"—in another child. *B*, Pseudofracture of distal tibia and fibula. Hypertrophy of toe in relation to the hamartomatous process in that area.

McCUNE-ALBRIGHT SYNDROME

(Osteitis Fibrosa Cystica)

Polyostotic Fibrous Dysplasia,
Irregular Skin Pigmentation, Sexual Precocity

McCune and Albright et al. described this condition in 1936 and 1937, respectively. More than 100 cases have been reported. The relative frequency of diagnosis in females versus males is 3:2.

ABNORMALITIES

Bone. Multiple areas of fibrous dysplasia, most commonly in long bones and pelvis; may also include cranium, facial bones (causing facial asymmetry), ribs, and occasionally the spine. May result in deformity, increased thickness of bone, or both.

Skin. Irregular brown pigmentation, most commonly over sacrum, buttocks, upper spine; unilateral in about 50 per cent of patients. The pattern of the pigmentary changes often follow the Blascho lines.

Endocrine. Precocious puberty. Hyperthyroidism, hyperparathyroidism. Pituitary adenomas secreting growth hormone. Acromegaly. Cushing syndrome. Hyperprolactinemia.

NATURAL HISTORY. The pigmentation is usually evident in infancy, and the bone dysplasia may progress during childhood, resulting in deformity, fracture, or both, most commonly in the upper femur. Thickening of bone in the calvarium can lead to cranial nerve compression with such serious consequences as blindness or deafness. The sexual precocity in the female is often unusual in character, with menstruation prior to development of breasts or pubic hair. The accelerated maturation coincident with sexual precocity may result in early attainment of full stature, so that adult height can be relatively short. Thyrotoxicosis occurs frequently and postoperative thyroid storm has occurred on rare occasions.

ETIOLOGY. Sporadic. It is most likely that this disorder is due to a somatic activating mutation of the gene encoding the α-subunit of the G protein. G proteins are involved in signal transduction pathways that affect the production of cyclic adenosine monophosphate (cAMP). An overactive cAMP pathway stimulates the growth and function of the gonads, adrenal cortex, specific pituitary-cell populations, osteoblasts, and melanocytes. This explains the observation that the endocrinologic abnormalities in McCune-Albright syndrome are the result of autonomous hyperfunction of the endocrine glands rather than centrally mediated.

References

McCune, D. J.: Osteitis fibrosa cystica. Am. J. Dis. Child., 52:745, 1936.

Albright, F., et al.: Syndrome characterized by osteitis fibrosa disseminata, area of pigmentation and endocrine dysfunction, with precocious puberty in females. Report of five cases. N. Engl. J. Med., 216:727, 1937.

Arlien-Soborg, U., and Iversen, T.: Albright's syndrome. A brief survey and report of a case in a seven year old girl. Acta Paediatr., 45:558, 1956.

DiGeorge, A. M.: Albright syndrome: Is it coming of age? J. Pediatr., 87:1018, 1975.

D'Armiento, M., et al.: McCune-Albright syndrome: Evidence for autonomous multiendocrine hyperfunction. J. Pediatr., 102:584, 1983.

Weinstein, L. S., et al.: Activating mutations of the stimulatory G protein in the McCune-Albright syndrome. N. Engl. J. Med., 325:1688, 1991.

Schwindinger, W. F., et al.: Identification of a mutation in the gene encoding the α subunit of the stimulatory G protein of adenyl cyclase in McCune-Albright syndrome. Proc. Natl. Acad. Sci. U. S. A., 89:5152, 1992.

Rieger, E., et al.: Melanotic macules following Blaschko's lines in McCune-Albright syndrome. Br. J. Dermatol., 130:215, 1994.

FIGURE 1. McCune-Albright syndrome. *A,* Irregular café au lait pigmentation over lower back. *B,* Dense, thick bone at the base of the skull.

VON HIPPEL-LINDAU SYNDROME

Retinal Angiomata, Cerebellar Hemangioblastoma

Lindau, in 1926, recognized this association of angiomatous retina (von Hippel disease) and angiomatous tumors of the cerebellum and other parts of the CNS. Well over 500 cases have been published. The disorder may well be underestimated, since as many as one half of affected individuals who carry the gene have only one symptomatic lesion and are therefore not recognized to have von Hippel-Lindau syndrome.

ABNORMALITIES

Eyes. Angioma, often peripheral, with "beaded" artery leading into it and tortuous dilated vein from it.

Cerebellum. Hemangioblastoma, sometimes with cyst, most commonly in cortical area of cerebellum, occasionally in spinal cord or elsewhere in brain. May calcify.

OCCASIONAL ABNORMALITIES.
Hemangiomata of face, adrenal, lung, and liver; multiple cysts of pancreas, kidney, and epididymis; renal cell carcinoma; hypernephromata; pheochromocytoma; pancreatic cancer; adenocarcinoma of ampulla of Vater; paragangliomas; polycythemia.

NATURAL HISTORY.
Retinal lesions usually not apparent until approximately 25 years of age, with subsequent visual impairment. Cerebellar signs may appear in third decade. Ninety-seven per cent of patients present by 60 years. Light coagulation or cryotherapy may be effective in treating the retinal angiomata and avoiding retinal detachment. There is about a 25 per cent risk of renal cancer, not uncommonly bilateral, for which renal transplantation merits consideration. The mean age for patients presenting with renal cell carcinoma is 46.5 years, with a range from 24 to 67. A regular screening protocol has been established by Maher et al. to detect complications in affected individuals at an early age and to determine if at-risk relatives are affected. This includes a yearly physical exam including funduscopic evaluation and urine testing, annual abdominal ultrasonography, and urinary catecholamine analysis, with cranial, renal, and abdominal CT scanning less frequently.

ETIOLOGY.
Autosomal dominant with varying expression. Based on genetic linkage analysis, the locus for the genetic alteration in von Hippel-Lindau syndrome has been assigned to the short arm of chromosome 3 at 3p25-p26. It has been suggested that the altered gene is a tumor suppressor gene. Tumor development requires mutation of both alleles. An inherited mutation leads to inactivation of one allele and an acquired somatic mutation or chromosomal aberration to the inactivation or loss of the other.

References

Lindau, A.: Studien über Kleinhirnsystem. Bon Pathogenese und Beziehungen zur Angiomatosis retinae. Acta Pathol. Microbiol. Scand. Suppl., *1*:1, 1926.

Christoferson, L. A., Gustafson, M. B., and Petersen, A. G.: Von Hippel-Lindau's disease. J. A. M. A., *178*: 280, 1961.

Petersen, G. J., et al.: Renal transplantation in Lindau-von Hippel disease. Arch. Surg., *112*:841, 1977.

Seizinger, B. R., et al.: Von Hippel-Lindau disease maps to the region of chromosome 3p associated with renal cell carcinoma. Nature, *332*:268, 1988.

Maher, E. R., et al.: Clinical features and natural history of Von Hippel-Lindau disease. Q. J. Med., *283*: 1151, 1990.

Maher, E. R., et al.: Mapping of the Von Hippel-Lindau disease locus to a small region of chromosome 3p by genetic linkage analysis. Genomics, *10*:957, 1991.

Neumann, H. P. H., and Wiestler, O. D.: Clustering of features of Von-Hippel-Lindau syndrome: Evidence for a complex genetic locus. Lancet, *337*:1052, 1991.

KLIPPEL-TRENAUNAY-WEBER SYNDROME

Asymmetric Limb Hypertrophy, Hemangiomata

This entity was originally reported by Klippel and Trenaunay in 1900. Parkes-Weber added the infrequent finding of arteriovenous fistula in 1907. Numerous cases have been published.

ABNORMALITIES

Limbs. Congenital or early childhood hypertrophy of usually one, but occasionally more than one, limb. The condition involves one leg in about 75 per cent of cases. The hypertrophy may not necessarily coincide with the area of hemangiomatous involvement.

Skin. The vascular lesions vary greatly and include the following types: capillary and cavernous hemangiomas, phlebectasia, and varicosities. These lesions can occur in any area, but are more commonly located on the legs, buttocks, abdomen, and lower trunk. Unilateral distribution predominates, but bilateral involvement is not uncommon.

OCCASIONAL ABNORMALITIES

Limbs. Arteriovenous fistula, lymphangiomatous anomalies, atrophy.

Hands and Feet. Macrodactyly, disproportionate growth of the digits whether large or small, syndactyly, polydactyly, oligodactyly.

Skin. Hyperpigmented nevi and streaks, neonatal and childhood ulcers and vesicles, cutis marmorata, telangiectasia.

Craniofacial. Asymmetric facial hypertrophy, hemangiomata, microcephaly, macrocephaly due to a large brain, intracranial calcifications, and eye abnormalities such as glaucoma, cataracts, heterochromia, and a Marcus Gunn pupil.

Viscera. Visceromegaly; hemangiomata of the intestinal tract, urinary system, mesentery, and pleura; aberrant major blood vessels, lymphectasia.

Performance. Mental deficiency and/or seizures, usually only in patients having facial hemangiomatosis.

Growth. Small stature, tall stature.

Other. Enlargement of the genitalia, intravascular clotting problems, lipodystrophy. Absence of inferior vena cava.

NATURAL HISTORY. The usual patient with this syndrome does relatively well without any treatment or with elastic compression only. There may be disproportionate growth, which requires epiphyseal fusion or removal of the appropriate phalanx. Joint discomfort is not uncommon, and arthritic-type problems may develop. Leg swelling can be bothersome, and ulcers and other chronic skin difficulties may occur. Clinically significant arteriovenous shunting almost never occurs. Surgical intervention is almost never needed. However, in the rare situation in which the extremity reaches gigantic proportions or secondary clotting difficulties occur, amputation is necessary. Hemangiomata of the viscera, brain, eyes, urinary and gastrointestinal tracts, and other areas should always be looked for in this extremely variable disorder. Magnetic resonance imaging is the best noninvasive imaging technique to evaluate patients with vascular malformations.

ETIOLOGY. Unknown. Sporadic occurrence.

References

Klippel, M., and Trenaunay, P.: Du naevus variqueux osteohypertrophique. Arch. Gen. Med., *185*:641, 1900.

Parkes-Weber, F.: Angioma formation in connection with hypertrophy of limbs and hemi-hypertrophy. Br. J. Dermatol., *19*:231, 1907.

Kuffer, F. R., et al.: Klippel-Trenaunay syndrome, visceral angiomatosis, and thrombocytopenia. J. Pediatr. Surg., *3*:65, 1968.

Furukawa, T., et al.: Sturge-Weber and Klippel-Trenaunay syndrome with nevus of Ota and Sto. Arch. Dermatol., *102*:640, 1970.

Lindenauer, S. M.: Congenital arteriovenous fistula and the Klippel-Trenaunay syndrome. Ann. Surg., *174*:248, 1971.

Stephan, M. J., et al.: Macrocephaly in association with unusual cutaneous angiomatosis. J. Pediatr., *87*:353, 1975.

Baskerville, P. A., et al.: The Klippel-Trenaunay syndrome: Clinical, radiological and haemodynamic features and management. Br. J. Surg., *72*:232, 1985.

Gloviczki, P., et al.: Klippel-Trenaunay syndrome: The risks and benefits of vascular interventions. Surgery, *110*:469, 1991.

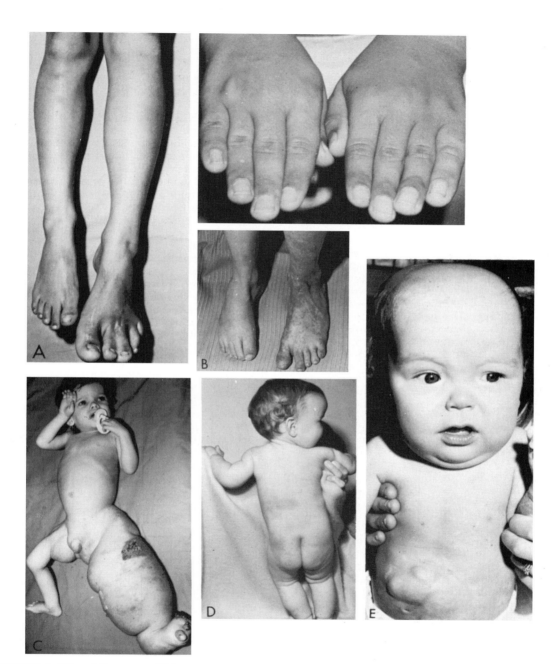

FIGURE 1. Klippel-Trenaunay-Weber syndrome. *A*, A 14-year-old showing asymmetric hypertrophy in legs, hands (note left fifth finger), and feet, with abnormal vasculature, as is evident in the dorsum of the left foot. *B*, Feet of a mentally deficient microcephalic boy showing left-sided hemangiomatous involvement and macrodactyly. *C*, Mentally normal girl with involvement of clitoris and right thigh and severe involvement of left leg with secondary intravascular clotting. The left leg was amputated, plastic surgery was done in the other involved areas, and the patient is vastly improved. *D*, Mentally normal girl with macrocephaly and hemangiomata in left trunk and lower limb. *E*, Young, normally functioning infant with macrocephaly and cavernous hemangioma in right upper abdomen.

PROTEUS SYNDROME

Hemihypertrophy, Subcutaneous Tumors, Macrodactyly

Initially described in 1979 by Cohen and Hayden, this disorder was set forth as a clinical entity in 1983 by Wiedemann, who utilized the term "proteus" (after the Greek God Proteus, the polymorphous) to characterize the variable and changing phenotype of this condition. It has been suggested by Dr. Michael Cohen, Dalhousie University, Halifax, Nova Scotia, that John Merrick, the elephant man, most likely had the Proteus syndrome.

ABNORMALITIES

Growth. Overgrowth may involve the whole body, it may be unilateral involving one limb, or it may be localized involving a digit or any combination of the above. Increased stature. Weight decreased for height age. Macrocephaly.

Skin and Subcutaneous Tissue. Generalized thickening. Hyperpigmented areas that appear to represent epidermal nevi. Lipomata, lymphangiomata, and hemangiomata with a predilection for the thorax and upper abdomen.

Skeletal. Hemihypertrophy. Bony prominences over skull. Angulation defects of knees. Scoliosis. Kyphosis. Hip dislocation. Valgus deformities of halluces and feet. Clinodactyly. Dysplastic vertebrae. Coarse ribs and scapula.

Hands and Feet. Macrodactyly. Soft tissue hypertrophy, which may appear as gyriform, changes particularly over plantar surfaces of feet and less commonly the hands.

OCCASIONAL ABNORMALITIES. Elonga-
tion of neck and trunk. Craniosynostosis. Broad, depressed nasal bridge. Gyriform hyperplasia over side of nose or in the other locations. Ptosis. Strabismus. Epibulbar dermoid. Enlarged eyes. Microphthalmia. Myopia. Cataracts. Nystagmus. Submucous cleft palate. Pectus excavatum. Elbow ankylosis. Mental deficiency. Seizures. Cyst-like alterations of lungs. Muscle atrophy. Abdominal and pelvic lipomatosis. Café-au-lait spots. Exostosis of external auditory canals and on alveolar ridges. Hyperostosis of nasal bridge. Fibrocystic diseases of breast. Adenoma of parotid gland. Yolk sac tumor of testes. Papillary adenoma of the epididymis. Goiter. Enlarged penis. Macro-orchidism. Hypertrophic cardiomyopathy and cardiac conduction defects. Renal abnormalities including enlarged kidneys with cysts, hemangiomas, and hydronephrosis.

NATURAL HISTORY. Frequently normal at birth, although birth weight is frequently increased and a few patients have had the characteristic features in the immediate newborn period. The characteristic features become obvious over the first year of life. Generally progressive throughout childhood, growth of the hamartomata and the generalized hypertrophy usually cease after puberty. Moderate mental deficiency in 20 per cent of cases. Morbidity is significant. Of 11 patients evaluated by Clark et al., 2 required amputation of a leg, 6 had fingers or toes removed, and 2 women had breast implants and reconstruction. Spinal stenosis and neurologic sequelae may develop due to vertebral anomalies or tumor infiltration. Cystic emphysematous pulmonary disease may be associated with severe morbidity and in some cases death. Affected individuals should be carefully monitored for the development of all types of neoplasms, since the full spectrum of this disorder is not known.

ETIOLOGY. Unknown. All cases have been sporadic events in otherwise normal families. Recent reports have suggested that this disorder is due to somatic mosaicism.

References

Cohen, M. M., and Hayden, P. W.: A newly recognized hamartomatous syndrome. Birth Defects, 15(5B): 291, 1979.

Wiedemann, H. R., et al.: The proteus syndrome: Partial gigantism of the hands and/or feet, nevi, hemihypertrophy, subcutaneous tumors, macrocephaly or other skull anomalies and possible accelerated growth and visceral affections. Eur. J. Pediatr., 140:5, 1983.

Burgio, G. R., and Wiedemann, H. R.: Further and new details on the proteus syndrome. Eur. J. Pediatr., 143:71, 1984.

Clark, R. D., et al.: Proteus syndrome: An expanded phenotype. Am. J. Med. Genet., 27:99, 1987.

Cohen, M. M.: Understanding Proteus syndrome, unmasking the elephant man, and stemming elephant fever. Neurofibromatosis, 1:260, 1988.

Cohen, M. M.: Proteus syndrome: Clinical evidence for somatic mosaicism and selective review. Am. J. Med. Genet., 47:645, 1993.

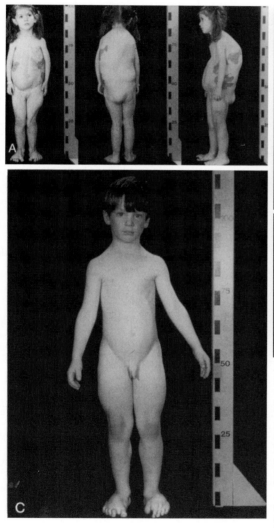

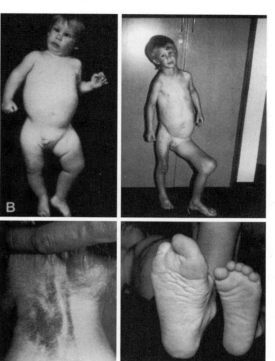

FIGURE 1. Proteus syndrome. *A*, A 4⁶/₁₂-year-old girl with Proteus syndrome. Note the large, simple ears; the soft tissue masses, which have distorted the abdomen, left thigh, and back; and the splayed toes. The hemangiomata over the abdomen are flat, but dark vesicles are erupting. *B*, A boy with Proteus syndrome at 8 months and at 4⁸/₁₂ years of age. Note the progression of the soft tissue tumors and leg asymmetry. Note also the linear sebaceous nevus on the back of the neck, the hypertrophied, overlapping toes, and the thickened, rugated plantar surface. *C*, A 5-year-old mildly affected boy with increased subcutaneous tissue over the thighs and broad feet with splayed toes. (From Clark, R. D., et al.: Am. J. Med. Genet., 27:99, 1987, with permission.)

ENCEPHALOCRANIOCUTANEOUS LIPOMATOSIS

Unilateral Craniofacial Lipomas,
Ipsilateral Cerebral Atrophy, Focal Areas of Alopecia

This disorder was initially described by Haberland and Peron in 1970. Subsequently, 15 additional cases have been reported.

ABNORMALITIES

Performance. Marked developmental delay. Mental retardation. Seizures. Spasticity.

Brain. Unilateral porencephalic cyst with cortical atrophy and calcification of the cerebral cortex overlying the cyst. Defective lamination of the cerebrum. Micropolygyria. Lipomas in the meninges covering the affected cerebral hemisphere.

Craniofacies. Asymmetry of the skull and face due to unilateral lipomatous involvement of the dermis of the skin covering the face and head and the diploic space of the frontal bone on the same side as the brain defect. Focal areas of alopecia overlying the lipomas.

Eyes. Hard pedunculated outgrowths attached to margin of upper lid that are made up of connective tissue. Epibulbar dermoid.

OCCASIONAL ABNORMALITIES.

Microphthalmia. Iris dysplasia including coloboma. Cloudy cornea. Areas of skin hypoplasia overlaying the craniofacial lipomas. Hydrocephalus. Arachnoid cyst. Spinal cord lipomatosis. Skull defect overlaying the cerebral defect. Lipomas of the heart.

NATURAL HISTORY. Seizures develop during childhood in the vast majority of cases. The degree of mental retardation is variable. Insufficient numbers of patients have been documented to provide adequate information regarding long-term follow-up.

ETIOLOGY. Unknown. All affected patients have been sporadic.

COMMENT. There is some controversy as to whether this represents a distinct disorder or a more localized unilateral form of Proteus syndrome.

References

Haberland, C., and Peron, M.: Encephalocranio-cutaneous lipomatosis. Arch. Neurol., 22:144, 1970.

Wiedemann, H. R., and Burgio, G. R.: Encephalocraniocutaneous lipomatosis and Proteus syndrome. Am. J. Med. Genet., 25:403, 1986.

Bamforth, J. S. G., et al.: Encephalocraniocutaneous lipomatosis: Report of two cases and a review of the literature. Neurofibromatosis, 2:166, 1989.

Kodsi, S. R., et al.: Ocular and systemic manifestations of encephalocraniocutaneous lipomatosis. Am. J. Ophthalmol., 118:77, 1994.

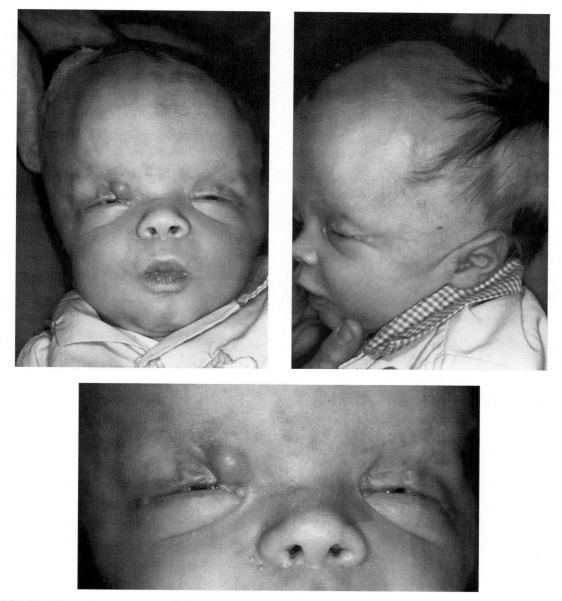

FIGURE 1. Note the focal areas of alopecia and the pedunculated outgrowths attached to the margin of the eyelids. (Courtesy of Dr. David Viskochil, University of Utah, Salt Lake City, Utah.)

MAFFUCCI SYNDROME

Enchondromatosis, Hemangiomata

Maffucci, in 1881, described a patient with dyschondroplasia and multiple cutaneous hemangiomata. Approximately 170 cases have been recorded subsequently.

ABNORMALITIES. Onset from the neonatal period to adolescence.

Skeletal. Variable early bowing of the long bones, with asymmetric retarded growth. Enchondromata (40 per cent unilateral) primarily in the hands, feet, and tubular long bones.

Vascular. Hemangiomata, most frequently located in the dermis and subcutaneous fat adjacent to the areas of enchondromatosis, but may occur anywhere. Types of hemangiomata are capillary, cavernous, and especially phlebectasia, which often have a grape-like appearance. Thrombosis of the dilated blood vessels with phlebolith formation occurs in 43 per cent of cases.

OCCASIONAL ABNORMALITIES. Lymphangiectasis, lymphangiomata, hemangiomata of the mucous membranes and gastrointestinal tract, other tumors, both malignant and benign and of mesodermal and nonmesodermal origin. Intracranial tumors, usually of cartilaginous origin, in approximately 15 per cent.

NATURAL HISTORY. The patients usually appear normal at birth, but within the first 4 years, hemangiomata appear, 25 per cent during the first year. Subsequent enchondromata formation is noted by adolescence. The disorder can be mild, but it is often severe enough to require multiple surgical procedures and occasionally amputation. About 26 per cent have fractures related to enchondromata. The risk of chondrosarcomatous change is about 15 per cent.

ETIOLOGY. Unknown. Sporadic occurrence.

References

Maffucci, A.: Di un caso di encondroma ed angioma multiplo: Contribuzione alla genesi embrionale dei tumor. Movimento Med. Chir., 3:399, 1881.

Bean, W. B.: Dyschondroplasia and hemangiomata (Maffucci's syndrome) II. Arch. Intern. Med., 102: 544, 1958.

Lewis, R. J., and Ketcham, A. S.: Maffucci's syndrome. J. Bone Joint Surg. [Am.], 55:1465, 1973.

Sun, Te-Ching, et al.: Chondrosarcoma in Maffucci's syndrome. J. Bone Joint Surg. [Am.], 67-A:1214, 1985.

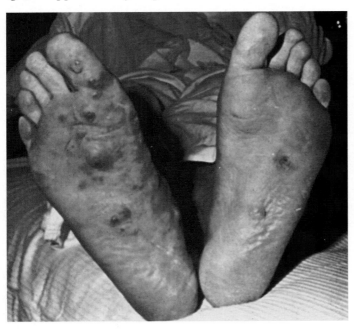

FIGURE 1. Maffucci syndrome. Note the enlarged right foot and the vascular lesions. These pictures were taken just following the removal of this man's right arm because of chondrosarcomatous change in an area of enchondromata. He had also had gastrointestinal bleeding episodes secondary to lower intestinal hemangiomata.

OSTEOCHONDROMATOSIS SYNDROME

(Ollier Disease, Enchondromatosis)

Asymmetric Enchondromata With Local Growth Deficiency

Ollier described this disorder in 1899, and well over 100 cases have been reported.

ABNORMALITIES
Skeletal. Rounded masses of hyaline cartilage lead to fan-like radiolucencies in metaphyses, later diaphyses, and sometimes epiphyses. Usually bilateral but asymmetric, with limited growth of affected bones, which are most commonly the tubular long bones and sometimes the pelvis. Skull involvement is very uncommon.

Other. Granulosa cell tumors of the ovary have occurred but only rarely.

NATURAL HISTORY. The extremity may be short at birth, with no evidence of enchondromata. Asymmetric growth usually first noted at 1 to 4 years of age, with little progression after adolescence. The patients are prone to fractures. An unknown, probably low risk of developing chondrosarcoma exists. Reactivation of growth in adult life should raise concern regarding malignant degeneration.

ETIOLOGY. Unknown. Usually sporadic, but does occur rarely in more than one member of a family.

References

Ollier, L.: De la Dyschondroplasia. Bull. Soc. Chir. (Lyon), *3*:22, 1899.

Margolis, J.: Ollier's disease. Arch. Intern. Med., *103*: 279, 1959.

Mainzer, F., Minagi, H., and Steinbach, H. L.: The variable manifestations of multiple enchondromatosis. Radiology, *99*:377, 1971.

Vaz, R. M., and Turner, C.: Ollier disease (enchondromatosis) associated with ovarian juvenile granulosa cell and precocious pseudopuberty. J. Pediatr., *108*:945, 1986.

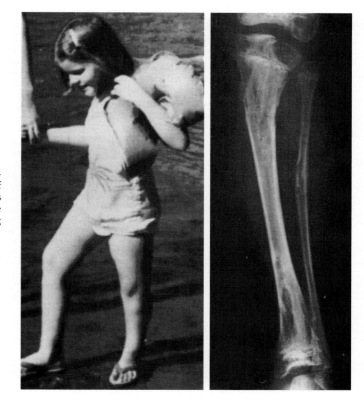

FIGURE 1. Osteochondromatosis syndrome. A 6-year-old and roentgenogram of her left tibia. She had onset of leg shortness at 2 years of age. By 16 years of age she had suffered several fractures of the left leg and had developed scoliosis.

PEUTZ-JEGHERS SYNDROME

Mucocutaneous Pigmentation, Intestinal Polyposis

In 1896, Hutchinson described the pigmentary changes in an individual who later died of intussusception. Peutz clearly set forth the disease in 1921, and Jeghers et al. further established this disease entity in 1949. Many cases have been documented.

ABNORMALITIES

Pigmentation. Vertical bands of epidermal pigment presenting as blue-gray or brownish spots on lips, buccal mucous membrane, perioral area, and sometimes digits and elsewhere.

Polyposis. Hamartomatous muscularis mucosae polyps in the stomach; small bowel (jejunum and duodenum more frequently than ileum) and colon; and occasionally in nasopharynx, bladder, biliary tract, and bronchial mucosa. Polyps are usually multiple. They are not premalignant. However, there is an increased risk for adenomas and adenocarcinomas, which may develop in any area of gastrointestinal tract lined by columnar epithelium.

Other Tumors. Approximately 35 per cent of patients have extraintestinal malignancies including bronchogenic carcinomia, benign and malignant neoplasms of the thyroid, gallbladder, and biliary tract. Breast cancer, usually ductal. Pancreatic cancer. Malignant tumors of the reproductive tract including malignant adenoma of the cervix, unique ovarian sex cord tumors, Sertoli cell testicular tumors that produce estrogen and thus cause gynecomastia.

NATURAL HISTORY. The pigmentary spots appear from infancy through early childhood and tend to fade in the adult. Seventy per cent of patients have some gastrointestinal problem by age 20 years, most commonly colicky abdominal pain (60 per cent), intestinal bleeding (25 per cent), or both. Intussusception, which may spontaneously recede, is the most serious complication, and iron deficiency anemia may result from chronic blood loss. Approximately 50 per cent of affected patients develop an intestinal or extraintestinal cancer. Almost one half of the patients with malignancy have been younger than 30 years of age. Clubbing of the fingers may occasionally occur in this disease. Screening of affected patients as well as potentially affected family members should include colonoscopy, an upper gastrointestinal series with small bowel follow-through, pelvic ultrasonography in females, and careful examination of testicles in males.

ETIOLOGY. Autosomal dominant with a high degree of penetrance.

References

Hutchinson, J.: Pigmentation of the lips and mouth. Arch. Surg., 7:290, 1896.

Peutz, J. L. A.: Very remarkable case of familial polyposis of mucous membrane of intestinal tract and nasopharynx accompanied by peculiar pigmentation of skin and mucous membrane. Ned. Maanschr. Geneesk., 10:134, 1921.

Jeghers, H., McKusick, V. A., and Katz, K. H.: Generalized intestinal polyposis and melanin spots of the oral mucosa, lips, and digits. A syndrome of diagnostic significance. N. Engl. J. Med., 241:993, 1949.

Bartholomew, L. G., et al.: Intestinal polyposis associated with mucocutaneous pigmentation. Surg. Gynecol. Obstet., 115:1, 1962.

Tovar, J. A., et al.: Peutz-Jeghers syndrome in children: Report of two cases and review of the literature. J. Pediatr. Surg., 18:1, 1983.

Buck, J. L.: From the archives of AFIP. Peutz-Jeghers syndrome. Radiographics, 12:365, 1992.

Rustgi, A. K.: Hereditary gastrointestinal polyposis and nonpolyposis syndromes. N. Engl. J. Med., 331:1694, 1994.

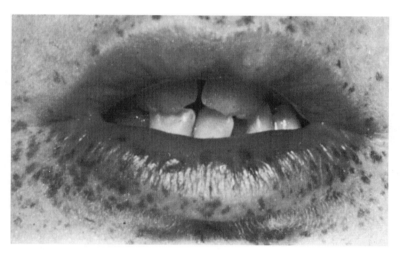

FIGURE 1. Peutz-Jeghers syndrome. Spotty pigmentation of lips and periorbital area in a child with intestinal polyps. (From Sheward, J. D.: Br. Med. J., 1:921, 1962, with permission.)

BANNAYAN-RILEY-RUVALCABA SYNDROME

(Ruvalcaba-Myhre Syndrome,
Riley-Smith Syndrome, Bannayan Syndrome)

*Macrocephaly, Polyposis of Colon,
Pigmentary changes of the Penis*

In 1986, Saul and Stevenson proposed that Bannayan syndrome and Ruvalcaba-Myhre syndrome were the same disorder. Subsequently, Dvir et al. added Riley-Smith syndrome and suggested that all three of these conditions represent one etiologic entity, which Cohen referred to as Bannayan-Riley-Ruvalcaba syndrome.

ABNORMALITIES

Growth. Birth weight greater than 4 kg and birth length greater than 97th percentile. Normal adult stature.

Performance. Hypotonia, gross motor delay, speech delay, and/or mild to severe mental deficiency in 50 per cent. Seizures (25 per cent).

Craniofacies. Macrocephaly, with ventricles of normal size. Down-slanting palpebral fissures (60 per cent). Strabismus or amblyopia (15 per cent). Prominent Schwalbe lines and prominent corneal nerves (35 per cent).

Intestines. Ileal and colonic hamartomatous polyps (45 per cent).

Neoplasms. Hamartomas that are lipomas in 75 per cent, hemangiomas in 10 per cent, and mixed type in 20 per cent. Most are subcutaneous, although they can be cranial (20 per cent) or osseous (10 per cent).

Penis. Tan, nonelevated spots on glans penis, and shaft.

Other. Myopathic process in proximal muscles (60 per cent). Cutaneous angiolipomas, encapsulated or diffusely infiltrating, in 50 per cent. Joint hyperextensibility, pectus excavatum, and scoliosis in 50 per cent.

OCCASIONAL ABNORMALITIES.

Pseudopapilledema, diabetes, Hashimoto thyroiditis, acanthosis nigricans lymphangiomyomas, angiokeratomas, verruca vulgaris–type facial skin changes, café au lait spots, tongue polyps, supernumerary nipples, enlarged testes, enlarged penis.

NATURAL HISTORY. Although overgrowth is usually present in the newborn period, final adult height is within the normal range. The ileal and colonic polyps often present in childhood with intussusception and rectal bleeding; sometimes they do not become evident until middle age. Lipomas can be extremely large.

ETIOLOGY. Autosomal dominant.

COMMENT. Muscle biopsy in a number of patients has revealed a lipid storage myopathy primarily in enlarged type I skeletal muscle fibers. Type II fibers are smaller than usual and contain less fat. The myopathy has been treated successfully with carnitine.

References

Riley, H. D., and Smith, W. R.: Macrocephaly, pseudopapilledema, and multiple hemangiomata. Pediatrics, 26:293, 1960.

Bannayan, G. A.: Lipomatosis, angiomatosis and macrocephaly: A previously undescribed congenital syndrome. Arch. Pathol., 92:1, 1971.

Ruvalcaba, R. H. A., Myhre, S., and Smith, D. W.: A syndrome with macrencephaly, intestinal polyposis and pigmentary penile lesions. Clin. Genet., 18:413, 1980.

DiLiberti, J. H., et al.: A new lipid storage myopathy observed in individuals with the Ruvalcaba-Myhre-Smith syndrome. Am. J. Med. Genet., 18:163, 1984.

Gorlin, R. J., et al.: Bannayan-Riley-Ruvalcaba syndrome. Am. J. Med. Genet., 44:307, 1992.

DiLiberti, J. H.: Correlation of skeletal muscle biopsy with phenotype in the familial macrocephaly syndromes. Am. J. Med. Genet., 29:46, 1992.

Powell, B. R., et al.: Dominantly inherited megalencephaly, muscle weakness, myoliposis: A carnitine-deficient myopathy within the spectrum of Ruvalcaba-Myhre-Smith syndrome. J. Pediatr., 123:70, 1993.

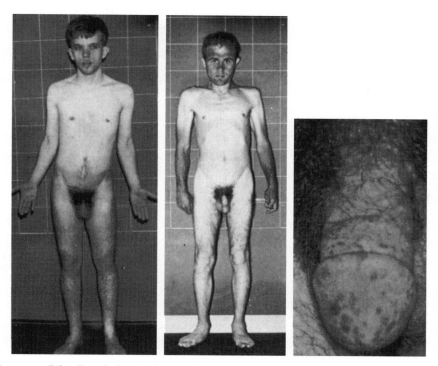

FIGURE 1. Bannayan-Riley-Ruvalcaba syndrome. Two unrelated affected males in their twenties, showing macrocephaly, supernumerary nipples (*left*), scar from early colectomy (*left*), and pigmentary skin lesions. (From Ruvalcaba, R. H. A., et al.: Clin. Genet. *18*:413, 1980, with permission.)

OSLER HEMORRHAGIC TELANGIECTASIA SYNDROME
(Hereditary Hemorrhagic Telangiectasia)

Epistaxes, Multiple Telangiectases

This entity was set forth in 1901 by Osler. The telangiectases contain dilated vessels having only an endothelial wall with no elastic tissue and a tendency toward arteriovenous fistulae. Many affected families have been reported, and the incidence is about 1 in 50,000.

ABNORMALITIES

Vessels. Pinpoint, spider, and/or nodular telangiectases most commonly on tongue, mucosa of lips, face, conjunctiva, ears, fingertips, nail beds, and nasal mucous membrane; occasionally in gastrointestinal tract, bladder, vagina, uterus, lungs, liver, and/or brain. Cutaneous telangiectases usually not evident until second or third decade.

OCCASIONAL ABNORMALITIES. Arteriovenous fistulae in lungs (15 per cent) and liver. Mucosal and submucosal arteriovenous malformations of the gastrointestinal tract. Arterial aneurysms, venous varicosities, and arteriovenous fistulas of celiac and mesenteric vessels. Cirrhosis of liver. Cavernous angiomata. Port-wine stain. Vascular anomalies in brain and spinal cord. Duodenal ulcer.

NATURAL HISTORY. Epistaxis, which often occurs in childhood, is the most common form of bleeding followed by gastrointestinal, genitourinary, pulmonary, and intracerebral. Intraocular hemorrhage is rare. Ten per cent of patients never bleed, while approximately one third require hospitalization for bleeding. Neurologic complications occur at any age, with a peak incidence in the third decade, and result from pulmonary arteriovenous fistula (60 per cent), vascular malformation of the brain (28 per cent), and spinal cord (8 per cent) and portosystemic encephalopathy (3 per cent). Of major concern is the potential for brain abscess, cerebral embolism, and hypoxemia secondary to the pulmonary arteriovenous fistulas. Hepatic arteriovenous fistula can cause hepatomegaly, right upper quadrant pain, pulsatile mass, a thrill, and/or bruit. Left to right shunting through the fistula can lead to high-output congestive heart failure. Bleeding is generally aggravated by pregnancy. Fewer than 10 per cent of patients die of associated complications. Oral iron supplementation is almost always necessary. Oral estrogen and septal dermoplasty have been used to successfully manage the epistaxis in some cases. Examinations for pulmonary arteriovenous fistulas and for retinal telangiectases should be performed periodically.

ETIOLOGY. Autosomal dominant with varying expression. The gene has been mapped, by linkage analysis, to 9q33-34.

References

Osler, W.: On a family form of recurring epistaxis, associated with multiple telangiectases of skin and mucous membrane. Bull. Hopkins Hosp., *12*:333, 1901.

Bird, R. M., et al.: Family reunion study of hereditary hemorrhagic telangiectasia. N. Engl. J. Med., *257*: 105, 1957.

Schaumann, B., and Alter, M.: Cerebrovascular malformations in hereditary hemorrhagic telangiectasia. Minn. Med., *56*:951, 1973.

Peery, W. H.: Clinical spectrum of hereditary hemorrhagic telangiectasia (Osler-Weber-Rendu disease). Am. J. Med., *82*:989, 1987.

McDonald, M. T., et al.: A disease locus for hereditary haemorrhagic telangiectasia maps to chromosome 9q33-34. Nat. Genet., *6*:197, 1994.

Guttmacher, A. E., et al.: Hereditary hemorrhagic telangiectasia. N. Engl. J. Med. *333*:918, 1995.

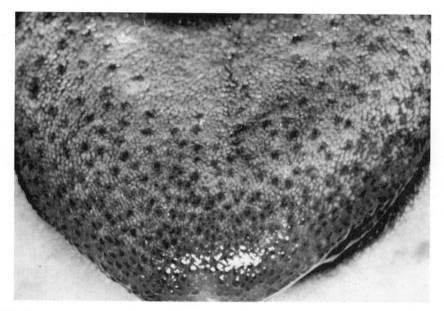

FIGURE 1. Osler hemorrhagic telangiectasia syndrome. Small telangiectases in the tongue of a girl who presented with cyanotic plethora secondary to multiple arteriovenous fistula in the lung.

MULTIPLE NEUROMA SYNDROME
(Multiple Endocrine Neoplasia, Type 2b)

*Multiple Neuromata of Tongue,
Lips With or Without Medullary Thyroid
Carcinoma, With or Without Pheochromocytoma*

This disorder represents one of the three different forms of multiple endocrine neoplasia type 2 (MEN2). The other two forms, MEN2A and MTC-only are associated with normal physical appearance. MEN2A is characterized by medullary thyroid carcinoma; parathyroid hyperplasia, and pheochromocytoma, while the MTC-only syndrome or FMTC represents familial medullary thyroid carcinoma without other components of MEN2A. MEN2B is the only one of these three disorders associated with a pattern of malformation.

ABNORMALITIES
Mucosa. Ganglioneuromatosis extending from lips to rectum and manifest by prominent lips, nodular tongue, involvement of nasal, laryngeal, and intestinal mucous membranes; thickened, anteverted eyelids.
Other Tumors. Medullary thyroid carcinoma, pheochromocytoma.
Skeletal. Marfanoid habitus, pes cavus, slipped femoral capital epiphyses, pectus excavatum, kyphosis, lordosis, scoliosis, increased joint laxity, weakness of proximal extremity muscles.
Other. Tendency toward coarse-appearing facies.

OCCASIONAL ABNORMALITIES. Slit lamp examination may reveal medullated nerve fibers in the cornea. Subconjunctival neuromas, cutaneous neuromata, and/or neurofibromata. Parathyroid hyperplasia; hypotonia. Developmental delay.

NATURAL HISTORY. Oral neuromata are usually evident in childhood, with medullary thyroid carcinoma and/or pheochromocytoma becoming serious risks after adolescence. When medullary thyroid carcinoma is implicated, a total thyroidectomy should usually be done because the lesion is often multicentric. When pheochromocytoma is implicated, a thorough exploration should be accomplished, since it is often bilateral and may also be extra-adrenal. Constipation with megacolon often severe enough to suggest Hirschsprung disease and/or diarrhea frequently develop before the endocrine neoplasms are detected. An annual screening evaluation of all at-risk family members should be performed in order to identify and treat presymptomatic individuals.

ETIOLOGY. Autosomal dominant. The gene has been mapped to the long arm of chromosome 10 in band q11.2. Mutations in the RET proto-oncogene account for the clinical phenotype.

COMMENT. An abnormal response to histamine skin test possibly related to diffuse enlargement of cutaneous nerves has been reported in patients with this disorder.

References

Gorlin, R. J., et al.: Multiple mucosal neuromas, pheochromocytoma and medullary carcinoma of the thyroid—a syndrome. Cancer, 22:293, 1968.

Schimke, R. N., et al.: Syndrome of bilateral pheochromocytoma, medullary thyroid carcinoma and multiple neuromas. N. Engl. J. Med., 279:1, 1968.

Carney, J. A., et al.: Alimentary tract ganglioneuromatosis. A major component of the syndrome of multiple endocrine neoplasia, type 2b. N. Engl. J. Med., 295:1287, 1976.

Carney, J. A., et al.: Abnormal cutaneous innervation in multiple endocrine neoplasia, type 2b. Ann. Intern. Med., 94:362, 1981.

Hofstra, R. M. W., et al.: A mutation in the RET proto-oncogene associated with multiple endocrine neoplasia type 2B and sporadic medullary thyroid carcinoma. Nature, 367:375, 1994.

Raue, F., et al.: Multiple endocrine neoplasia type 2: Clinical features and screening. Endocrinol. Metab. Clin. North Am., 23:137, 1994.

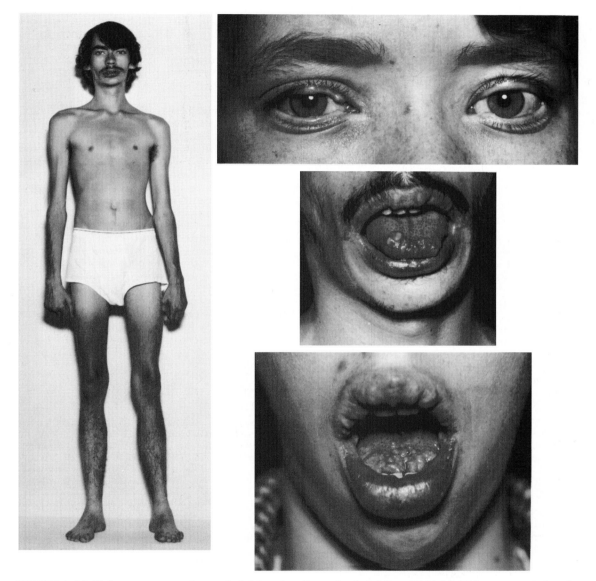

FIGURE 1. Multiple neuroma syndrome. *Left*, Note the slim asthenic habitus. *Right*, Multiple neuromata involving the conjunctiva and tongue and contributing to the prominent lips. (Courtesy of A. B. Hayles, Mayo Clinic, Rochester, Minn.)

GORLIN SYNDROME
(Nevoid Basal Cell Carcinoma Syndrome)

Basal Cell Carcinomas, Broad Facies, Rib Anomalies

Though this condition had been previously described, it was Gorlin and Goltz who recognized the full extent of this pattern of malformation in 1960. Subsequently, well over 500 cases have been reported.

ABNORMALITIES
Craniofacial. Macrocephaly (80 per cent). Frontoparietal bossing (66 per cent). Broad nasal bridge (59 per cent). Well-developed supraorbital ridges. Heavy, often fused eyebrows. Mild hypertelorism. Prognathism (33 per cent). Hyperpneumatization of paranasal sinuses. Bony bridging of sella turcica (60 to 80 per cent).
Dentition. Odontogenic keratocysts of jaws (75 per cent). Misshapen and/or carious teeth.
Hands. Short metacarpals, especially the fourth (29 per cent).
Thorax. Bifid, synostotic, and/or partially missing ribs (60 per cent). Scoliosis. Sloping, narrow shoulders (41 per cent). Thoracic or cervical vertebral anomalies (40 per cent).
Skin. Nevoid basal cell carcinomas over neck, upper arms, trunk, and face. Epidermal cysts. Punctate dyskeratotic pits on palms (65 per cent), soles (68 per cent), or both (58 per cent). Milia, especially facial (52 per cent).
Ectopic Calcification. Falx cerebri (85 per cent), falx cerebelli (40 per cent), petroclinoid ligament (20 per cent), dura, pia, and choroid plexus.
Ovaries. Development of calcified ovarian fibromata (14 per cent).

OCCASIONAL ABNORMALITIES. Mental deficiency, agenesis of corpus callosum, anosmia, hydrocephalus, hypertelorism, telecanthus, inner canthal folds, highly arched eyebrows, cataract, coloboma of iris, prominent medullated retinal nerve fibers, retinal atrophy, glaucoma, chalazion, strabismus, cleft lip with or without cleft palate, low-pitched female voice, pectus excavatum/carinatum, Sprengel deformity, "marfanoid" build, arachnodactyly, pre- or postaxial polydactyly, immobile thumbs, pseudocystic lytic lesions of bones, lumbarization of sacrum, hypogonadism in males, subcutaneous calcifications of skin. Renal anomalies. Other neoplasms including medulloblastoma, meningioma, fibromata, lipomata, melanoma, neurofibromata of skin, cardiac tumor, eyelid carcinomas, breast cancer, lung cancer, chronic lymphoid leukemia, non-Hodgkin lymphoma, ovarian dermoid, lymphomesenteric cysts that tend to calcify.

NATURAL HISTORY. Although they have occurred in 2-year-olds, the nevoid basal cell carcinomas usually appear between puberty and 35 years with a mean age of about 20 years. Before puberty the lesions are harmless. Thereafter, concern should be raised when the lesions begin to grow, ulcerate, bleed, or crust. The jaw cysts enlarge, especially in later childhood, and may recur following curettage. Mean age of onset is about 15 years. A constant vigil must be maintained in order to detect other tumors that are a common feature of this syndrome. Palmar pitting can be made more obvious by immersion of the hands in water for 15 minutes.

ETIOLOGY. Autosomal dominant. The gene has been mapped to chromosome 9q23.1-q31 and most likely functions as a tumor suppressor gene. Older paternal age is a factor in fresh mutational cases.

References

Binkley, G. W., and Johnson, H. H., Jr.: Epithelioma adenoides cysticum: Basal cell nevi, agenesis of the corpus callosum and dental cysts. A clinical and autopsy study. Arch. Dermatol., 63:73, 1951.

Gorlin, R. J., and Goltz, R. W.: Multiple nevoid basal-cell epithelioma, jaw cysts, and bifid ribs. A syndrome. N. Engl. J. Med., 262:908, 1960.

Gorlin, R. J., et al.: The multiple basal-cell nevi syndrome. Cancer, 18:89, 1965.

Ferrier, P. E., and Hinrichs, W. L.: Basal-cell carcinoma syndrome. Am. J. Dis. Child., 113:538, 1967.

Gorlin, R. J.: Nevoid basal-cell carcinoma syndrome. Medicine, 66:98, 1987.

Gailani, M. R., et al.: Developmental defects in Gorlin syndrome related to a putative tumor suppressor gene on chromosome 9. Cell, 69:111, 1992.

Evans, D. G. R., et al.: Complications of the naevoid basal cell carcinoma syndrome: Results of a population based study. J. Med. Genet., 30:460, 1993.

Shanley, S., et al.: Nevoid basal cell carcinoma syndrome: Review of 118 affected individuals. Am. J. Med. Genet., 50:282, 1994.

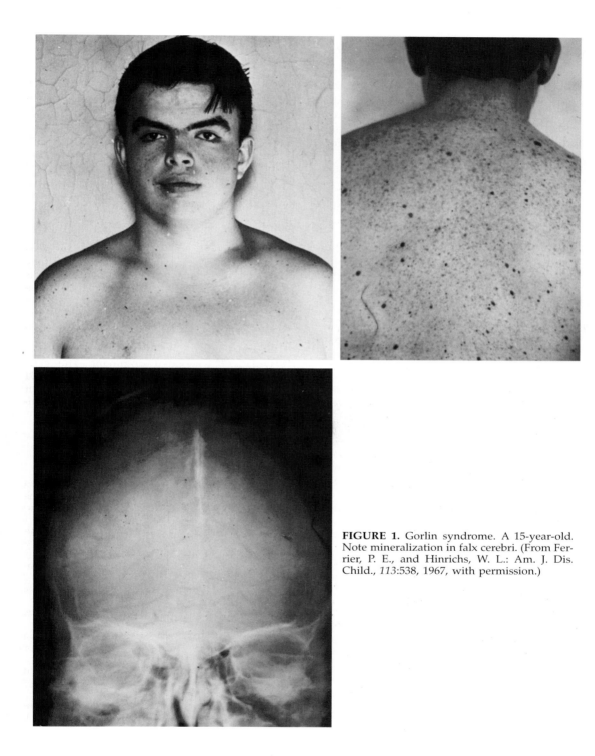

FIGURE 1. Gorlin syndrome. A 15-year-old. Note mineralization in falx cerebri. (From Ferrier, P. E., and Hinrichs, W. L.: Am. J. Dis. Child., *113*:538, 1967, with permission.)

MULTIPLE LENTIGINES SYNDROME

(LEOPARD Syndrome)

Multiple Lentigines, Pulmonic Stenosis, Mild Hypertelorism, Deafness

Gorlin et al. recognized the multiple defect nature of this disorder and utilized the acronym LEOPARD to denote the *l*entigines, *E*KG abnormalities, *o*cular hypertelorism, *p*ulmonic stenosis, *a*bnormalities of genitalia, *r*etardation of growth, and *d*eafness. More than 70 cases have been described.

ABNORMALITIES

Cutaneous. Multiple 1- to 5-mm dark lentigines, especially on neck and trunk.

Cardiac. Mild pulmonic stenosis. Hypertrophic obstructive cardiomyopathy. Electrocardiographic changes of prolonged P-R and QRS, abnormal P waves.

Other. Mild growth deficiency, mild ocular hypertelorism, prominent ears, mild to moderate sensorineural deafness, winged scapulae, pectus excavatum or carinatum, late adolescence. Cryptorchidism.

OCCASIONAL ABNORMALITIES.

Mental deficiency, cleft palate, mandibular prognathism, café au lait spots, unilateral renal and/or gonadal agenesis or hypoplasia. Hypogonadism, hypospadias, hyposmia, subaortic stenosis. Kyphoscoliosis.

NATURAL HISTORY.

Lentigines differ from freckles in being darker of color, usually present at birth, and not related to sunlight exposure. They often increase in number with age and may occur in any cutaneous area. Many of the other features of the disorder are not readily apparent and must be searched for; examples are the deafness and cardiac findings. Hypogonadism may be secondary to hypogonadotropism; hence, these individuals should be followed closely at the age of adolescence in order to determine whether sex hormone replacement therapy is indicated.

ETIOLOGY. Autosomal dominant with wide variability in expression, including lack of lentigines in an occasional patient.

References

Gorlin, R. J., Anderson, R. C., and Blaw, M.: Multiple lentigines syndrome. Am. J. Dis. Child., *117*:652, 1969.

Sommer, A., et al.: A family study of the LEOPARD' syndrome. Am. J. Dis. Child., *121*:520, 1971.

Swanson, S. L., Santen, R. J., and Smith, D. W.: Multiple lentigines syndrome. J. Pediatr., *78*:1037, 1971.

Voron, D. A., Hatfield, H. A., and Kalkhoff, R. K.: Multiple lentigines syndrome. Case report and review of the literature. Am. J. Med., *60*:447, 1976.

St. John Sutton, M. G., et al.: Hypertrophic obstructive cardiomyopathy and lentiginosis: A little known neural ectodermal syndrome. Am. J. Cardiol., *47*: 214, 1981.

Peter, J. R., and Kemp, J. S.: Leopard syndrome: Death because of chronic respiratory insufficiency. Am. J. Med. Genet., *37*:340, 1990.

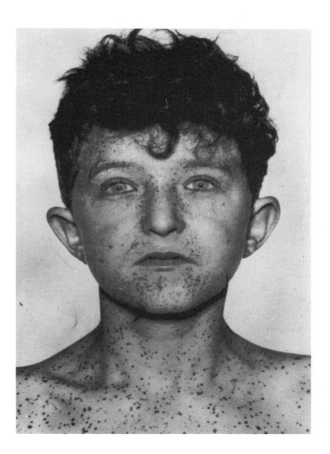

FIGURE 1. Multiple lentigines syndrome. Adolescent boy showing lentigines, prominent ears, and mild ocular hypertelorism. (From Gorlin, R. J., et al.: Am. J. Dis. Child., *117*:652, 1969, with permission.)

GOLTZ SYNDROME

Poikiloderma With Focal Dermal Hypoplasia, Syndactyly, Dental Anomalies

This mesoectodermal disorder was recognized as a distinct entity by Goltz et al. in 1962, although well-described cases had been reported prior to that time. More than 175 cases have been documented.

ABNORMALITIES

Skin. Pink or red, atrophic macules that may be slightly raised or depressed and have a linear and asymmetric distribution. Mainly on thighs, forearm, and cheeks. Telangiectasis. Lipomatous nodules projecting through localized areas of skin atrophy. Angiofibromatous nodules around lips, in vulval and perianal areas, around the eyes, the ears (on pinnae and in middle ear), the fingers and toes, the groin and umbilicus, inside the mouth, and in esophagus.

Nails. Dystrophic nails, narrow and/or hypoplastic.

Hair. Sparse and brittle. Localized areas of alopecia in head and pubic.

Dentition. Hypoplasia of teeth, anodontia, enamel hypoplasia, late eruption, irregular placement, malocclusion, and/or notched incisors.

Skeletal. Asymmetric involvement of hands and feet in 60 per cent including syndactyly, absence or hypoplasia of digits, ectrodactyly, polydactyly, and absence of an extremity. Scoliosis (20 per cent). Longitudinal striations in the metaphyses of long bones. Spina bifida occulta. Clavicular dysplasia. Failure of pubic bone fusion. Skeletal asymmetry.

Face. Asymmetry with mild hemihypertrophy. Narrow nasal bridge and broad tip sometimes with unilateral notch of ala nasi. Thin, protruding, simple low-set ears. Pointed chin.

Eyes. Strabismus, coloboma of the iris and aniridia, microphthalmos, anophthalmos, choroidoretinal coloboma. Involvement is frequently unilateral.

Other. Horseshoe kidney. Cystic dysplasia of kidney. Umbilical, inguinal, and/or epigastric herniae. Hiatus hernia.

OCCASIONAL ABNORMALITIES. Moderate short stature, joint hypermotility, mental retardation (15 per cent), hearing impairment, microcephaly, bulbar angiofibroma of eye, congenital heart defects, hernia. Expansile, tumor-like bone lesions.

NATURAL HISTORY. The skin lesions are usually present at birth, although the skin lipomata and the lip and anal papillomata may develop later. No effective therapy is known except plastic surgery for the syndactyly and removal of the papillomata when indicated. However, the latter may recur. Despite serious structural anomalies of the eyes, acuity may be surprisingly good.

ETIOLOGY. The vast majority of cases have been sporadic and female. X-linked dominant inheritance with lethality in hemizygous males is the most likely mode of inheritance. Most cases represent fresh mutations. Because of combined partial phenotypes of both Goltz and Aicardi syndromes in some patients with terminal deletions of Xp, it has been suggested that the critical genes for both syndromes might be contiguous at the Xp terminal region.

References

Jenner, M.: Naeviforme, Poikilodermie—artige Hautveränderungen mit Missbildungen-(Schwimmhautbildungen an den Fingern, Papillome am Anus). 2 bl. Hautkr., 27:468, 1928.

Wodniansky, P.: Über die Formen der congenitalen Poikilodermie. Arch. Klin. Exp. Dermatol., 205:331, 1957.

Goltz, R. W., et al.: Focal dermal hypoplasia. Arch. Dermatol., 86:708, 1962.

Gorlin, R. J., et al.: Focal dermal hypoplasia syndrome. Acta Dermatovener. (Stockholm), 43:421, 1963.

Holden, J. D., and Akers, W. A.: Goltz's syndrome: Focal dermal hypoplasia. A combined mesoectodermal dysplasia. Am. J. Dis. Child., 114:292, 1967.

Temple, I. K., et al.: Focal dermal hypoplasia (Goltz syndrome). J. Med. Genet., 27:180, 1990.

Naritomi, K., et al.: Combined Goltz and Aicardi syndromes in a terminal Xp deletion: Are they a contiguous gene syndrome? Am. J. Med. Genet., 43:839, 1992.

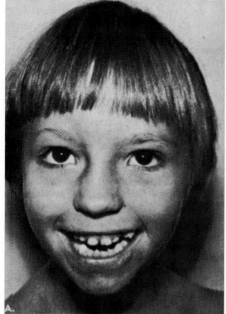

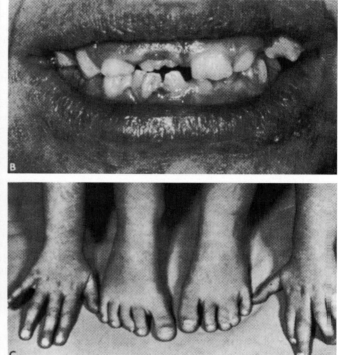

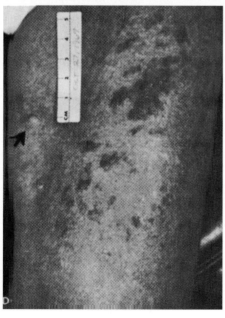

FIGURE 1. Goltz syndrome. *A,* An 11-year-old girl. *B,* Late eruption of teeth with dental hypoplasia and malformation. *C,* Note the syndactyly of the left hand and foot. *D,* Thigh, showing irregular areas of altered pigmentation and of fatty herniation through loci of focal dermal hypoplasia (*arrow*).

AICARDI SYNDROME

Infantile Spasms, Agenesis
of Corpus Callosum, Chorioretinal Lacunae

This disorder was initially described in 1965 by Aicardi et al. Subsequently, over 200 cases have been reported. With the exception of one male with a XXY karyotype, all have been females.

ABNORMALITIES

Brain. Microcephaly. Partial or total agenesis of corpus callosum. Deformed ventricular system with enlargement and irregularity of the lateral and third ventricles. Cortical and subependymal heterotopias of gray matter. Pachygyria. Hypoplastic cerebellar vermis and cystic dilatation of fourth ventricle.

Neurologic. Infantile spasms. Typical EEG consisting of generalized background disorganization with high-amplitude slowing and burst suppression activity. Of greatest significance is the independent activity of each hemisphere. Mental deficiency. Hypotonia.

Ocular. Bilateral chorioretinopathy consisting of discrete yellow-white holes or "lacunae" with sharp borders and little pigmentary change in surrounding retina. Microphthalmia. Optic nerve colobomata. Diminished size of optic nerves and chiasma.

Costovertebral. Hemivertebrae, butterfly and block vertebrae. Spina bifida. Scoliosis. Absent, extra, fused, or bifid ribs.

OCCASIONAL ABNORMALITIES. Postnatal growth deficiency. Cleft lip and palate. Proximally placed thumbs. Papilloma of choroid plexus. Hepatoblastoma. Benign teratoma. Embryonal carcinoma. Lipoma and metastatic angiosarcoma. Retrobulbar cysts. Retinal detachment. Cataract. Nystagmus. Deficient growth hormone and cortisol levels.

NATURAL HISTORY. Infantile spasms are usually the presenting sign beginning anytime during the first year (frequently before 3 months) and usually ceasing before 2 years, at which time other types of seizures develop. Death prior to adolescence or early adulthood occurs in the majority of cases usually the result of pneumonia frequently aggravated by kyphoscoliosis, the poor neurologic status, or an immunodeficiency state, which has been reported in one patient. Profound mental retardation and intractable seizures occur in the survivors. Some degree of vision is usually present. Magnetic resonance imaging is often necessary to document the defects in brain development. A more favorable prognosis has been documented in a few patients.

ETIOLOGY. X-linked dominant lethal in the hemizygous male. No affected siblings have been documented, suggesting that all cases represent fresh gene mutations.

COMMENT. Similar clinical findings are present in Aicardi syndrome, Goltz syndrome, and microphthalmia-linear skin defects syndrome. The latter has been shown to be due to del Xp22.3. It has been suggested that gene disruption at Xp22 may lead to all three of these X-linked dominant male lethal conditions.

References

Aicardi, J., et al.: Spasms in flexion, callosal agenesis, ocular abnormalities: A new syndrome. Electroencephalogr. Clin. Neurophysiol., 19:609, 1965.

Donnenfeld, A. E., et al.: Clinical, cytogenetic, and pedigree findings in 18 cases of Aicardi syndrome. Am. J. Med. Genet., 32:461, 1989.

Donnenfeld, A. E., et al.: Microphthalmia and chorioretinal lesions in a girl with an Xp22.2 pter deletion and partial 3p trisomy: Clinical observations relevant to Aicardi syndrome gene localization. Am. J. Med. Genet., 37:182, 1990.

Carney, S. H., et al.: Aicardi syndrome: More than meets the eye. Surv. Ophthalmol., 37:419, 1993.

Ohtsuka, Y., et al.: Aicardi syndrome: A longitudinal clinical and electroencephalographic study. Epilepsia, 34:627, 1993.

Tsao, C. Y., et al.: Aicardi syndrome, metastatic angiosarcoma of the leg, and scalp lipoma. Am. J. Med. Genet., 45:594, 1993.

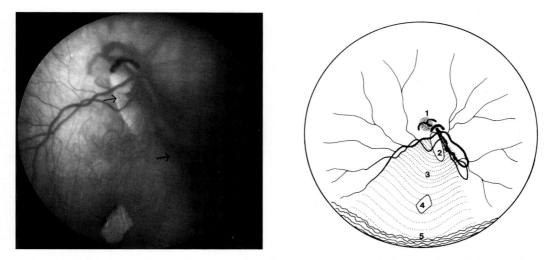

FIGURE 1. *Right*, Schematic of retinal malformations depicted in the retinal photograph on left. *1*, Optic disk; *2*, peripapillary chorioretinal lacuma; *3*, retinal excavatum; *4*, midperipheral chorioretinal lacuma; *5*, fibrous ridge. (From Carney, S. H., et al.: Surv. Ophthalmol., *37*:419, 1993, with permission.)

MICROPHTHALMIA–LINEAR SKIN DEFECTS SYNDROME

Al-Gazali et al. described two females with this disorder in 1988 and 1990. An additional ten patients have been reported.

ABNORMALITIES

Eyes. Microphthalmia; sclerocornea.
Skin. Dermal aplasia, without herniation of fatty tissue, usually involving face, scalp, and neck but occasionally upper part of the thorax.

OCCASIONAL ABNORMALITIES. Microcephaly: CNS defects including agenesis of corpus callosum and absence of septum pellucidium; additional eye abnormalities including anterior chamber defects, cataracts, iris coloboma, pigmentary retinopathy, and orbital cysts; structural cardiac defects (atrial septal defect, ventricular septal defect, overriding aorta); cardiac conduction defects; diaphragmatic hernia.

NATURAL HISTORY. Developmental milestones are reached at an appropriate age when the severe visual handicap is taken into consideration. Death occurred in the first year of life in two children, presumably secondary to cardiac arrhythmias.

ETIOLOGY. All patients have been females, suggesting an X-linked mutation lethal in males. Most have had a gross deletion or a translocation involving the short arm of the X chromosome resulting in monosomy for Xp22.3.

References

Al-Gazali, L. I., et al.: An XX male and two t (X;Y) females with linear skin defects and congenital microphthalmia: A new syndrome at Xp22.3. J. Med. Genet., 25:638, 1988.

Al-Gazali, L. I., et al.: Two 46XX, t (X;Y) females with linear skin defects and congenital microphthalmia: A new syndrome at Xp22.3. J. Med. Genet., 27:59, 1990.

Linder, N. M., et al.: Xp22.3 Microdeletion syndrome with microphthalmia, sclerocornea, linear skin defects, and congenital heart defects. Am. J. Med. Genet., 44:61, 1992.

Happle, R., et al.: MIDAS syndrome (microphthalmia, dermal aplasia, and sclerocornea): An X-linked phenotype distinct from Goltz syndrome. Am. J. Med. Genet., 47:710, 1993.

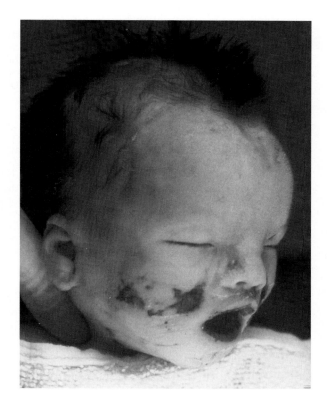

FIGURE 1. Newborn female. Note the irregular areas of skin hypoplasia. (Courtesy of Dr. Judith Allanson, Children's Hospital of Eastern Ontario, Ottawa, Ontario.)

DYSKERATOSIS CONGENITA SYNDROME

Hyperpigmentation of Skin,
Leukoplakia, Nail Dystrophy, Pancytopenia

Cole originally described this condition in 1930 and later summarized the findings. Over 100 cases have been reported.

ABNORMALITIES. Although hyperpigmentation of the skin may be present from birth, most of the abnormalities become apparent between 5 and 15 years of age. Growth deficit is mentioned but poorly documented.

Skin. Irregular reticular brownish gray pigmentation, which may be telangiectatic. The neck, upper chest, and upper arms are primarily affected. The recticular pigmentation often surrounds atrophic areas of hypopigmentation. Hyperkeratosis and hyperhidrosis of palms and soles. May have bullae.

Mucous Membranes. Premalignant leukoplakia may be found on lips, mouth, anus, urethra, and conjunctiva.

Eyes. Blepharitis, conjunctivitis, ectropion, and nasolacrimal obstruction with excessive tearing.

Nails. Dystrophy, which may progress to absence of nail.

Dentition. Caries, gingival recession, short-blunted roots, tooth mobility, and severe alveolar bone loss.

Hair. Tends to be sparse and fine; occasionally premature graying.

Hematologic. Pancytopenia.

Bone. Osteoporosis, possibly with relative fragility. Avascular necrosis.

Genitalia. Testicular hypoplasia.

Other. Esophageal nasopharyngeal, anal, urethral, ureteral, and vaginal strictures and stenosis.

OCCASIONAL ABNORMALITIES. Mental deficiency. Intracranial calcifications. Hepatic cirrhosis. Immunologic abnormalities, including reduced antibody, failure to respond to skin sensitization, primary thymic dysplasia, hypogammaglobulinemia, impaired rosette formation by lymphocytes, and/or decreased lymphocytic response to mitogenic substances. Hodgkin's disease, adenocarcinoma of pancreas, esophageal cancer, Hodgkin lymphoma, squamous cell carcinoma of the skin or mucosa, deafness.

NATURAL HISTORY. The problem in affected tissues tends to become more severe with age,

and most patients die before the fourth decade as a consequence of either pancytopenia (20 per cent), malignant transformation in the mucous membranes (30 per cent), or opportunistic infections (50 per cent). The mean age at death is 24 years (range, 8 to 50). When present, leukoplakia lesions should be excised as representing premalignant change.

ETIOLOGY. X-linked recessive inheritance in majority of familial cases. Linkage analysis has assigned the locus to Xq28. However, genetic heterogeneity has been suggested for this disorder based on a family in which male-to-male transmission has been documented, suggesting autosomal dominant inheritance in some cases.

COMMENT. The dermatologic term dyskeratosis congenita obviously depicts only one feature of this abiotrophic type of disease with hamartomatous features, in which the affected individual develops hypoplasia and dysplasia in the skin, mucous membranes, marrow, and other tissues. The sibling of one patient and the niece of another patient died of leukemia, the latter case raising the question of whether there may be an increased likelihood of leukemia in the heterozygote carrying this mutant gene.

References

Cole, H. N., Cole, H. N., Jr., and Lascheid, W. P.: Dyskeratosis congenita. Relationship to poikiloderma atrophicans vasculare and to aplastic anemia of Fanconi. Arch. Dermatol., 76:712, 1957.

Addison, J., and Rise, M. S.: The association of dyskeratosis congenita and Fanconi's anemia. Med. J. Aust., 1:797, 1965.

Georgouras, K.: Dyskeratosis congenita. Aust. J. Dermatol., 8:36, 1965.

Connor, J. M., and Teague, R. H.: Dyskeratosis congenita. Report of a large kindred. Br. J. Dermatol., 105:321, 1981.

Davidson, H. R., and Connor, J. M.: Dyskeratosis congenita. J. Med Genet., 25:843, 1988.

Shashidhar, Pai, G., et al.: Etiologic heterogeneity in dyskeratosis congenita. Am. J. Med. Genet., 32:63, 1989.

Arngrimsson, R., et al.: Dyskeratosis congenita: Three additional families show linkage to a locus in Xq28. J. Med. Genet., 30:618, 1993.

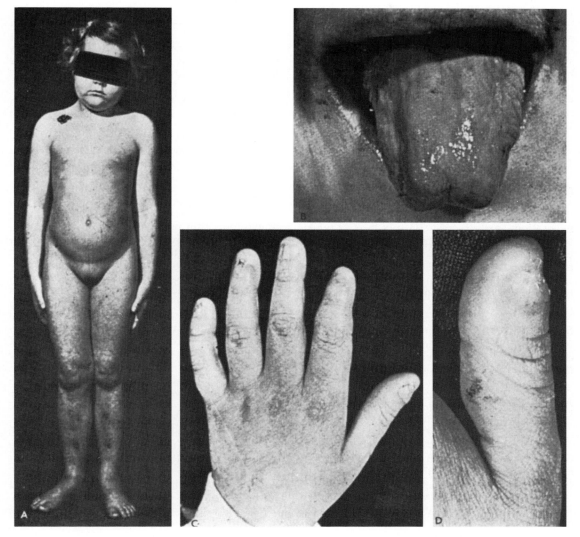

FIGURE 1. Dyskeratosis congenita syndrome. An 8-year-old patient showing reticulated skin pigmentation (*A*), smooth tongue without leukoplakia as yet (*B*), and nail hypoplasia to aplasia (*C* and *D*). (Courtesy of K. Georgouras, Sydney Australia.)

Q

Q. ECTODERMAL DYSPLASIAS

HYPOHIDROTIC ECTODERMAL DYSPLASIA SYNDROME

Defect in Sweating, Alopecia, Hypodontia

There are a number of ectodermal dysplasia syndromes, of which only a few are represented in this text. The division into hypohidrotic and hidrotic categories on the basis of the extent of the deficit of sweat glands is in no way absolute. Just as there is variable hypoplasia of hair follicles, there is variable hypoplasia of sweat glands.

Thurman described this entity in 1848. In 1875, Charles Darwin set forth the following concise commentary about this disease: "I may give an analogous case, communicated to me by Mr. W. Wedderhorn of a Hindoo family in Scinde, in which ten men, in the course of four generations, were furnished, in both jaws taken together, with only four small and weak incisor teeth and with eight posterior molars. The men thus affected have very little hair on the body, and became bald early in life. They also suffer much during hot weather from excessive dryness of the skin. It is remarkable that no instance has occurred of a daughter being thus affected." In 1929, Weech clearly separated this condition from other clinical problems having ectodermal dysplasia as a feature. Over 130 cases had been reported by 1956.

ABNORMALITIES

Skin. Thin and hypoplastic, with decreased pigment and tendency toward papular changes on face; periorbital wrinkling and hyperpigmentation. Scaling or peeling of skin in immediate newborn period.

Skin Appendages. Hair: fine, dry, and hypochromic; sparse to absent. Sweat glands: hypoplasia to absence of eccrine glands; apocrine glands more normally represented. Sebaceous glands: hypoplasia to absence.

Mucous Membranes. Hypoplasia, with absence of mucous glands in oral and nasal membranes. Mucous glands may also be absent from bronchial mucosa.

Dentition. Hypodontia to anodontia resulting in deficient alveolar ridge. Anterior teeth tend to be conical in shape.

Craniofacial. Low nasal bridge, small nose with hypoplastic alae nasi, full forehead, prominent supraorbital ridges. Prominent lips.

OCCASIONAL ABNORMALITIES. Hoarse voice, hypoplasia to absence of mammary glands and/or nipples, absence of tears, failure to develop nasal turbinates, mild to moderate nail dystrophy, eczematous change in skin, asthmatic symptoms.

NATURAL HISTORY. Hyperthermia as a consequence of inadequate sweating not only is a serious threat to life but may be the cause of mental deficiency, which is an occasional feature of this disease. Living in a cool climate and cooling by water when overheated are important measures. The hypoplasia of mucous membranes plus thin nares may require frequent irrigation of the nares to limit the severity of purulent rhinitis. Otitis media and lung infection may also be consequences of the mucous membrane defect. Mucous glands have been hypoplastic to absent not only in the respiratory tract but in esophageal and colonic mucosa as well. Early roentgenographic evaluation may reveal the extent of dental deficit, and dentures are indicated. Though the patient is often hairless at birth, some hair may develop. Short stature should not be considered a feature of this disorder. Therefore, affected males with growth deficiency should be evaluated for other causes such as endocrine deficiencies.

ETIOLOGY. X-linked recessive. The gene has been localized within the region Xq11-21.1 by linkage analysis. It has been estimated that approximately 90 per cent of female carriers can be identified by dental examination and sweat testing. The latter uses an iodine-in-alcohol followed by corn starch–in–castor oil application to identify streaks devoid of sweat glands along the lines of Blaschko, forming a V-shape over the back of carrier females. Linkage analysis using closely linked flanking markers can determine the carrier status of many at-risk females as well as the prenatal diagnosis of affected males during the first trimester of pregnancy.

COMMENT. An autosomal recessive type of hypohidrotic ectodermal dysplasia has been described. The clinical features have not been distinguishable from the X-linked hypohidrotic ectodermal dysplasia, except for the fact that females are as severely affected as males. The natural history is similar to that of X-linked hypohidrotic ectodermal dysplasia, although the patients may have a greater problem with ozena (foul, purulent nasal discharge). The parents have been normal.

References

Thurman, J.: Two cases in which the skin, hair and teeth were very imperfectly developed. Medico-Chir. Trans., 31:71, 1848.

Darwin, C.: The Variations of Animals and Plants under Domestication, 2nd ed. London, John Murray, 1875.

Weech, A. A.: Hereditary ectodermal dysplasia (congenital ectodermal defect). A report of two cases. Am. J. Dis. Child., 37:766, 1929.

Passarge, E., Nuzum, C. T., and Schubert, W. K.: Anhidrotic ectodermal dysplasia as autosomal recessive trait in an inbred kindred. Humangenetik, 3: 181, 1966.

Gorlin, R. J., Old, T., and Anderson, V. E.: Hypohidrotic ectodermal dysplasia females. A critical analysis and argument for genetic heterogeneity. Z. Kinderheilkd., 108:1, 1970.

Clarke, A.: Hypohidrotic ectodermal dysplasia. J. Med. Genet., 24:659, 1987.

Zonana, J., et al.: X-linked hypohidrotic ectodermal dysplasia: Localization within the region Xq11-21.1 by linkage analysis and implications for carrier detection and prenatal diagnosis. Am. J. Hum. Genet., 43:75, 1988.

Zonana, J., et al.: Prenatal diagnosis of X-linked hypohidrotic ectodermal dysplasia by linkage analysis. Am. J. Med. Genet., 35:132, 1990.

Crawford, P. J. M., et al.: Clinical and radiographic dental findings in X-linked hypohidrotic ectodermal dysplasia. J. Med. Genet., 28:181, 1991.

Clark, A., and Burn, J.: Sweat testing to identify female carriers of X-linked hypohidrotic ectodermal dysplasia. J. Med. Genet., 28:330, 1991.

Zonana, J., et al.: Detection of de novo mutations and analysis of their origin in families with X-linked hypohidrotic ectodermal dysplasia. J. Med. Genet., 31: 287, 1994.

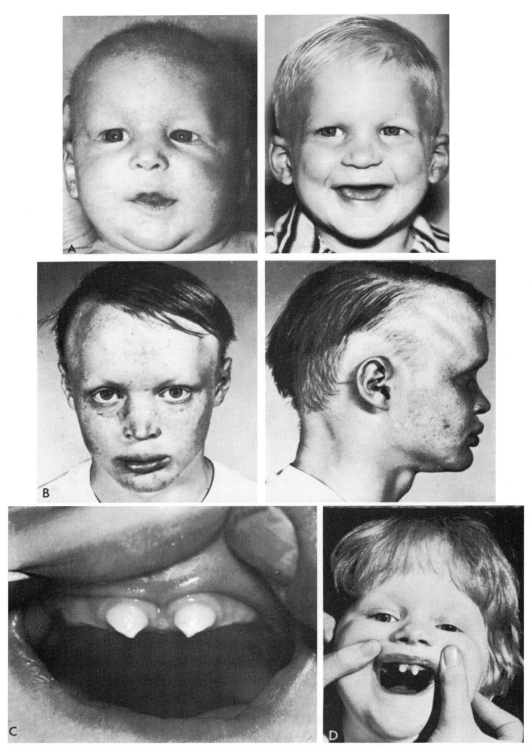

FIGURE 1. Hypohidrotic ectodermal dysplasia syndrome. *A,* Young infant; diagnosis made after hyperthermic episode. Same boy at 2 years of age. *B,* Older boy. The hypoplasia of the skin contributes to the prominent appearance of the lips. Note the midfacial hypoplasia. *C,* Hypoplasia of alveolar ridge in a 2-year old. Hypoplastic conical incisors. *D,* Partial expression in a female.

RAPP-HODGKIN ECTODERMAL DYSPLASIA SYNDROME

(Hypohidrotic Ectodermal Dysplasia, Autosomal Dominant Type)

Hypohidrosis, Oral Clefts, Dysplastic Nails

Rapp and Hodgkin reported three affected individuals in 1968, and Summitt and Hiatt added one additional case. Approximately 25 cases have been reported.

ABNORMALITIES
Skin. Thin, with decreased number of sweat pores. Sparse, fine hair. Pili canaliculi.
Nails. Small.
Dentition. Hypodontia with small, conical teeth.
Face. Low nasal bridge, narrow nose with hypoplastic ala nasi, maxillary hypoplasia. High forehead.
Mouth. Small. Cleft lip with or without cleft palate, cleft palate alone, cleft uvula, velopharyngeal incompetence.
Genitalia. Hypospadias.

OCCASIONAL ABNORMALITIES.
Short stature. Ptosis. Atretic ear canals. Hearing loss. Absent lacrimal puncta. Labial anomalies. Hypothelia. Syndactyly.

NATURAL HISTORY.
Liable to have hyperthermia in early childhood. Thereafter, although reduced sweating is described, heat intolerance is not usually a problem. Frequent occurrence of purulent conjunctivitis and otitis media, the latter presumably related to palatal incompetence. Speech difficulties are common. Deficient mucous coating of vocal cords can affect vocal quality.

ETIOLOGY.
Autosomal dominant, although X-linked dominant inheritance is not excluded. Sweat pores present, but markedly reduced in number on the palms.

References

Rapp, R. S., and Hodgkin, W. E.: Anhidrotic ectodermal dysplasia: Autosomal dominant inheritance with palate and lip anomalies. J. Med. Genet., 5:269, 1968.

Summitt, R. L., and Hiatt, R. L.: Hypohidrotic ectodermal dysplasia with multiple associated anomalies. Birth Defects, 7(8):121, 1971.

Wannarachue, N., Hall, B. D., and Smith, D. W.: Ectodermal dysplasia and multiple defects (Rapp-Hodgkin type). J. Pediatr., 81:1217, 1972.

Schroeder, H. W., and Sybert, V. P.: Rapp-Hodgkin ectodermal dysplasia. J. Pediatr., 110:72, 1987.

Salinas, C. F., and Montes-G, G. M.: Rapp-Hodgkin syndrome: Observations on ten cases and characteristic hair changes (pili canaliculi). Birth Defects, 24:149, 1988.

O'Donnell, B. P., and James, W. D.: Rapp-Hodgkin ectodermal dysplasia. J. Am. Acad. Dermatol., 27:323, 1992.

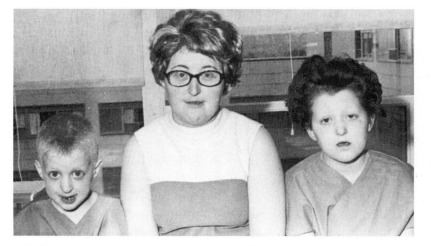

FIGURE 1. Rapp-Hodgkin ectodermal dysplasia syndrome. Affected mother and children in family reported by Rapp and Hodgkin. The mother is wearing a wig. Note the narrow nose, small mouth, and features of ectodermal dysplasia. (From Rapp, R. S., and Hodgkin, W. E.: J. Med. Genet., 5:269, 1968, with permission.)

TRICHO-DENTO-OSSEOUS SYNDROME

(TDO Syndrome)

Kinky Hair, Enamel Hypoplasia, Sclerotic Bone

Lichtenstein et al. defined this disorder in 107 individuals from one large kindred in 1972. Robinson et al. had previously described an autosomal dominant disorder with curly hair and enamel hypoplasia, with or without nail hypoplasia. Although it is not possible to be certain from the reported cases, the overall similarities suggest that they are the same disorder.

ABNORMALITIES

Hair. Kinky at birth.

Dentition. Small, widely spaced, pitted teeth with poor enamel, increased pulp chamber size (taurodontism).

Facies. Frontal bossing, dolichocephaly, squarish jaw.

Bone. Mild to moderate increased bone density, most evident in lateral roentgenograms of skull but also in the long bones and spine.

Nails. Brittle, with superficial peeling (about 50 per cent).

OCCASIONAL ABNORMALITY. Partial craniosynostosis.

NATURAL HISTORY. The hair sometimes straightens with age. The teeth become eroded and discolored, are prone to periapical abscesses, and are lost by the second to third decade. The sclerotic bone appears to be secondary to closely compacted lamellae and is rarely associated with any clinical symptomatology.

ETIOLOGY. Autosomal dominant. Elevated serum acid phosphatase level has been documented, although the significance of the finding is unknown.

COMMENT. It has been suggested that two types of tricho-dento-osseous syndrome can be distinguished. TDO-I, the disorder described above, and TDO-II. The latter condition is characterized by curly hair and pitted dysplastic teeth identical to that seen in TDO-I. However, unlike TDO-I, there is microcephaly, increased thickness of the calvaria, obliterated diploë, poorly pneumatized mastoids, and obliterated frontal sinuses. In addition, the enamel is not discolored, there is no evidence of increased density of long bones or premature closure of sutures, and the clavicles are undertubulated. TDO-II is also inherited as an autosomal dominant disorder.

References

Robinson, G. C., Miller, J. R., and Worth, H. M.: Hereditary enamel hypoplasia, its association with characteristic hair structure. Pediatrics, 37:489, 1966.

Lichtenstein, J., et al.: The tricho-dento-osseous (TDO) syndrome. Am. J. Hum. Genet., 24:569, 1972.

Shapiro, S. D., et al.: Tricho-dento-osseous syndrome. Am. J. Med. Genet., 16:225, 1983.

Wright, J. R., et al.: Tricho-dento-osseous syndrome. Features of the hair and teeth. Oral Surg. Oral Med. Oral Pathol., 77:487, 1994.

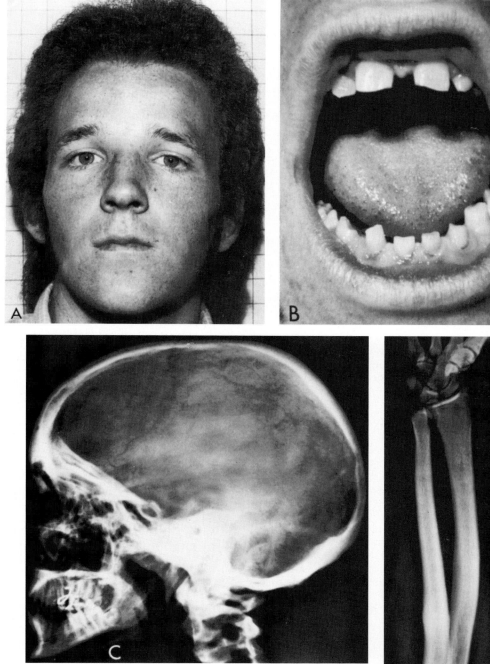

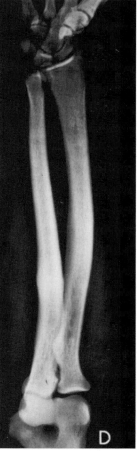

FIGURE 1. Tricho-dento-osseous syndrome. *A* to *D*, Young adult. Note the kinky hair, hypodontia, and increased bone density, especially at the base of the skull. (From Lichtenstein, J. R., et al.: Am. J. Hum. Genet., 24:569, 1972, with permission.)

CLOUSTON SYNDROME

*Nail Dystrophy, Dyskeratotic
Palms and Soles, Hair Hypoplasia*

Clouston in 1939 reported 119 individuals in a French-Canadian family. Rajagopalan and Tay described an affected Chinese pedigree in 1977. Over 200 instances have been described.

ABNORMALITIES

Skin. Thick dyskeratotic palms and soles. Hyperpigmentation over knuckles, elbows, axillae, areolae, and pubic area.

Hair. Hypoplasia to alopecia (61 per cent). Deficiency of eyelashes and eyebrows.

Nails. Hypoplasia to aplasia, dysplasia.

Eyes. Strabismus.

OCCASIONAL ABNORMALITIES. Cataract, photophobia, dull mentality, short stature, thickened skull, tufting of terminal phalanges.

ETIOLOGY. Autosomal dominant.

References

Joachim, H.: Hereditary dystrophy of the hair and nails in six generations. Ann. Intern. Med., *10*:400, 1936.

Clouston, H. R.: The major forms of hereditary ectodermal dysplasia (with an autopsy and biopsies on the anhidrotic type). Can. Med. Assoc. J., *40*:1, 1939.

Wilkey, W. D., and Stevenson, G. H.: A family with inherited ectodermal dystrophy. Can. Med. Assoc. J., *53*:226, 1945.

Gold, R. J. M., and Scriver, C. R.: Properties of hair keratin in an autosomal dominant form of ectodermal dysplasia. Am. J. Hum. Genet., *24*:549, 1972.

Rajagopalan, K. V., and Tay, C. H.: Hydrotic ectodermal dysplasia: Study of a large Chinese pedigree. Arch. Dermatol., *113*:481, 1977.

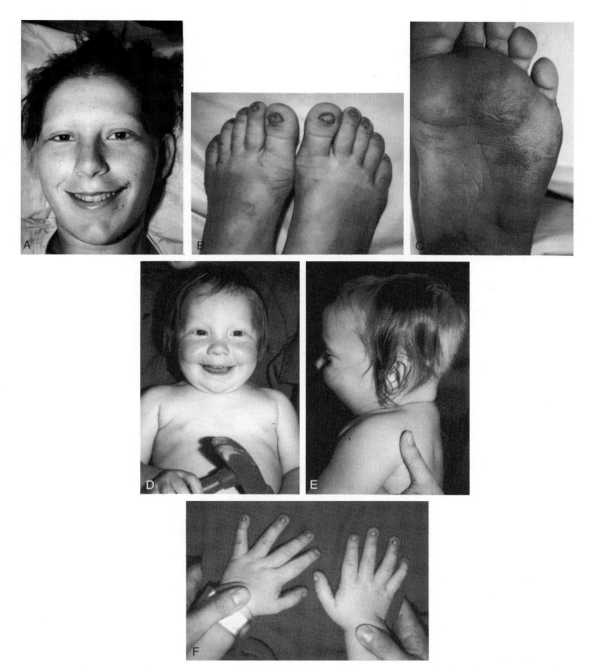

FIGURE 1. Clouston syndrome. *A* to *F*, A 19-year-old mother and her 22-month-old daughter. Note the sparse hair, dysplastic nails, and dyskeratotic soles.

PACHYONYCHIA CONGENITA SYNDROME

Thick Nails, Hyperkeratosis, Foot Blisters

Pachyonychia congenita is an ectodermal dysplasia described by Jadassohn and Lewandowsky, in which there is hypertrophic dystrophy of the distal nails.

ABNORMALITIES
Nails. Progressive thickening, yellow-brown discoloration, pinched margins, and an upward angulation of distal tips. The nails may eventually be hypoplastic or even absent.

Skin. Patchy to complete hyperkeratosis of palms and soles, callosities of feet, palmar and plantar bullae formation in areas of pressure that are often painful. Keratosis pilaris with tiny cutaneous horny excrescences, particularly on the extensor surfaces of the arms and legs and on the buttocks. Epidermal cysts filled with loose keratin on face, neck, and upper chest. Verrucous lesions on the elbows, knees, and lower legs.

Mucous Membranes. Leukokeratosis of mouth and tongue, especially in positions of increased trauma. Scalloped tongue edge.

Dentition. Erupted teeth at birth, lost by 4 to 6 months. Early eruption of primary teeth and early loss of secondary teeth due to severe caries.

OCCASIONAL ABNORMALITIES.
Mental deficiency. Corneal thickening, cataracts, thickening of tympanic membrane, hyperhidrosis, particularly of palms and soles. Dry and sparse hair. Osteomata of frontal bones. Intestinal diverticula. Large joint arthritis. Bushy eyebrows. Hoarseness secondary to laryngeal leukokeratosis. Malformed teeth and twinning of the incisors.

NATURAL HISTORY.
Clinical manifestations are present at birth or by 6 months of age in approximately 80 per cent of patients. Usually the nails are grossly thickened by 1 year of age. Complete surgical removal of the nails is sometimes merited, although any matrix left behind will reform abnormal nails. Severe recurrent upper respiratory symptoms has occurred in those with severe laryngeal involvement. Areas of chronic bullous formation should be followed carefully for development of possible skin malignancy. An abnormality of cell-mediated immunity leading to a deficiency in the recognition and processing of candida can result in recurrent oral and cutaneous candidiasis, which can compound the nail problems.

COMMENT.
Two major forms of this disorder have been described: The Jadossohn-Lewandowsky form characterized by pachyonychia, palmoplantar hyperkeratosis, hyperhidrosis, occasional blistering, follicular keratosis, and oral leukokeratosis; and a rarer form defined by Jackson and Lawler characterized by pachyonychia, multiple epidermal cysts, recurrent flexural infections, natal teeth, and straight bushy eyebrow hair. Oral leukokeratosis is not a feature of this latter form.

ETIOLOGY.
Autosomal dominant. Mutations in two different keratin genes located at chromosome 17q12-q21 are responsible for the two major forms of pachyonychia congenita. The Jadassohn-Lewandowsky form is caused by mutations in keratin 16 and the Jackson-Lawler type by mutations in keratin 17.

References

Jadassohn, J., and Lewandowsky, F.: Pachyonychia congenita, keratosis disseminata circumscripta (folliculosis): Tylomata; leukokeratosis linguae. Ikonographia Dermatologica, Tab., *629*, 1906.

Soderquist, N. A., and Reed, W. B.: Pachyonychia congenita with epidermal cysts and other congenital dyskeratoses. Arch. Dermatol., *97*:31, 1968.

Young, L. L., and Lenox, J. A.: Pachyonychia congenita. A long-term evaluation. Oral Surg., *36*:663, 1973.

Stieglitz, J. B., and Centerwall, W. R.: Pachyonychia congenita. (Jadassohn-Lewandowsky syndrome): A seventeen-member, four-generation pedigree with unusual respiratory and dental involvement. Am. J. Med. Genet., *14*:21, 1983.

Su, W. P. D., et al.: Pachyonychia congenita: A clinical study of 12 cases and review of the literature. Pediatr. Dermatol., *7*:32, 1990.

Rohold, A. E., and Brandrup, F.: Pachyonychia congenita: Therapeutic and immunologic aspects. Pediatr. Dermatol., *7*:307, 1990.

McLean, W. H. I., et al.: Keratin 16 and keratin 17 mutations cause pachyonychia congenita. Nat. Genet., *9*:273, 1995.

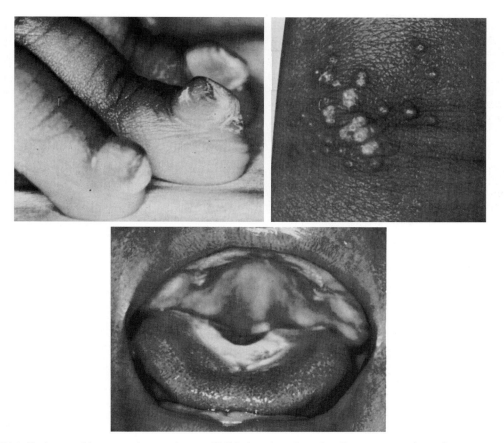

FIGURE 1. Pachyonychia congenita syndrome. Child showing altered nails, cutaneous hyperkeratoses at knee, and leukokeratotic lesions on tongue and lateral palate.

PACHYDERMOPERIOSTOSIS SYNDROME

Thick Coarse Skin, Clubbing

This disorder was originally described by Friedreich in 1868 and further clarified by Touraine et al. in 1935.

ABNORMALITIES

Skin. Development of coarse, thick, oily skin, especially over upper face and scalp, with secondary cutis verticis gyrata and sometimes ptosis of the eyelids. Hyperhidrosis of hands and feet, peripheral vascular stasis. Seborrheic hyperplasia with thick stratum corneum.

Limbs. Clubbing with periostosis, most pronounced at tendinous insertions. Joint and muscle discomfort.

OCCASIONAL ABNORMALITIES. Papular mucinosis, large keloids. Resorption of distal phalanges of hands and feet.

NATURAL HISTORY. Earliest age of onset is about 3 years, with accentuation at adolescence and for a decade or so thereafter; more severe in males.

ETIOLOGY. Autosomal dominant, with wide variance in expression.

References

Friedreich, N.: Hyperostose des gesammten Skelettes. Virchows Arch. Pathol. Anat., 43:83, 1868.

Touraine, A., Solente, G., and Golé, L.: Un syndrome ostéodermopathique: La pachydermie plicaturée avec pachypériostose des extrémités. Presse Med., 43:1820, 1935.

Rimoin, D. L.: Pachydermoperiostosis (idiopathic clubbing and periostosis). Genetic and physiologic considerations. N. Engl. J. Med., 272:923, 1965.

Hedayati, H., Barmada, R., and Skosey, J. L.: Acrolysis in pachydermoperiostosis. Arch. Intern. Med., 140: 1087, 1980.

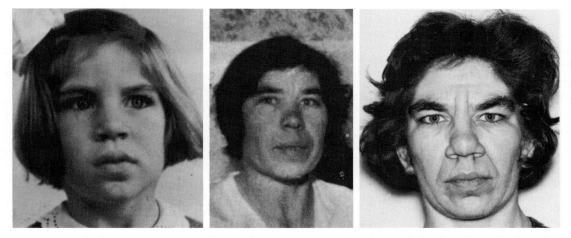

FIGURE 1. Pachydermoperiostosis syndrome. Child who showed evidence of the disorder at birth with an "acromegal" appearance. Although she was large as a child, her adult height was 5 feet, 6 inches. She had amenorrhea with a rudimentary uterus and small ovaries. The middle photo shows her at 30 years of age, with progression in the thickening of skin and hirsutism. Her mother, shown to the right, was similarly but less severely affected. (From Ursing, B.: Acta Med. Scand., *188*:157, 1970, with permission.)

XERODERMA PIGMENTOSA SYNDROME

Undue Sunlight Sensitivity, Atrophic and Pigmentary Skin Changes, Actinic Skin Tumors

Xeroderma pigmentosa occurs in about 1 in 250,000 individuals. Nearly 1000 cases have been reported.

ABNORMALITIES

Skin. Sunlight sensitivity with first exposure. Freckling. Progressive skin atrophy with irregular pigmentation. Cutaneous telangiectasia. Angiomata. Keratoses. Development of basal cell and squamous cell carcinoma, and less often keratocanthoma, adenocarcinoma, melanoma, neuroma, sarcoma, and angiosarcoma.

Eye. Photophobia. Recurrent conjunctival injection. Corneal abnormalities consisting of exposure keratitis leading to corneal clouding and/or vascularization. Neoplasms involving conjunctiva, cornea, and eyelids.

Oral. Atrophic skin of mouth sometimes leading to difficulty opening mouth. Squamous cell carcinoma of tongue tip, gingiva, and/or palate.

Neurologic. Slowly progressive neurologic abnormalities sometimes associated with mental deterioration. Microcephaly. Cerebral atrophy. Choreoathetosis, ataxia, and spasticity. Impaired hearing. Abnormal speech. Abnormal EEG.

OCCASIONAL ABNORMALITIES. Primary internal neoplasms including brain tumors, lung tumors, and leukemia. Immune abnormalities. Frequent infections.

NATURAL HISTORY. Cutaneous symptoms have onset at median age of between 1 and 2 years. The mean age of first nonmelanoma skin cancer is 8 years. Ninety-seven per cent of squamous cell and basal cell cancers occur on face, head, or neck, indicating the important role that sun exposure has in the induction of these neoplasms. Four per cent of squamous cell carcinomas metastasize. Seventy per cent probability of survival has been documented at age 40 years. Thirty-three per cent of deaths are due to cancer and 11 per cent to infection.

ETIOLOGY. Autosomal recessive. The majority of affected patients have a defect in the excision repair of ultraviolet radiation–induced DNA damage. Xp patients fall into one of ten complementation groups (A through I plus a variant).

Groups A, C, and D are most common. Neurologic problems are generally found in groups A and D patients, who show the lowest level of DNA repair, whereas group C patients, who show the highest level of repair, are usually without overt neurologic disorders and have a longer life span. The severity of the skin and eye lesions relates more to the degree of sun exposure. The defect can be identified in cultured fibroblasts from amniocentesis.

COMMENT. The DeSanctis-Cacchione syndrome is a subgroup of xeroderma pigmentosa with neurologic involvement that includes xeroderma pigmentosa, progressive mental deterioration, growth deficiency, microcephaly, and hypogonadism probably secondary to hypothalamic insufficiency. Natural history includes slow developmental progress and growth, with variable neurologic dysfunction, including seizures from early childhood, spasticity, ataxia, peripheral neuropathy, and sometimes sensorineural deafness. Progressive skin deterioration occurs especially related to exposure to the sun. Shortened life expectancy has been documented due to CNS deterioration and/or malignancy. The disorder is the result of a pair of autosomal recessive genes. Patients with DeSanctis-Cacchione syndrome usually belong to complementation groups A or D.

References

DeSanctis, C., and Cacchione, A.: L'idiozia xerodermia. Riv. Spec. Freniatr., 56:269, 1932.

Rook, A., Wilkinson, D. S., and Ebling, F. J. G. (eds.): Textbook of Dermatology. Oxford and Edinburgh, Blackwell Scientific Publications, 1968.

Regan, J. D., et al.: Xeroderma pigmentosa: A rapid sensitive method for prenatal diagnosis. Science, 174:147, 1971.

Pawsey, S. A., et al.: Clinical, genetic and DNA repair studies on a consecutive series of patients with xeroderma pigmentosa. Q. J. Med., 48:179, 1979.

Kraemer, K. H., et al.: Xeroderma pigmentosa: Cutaneous, ocular and neurologic abnormalities in 830 published cases. Arch. Dermatol., 123:241, 1987.

Greenhaw, G. A., et al.: Xeroderma pigmentosum and Cockayne syndrome: Overlapping clinical and biochemical phenotypes. Am. J. Hum. Genet., 50:677, 1992.

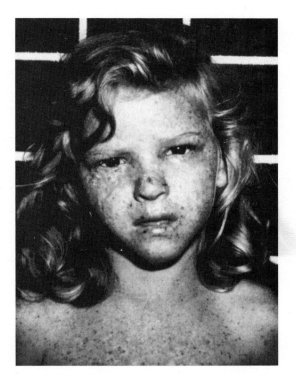

FIGURE 1. A 7-year-old of normal intelligence and light-sensitive xeroderma pigmentosa. (Courtesy of Dr. Robert Summitt, University of Tennessee College of Medicine, Memphis, Tenn.)

SENTER-KID SYNDROME

Ichthyosiform Erythroderma, Sensorineural Deafness

Initially reported by Burns in 1915, this disorder was further delineated by Senter et al., who reported an affected child in 1978 and recognized 12 similar patients from the literature. Skinner et al. introduced the acronym KID (*ker*atitis, *i*chythyosis, *d*eafness) syndrome to highlight the principal features.

ABNORMALITIES

Performance. Sensorineural deafness.

Growth. Ichthyosiform erythroderma with mild lamellar ichthyosis and hyperkeratosis of the skin of the palms, soles, elbows, and knees. Variable alopecia. Decreased sweating.

Nails. Variable nail dystrophy.

Dentition. Variable malformations of teeth.

Eyes. Corneal dystrophy manifest by progressive vascularization with photophobia and tearing leading to corneal destruction with the development of keratodermia (a pannus of vascular or fibrotic tissue) progressing to occlusion of vision.

Other. Cryptorchidism. Variable flexion contractures. Tight heel cords. Oral abnormalities including leukokeratosis, erythematous lesions, and scrotal tongue.

OCCASIONAL ABNORMALITIES.
Squamous cell carcinoma of skin and tongue. Hirschprungs disease. Mental deficiency. Breast hypoplasia. Cochleosaccular abnormality of temporal bone.

NATURAL HISTORY.
The corneal dystrophy, which occurs in 83 per cent of patients, is the most serious aspect because it can lead to blindness. Life-long ophthalmologic examinations are indicated. Early evaluation of hearing is necessary. Mycotic and bacterial skin infections have occurred in more than one half of the cases.

ETIOLOGY.
Autosomal dominant. Most cases are sporadic and thus represent a fresh gene mutation. An autosomal recessive form has been described in three affected siblings and one sporadic case. The principal features of that form include hepatic disease, growth failure, and/or mental deficiency, in addition to the other features of the autosomal dominant type.

References

Burns, F. S.: A case of generalized congenital erythroderma. J. Cutan. Dis., *33*:255, 1915.

Senter, T. P., et al.: Atypical ichthyosiform erythroderma and congenital sensorineural deafness—a distinct syndrome. J. Pediatr., *92*:68, 1978.

Cram, D. L., Resneck, J. S., and Jackson, W. B.: A congenital ichthyosiform syndrome with deafness and keratitis. Arch. Dermatol., *115*:467, 1979.

Skinner, B. A., et al.: The Keratitis, ichthyosis, and deafness (KID) syndrome. Arch. Dermatol., *117*:285, 1981.

Langer, K., et al.: Keratitis, ichthyosis and deafness (KID) syndrome: Report of three cases and a review of the literature. Br. J. Dermatol., *122*:689, 1990.

Nazzaro, V., et al.: Familial occurrence of KID (keratitis, ichthyosis, deafness) syndrome. J. Am. Acad. Dermatol., *23*:385, 1990.

Wilson, G. N., et al.: Keratitis, hepatitis, ichthyosis, and deafness: Report and review of KID syndrome. Am. J. Med. Genet., *40*:255, 1991.

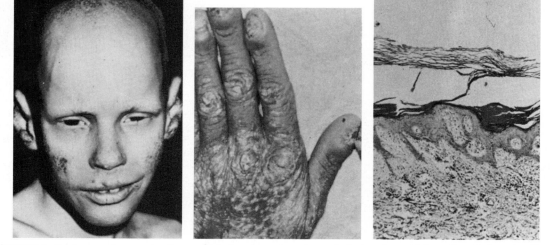

FIGURE 1. Senter syndrome. An 8-year-old showing alopecia, nail dystrophy, and lamellar ichthyosis. (From Senter, T. P., et al.: J. Pediatr., *92*:68, 1978, with permission.)

R

R. ENVIRONMENTAL AGENTS

FETAL ALCOHOL SYNDROME

Prenatal Onset Growth Deficiency, Microcephaly, Short Palpebral Fissures

In 1968, Lemoine of Nantes, France, recognized the multiple effects that alcohol can have on the developing fetus, including the more severe end of the spectrum, the fetal alcohol syndrome. Lemoine's report was not well accepted, and the disorder was independently rediscovered in 1973 by Jones et al. in the offspring of chronically alcoholic women. It is now appreciated as the most common major teratogen to which the fetus is liable to be exposed. In Gothenburg, Sweden, the studies of Olegaard et al. have shown that 1 in 300 babies is born with the prenatal effects of alcohol, with one half of these having the fetal alcohol syndrome. They estimate that 10 to 20 per cent of mental deficiency with an I.Q. in the 50 to 80 range is a result of alcohol, and one in six cases of cerebral palsy is the result of heavy alcohol exposure in utero. Studies in Seattle and in Northern France have shown the incidence to be greater than 1 in 1000 babies born. Hence, ethanol is of major public health concern as a teratogen.

In 1973, Jones et al. delineated this disorder in eight unrelated children, all born to women who were severe chronic alcoholics prior to and during their pregnancy. Additional studies have confirmed the initial observations.

ABNORMALITIES. Variable features from among the following:

Growth. Pre- and postnatal onset growth deficiency.

Performance. Average I.Q. of 63. Fine motor dysfunction manifested by weak grasp, poor eye-hand coordination, and/or tremulousness. Irritability in infancy, hyperactivity in childhood.

Craniofacial. Mild to moderate microcephaly, short palpebral fissures, maxillary hypoplasia. Short nose, smooth philtrum with thin and smooth upper lip.

Skeletal. Joint anomalies including abnormal position and/or function, altered palmar crease patterns. Small distal phalanges. Small fifth fingernails.

Cardiac. Heart murmur, frequently disappearing by 1 year of age. Ventricular septal defect most common, followed by auricular septal defect.

OCCASIONAL ABNORMALITIES. Ptosis of eyelid, frank microphthalmia, cleft lip with or without cleft palate, micrognathia, protruding auricles, mildly webbed neck, short neck, cervical vertebral malformations (10 to 20 per cent), rib anomalies, tetralogy of Fallot, coarctation of the aorta, strawberry hemangiomata, hypoplastic labia majora. Short fourth and fifth metacarpal bones. Meningomyelocele, hydrocephalus.

NATURAL HISTORY. There may be tremulousness in the early neonatal period. Postnatal linear growth tends to remain retarded, and the adipose tissue is thin. This often creates a "failure to thrive" interpretation. These individuals tend to be irritable as young infants, hyperactive as children, and more social as young adults. A 10-year follow-up of 8 of the 11 children initially diagnosed with this disorder indicates that four are mildly mentally retarded and are attending school in a combination of regular and remedial classes and four are severely handicapped. Problems with dental malalignment and malocclusion, eustachian tube dysfunction, and myopia have developed with time. The severity of the maternal alcoholism and the extent and severity of the pattern of malformation seem to be most predictive of ultimate prognosis. The average academic functioning was at the fourth grade level with arithmetic deficits most characteristic in a group of adolescents and adults with a mean age of 18 years. Abnormal behavior such as poor judgment, distractibility, and difficulty recognizing social cues were common.

ETIOLOGY. Ethanol or its by-products. The least significant effect recognized at two drinks per day has been slightly smaller birth size (approximately 160 g smaller than average). It is not until four to six drinks per day are consumed that additional subtle clinical features begin to become evident. Most of the children believed to have fetal alcohol syndrome have been born of frankly alcoholic women whose intake is eight to ten drinks or more per day. The risk of a serious problem in the offspring of a chronically alcoholic woman has been estimated to be 30 to 50 per cent, the greatest risk being for varying degrees of mental deficiency.

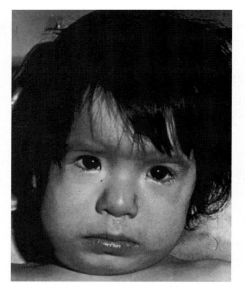

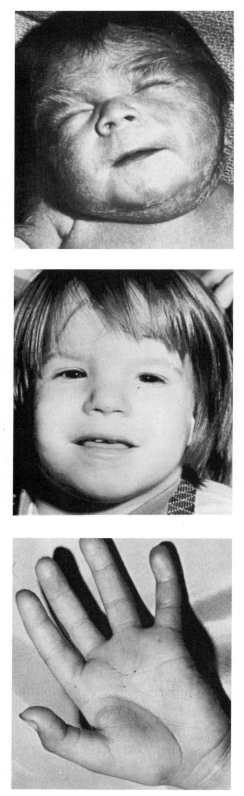

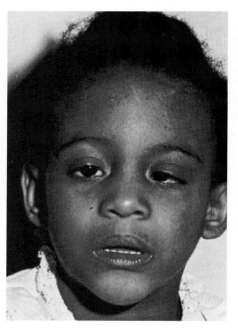

FIGURE 1. Fetal alcohol syndrome. Affected children of chronic alcoholic women; at birth (A), 1 year (B), 2⁶/₁₂ years (C), and 3⁹/₁₂ years (D). Note the short palpebral fissures for all children, strabismus (B and D), ptosis of the eyelid (D), and facial hirsutism in the newborn (A). The hand shows mildly altered upper palmar crease patterning (E). (A from Jones, K. L., and Smith, D. W.: Lancet, 2:999, 1973; B to E from Jones, K. L., et al.: Lancet, 1:1267, 1973, with permission.)

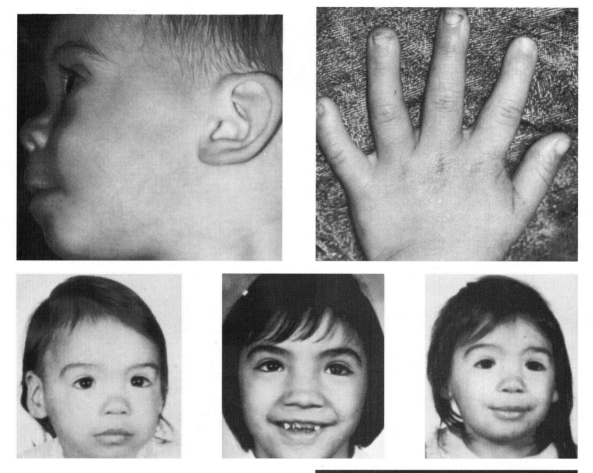

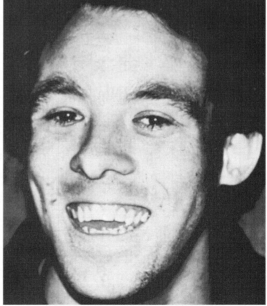

FIGURE 2. Fetal alcohol syndrome. *Upper,* Profile of an infant, showing short, upturned nose; thin upper lip; relatively small mandible; and prominent crus across concha of ear. There may be small nails, mild syndactyly, and relatively short fourth and fifth metacarpals. *Middle,* Change in facies in the same child from 18 months to 2⁶/₁₂ years to 7 years of age. *Lower,* A 22-year-old with fetal alcohol syndrome, still showing short palpebral fissures, smooth philtrum, and smooth upper lip. He is a pleasant individual, with an I.Q. of 65.

COMMENT. The most serious consequence of heavy prenatal alcohol exposure is the problem of brain development and function. Beyond diminished brain cell number and intelligence, there can be problems of malformation, which include heterotopias (faulty migration) of neurons and frank malformation of early brain.

References

Lemoine, P., et al.: Les enfants de parents alcoholiques. Ovest. Med., 21:476, 1968.

Jones, K. L., et al.: Pattern of malformation in offspring of chronic alcoholic mothers. Lancet, 1:1267, 1973.

Jones, K. L., and Smith, D. W.: Recognition of the fetal alcohol syndrome in early infancy. Lancet, 2:999, 1973.

Jones, K. L., et al.: Outcome in offspring of chronic alcoholic women. Lancet, 1:1076, 1974.

Majewski, F., et al.: Zur Klinik und Pathogenese der Alkohol-Embryo. Bericht über 68 Fälle, Munch. Med. Wochenschr., 118:1635, 1976.

Clarren, S. K., and Smith, D. W.: The fetal alcohol syndrome; a review of the world literature. N. Engl. J. Med., 198:1063, 1978.

Olegaard, R., et al.: Effects on the child of alcohol abuse during pregnancy. Acta Paediatr. Scand., 275(Suppl.):112, 1979.

Smith, D. W.: The fetal alcohol syndrome. Hosp. Pract., 10:121, 1979.

Jones, K. L.: Fetal alcohol syndrome. Pediatr. Rev., 8: 122, 1986.

Streissguth, A. P., et al.: Fetal alcohol syndrome in adolescents and adults. J. A. M. A., 265:1961, 1991.

FETAL HYDANTOIN SYNDROME
(Fetal Dilantin Syndrome)

Although data suggesting the possible teratogenic effects of anticonvulsants were first presented by Meadow in 1968, convincing epidemiologic evidence of the association between hydantoins and congenital abnormalities awaited the studies of Fedrick and of Monson et al. Further studies by Speidel and Meadow and by Hill et al. have revealed a pattern of malformation that may include digit and nail hypoplasia, unusual facies, and growth and mental deficiencies.

ABNORMALITIES. Varying combinations of the following, with the fetal hydantoin syndrome representing the broader, more severe end of the spectrum.

Growth. Mild to moderate growth deficiency, usually of prenatal onset, but may be accentuated in the early postnatal months.

Performance. Occasional borderline to mild mental deficiency. Performance in childhood may be better than that anticipated from progress in early infancy.

Craniofacial. Wide anterior fontanel; metopic ridging; ocular hypertelorism; broad, depressed nasal bridge; short nose with bowed upper lip; broad alveolar ridge; cleft lip and palate.

Limbs. Hypoplasia of distal phalanges with small nails, especially postaxial digits; low arch dermal ridge patterning of hypoplastic fingertips; digitalized thumb; dislocation of hip.

Other. Short neck, rib anomalies, widely spaced small nipples, umbilical and inguinal hernias, pilonidal sinus, coarse profuse scalp hair, hirsutism, low-set hairline, abnormal palmar crease. Strabismus.

OCCASIONAL ABNORMALITIES. Microcephaly, brachycephaly, positional foot deformities, strabismus, coloboma, ptosis, slanted palpebral fissures, webbed neck, pulmonary or aortic valvular stenosis, coarctation of aorta, patent ductus arteriosus, cardiac septal defects, single umbilical artery, pyloric stenosis, duodenal atresia, anal atresia, renal malformation, hypospadias, micropenis, ambiguous genitalia, cryptorchidism, symphalangism, syndactyly, holoprosencephaly malformation sequence.

NATURAL HISTORY. The infants not uncommonly have relative failure to thrive during the early months for reasons unknown. Some improvement may be seen in the growth of nails and distal phalanges. The mild degrees of mental deficiency are the greatest concern. Those with the fetal hydantoin syndrome who show multiple hydantoin effects have an average I.Q. of 71.

ETIOLOGY. Phenytoin (Dilantin) or one of its metabolites. It appears that similar craniofacial features referred to as the "anticonvulsant facies" are associated with prenatal exposure to carbamazepine, valproic acid, mysoline, and phenobarbital. Furthermore, there is evidence that exposure to a combination of the anticonvulsants may increase the risk to the fetus. The risk of the hydantoin-exposed fetus having the fetal hydantoin syndrome is about 10 per cent, and the risk for having some effects of the disorder is an additional 33 per cent. No dose-response curve has been demonstrated, nor has a "safe" dose been found below which there is no increased teratogenic risk. Numerous studies now suggest that susceptibility of the fetus to the teratogenic effects of hydantoins depends on the fetal genotype. Inherited defects in phenytoin arene oxide detoxification may contribute.

References

Meadow, S. R.: Anticonvulsant drugs and congenital abnormalities. Lancet, 2:1296, 1968.

Aase, J. M.: Anticonvulsant drugs and congenital abnormalities. Am. J. Dis. Child., 127:758, 1970.

Speidel, B. D., and Meadow, S. R.: Maternal epilepsy and abnormalities of the fetus and newborn. Lancet, 2:839, 1972.

Fedrick, J.: Epilepsy and pregnancy: A report from the Oxford Record Linkage Study. Br. Med. J., 2:442, 1973.

Monson, R. R., et al.: Diphenylhydantoin and selected congenital malformations. N. Engl. J. Med., 289:1049, 1973.

Hill, R. M., et al.: Infants exposed in utero to antiepileptic drugs. Am. J. Dis. Child., 127:645, 1974.

Hanson, J. W., and Smith, D. W.: The fetal hydantoin syndrome. J. Pediatr., 87:285, 1975.

Hanson, J. W., et al.: Risks to the offspring of women treated with hydantoin anticonvulsant, with emphasis on the fetal hydantoin syndrome. J. Pediatr., 89:662, 1976.

Phelen, M. C., Pellock, J. M., and Nance, W. E.: Discordant expression of fetal hydantoin syndrome in heteropaternal dizygotic twins. N. Engl. J. Med., 307:99, 1982.

Finnell, R. H., and Chernoff, G. F.: Editorial comment: Genetic background: The elusive component in the fetal hydantoin syndrome. Am. J. Med. Genet., 19:459, 1984.

Strickler, S. M., et al.: Genetic predisposition to phenytoin-induced birth defects. Lancet, 2:746, 1985.

Jones, K. L., et al.: Pattern of malformation in the children of women treated with carbamazepine during pregnancy. N. Engl. J. Med., 320:1661, 1989.

Buehler, B. A., et al.: Prenatal prediction of risk of the fetal hydantoin syndrome. N. Engl. J. Med., 322:1567, 1990.

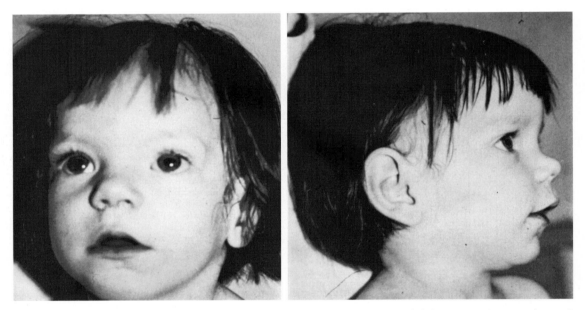

FIGURE 1. Fetal hydantoin syndrome. A 15-month-old with growth and mental deficiencies whose mother took diphenylhydantoin and phenobarbital throughout pregnancy. Note the hypoplastic nails and phalanges, mild ptosis, relatively low and broad nasal bridge, and coarse hair. (Courtesy of J. Hanson, University of Iowa, Iowa City, Iowa.)

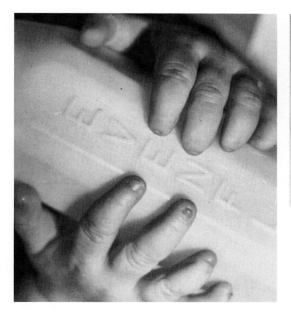
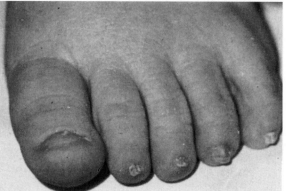

FIGURE 1. *Continued.*

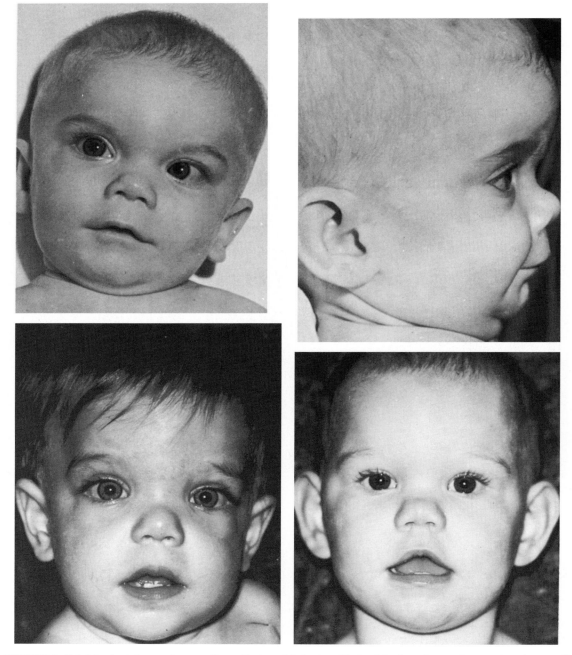

FIGURE 2. Fetal hydantoin syndrome. *Above,* Facies of infants with fetal hydantoin syndrome, showing small nose, low nasal bridge with hypertelorism, strabismus, and bowed upper lip. The child in the lower right was exposed to high levels of both alcohol and hydantoin.

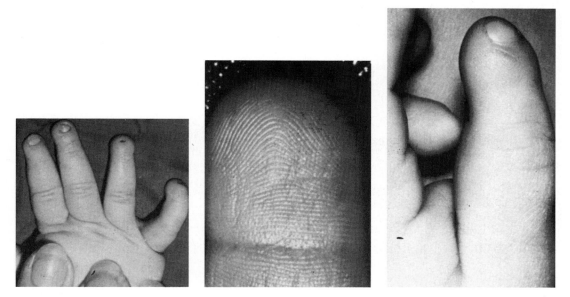

FIGURE 3. Fetal hydantoin syndrome. Nail hypoplasia, most severe on ulnar side, low arch dermal ridge patterning, and occasional finger-like thumb.

FETAL TRIMETHADIONE SYNDROME

(Tridione Syndrome)

In 1970, German et al. reported significant abnormalities among the offspring of four women treated with trimethadione or paramethadione. Feldman et al. summarized the results of 53 pregnancies in which the mother was treated during the first trimester with either trimethadione or paramethadione.

ABNORMALITIES. Varying features from among the following:

Performance. Mental deficiency, speech disorders.

Growth. Prenatal onset growth deficiency.

Craniofacial. Mild brachycephaly. Mild midfacial hypoplasia, short upturned nose with broad and low nasal bridge, prominent forehead, mild synophrys with unusual upslant to eyebrows. Strabismus, ptosis, epicanthal folds. Cleft lip and palate, high arched palate, micrognathia. Poorly developed rectangular or cupped and overlapping helix.

Cardiovascular. Septal defects, tetralogy of Fallot.

Genitourinary. Ambiguous genitalia, hypospadias, clitoral hypertrophy.

Limbs. Simian crease.

OCCASIONAL ABNORMALITIES. Facial hemangiomata, webbed neck, scoliosis, transposition of the great vessels, hypoplastic heart, pyloric stenosis, renal anomalies, umbilical and inguinal hernias, hearing and visual deficits, dislocated hip.

NATURAL HISTORY. Mental deficiency and serious cardiac defects give many cases a poor prognosis.

ETIOLOGY. Both trimethadione and its congener paramethadione have been associated with a similar constellation of defects. Of the 53 pregnancies reviewed by Feldman et al., 13 resulted in spontaneous abortion, and 83 per cent of the live-born infants had at least one major malformation, 14 of which led to death.

COMMENT. The frequency and severity of defects associated with maternal use of these drugs during pregnancy are high enough to warrant consideration of early elective termination of pregnancy.

References

German, J., Lowal, A., and Ehlers, K. H.: Trimethadione and human teratogenesis. Teratology, 3:349, 1970.

Zackai, E., et al.: The fetal trimethadione syndrome. J. Pediatr., 87:280, 1975.

Feldman, G. L., Weaver, D. D., and Lovrien, E. W.: The fetal trimethadione syndrome. Am. J. Dis. Child., 131:1389, 1977.

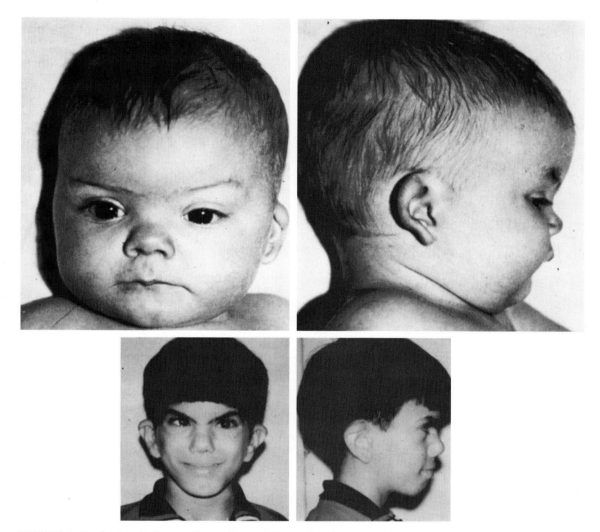

FIGURE 1. Fetal trimethadione effects. *Above*, A 5-month-old with tetralogy of Fallot whose mother took trimethadione throughout pregnancy. Note ear malformation, hypoplastic midface, and unusual eyebrow configuration. (Courtesy of J. Hanson, University of Iowa, Iowa City, Iowa.) *Below*, A 10-year-old with speech delay whose mother took trimethadione during pregnancy. Note ear malformation, unusual slant to eyebrows, and strabismus. (Courtesy of E. Zackai, Philadelphia Children's Hospital, Philadelphia, Pa.)

FETAL VALPROATE SYNDROME

Concern was raised regarding prenatal valproic acid exposure in 1982 by Robert and Guiband, who documented an association between maternal ingestion of valproic acid and meningomyelocele in the offspring. DiLiberti et al. and Hanson et al. set forth a broader pattern of malformation in 1984.

ABNORMALITIES

Craniofacies. Narrow bifrontal diameter. High forehead. Epicanthal folds connecting with an infraorbital crease or groove; telecanthus; broad, low nasal bridge with short nose and anteverted nostrils. Midface hypoplasia. Long philtrum with a thin vermilion border. Relatively small mouth.

Cardiovascular. Aortic coarctation. Hypoplastic left heart. Aortic valve stenosis. Interrupted aortic arch. Secundum type atrial septal defect. Pulmonary atresia without ventricular septal defect. Perimembranous ventricular septal defect.

Limbs. Long, thin fingers and toes. Hyperconvex fingernails.

Other. Meningomyelocele. Cleft lip.

OCCASIONAL ABNORMALITIES. Growth and mental deficiencies. Supernumerary nipples. Hypospadias. Inguinal and umbilical hernias. Broad chest. Bifid rib. Postaxial polydactyly. Radial ray reduction defects. Preaxial defects of feet. Triphalangeal thumbs.

NATURAL HISTORY. Insufficient data are available to make any definitive conclusions regarding the long-term prognosis relative to intellectual performance in children prenatally exposed to valproic acid. However, among a group of fetuses exposed to valproic acid, 5 out of 92 (5.4 per cent) had an open (lumbo) sacral spina bifida.

ETIOLOGY. Prenatal valproic acid exposure. In a study of 14 prospectively ascertained infants exposed prenatally to valproic acid alone, almost half were distressed during labor, and 28 per cent had low Apgar scores. Four of the 14 had a pattern of malformation consistent with the fetal valproate syndrome.

References

Robert, E., and Guiband, P.: Maternal valproic acid and congenital neural tube defects. Lancet, 2:934, 1982.

DiLiberti, J. H., et al.: The fetal valproate syndrome. Am. J. Med. Genet., 19:473, 1984.

Hanson, J. W., et al.: Effects of valproic acid on the fetus. Pediatr. Res., 18:306A, 1984.

Ardinger, H. H., Clark, E. B., and Hanson, J. W.: Cardiac malformations associated with fetal valproic acid exposure. Proc. Greenwood Genet. Center, 5: 162, 1986.

Jager-Roman, E., et al.: Fetal growth, major malformations, and minor anomalies in infants born to women receiving valproic acid. J. Pediatr., 108:997, 1986.

Sharony, R., et al.: Preaxial ray reduction defects as part of valproic acid embryofetopathy. Prenat. Diagn., 13:909, 1991.

Omtzigt, J. G. C., et al.: The risk of spina bifida aperta after first-trimester exposure to valproate in a prenatal cohort. Neurology, 42(Suppl. 5):119, 1992.

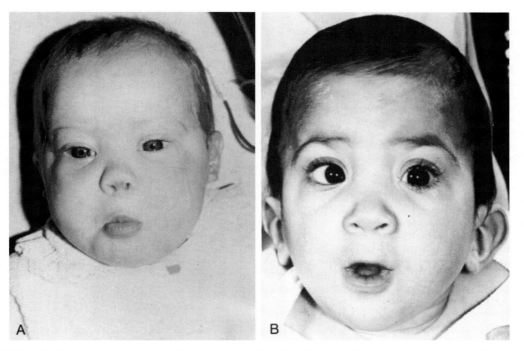

FIGURE 1. Fetal valproate syndrome. *A*, A 7-month-old girl with epicanthal folds that connect with an infra-orbital crease, short nose, long philtrum, and small mouth. *B*, A 10-month-old boy with a short nose, long philtrum with a thin vermilion border, and a relatively small mouth. (From Diliberti, J. H., et al.: Am. J. Med. Genet., *19*:473, 1984, with permission.)

FETAL WARFARIN SYNDROME

(Warfarin Embryopathy, Fetal Coumarin Syndrome)

Nasal Hypoplasia, Stippled Epiphyses, Coumarin Derivative Exposure in First Trimester

Isolated reports of infants who, in retrospect, were affected by warfarin were followed in 1975 by simultaneous recognition of this association in five infants. A number of infants are known to have been affected.

ABNORMALITIES

Facies. Nasal hypoplasia and depressed nasal bridge, often with a deep groove between the alae nasi and nasal tip.

Skeletal. Stippling of uncalcified epiphyses, particularly of axial skeleton, at the proximal femora and in the calcanei; stippling disappears after the first year.

Limbs. Mild hypoplasia of the nails and shortened fingers.

Growth. Low birth weight; most demonstrate catch-up growth.

Performance. Significant mental retardation. Seizures.

OCCASIONAL ABNORMALITIES. CNS and eye abnormalities, including microcephaly, hydrocephalus, Dandy-Walker malformation, agenesis of corpus callosum; optic atrophy, microphthalmia, Peter anomaly of eye. Severe rhizomelia, scoliosis, congenital heart defect.

NATURAL HISTORY. Infants often present with upper airway obstruction, which is relieved by the placement of an oral airway. Seven infants have died and five are significantly retarded; the others have done well except for persistent cosmetic malformation of the nose. The stippling is incorporated into the calcifying epiphyses and has resulted in few problems.

ETIOLOGY. Although the critical period of coumarin exposure is between 6 and 9 weeks' gestation, controversy exists regarding second- and third-trimester exposure. Previous studies have suggested that the CNS abnormalities are associated with exposure limited to the second or third trimester and are related to secondary disruption of CNS architecture most likely due to hemorrhage. However, a case report suggests that prenatal coumarin exposure between the eighth and twelfth weeks of gestation can lead to CNS abnormalities, indicating a direct teratogenic effect on CNS morphogenesis. Furthermore, three prospective studies of children exposed during the second and third trimesters revealed no evidence of CNS or eye abnormalities, suggesting that the incidence of CNS problems in babies born to women receiving coumarin limited to the later two trimesters must be exceedingly low.

COMMENT. An estimate of the overall risk in pregnancies in which coumarin derivatives are used is that about two thirds will have a normal outcome, with the others ending in the birth of infants with fetal warfarin syndrome and CNS effects or in spontaneous abortion. The similarity between this disorder and X-linked recessive chondrodysplasia punctata (CDPX) has suggested a common pathogenesis for these two disorders. Recent evidence that warfarin appears to inhibit arylsulfatase E (ARSE), a genetically determined deficiency which is responsible for CDPX, provides support for this concept.

References

DiSaia, P. J.: Pregnancy and delivery of a patient with a Starr-Edwards mitral valve prosthesis. Report of a case. Obstet. Gynecol., 28:469, 1966.

Kerber, I. J., Warr, O. S., and Richardson, C.: Pregnancy in a patient with a prosthetic mitral valve. J. A. M. A., 203:223, 1968.

Becker, M. H., et al.: Chondrodysplasia punctata. Is maternal warfarin a factor? Am. J. Dis. Child., 129:356, 1975.

Pettifor, J. M., and Benson, R.: Congenital malformations associated with the administration of oral anticoagulants during pregnancy. J. Pediatr., 86:459, 1975.

Shaul, W. L., Emergy, H., and Hall, J. G.: Chondrodysplasia punctata and maternal warfarin use during pregnancy. Am. J. Dis. Child., 129:360, 1975.

Hall, J. G., Pauli, R. M., and Wilson, K. M.: Maternal and fetal sequelae of anticoagulation during pregnancy. Am. J. Med., 68:122, 1980.

Kaplan, L. C.: Congenital Dandy Walker malformation associated with first trimester warfarin: A case report and literature review. Teratology, 32:333, 1985.

Iturbe-Alessio, I., et al.: Risks of anticoagulant therapy in women with artificial heart valves. N. Engl. J. Med., 315:1390, 1986.

Francho, B., et al.: A cluster of sulfatase genes on Xp22.3: Mutations in chondrodysplasia punctata (CDPX) and implications for warfarin embryopathy. Cell, 81:15, 1995.

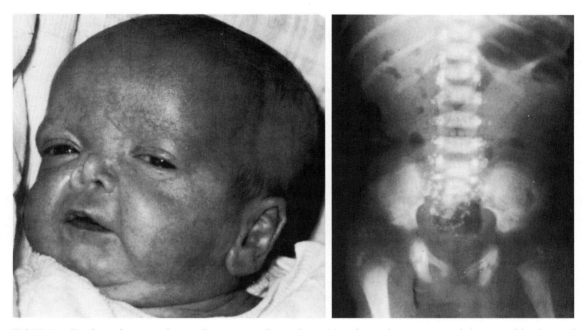

FIGURE 1. Fetal warfarin syndrome. Patient at 5 days of age. Note hypoplastic nose with low nasal bridge and broad, flat face. Roentgenogram at 1 day of age showing stippling along the vertebral column, in the sacral area, and in proximal femurs. Stippling was also noted in the cervical vertebrae, acromion process, and tarsal bones. (From Shaul, W. L., Emery, H., and Hall, J. G.: Am. J. Dis. Child., *129*:360, 1975, with permission.)

FETAL AMINOPTERIN/METHOTREXATE SYNDROME

Cranial Dysplasia, Broad Nasal Bridge, Low-Set Ears

The folic acid antagonist aminopterin has occasionally been utilized as an abortifacient during the first trimester of pregnancy. Thiersch first noted abnormal morphogenesis in three abortuses and one full-term offspring of mothers who received aminopterin from 4 to 9 weeks following the presumed time of conception. Subsequently, other cases have been published, including an account of teratogenicity secondary to methotrexate, the methyl derivative of aminopterin that is frequently used for the treatment of rheumatoid arthritis and psoriasis as well as being an abortifacient.

ABNORMALITIES
Growth. Prenatal onset growth deficiency. Microcephaly.
Craniofacial. Severe hypoplasia of frontal bone, parietal bones, temporal or occipital bones, wide fontanels, and synostosis of lambdoid or coronal sutures. Upsweep of frontal scalp hair. Broad nasal bridge, shallow supraorbital ridges, prominent eyes, micrognathia, low-set ears, maxillary hypoplasia, epicanthal folds.
Limbs. Relative shortness, especially of forearm (mesomelia). Talipes equinovarus, hypodactyly, syndactyly.

OCCASIONAL ABNORMALITIES.
Cleft palate, neural tube closure defect, dislocation of hip, retarded ossification of pubis and ischium, rib anomalies, short thumbs, single crease on fifth finger, dextroposition of the heart, hypotonia.

NATURAL HISTORY. Although fetal or early postnatal death does occur, a number of patients have survived beyond the first year of age. Postnatal growth deficiency occurs frequently. However, mental and motor performance usually has been described as normal. E. B. Shaw of San Francisco has observed a 17-year-old affected girl with normal intelligence.

ETIOLOGY. Aminopterin and/or methotrexate, its methyl derivative. It has been suggested that a critical period for exposure exists at 6 through 8 weeks after conception and that a maternal methotrexate dose above 10 mg/week is necessary to produce defects in the fetus.

References

Thiersch, J. B.: Therapeutic abortions with a folic acid antagonist, 4-aminopteroylglutamic acid (4-amino P.G.A.) administered by the oral route. Am. J. Obstet. Gynecol., 63:1298, 1952.

Milunsky, A., Graef, J. W., and Gaynor, M. F., Jr.: Methotrexate induced congenital malformations with a review of the literature. J. Pediatr., 72:790, 1968.

Shaw, E. B., and Steinbach, H. L.: Aminopterin-induced fetal malformation. Am. J. Dis. Child., 115: 477, 1968.

Feldkamp, M., and Carey, J. C.: Clinical teratology counseling and consultation case report: Low dose methotrexate exposure in the early weeks of pregnancy. Teratology, 47:533, 1993.

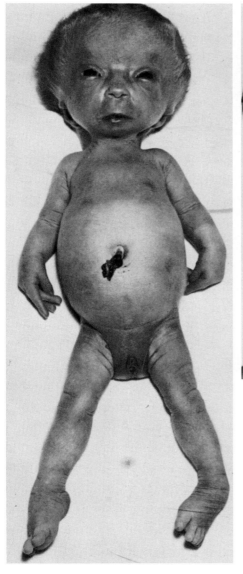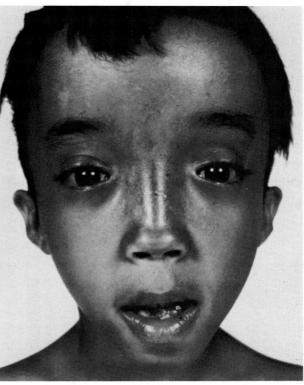

FIGURE 1. Fetal aminopterin syndrome. *Left*, Affected newborn weighing 1.3 kg at 42 weeks' gestation (From Warkany, J., et al.: Am. J. Dis. Child., *97*:274, 1959, with permission.) *Right*, Affected boy. (Courtesy of Dr. Noreen L. Rudd, Toronto, Ontario.)

RETINOIC ACID EMBRYOPATHY
(Accutane Embryopathy)

Central Nervous System Defects, Microtia, Cardiac Defects

First licensed in the United States in September, 1982, with the brand name Accutane, isotretinoin (13-*cis*-retinoic acid) was initially recognized to be a human teratogen 1 year later. In 1985, Lammer et al. set forth the spectrum of structural defects. Of 21 affected infants, 17 had defects of the craniofacies, 12 had cardiac defects, 18 had altered morphogenesis of the CNS, and 7 had anomalies of thymic development.

ABNORMALITIES
Craniofacial. Mild facial asymmetry. Bilateral microtia and/or anotia with stenosis of the external ear canal. Posterior helical pits. Facial nerve paralysis ipsilateral to malformed ear. Accessory parietal sutures. A narrow sloping forehead. Micrognathia. Hair pattern abnormalities. Flat depressed nasal bridge and ocular hypertelorism. Abnormal mottling of teeth.
Cardiovascular. Conotruncal malformations, including transposition of the great vessels, tetralogy of Fallot, double-outlet right ventricle, truncus arteriosus communis, and supracristal ventricular septal defect. Aortic arch interruption (type B). Retroesophageal right subclavian artery. Aortic arch hypoplasia. Hypoplastic left ventricle.
Central Nervous System. Hydrocephalus. Microcephaly. Structural errors of cortical and cerebellar neuronal migration and gross malformations of posterior fossa structures, including cerebellar hypoplasia, agenesis of the vermis, cerebellar microdysgenesis, and megacisterna.
Performance. Subnormal range of intelligence.
Other. Thymic and parathyroid abnormalities.

OCCASIONAL ABNORMALITIES. Cleft palate.

NATURAL HISTORY. Among the 21 affected infants evaluated by Lammer et al., 3 were still-born and 9 were live-born infants who died secondary to cardiac defects, brain malformations, or combinations of the two. Information regarding the nine affected infants who survived the neonatal period is unknown. However, in an ongoing study, designed to determine natural history, 19 per cent of 31 prospectively ascertained 5-year-olds prenatally exposed to isotretinoin had a full-scale I.Q. less than 70 and an additional 28 per cent had I.Q.s between 71 and 85. Although each of the five patients whose I.Q. was less than 70 had major malformations, six of the ten patients with an I.Q. in the borderline range did not have major malformations, indicating that the lack of major structural abnormalities does not necessarily predict normal intellectual performance.

ETIOLOGY. Isotretinoin (Accutane). A 35 per cent risk for the Accutane embryopathy exists in the offspring of women who continue to take Accutane beyond the 15th day following conception. There have been no affected babies born to women who stopped taking Accutane prior to the 15th day following conception. Furthermore, there is no evidence to suggest that maternal use of the drug prior to conception is teratogenic. Daily dosage of Accutane from 0.5 to 1.5 mg/kg of maternal body weight is felt to be teratogenic.

References

Rosa, F. W.: Teratogenicity of isotretinoin. Lancet, 2: 513, 1983.

Fernoff, P. M., and Lammer, E. J.: Craniofacial features of isotretinoin embryopathy. J. Pediatr., *105*:595, 1984.

Lott, I. T., et al.: Fetal hydrocephalus and ear anomalies associated with maternal use of isotretinoin. J. Pediatr., *105*:597, 1984.

Lammer, E. J., et al.: Retinoic acid embryopathy. N. Engl. J. Med., *313*:837, 1985.

Lammer, E. J., et al.: Risk for major malformations among human fetuses exposed to isotretinoin (13-*cis*-retinoic acid). Teratology, *35*:68A, 1987.

Teratology Society: Recommendations for isotretinoin use in women of childbearing potential. Teratology, 44:1, 1991.

Adams, J., and Lammer, E. J.: Neurobehavioral teratology of isotretinoins. Reprod. Toxicol., *7*:175, 1993.

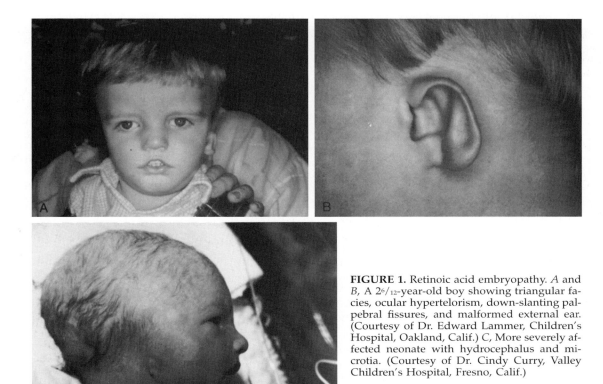

FIGURE 1. Retinoic acid embryopathy. *A* and *B*, A 2⁶/₁₂-year-old boy showing triangular facies, ocular hypertelorism, down-slanting palpebral fissures, and malformed external ear. (Courtesy of Dr. Edward Lammer, Children's Hospital, Oakland, Calif.) *C*, More severely affected neonate with hydrocephalus and microtia. (Courtesy of Dr. Cindy Curry, Valley Children's Hospital, Fresno, Calif.)

FETAL RUBELLA EFFECTS

(Fetal Rubella Syndrome)

Deafness, Cataracts, Patent Ductus Arteriosus

Gregg, in 1941, first called attention to the permanent residua of fetal rubella acquired from the mother during the first trimester of gestation. Culture of the viral agent during the severe 1964 epidemic resulted in an appreciation of the "expanded rubella syndrome" as the consequence of widespread chronic disease. The effects range from deafness, one of the most common residua, to the more complete fetal rubella syndrome.

ABNORMALITIES. Fetal death may occur. The following are the tissues that are affected and the consequent abnormalities noted in the 1964 epidemic. The asterisks (*) indicate permanent residua.

Tissue	Abnormalities
General hypoplasia	Growth deficiency
Central nervous system	*Mental deficiency, microcephaly
Cochlea	*Deafness
Lens	*Cataract
Other parts of eye	*Glaucoma, corneal opacity, chorioretinitis, microphthalmia, strabismus
Blood vessels	*Patent ductus arteriosus, peripheral pulmonic stenosis, fibromuscular proliferation with thickened intima of medium and large arteries
Myocardium	*Septal defects, myocardial disease

Early Infancy

Tissue	Abnormalities
Marrow elements	Thrombocytopenia, anemia
Reticuloendothelial	Hepatosplenomegaly
Liver	Obstructive jaundice
Bone	Osteolytic metaphyseal lesions
Lung	Interstitial pneumonia

OCCASIONAL ABNORMALITIES. Renal disease, hemolytic anemia, large anterior fontanel, late eruption of teeth, hypospadias, cryptorchidism, meningocele, dermatoglyphic alterations. Diabetes mellitus. Hypopituitarism.

NATURAL HISTORY. The frequency of fetal infection from mothers having rubella during the first trimester is about 50 per cent. The risks associated with rubella still exist in the second trimester, especially growth deficiency, deafness, mental deficiency, and peripheral pulmonic stenosis. Cultures for rubella virus in the excretions of patients were positive in 63 per cent of neonates with evidence of the rubella syndrome; 31 per cent of the cultures were still positive at 5 to 7 months, 7 per cent at 10 to 13 months, and none past the age of 3 years. However, rubella virus was recovered from a cataract removed from a 3-year-old child. Thus, the disease is chronic, and although the neonate has prenatal antibodies to rubella, the intracellular rubella virus may persist for a long period of time.

The occurrence of residual defects, especially of mental deficiency (60 per cent have I.Q.s below 90 and 20 per cent below 70), was much higher in the 1964 epidemic than in those of the past, in which deafness was the most common residuum of fetal rubella (31 per cent).

Prevention of maternal rubella by widespread administration of attenuated rubella vaccine is completely merited. Beyond this, the occurrence of validated maternal rubella during the first half of pregnancy should induce serious consideration of early termination of that pregnancy.

ETIOLOGY. Rubella virus. The agent may remain in the tissues and cause pathology years after birth. One example is the later development of diabetes mellitus due to long-term, chronic viropathy in the islets of Langerhans of the pancreas.

References

Gregg, N. M.: Congenital cataract following German measles in the mother. Trans. Ophthalmol. Soc. Aust., 3:35, 1941.

Cooper, L. Z., and Krugman, S.: Diagnosis and management: Congenital rubella. Pediatrics, 37:335, 1966.

Menser, M. A., Dods, L., and Harley, J. D.: A twenty-five-year follow-up of congenital rubella. Lancet, 2: 1347, 1967.

Hardy, J. B.: Clinical and developmental aspects of congenital rubella. Arch. Otolaryngol., 98:230, 1973.

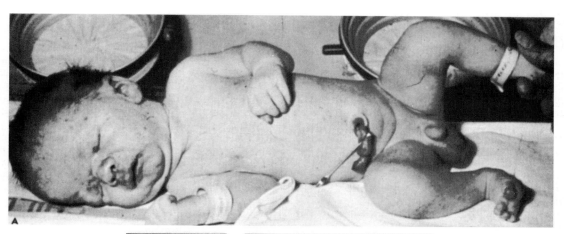

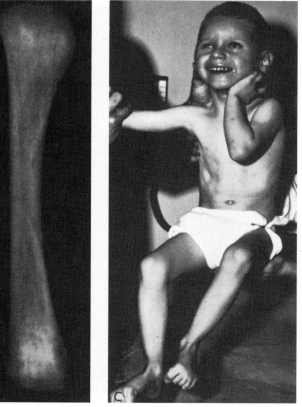

FIGURE 1. Fetal rubella effects. *A*, Neonate, clinically sick with lethargy, petechiae, and hepatosplenomegaly. (From Smith D. W.: J. Pediatr., 70:517, 1967, with permission.) *B*, Osseous lesions in the femur of 5-day-old baby. Note coarse trabecular pattern and subperiosteal rarefaction. *C*, Child, $3^{9}/_{12}$ years old, with height age of $2^{9}/_{12}$ years and mental deficiency. The patient has cataracts, chorioretinitis, hearing impairment, and cryptorchidism—all the apparent residua of congenital rubella.

FETAL VARICELLA EFFECTS

Cicatricial Skin, Limb Hypoplasia, Mental Deficiency With Seizures

LaForet and Lynch first described defects in the child of a woman who had varicella during early gestation. Strabstein et al. summarized five cases, and Dudgeon has personally evaluated at least eight additional cases. Many additional cases have been reported.

ABNORMALITIES

Performance. Mental deficiency with or without seizures in the majority, with cortical atrophy.

Growth. Variable prenatal growth deficiency. Microcephaly.

Eyes. Chorioretinitis.

Limbs. Hypoplasia of limb, with or without rudimentary digits, with or without paralysis with atrophy of limb. Club foot.

Skin. Cutaneous scars.

OCCASIONAL ABNORMALITIES.
Cataracts, microphthalmia, atrophy and hypoplasia of optic disk, and nystagmus. Horner syndrome. Underdeveloped clavicle, scapula, and rib. Anal/vesicle sphincter dysfunction. Scoliosis.

NATURAL HISTORY.
50 per cent of affected have died in early infancy. Although it has previously been suggested that the majority of the survivors have had mental deficiency with seizures, prospective studies indicate that a wide spectrum of severity exists for this disorder. One of the two affected patients reported by Jones et al. had mild cutaneous scars on the face, arms, and legs, a left Horner syndrome, and a retinal scar, while the other had a pendular nystagmus.

ETIOLOGY.
Most cases have occurred in the wake of maternal varicella during the period of 8 to 20 weeks' gestation. The incidence of problems in the offspring of women infected with varicella prior to the 20th week of pregnancy is between 1 and 2 per cent.

References

LaForet, E. G., and Lynch, C. L., Jr.: Multiple congenital defects following maternal varicella. N. Engl. J. Med., 236:534, 1947.

Strabstein, J. C., et al.: Is there a congenital varicella syndrome? J. Pediatr., 64:239, 1974.

Higa, K., et al.: Varicella-zoster virus infections during pregnancy: Hypothesis concerning the mechanisms of congenital malformations. Obstet. Gynecol., 69:214, 1987.

Lambert, S. R., et al.: Ocular manifestations of the congenital varicella syndrome. Arch. Ophthalmol., 107:52, 1989.

Jones, K. L., et al.: Offspring of women infected with varicella during pregnancy: A prospective study. Teratology, 49:29, 1994.

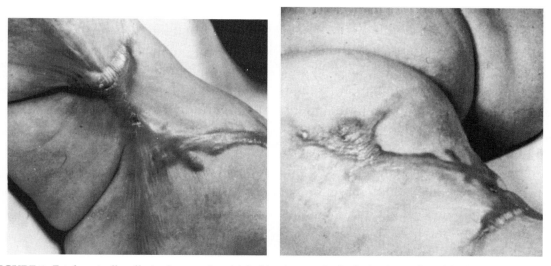

FIGURE 1. Fetal varicella effects. Severe cicatricial skin changes in limbs in the wake of fetal varicella may be not only of cosmetic concern but also associated with tissue deficits in the surrounding region. (Courtesy of Dr. Phillip Dudgeon, The Hospital for Sick Children, London.)

HYPERTHERMIA-INDUCED SPECTRUM OF DEFECTS

A number of animal studies, the most extensive of which have been those of Edwards on the guinea pig, have shown severe maternal hyperthermia during the first one third to one half of gestation to be teratogenic.

Although studies in the human are limited, problems of growth, development, and dysfunction of the brain similar to those seen in the animal studies have been documented. The nature of the defects relates to the timing and extent of the hyperthermia rather than to its cause. Most of the relevant cases have been tentatively related to febrile illness, with the patient having a temperature of a 38.9°C or higher, most commonly 40°C or above. The duration of the high fever has been 1 day or more, usually several days, which is unusual in the first third of gestation. The illness has varied, with influenza, pyelonephritis, and streptococcal pharyngitis being the most common. Two cases were considered secondary to severe hyperthermia induced by prolonged sauna bathing (30 to 45 minutes), and one case was thought to be related to very prolonged hot tub bathing. The latter three cases are extraordinary in the duration of heat exposure.

Retrospective human studies of more than 170 cases of neural tube defect, including anencephaly, meningomyelocele, and occipital encephalocele, have disclosed an overall history of maternal hyperthermia during the week of neural tube closure (21 to 28 days) in approximately 10 per cent of the cases, whereas no such history was determined in the controls. These findings are compatible with the hypothesis that hyperthermia is one cause for neural tube defects in the human.

A 14 per cent incidence of "febrile" illness during early pregnancy in the mothers of 113 embryos with neural tube defects who were aborted therapeutically was documented. The embryos were obtained through the Congenital Anomaly Research Center of Kyoto University. The history of maternal fever was documented before or immediately after the fetal loss, before the neural tube defect was documented.

In addition, a number of craniofacial anomalies including microcephaly, small midface, microphthalmia, micrognathia, and occasionally cleft lip and/or palate and ear anomalies as well as mental deficiency and hypotonia have been seen. To date there has not been an adequate prospective study from which one could derive risk data concerning the developing offspring subjected to a given level of hyperthermia at a given time of gestation.

In addition to potential dysmorphogenesis in early gestation, maternal hyperthermia has been associated with an increase in spontaneous abortion, stillbirth, and prematurity.

References

Edwards, M. J.: Congenital defects in guinea pigs following induced hyperthermia during gestation. Arch. Pathol., 84:42, 1967.

Edwards, M. J.: Congenital defects in guinea pigs: Prenatal retardation of brain growth of guinea pigs following hyperthermia during gestation. Teratology, 2:239, 1969.

Edwards, M. J.: The experimental production of arthrogryposis multiplex congenita in guinea pigs by maternal hyperthermia during gestation. J. Pathol., 104:221, 1971.

Miller, P., Smith, D. W., and Shepard, T.: Maternal hyperthermia as a possible cause of anencephaly. Lancet, 1:519, 1978.

Chance, P. I., and Smith, D. W.: Hyperthermia and meningomyelocele and anencephaly. Lancet, 1:769, 1978.

Halperin, L. R., and Wilroy, R. S.: Maternal hyperthermia and neural tube defects. Lancet, 2:212, 1978.

Smith, D. W., Clarren, S. K., and Harvey, M. A.: Hyperthermia as a possible teratogenic agent. J. Pediatr., 92:878, 1978.

Clarren, S. K., et al.: Hyperthermia—a prospective evaluation of a possible teratogenic agent in man. J. Pediatr., 95:81, 1979.

Shiota, K.: Neural tube defects and maternal hyperthermia in early pregnancy: Epidemiology in a human embryo population. Am. J. Med. Genet., 12: 281, 1982.

Milunsky, A., et al.: Maternal heat exposure and neural tube defects. J. A. M. A., 268:882, 1992.

Lynberg, M. C.: Maternal flu, fever and the risk of neural tube defects: A population based case-control study. Am. J. Epidemiol., 140:244, 1994.

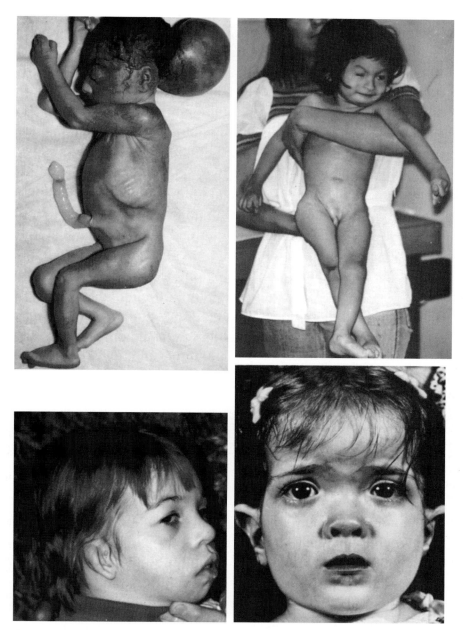

FIGURE 1. Hyperthermia-induced defects. *Upper left,* Encephalocele; maternal history of high fever between days 23 and 25 of gestation. *Upper right,* An 18-month-old severely retarded boy with hypotonic diplegia, micropenis, unilateral microphthalmia, cleft palate, and micrognathia. Maternal fever of 40° to 41°C between the fourth and fifth weeks of gestation. *Lower left,* A 12-year-old severely retarded girl with hypotonic diplegia, midface hypoplasia, micrognathia, incomplete ear morphogenesis, and a cardiac defect. Maternal "flu" with high fever between the sixth and eighth weeks of gestation. *Lower right,* A 14-month-old with moderate hypotonic diplegia and developmental deficiency, who has a hypoplastic midface with mild ocular hypertelorism, low nasal bridge, and prominent auricles. Maternal fever of 40°C between the seventh and eighth weeks of gestation. (*Lower right* from Pleet, H., Graham, J. M. Jr., and Smith, D. W.: J. Pediatr., *67:*785, 1981, with permission.)

MATERNAL PKU FETAL EFFECTS

Mental Deficiency, Microcephaly, Retarded Growth, Increased Incidence of Structural Defects

In 1963, Mabry et al. reported maternal phenylketonuria (PKU) as a cause of mental retardation. Affected children have normal phenylalanine hydroxylase activity but are presumably damaged during pregnancy by the elevated phenylalanine level in their mothers. The actual mechanism by which the imbalanced prenatal amino acid environment produces these defects is still a matter of speculation.

The majority of the structural defects, including growth deficiency, probably occur during organogenesis and appear to result from the toxic effect of an abnormally high phenylalanine level, which is concentrated on the fetal side of the placenta to a gradient of 3:2. During the later stage of gestation, there is interference with CNS myelination and maturation. Controlled phenylalanine intake during pregnancy is being attempted with varied results.

ABNORMALITIES

Performance. Mental deficiency in the vast majority, with I.Q.s often below 50.

Central Nervous System. Frequent mild manifestations of dysfunction. Increased muscle tone with pigeon-toed gait.

Growth. Pre- and postnatal growth deficiency.

Craniofacial. Mild to moderate microcephaly is seen in most cases, and at times, there is characteristic round facies with prominent glabella and epicanthal folds. Short palpebral fissures. Strabismus. Long, underdeveloped philtrum with thin upper lip, small upturned nose, and maxillary and mandibular hypoplasia.

Cardiac. Variable defects in 15 per cent of patients.

The findings of Lenke and Levy confirm earlier impressions and are delineated in Table 1–1.

OCCASIONAL ABNORMALITIES.
Cervical and sacral spine anomalies, cleft lip and palate, esophageal atresia, microphthalmia, irritability, overactivity.

ETIOLOGY.
The toxic effect of excess phenylalanine. The frequencies of teratogenic features

TABLE 1–1. ABNORMALITIES CAUSED BY MATERNAL PKU EFFECTS

Abnormality	20 mg/dl or more	16–19 mg/dl
Spontaneous abortions	24% (297)*	30% (66)
Mental retardation in the offspring	92% (172)	73% (37)
Microcephaly	73% (138)	68% (44)
Congenital heart disease	12% (225)	15% (46)
Birthweight, 2500 g or less	40% (89)	52% (33)

*Size of sample is indicated in parentheses.
1 mmol/l = 16.6 mg/dl.

are directly related to the maternal phenylalanine level. It is important that the phenylalanine level be controlled prior to conception. The diagnosis is confirmed by finding an elevated phenylalanine level in maternal blood.

COMMENT. An increasing number of women of normal intelligence with treated PKU are entering childbearing age, and there is growing concern about the effects of maternal metabolic dysfunction upon the fetus. There is some evidence that the fetus may be affected when the maternal phenylalanine level is as low as 4 to 10 mg/dl. The severity of the effects parallels the increasing levels of phenylalanine in maternal blood.

References

Mabry, C. C., et al.: Maternal phenylketonuria: Cause of mental retardation in children without the metabolic defect. N. Engl. J. Med., 269:1404, 1963.

Zaleski, L. A., Casey, R., and Zaleski, W. A.: Maternal phenylketonuria: Dietary treatment during pregnancy. Can. Med. Assoc. J., 121:1591, 1979.

Lenke, R. R., and Levy, H. L.: Maternal phenylketonuria and hyperphenylalaninemia; International survey of treated and untreated pregnancies. N. Engl. J. Med., 303:1202, 1980.

Lipson, A., et al.: Maternal hyperphenylalaninemia fetal effects. J. Pediatr., 104:216, 1984.

Koch, R., et al.: The North American Collaborative Study of Maternal Phenylketonuria (PKU): Status report 1993. Am. J. Dis. Child., 147:1224, 1993.

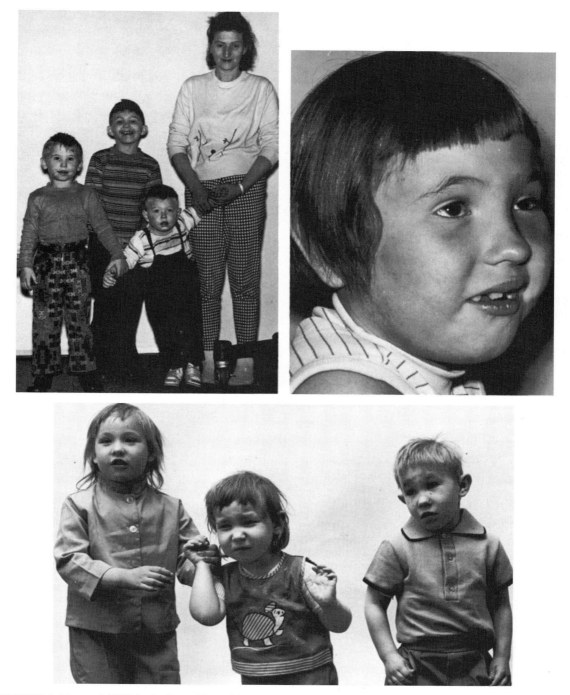

FIGURE 1. Maternal PKU fetal effects. *Upper left*, Mother with PKU and three affected offspring, none with PKU. *Upper right*, Affected girl. *Lower*, Three affected siblings of PKU mother. In addition to the relative microcephaly, note the subtle similarity in the facies, including the poorly defined philtrum. (Courtesy of Dr. Witheld Zaleski, University of Saskatoon, Department of Pediatrics, Saskatoon, Saskatchewan.)

S

S. MISCELLANEOUS SYNDROMES

COFFIN-SIRIS SYNDROME

*Hypoplastic to Absent Fifth
Finger and Toenails, Coarse Facies*

Coffin and Siris reported three patients with this disorder in 1970, and Weiswasser et al. reported an additional case in 1973. Also, several of the patients described by Senior might represent examples of this syndrome. More than 30 cases have been reported.

ABNORMALITIES
Growth. Prenatal onset of mild to moderate growth deficiency.
Performance. Mental deficiency, described as severe in 50 per cent of cases. Moderate to severe hypotonia.
Craniofacial. Mild microcephaly. Coarse facies. A wide mouth with full lips. Flat nasal bridge. Broad nasal tip. Long philtrum. Bushy eyebrows. Long eyelashes.
Limbs. Hypoplastic to absent fifth finger and toenails, with lesser hypoplasia in other digits. Absence of terminal phalanges (particularly of the fifth digit). Lax joints with radial dislocation at elbow. Coxa valga. Small patellae.
Hair. General hirsutism with tendency to have sparse scalp hair.

OCCASIONAL ABNORMALITIES.
Ptosis of eyelids, hypotelorism, preauricular skin tag, choanal atresia, hemangioma, cryptorchidism, umbilical or inguinal hernias, short sternum, cardiac defect (patent ductus arteriosus, ventricular septal defect, atrial septal defect, tetralogy of Fallot, patent foramen ovale with aberrant pulmonary vein). Gastrointestinal anomalies (gastric and duodonal ulcer, neonatal intussusception, intestinal malrotation, gastric outlet obstruction secondary to redundant gastric mocosa). Short forearm, vertebral anomalies, cleft palate, Dandy-Walker anomaly of brain, hypoplasia or partial agenesis of corpus collosum, and in one patient abnormal olivae and arcuate nuclei and cerebellar heterotopias. Renal anomalies (hydronephrosis, microureters with stenosis of the vesicoureteral junction, ectopic kidney).

NATURAL HISTORY. Feeding problems and recurrent upper and lower respiratory tract infections are frequent during early life. The coarse facies may not be present at birth. The sparse scalp hair improves with age.

ETIOLOGY. Occurrence in siblings of unaffected parents has raised the question of autosomal recessive inheritance. Similar nail hypoplasia has been noted in some babies born of women who received phenytoin (Dilantin) therapy during pregnancy.

COMMENT. The majority of affected individuals have been females.

References

Coffin, G. S., and Siris, E.: Mental retardation with absent fifth fingernail and terminal phalanx. Am. J. Dis. Child., *119*:433, 1970.
Senior, B.: Impaired growth and onychodysplasia. Short children with tiny toenails. Am. J. Dis. Child., *122*:7, 1971.
Weiswasser, W. H., et al.: Coffin-Siris syndrome: Two new cases. Am. J. Dis. Child., *125*:838, 1973.
Carey, J. C., and Hall, B. D.: The Coffin-Siris syndrome. Am. J. Dis. Child., 132:667, 1978.
DeBassio, W. A., Kemper, T. L., and Knoelel, J. E.: Coffin-Siris syndrome: Neuropathologic findings. Arch. Neurol., 42:350, 1985.
Bodurtha, J., et al.: Distinctive gastrointestinal anomaly associated with Coffin-Siris syndrome. J. Pediatr., 109:1015, 1986.
Levy, P., and Baraitser, M.: Coffin-Siris syndrome. J. Med. Genet., 28:338, 1991.

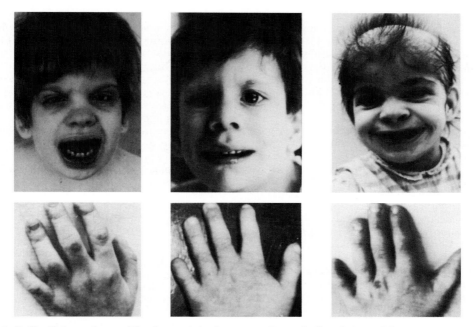

FIGURE 1. Coffin-Siris syndrome. The three original patients. (From Coffin, G. S., and Siris, E.: Am. J. Dis. Child., *119*:433, 1970, with permission.)

BÖRJESON-FORSSMAN-LEHMANN SYNDROME

Large Ears, Hypogonadism, Severe Mental Deficiency

In 1961, Börjeson et al. described an entity of X-linked mental deficiency, epilepsy, hypogonadism, obesity, and dysmorphic facies seen in three related males and three of their less severely affected female relatives. A total of five families have been reported.

ABNORMALITIES

Growth. Height usually less than 50th percentile. Moderate obesity may decrease in later life.

Performance. Severe mental deficiency, with an I.Q. of 10 to 40. Supraspinal hypotonia. Markedly abnormal EEG, with very poor alpha rhythms. Seizures may be present.

Craniofacial. Microcephaly. Coarse facies with prominent supraorbital ridges and deep-set eyes. Large (7.5 to 9 cm) but normally formed ears.

Eyes. Nystagmus, ptosis, and poor vision, with a variety of retinal and/or optic nerve abnormalities.

Genitalia. Small penis with small and soft or undescended testes and delayed secondary sexual characteristics. Hypogonadism appears to be hypogonadotropic.

Skeletal. Variable radiographic abnormalities: thick calvarium, small cervical spinal canal, mild scoliosis, kyphosis, Scheuermann-like vertebral changes, metaphyseal widening of the long bones and hands, hypoplastic distal and middle phalanges, thin cortices.

Other. Central nervous system anomalies are due to a primary abnormality of neuronal migration. Soft and fleshy hands with tapering fingers.

NATURAL HISTORY. From birth, these patients are hypotonic, with severe developmental delay. Walking may begin as late as 4 to 6 years and remains awkward. Speech is limited to a few phrases at most. There is no known unusual susceptibility to health problems, although bronchopneumonia was responsible for the demise of two of the original patients at the ages of 20 and 44 years. Life span is presumed to be normal. A sheltered environment is necessary because of severe limitations of nervous system performance.

ETIOLOGY. X-linked recessive inheritance. The gene for this disorder has been mapped to Xq26-27. Female heterozygotes fall into a spectrum of those without any observable features to those with the abnormalities of growth and craniofacial, ocular, and skeletal features characteristic of this syndrome. Performance ranges from moderate mental retardation (I.Q. of 56 to 70) to above-average intelligence in heterozygous females.

References

Börjeson, M., Forssman, H., and Lehmann, O.: Combination of idiocy, epilepsy, hypogonadism, dwarfism, hypometabolism, and morphologic peculiarities inherited as an X-linked recessive syndrome. Proc. 2nd Int. Congr. Ment. Retard., Vienna (1961), Part I, 1963, p. 188.

Börjeson, M., Forssman, H., and Lehmann, O.: An X-linked, recessively inherited syndrome characterized by grave mental deficiency, epilepsy, and endocrine disorder. Acta Med. Scand., *171:*13, 1962.

Brun, A., Börjeson, M., and Forssman, H.: An inherited syndrome with mental deficiency and endocrine disorder. A patho-anatomical study. J. Ment. Defic. Res., *18:*317, 1974.

Robinson, L. K., et al.: The Börjeson-Forssman-Lehmann syndrome. Am. J. Med. Genet., *15:*457, 1983.

Ardinger, H. H., Hanson, J. W., and Zellweger, H. U.: Börjeson-Forssman-Lehmann syndrome. Further delineation in five cases. Am. J. Med. Genet., *19:*653, 1984.

Turner, G., et al.: Börjeson-Forssman-Lehmann syndrome: Clinical manifestations and gene localization to Xq26-27. Am. J. Med. Genet., *34:*463, 1989.

Matthews, K. D., et al.: Linkage localization of Börjeson-Forssman-Lehmann syndrome. Am. J. Med. Genet., *34:*470, 1989.

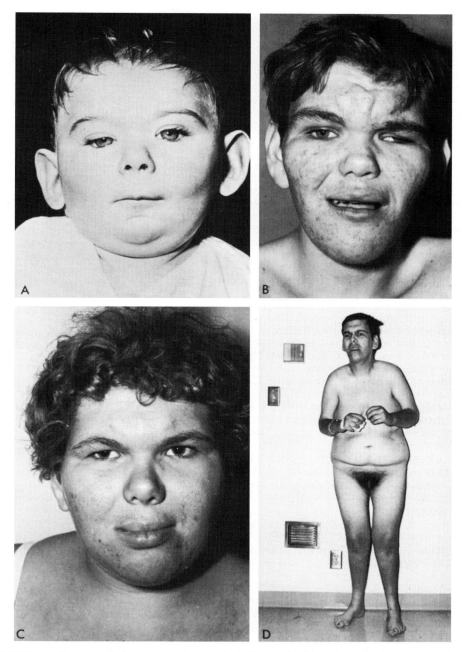

FIGURE 1. Börjeson-Forssman-Lehmann syndrome. *A*, A 10-month-old male with characteristic facial features and large ears. *B*, Unrelated 24-year-old male. *C*, A 23-year-old sister of patient shown in *B*, with mild mental deficiency and characteristic facies. *D*, A 27-year-old maternal cousin of patients shown in *B* and *C*, demonstrating obesity and hypogenitalism.

ARTERIOHEPATIC DYSPLASIA

(Alagille Syndrome)

Cholestasis, Peripheral Pulmonic Stenosis, Peculiar Facies

Initially described by Alagille et al. in 1969, this disorder was more completely delineated in 1973 by Watson and Miller, who reported five families with 21 affected individuals. Since that time, at least 80 more cases have been described. Males and females are affected equally.

ABNORMALITIES

General. Growth retardation (50 per cent).

Craniofacial. Typical facies (95 per cent) consisting of deep-set eyes, broad forehead, long straight nose with flattened tip, prominent chin, small, low-set or malformed ears.

Eyes. Posterior embryotoxon (abnormal prominence of the Schwalbe line, the line formed by the junction of the Descement membrane with the uvea at the anterior chamber angle causing the margin of the cornea to be opaque) in 88 per cent. Axenfeldt anomaly (iris strands).

Cardiac. Peripheral pulmonary artery stenosis with or without associated complex cardiovascular abnormalities (85 per cent).

Skeletal. Butterfly-like vertebral arch defects (87 per cent). Other vertebral defects, including hemivertebrae and spina bifida occulta. Rib anomalies.

Hepatic. Paucity of intrahepatic interlobular bile ducts. Chronic cholestasis (91 per cent). Hypercholesterolemia.

OCCASIONAL ABNORMALITIES

General. Mild mental retardation (16 per cent).

Eyes. Retinal degeneration including chorioretinal involvement and pigmentary clumping. Strabismus. Ectopic pupils. Choroidal folds. Anomalous optic disk or vessels and refractive errors.

Cardiac. Atrial septal defect. Ventricular septal defect. Patent ductus arteriosus. Coarctation of the aorta.

Hands. Short distal phalanges.

Liver. Extrahepatic biliary duct involvement (20 per cent). Primary hepatocellular cancer.

Renal. Structural and parenchymal abnormalities (10 per cent). Decreased creatinine clearance, increased blood urea nitrogen, increased serum uric acid. Histologic abnormalities consisting of mesangiolipidosis noted in 74 per cent.

Genitalia. Hypogonadism.

Endocrine. Decreased growth hormone. Increased testosterone. Hypothyroidism.

Other. Cleft palate. Shortened ulna. Spina bifida occulta. Lack of normal increase in interpedicular distance from L1–L5. Abnormalities of inner ear structures. Club feet. Thyroid cancer. High-pitched voice.

NATURAL HISTORY. Most patients present with neonatal jaundice. Cholestasis (elevated serum bile acids), which develops within the first 3 months in 44 per cent and between 4 months and 3 years in the remainder, is manifested by pruritus, acholic stools, xanthomata, or hepatomegaly. Although bile pigment excretion improves with time, most patients continue to have symptoms of liver involvement or abnormal liver function tests. Thirty-nine per cent develop periportal fibrotic changes. After 5 years of age, clinical signs of cholestasis tend to decrease, although biochemical signs remain. One quarter of patients die. Liver complications and cardiovascular defects were responsible for 19 and 29 per cent of the deaths, respectively. Long-term prognosis depends on severity and duration of early cholestasis, severity of cardiovascular defects, and liver status as it relates to liver failure or portal hypertension.

ETIOLOGY. Autosomal dominant. The disorder has been assigned to chromosome 20p within band 20p12.

References

Alagille, D., et al.: L'atrésie des voies biliaires intra-hépatiques avec voies biliaires extrahépatiques perméables chez l'enfant. J. Par. Pediatr., 301, 1969.

Watson, G. H., and Miller, V.: Arteriohepatic dysplasia: Familial pulmonary arterial stenosis with neonatal liver disease. Arch. Dis. Child., 48:459, 1973.

Alagille, D., et al.: Hepatic ductular hypoplasia associated with characteristic facies, vertebral malformations, retarded physical, mental and sexual development, and cardiac murmur. J. Pediatr., 86:63, 1975.

Bryne, J. L. B., et al.: Del(20p) with manifestations of arteriohepatic dysplasia. Am. J. Med. Genet., 24:673, 1986.

Alagille, D., et al.: Syndromic paucity of interlobular bile ducts (Alagille syndrome or arteriohepatic dysplasia): Review of 80 cases. J. Pediatr., 110:195, 1987.

Mueller, R. F.: The Alagille syndrome (arteriohepatic dysplasia). J. Med. Genet., 24:621, 1987.

Spinner, N. B., et al.: Cytogenetically balanced t(2;20) in a two-generation family with Alagille syndrome: Cytogenetic and molecular studies. Am. J. Hum. Genet., 55:238, 1994.

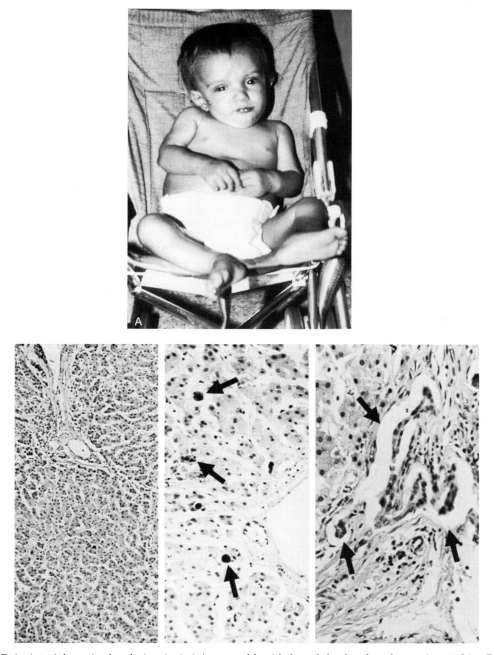

FIGURE 1. Arteriohepatic dysplasia. *A*, A 1⁶/₁₂-year-old with broad forehead and prominent chin. *B*, Three histologic sections of the liver from a patient with arteriohepatic dysplasia. On the left is a low-power view showing fine fibrosis and nodularity; higher power views in the middle and on the right reveal a paucity of intrahepatic bile ducts. The *arrows* denote bile stasis (*middle section*) and bile ducts (*right section*).

MELNICK-NEEDLES SYNDROME

Prominent Eyes, Bowing of Long Bones, Ribbon-like Ribs

This disorder was reported by Melnick and Needles in 1966, and subsequently approximately 35 cases have been documented.

ABNORMALITIES

Craniofacial. Small facies with prominent hirsute forehead and exophthalmos, mild hypertelorism, full cheeks, and small mandible with an obtuse angle and hypoplastic coronoid process. Late closure of fontanels, dense base of skull, lag in paranasal sinus development. Micrognathia. Malaligned teeth.

Limbs. Short upper arms and distal phalanges. Bowing of humerus, radius, ulna, and tibia. Metaphyseal flaring of long bones. Coxa valga. Genu valgum. Short distal phalanges with cone-shaped epiphyses.

Other Skeletal. Relatively small thoracic cage with irregular ribbon-like ribs and short clavicles with wide medial ends and narrow shoulders, short scapulae, and pectus excavatum. Tall vertebrae with anterior concavity in thoracic region. Iliac flaring. Kyphoscoliosis.

OCCASIONAL ABNORMALITIES.

Strabismus. Coarse hair. Cleft palate. Large ears. Hoarse voice. Ureteral stenosis leading to hydronephrosis. Hip dislocation. Club feet. Pes planus. Delayed motor development. Short stature. Muscle hypotonia. Limitations of elbow extension. Acro-osteolysis. Mitral and tricuspid valve prolapse. Hyperlaxity of skin in males.

NATURAL HISTORY.

Small face with prominent and hyperteloric-appearing eyes. Abnormal gait and bowing may be the first evident signs of the disorder. Dental malocclusion is frequent, and with time, osteoarthritis of the back and/or hip may become a problem. A contracted pelvis in the female may make vaginal delivery difficult. Stature is usually normal. Frequent respiratory infections may be due to the small thoracic cage. Pulmonary hypertension has occurred.

ETIOLOGY.

X-linked dominant inheritance. The vast majority of cases have been female. Three males with characteristic features of this disorder have been born to unaffected mothers and thus represent fresh gene mutations. However, early lethality, as well as a much more severe phenotype, has been documented in all four males that have been born to affected mothers. Characteristic features in those four cases include widely spaced, prominent eyes; severe micrognathia; omphalocele; hypoplastic kidneys; positional deformities of the hands and feet; cervicothoracic kyphosis; thoracolumbar lordosis; bowing of the long bones; and pseudoarthrosis of the clavicles.

References

Melnick, J. C., and Needles, C. F.: An undiagnosed bone dysplasia. Am. J. Roentgenol. Radium Ther. Nucl. Med., *97:*39, 1966.

Coste, F., Maroteaux, P., and Chouraki, L.: Osteoplasty (Melnick-Needles syndrome). Ann. Rheum. Dis., 27: 360, 1968.

von Oeyen, P., et al.: Omphalocele and multiple severe congenital anomalies associated with osteodysplasty (Melnick-Needles syndrome). Am. J. Med. Genet., *13:*453, 1982.

Krajewska-Walasek, M., et al.: Melnick-Needles syndrome in males. Am. J. Med. Genet., 27:153, 1987.

Eggli, K., et al.: Melnick-Needles syndrome. Four new cases. Pediatr. Radiol., 22:257, 1992.

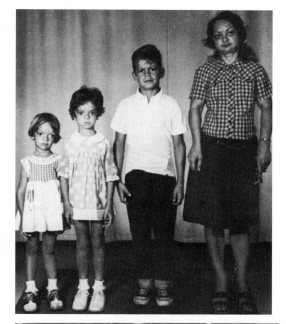

FIGURE 1. Melnick-Needles syndrome. *Left*, Affected mother and two daughters; note the facies and lower limbs. The boy is not affected. (Courtesy of Dr. William Nyhan, University of California, San Diego, Calif.) *Below*, Facies of an affected young woman. (Courtesy of Dr. Manuel Hernandez, Madrid, Spain.)

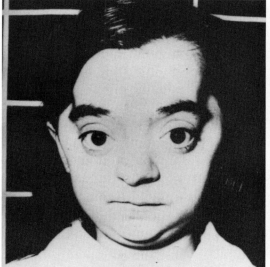
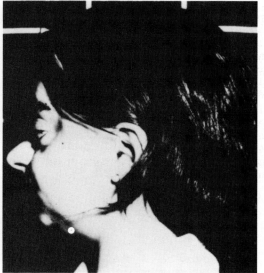

BARDET-BIEDL SYNDROME

Retinal Pigmentation, Obesity, Polydactyly

The variable manifestations of this syndrome were initially described by Bardet and Biedl in the 1920s. Subsequently, more than 300 cases have been reported. This disorder is clearly different from the condition described in 1865 by Laurence and Moon, although it was referred to as the Laurence-Moon-Biedl syndrome in the third edition of this book.

ABNORMALITIES
Growth. Obesity (83 per cent) with the majority below the 50th percentile for height.
Performance. Mental deficiency with verbal I.Q. of 79 or below in 77 per cent and performance I.Q. of 79 or below in 44 per cent. Inappropriate mannerisms and shallow affect are common. I.Q. correlates with visual handicap.
Ocular. Retinal dystrophy (100 per cent). Myopia (75 per cent). Astigmatism (63 per cent). Nystagmus (52 per cent). Glaucoma (22 per cent). Posterior capsular cataracts (44 per cent). Mature cataracts or aphakia (30 per cent). Typical retinitis pigmentosa (8 per cent).
Limbs. Postaxial polydactyly (58 per cent). Syndactyly. Brachydactyly of hands (50 per cent). Broad, short feet.
Kidney. Abnormal calyces (95 per cent). Communicating cysts or diverticulae (62 per cent). Fetal lobulations (95 per cent). Diffuse cortical loss (29 per cent). Focal scarring (24 per cent).
Hypogonadism. Small penis and testes (88 per cent).

OTHER ABNORMALITIES. Cardiac defects. Macrocephaly. Urologic anomalies. Diabetes mellitus. Diabetes insipidus. Clinodactyly of the fifth finger. Cystic dilatation of the intrahepatic and common bile ducts. Hirsutism. Ovarian stromal hyperplasia. Vaginal atresia.

NATURAL HISTORY. The mental deficiency is usually mild to moderate, and the retinal dystrophy generally results in problems with night vision during childhood, constricted visual fields, abnormalities of color vision, and extinguished or minimal rod-and-cone responses on ERG. Visual acuity deteriorates with age. Only about 15 per cent of patients show an atypical retinal pigmentation by 5 to 10 years of age. However, by age 20, 73 per cent of patients are blind. Most patients have mild problems in renal function with partial defects in urine concentration and renal tubular acidosis. Renal failure occurs, although infrequently. Hypertension is present in 60 per cent. Obesity is usually present from early infancy. The hypogonadism has been described as primary germinal hypoplasia and also as hypogonadotropic in type. Although no affected male has fathered a child, women have given birth to children. Normal development of secondary sexual characteristics is the rule in women. Irregular menstrual periods are common.

ETIOLOGY. Autosomal recessive. Marked variability of expression exists, even within families, for the mental retardation, polydactyly, degree of obesity, reproductive dysfunction, and functional abnormalities of the kidneys. However, the type of retinal dystrophy is consistent among affected family members. Three different loci, one on chromosome 16q21, a second on chromosome 11q, and a third on chromosome 3 have been identified by linkage analysis indicating the existence of nonallelic heterogeneity in this disorder.

References

Bardet, G.: Sur un syndrome d'obésité infantile avec polydactylie et rétinite pigmentaire. (Contribution à l'étude des formes cliniques de l'obesité hypophysaire.) Faculté de Medicine de Paris, Thesis, 470, 1920.

Biedl, A.: Ein Geschwisterpaar mit adiposo-genitaler Dystropie. Dtsch. Med. Wochenschr., 48:1630, 1922.

Klein, D., and Ammann, F.: The syndrome of Laurence-Moon-Bardet-Biedl and allied diseases in Switzerland: Clinical, genetic and epidemiological studies. J. Neurol. Sci., 9:479, 1969.

Hurley, R. M., et al.: The renal lesion of the Laurence-Moon-Beidl syndrome. J. Pediatr., 87:206, 1975.

Green, J. S., et al.: The cardinal manifestations of Bardet-Biedl syndrome, a form of Laurence-Moon-Biedl syndrome. N. Engl. J. Med., 321:1002, 1989.

Kwitek-Black, A. E., et al.: Linkage of Bardet-Biedl syndrome to chromosome 16q and evidence for non-allelic genetic heterogeneity. Nat. Genet., 5:392, 1993.

Elbedour, K., et al.: Cardiac abnormalities in the Bardet-Biedl syndrome. Echocardiographic studies of 22 patients. Am. J. Med. Genet., 52:164, 1994.

Leppert, M., et al.: Bardet-Biedl syndrome is linked to DNA markers on chromosome 11q and is genetically heterogeneous. Nat. Genet., 7:108, 1994.

Sheffield, V. C., et al.: Identification of a Bardet-Biedl syndrome locus on chromosome 3 and evaluation of an efficient approach to homozygosity mapping. Hum. Mol. Genet., 3:1331, 1994.

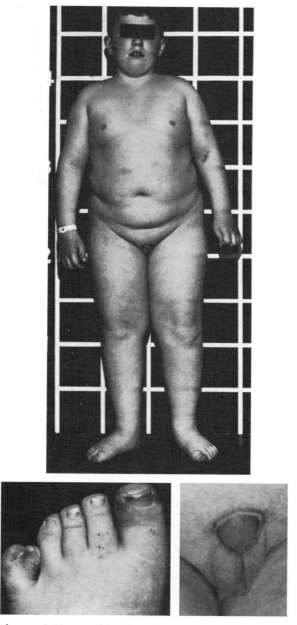

FIGURE 1. Bardet-Biedl syndrome. A 10-year-old male with retinal pigmentation and renal insufficiency. Obesity from birth. I.Q. of 52.

RIEGER SYNDROME

Iris Dysplasia, Hypodontia

In 1935, Rieger described the malformation of the anterior segment of the eye that now bears his name, the Rieger eye malformation. Subsequently, dental anomalies were observed in individuals with this defect and the combination has come to be known as the Rieger syndrome.

ABNORMALITIES
Ocular. Dysplasia of the iris (goniodysgenesis) including iris hypoplasia, strands of tissue connecting the iris to the posterior cornea, prominent Schwalbe line (posterior embryotoxon).
Facial. Broad nasal bridge, maxillary hypoplasia, thin upper lip, short philtrum.
Dentition. Hypodontia usually of upper incisors.
Other. Failure of involution of the periumbilical skin.

OTHER ABNORMALITIES. Glaucoma, abnormal placement of pupil. Hypospadias. Imperforate anus. Growth hormone deficiency.

COMMENT. The Rieger eye malformation, also known as the Axenfeld-Rieger anomaly or mesodermal dysgenesis of the iris, is a defect that can occur as an isolated manifestation or as one component of several distinct syndromes. These include the Rieger syndrome, several other mendelian conditions, and various chromosomal abnormalities including dup(3p), del(4p), del(4q), and del(13q). Regardless of the etiology, about 50 per cent of patients with the Rieger eye malformation will develop glaucoma during childhood or adolescence. Murray et al. mapped the gene for Rieger syndrome in three families to chromosome 4q25 based on the cases in the literature who had 4q deletion. Another family, however, who has the Rieger eye malformation without hypodontia did not map to that region, confirming heterogeneity.

ETIOLOGY. Autosomal dominant with variable expression.

References

Rieger, H.: Beiträge zur Kenntnis schener Missbildungen der Iris. Arch. Ophthalmol., *133*:602, 1935.
Fitch, N., and Kaback, M.: The Axenfeld syndrome and the Rieger syndrome. J. Med. Genet., *15*:30, 1978.
Jorgensen, R. J., et al.: The Rieger syndrome. Am. J. Med. Genet., 2:307, 1978.
Carey, J. C., et al.: Heterogeneity of the Rieger eye malformation. Clin. Res., *28*:116A, 1980.
Shields, M. B., et al.: Axenfeld-Rieger syndrome: A spectrum of developmental disorders. Ophthalmology, *29*:387, 1985.
Murray, J. C., et al.: Linkage of Rieger syndrome to the region of the epidermal growth factor gene on chromosome 4. Nat. Genet., 2:46, 1992.

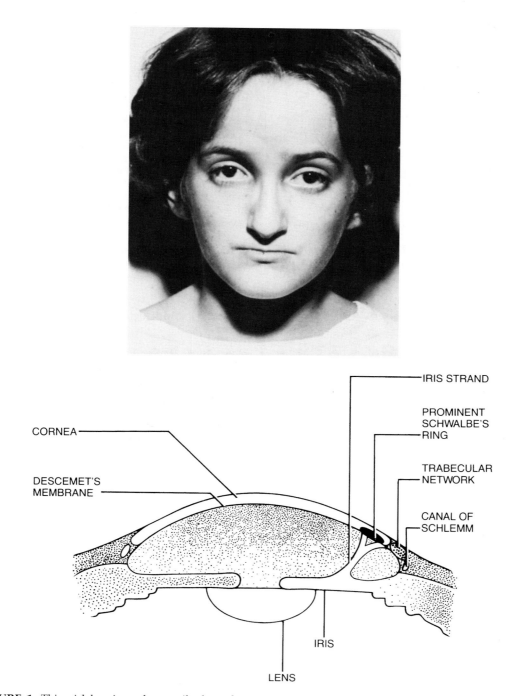

IRIS STRAND

PROMINENT
SCHWALBE'S
RING

TRABECULAR
NETWORK

CANAL OF
SCHLEMM

CORNEA

DESCEMET'S
MEMBRANE

IRIS

LENS

FIGURE 1. This girl has irregular pupils, hypodontia, maxillary hypoplasia with malocclusion, and a short philtrum. The diagram depicts the transverse section of the ocular anterior chamber with a normal angle on the left and the Rieger eye malformation on the right. Note the hypoplasia of the iris and the iris strands.

PETERS'-PLUS SYNDROME

*Peters Anomaly, Short Limb
Dwarfism, Mental Retardation*

This disorder was initially set forth in 1984 by Van Schooneveld, who described 11 affected individuals and introduced the term Peters'-Plus syndrome. Greater than 40 cases have now been reported.

ABNORMALITIES
Performance. Mental retardation varying from mild to severe in 80 per cent.
Growth. Prenatal onset growth deficiency. Birth length less than third percentile for gestational age in 82 per cent. Postnatal growth deficiency in 100 per cent, with adult height in females ranging from 128 to 151 cm and in males ranging from 141 to 155 cm.
Craniofacies. Round face in childhood. Prominent forehead. Hypertelorism. Long philtrum. Cupid-bow shape of upper lip. Thin vermilion border. Small, mildly malformed ears. Preauricular pits. Micrognathia. Broad neck.
Eyes. Peters anomaly or other anterior chamber cleavage disorder. Narrow palpebral fissures. Nystagmus. Glaucoma.
Limb. Short limbs primarily rhizomelic. Decreased range of motion at elbows. Hypermobility of other joints. Broad and short hands and feet. Fifth finger clinodactyly.
Other. Cardiac defects including atrial and ventricular septal defects and pulmonary stenosis. Hydronephrosis. Duplication of kidneys. Cryptorchidism.

OCCASIONAL ABNORMALITIES.
Cleft lip and palate. Short lingular frenulum. Microcephaly. Macrocephaly. Dilated lateral ventricles. Abnormal ossification of the skull. Up-slanting palpebral fissures. Cataract. Mild cutaneous syndactyly. Simian crease. Pes cavus. Seizures. Spastic diplegia. Hypoplastic labia majora. Hypoplastic clitoris. Hypospadias. Abnormal foreskin. Vertebral anomaly. Pectus excavatum. Agenesis of corpus callosum.

NATURAL HISTORY. Feeding problems often requiring prolonged gavage are common. All patients learn to speak and acquire simple skills, although developmental milestones are significantly delayed. The corneal opacities may diminish during the first 6 months of life, but they never clear enough to permit normal vision.

ETIOLOGY. Autosomal recessive.

COMMENT. Peters anomaly, a defect of the anterior chamber, includes central corneal opacity (leukoma), thinning of the posterior aspect of the cornea, and iridocorneal adhesions attached to the edges of the leukoma. Peters anomaly usually occurs as an isolated defect in an otherwise normal individual. However, it can occur as one feature of a multiple malformation syndrome such as Peters'-Plus syndrome.

References

Van Schooneveld, M. J., et al.: Peters'-Plus: A new syndrome. Ophthalmic Paediatr. Genet., 4:141, 1984.
Saal, H. M., et al.: Autosomal recessive Robinow-like syndrome with anterior chamber cleavage anomalies. Am. J. Med. Genet., 30:709. 1988.
Hennekam, R. C. M., et al.: The Peters'-Plus syndrome: Description of 16 patients and review of the literature. Clin. Dysmorphol., 2:283, 1993.
Thompson, E. M., et al.: Kivlin syndrome and Peters'-Plus syndrome: Are they the same disorder? Clin. Dysmorphol., 2:301, 1993.

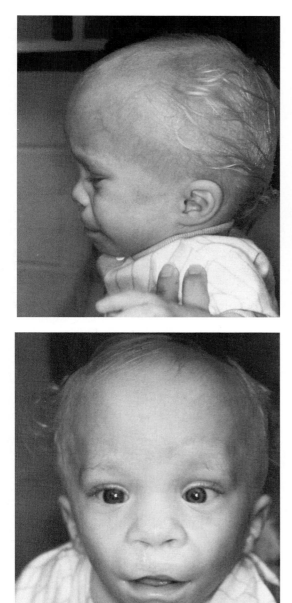

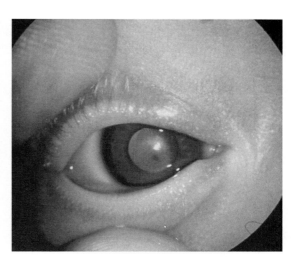

FIGURE 1. A 15-month-old male. Note the round face with prominent forehead, long philtrum with Cupid-bow shape of upper lip, and thin vermilion border. The corneal opacity noted in the right eye at 4 months was markedly decreased by 15 months. (From Hennekam, R. C. M., et al.: Clin. Dysmorphol., 2:283, 1993, with permission.)

CEREBRO-COSTO-MANDIBULAR SYNDROME

Rib-Gap Defect With Small Thorax, Severe Micrognathia

This disorder was initially described by Smith et al. in 1966, and over 30 cases have been reported.

ABNORMALITIES
Performance. Mental deficiency and speech difficulties are frequent among the survivors.
Growth. Postnatal growth deficiency.
Facies. Severe micrognathia with glossoptosis and short to cleft soft palate.
Thorax. Bell-shaped small thorax with gaps between posterior ossified rib and anterior cartilaginous rib, especially fourth to tenth ribs. Rudimentary ribs. Anomalous rib insertion to vertebrae.
Other. Inconsistent observations of pterygium colli, abnormal tracheal cartilaginous rings, vertebral anomalies, elbow hypoplasia, hearing loss, renal cyst and/or ectopia, club foot, and congenital hip dislocation.

OCCASIONAL ABNORMALITIES. Microcephaly. Fifth finger clinodactyly. Hypoplastic humerus. Sacral fusion. Flask-shaped configuration of pelvis. Hypoplastic sternum, clavicles, and pubic rami. Epiphyseal stippling of calcaneus. Ventricular septal defect. Porencephaly. Hydranencephaly. Meningomyelocele.

NATURAL HISTORY. Forty per cent die in the first year, one half of these in the first month due to respiratory insufficiency. Of those who survive, feeding and speech difficulties are common, as well as mental deficiency in 50 per cent of cases. The rib gap defects resolve into pseudoarthroses with time.

ETIOLOGY. Autosomal recessive inheritance is implied by the occurrence of offspring from normal parentage as well as consanguinity. However, parent-to-child transmission has been reported, suggesting autosomal dominant inheritance for some cases of this disorder.

References

Smith, D. W., Theiler, K., and Schachenmann, G.: Rib-gap defect with micrognathia, malformed tracheal cartilages, and redundant skin: A new pattern of defective development. J. Pediatr., 69:799, 1966.

Doyle, J. F.: The skeletal defects of the cerebro-costo-mandibular syndrome. Ir. J. Med. Sci., Ser. 7, 2:595, 1969.

McNicholl, B., et al.: Cerebro-costo-mandibular syndrome. A new familial developmental disorder. Arch. Dis. Child., 45:421, 1970.

Silverman, F. N., et al.: Cerebro-costo-mandibular syndrome. J. Pediatr., 97:406, 1980.

Tachibina, K., et al.: Cerebro-costo-mandibular syndrome. Hum. Genet., 54:283, 1980.

Leroy, J. G., et al.: Cerebro-costo-mandibular syndrome with autosomal dominant inheritance. J. Pediatr., 99:441, 1981.

Hennekam, R. C. M., et al.: The cerebro-costo-mandibular syndrome: Third report of familial occurrence. Clin. Genet., 28:118, 1985.

Burton, E. M., and Oestreich, A. E.: Cerebro-costo-mandibular syndrome with stippled epiphysis and cystic fibrosis. Pediatr. Radiol., 18:365, 1988.

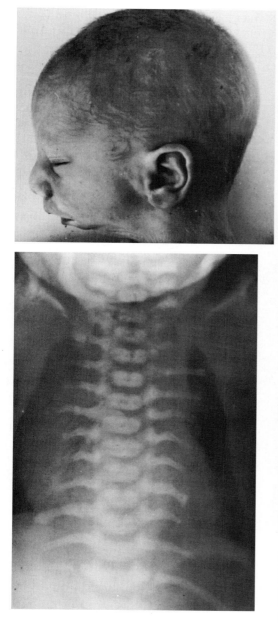

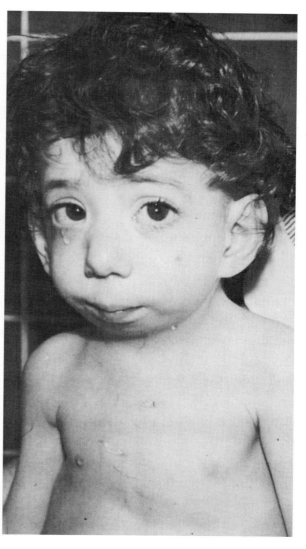

FIGURE 1. Cerebro-costo-mandibular syndrome. *Left*, Newborn showing severe micrognathia and incompletely ossified aberrant ribs. (From Smith, D. W., et al.: J. Pediatr., *69*:799, 1966, with permission.) *Right*, A 4-year-old. (From McNicholl, B., et al.: Arch. Dis. Child., *45*:421, 1970, with permission.)

JARCHO-LEVIN SYNDROME

(Spondylothoracic Dysplasia)

Jarcho and Levin described this disorder in 1938, and subsequently, at least 21 cases have been reported.

ABNORMALITIES

Growth. Short trunk dwarfism of prenatal onset.
Craniofacial. Prominent occiput; tendency to have broad forehead, wide nasal bridge, anteverted nares, and up-slant to palpebral fissures.
Thorax and Spine. Short thorax with "crab-like" rib cage associated with multiple vertebral defects and ribs that flare in a fan-like pattern. Posterior fusion and absence of ribs. Short neck and low posterior hairline. Pectus carinatum. Increased anteroposterior chest diameter. Lordosis. Kyphoscoliosis.
Limbs. Normal with impression of being long.
Other. Protuberant abdomen.

OCCASIONAL ABNORMALITIES.
Cleft palate. Cryptorchidism. Hernias. Hydronephrosis with ureteral obstruction. Bilobed bladder. Absent external genitalia. Anal and urethral atresia. Uterus didelphys. Cerebral polygyria. Neural tube defects (33 per cent). Single umbilical artery.

NATURAL HISTORY.
Although the majority of affected individuals die in early infancy as a result of recurrent pulmonary infection and respiratory insufficiency secondary to the small thoracic volume, a small number have lived beyond 1 year of age. One has survived to age 11. Although he has moderately severe restrictive pulmonary disease, he is active in sports and is doing well academically.

ETIOLOGY.
Autosomal recessive. Most reported cases have occurred in Puerto Rican individuals.

COMMENT.
A clinically similar disorder referred to as spondylocostal dysostosis is associated with vertebral and rib malformations but absence of fan-like flaring of the ribs on radiographs. Survival is much better and neural tube defects only rarely occur. Inheritance in most cases is autosomal recessive, although autosomal dominant inheritance has been described.

References

Jarcho, S., and Levin, P. M.: Hereditary malformations of the vertebral bodies. Johns Hopkins Med. J., *62*: 216, 1938.

Pérez-Comas, A., and Garcia-Castro, J. M.: Occipito-facial-cervico-thoracic-abdomino-digital dysplasia: Jarcho-Levin syndrome of vertebral anomalies. J. Pediatr., *85*:388, 1974.

Poor, M. A., et al.: Nonskeletal malformations in one of three siblings with Jarcho-Levin syndrome of vertebral anomalies. J. Pediatr., *103*:270, 1983.

Karnes, P. S., et al.: Jarcho-Levin syndrome: Four new cases and classification of subtypes. Am. J. Med. Genet., *40*:264, 1991.

McCall, C. P., et al.: Jarcho-Levin syndrome: Unusual survival in a classical case. Am. J. Med. Genet., *49*: 328, 1994.

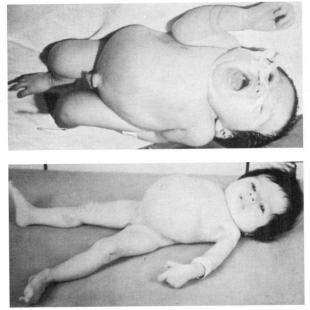
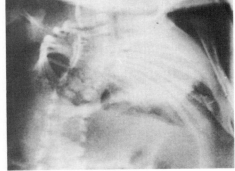

FIGURE 1. Jarcho-Levin syndrome. Affected neonate and young infant, with roentgenogram of the former. (From Pérez-Comas, A., and Garcia-Castro, J. M.: J. Pediatr., *85*:388, 1974, with permission.)

LEPRECHAUNISM SYNDROME

(Donohue Syndrome)

Prenatal Adipose Deficiency, Full Lips, Islet Cell Hyperplasia

This somewhat puzzling disorder was initially described as dysendocrinism by Donohue in 1948. Later, Donohue and Uchida reported two siblings under the term leprechaunism, and since then more than 30 cases have been recorded.

ABNORMALITIES

Growth. Prenatal and postnatal growth deficiency with retarded osseous maturation and marked lack of adipose tissue; mean birth weight, about 2.6 kg.

Facies. Small, with prominent eyes, wide nostrils, thick lips, large ears. Gingival hyperplasia.

Endocrine. Large phallus, breast hyperplasia (female), Leydig cell hyperplasia (male), follicular development with cystic ovary, hyperplasia of islets of Langerhans, hyperglycemia, hyperinsulinemia. Precocious puberty. Increased umbilical cord human chorionic gonadotropin.

Other. Body and facial hirsutism. Acanthosis nigricans. Nail dysplasia. Wrinkled, loose skin. Pachyderma. Rugation of orifices. Hyperkeratosis. Prominent nipples. Apparent motor and mental retardation. Abdominal distention. Relatively large hands and feet.

NATURAL HISTORY. Usually severe failure to thrive and frequent infections, with death in early infancy. One patient survived to $2^{3}/_{12}$ years of age. Hypoglycemia occurs following prolonged fast.

ETIOLOGY. Autosomal recessive inheritance. Mutations of the insulin receptor gene located on chromosome 19p13.2 have been documented. The resultant severe insulin resistance leads to many of the features of this disorder including the growth deficiency, hyperglycemia, hyperinsulinemia, and hyperplasia of the islets of Langerhans.

References

Donohue, W. L.: Dysendocrinism. J. Pediatr., 32:739, 1948.

Donohue, W. L., and Uchida, I.: Leprechaunism. A euphemism for a rare familial disorder. J. Pediatr., 45: 505, 1954.

D'Ercole, J. A., et al.: Leprechaunism: Studies on the relationship between hyperinsulinism, insulin resistance, and growth retardation. J. Clin. Endocrinol. Metab., 48 495, 1979.

Elsas, L. J., et al.: Leprechaunism: An inherited defect in a high-affinity insulin receptor. Am. J. Hum. Genet., 37:73, 1985.

Kadowaki, T., et al.: Two mutant alleles of the insulin receptor gene in a patient with extreme insulin resistance. Science, 240:787, 1988.

Taylor, S. I., et al.: Mutations in the insulin receptor. Endocr. Rev., 13:566, 1992.

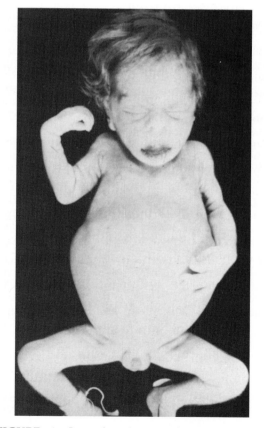

FIGURE 1. Leprechaunism syndrome. Necropsy photo of neonate with hyperglycemia and hyperinsulinemia who showed cellular unreponsiveness to insulin and who had islet cell hyperplasia at necropsy. (Courtesy of Dr. J. A. D'Ercole and Dr. Louis Underwood, University of North Carolina of Medicine, Chapel Hill, N.C.)

BERARDINELLI LIPODYSTROPHY SYNDROME

(Generalized Lipodystrophy)

Lipoatrophy, Phallic Hypertrophy, Hepatomegaly, Hyperlipemia

Berardinelli reported this unusual lipodystrophic syndrome in 1954. Although many cases have been recorded subsequently, the metabolic defect responsible for this inborn error of metabolism has not been determined.

ABNORMALITIES

Performance. Mental deficiency as a variable feature.

Growth. Accelerated growth and maturation, enlargement of hands and feet, phallic enlargement, hypertrophy of muscle with excess glycogen, lack of metabolically active adipose from early life with sparing of mechanical adipose tissue (i.e., in orbits, palms and soles, crista galli, buccal region, tongue, scalp, breasts, perineum, periarticular regions, and epidural areas).

Skin. Coarse with hyperpigmentation, especially in axillae. Variable acanthosis nigricans.

Hair. Hirsutism with curly scalp hair.

Vascular. Large superficial veins.

Liver. Hepatomegaly with excess neutral fat and glycogen and eventual cirrhosis.

Plasma. Hyperlipidemia. Hypertriglyceridemia. Insulin-resistant diabetes.

OCCASIONAL ABNORMALITIES. Cardiomegaly, corneal opacities, hyperproteinemia, hyperinsulinemia. Polycystic ovarian disease. Percussion myxedema.

NATURAL HISTORY. The accelerated growth and hyperlipemia are most prominent in early childhood, and hyperglycemia may develop in later childhood. Cirrhosis of the liver with esophageal varices may become a fatal complication.

COMMENT. Although the accelerated growth and maturation plus the muscle hypertrophy and enlargement of the phallus are suggestive of androgen effect, neither androgens nor gonadotropins are elevated, and the hirsutism does not include pubic and axillary hair. Oserd et al. found that mononuclear leukocytes from affected patients bound less insulin than cells from controls, suggesting that altered insulin receptors are responsible for the insulin resistance and decreased synthesis of triglycerides.

ETIOLOGY. Autosomal recessive, as indicated by sibship occurrence and parental consanguinity. Ineffective insulin action is a major factor in the pathogenesis of this disorder.

References

Berardinelli, W.: An undiagnosed endocrinometabolic syndrome: Report of two cases. J. Clin. Endocrinol. Metab., *14*:193, 1954.

Seip, M., and Trygstad, O.: Generalized lipodystrophy. Arch. Dis. Child., *38*:447, 1963.

Senior, B., and Gellis, S. S.: The syndromes of total lipodystrophy and of partial lipodystrophy. Pediatrics, *33*:593, 1964.

Oserd, S., et al.: Decreased binding of insulin to its receptor in patients with congenital generalized lipodystrophy. N. Engl. J. Med., *296*:245, 1977.

Garg, A., et al.: Peculiar distribution of adipose tissue in patients with congenital generalized lipodystrophy. J. Clin. Endocrinol. Metab., *75*:358, 1991.

Klein, S., et al.: Generalized lipodystrophy: In vivo evidence of hypermetabolism and insulin-resistant lipid, glucose and amino acid kinetic. Metabolism, *41*:893, 1992.

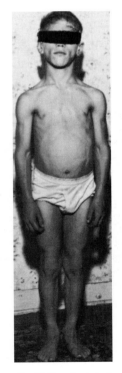

FIGURE 1. Berardinelli lipodystrophy syndrome. Preadolescent-age boy showing hypetrophied muscle and relative lack of subcutaneous fat. (Courtesy of Central Wisconsin Colony and Training School.)

DISTICHIASIS-LYMPHEDEMA SYNDROME

Double Row of Eyelashes, Lymphedema

ABNORMALITIES

Eyes. Distichiasis, an extra row of eyelashes, replacing meibomian glands (100 per cent).

Limbs. Lymphedema, predominantly from knee downward (66 per cent).

Other. Vertebral anomalies (62 per cent). Epidural cysts (46 per cent). Cardiac defects (38 per cent).

OCCASIONAL ABNORMALITIES.

Short stature. Ptosis. Microphthalmia. Strabismus. Partial ectropion of lower lid. Epicanthal folds. Pterygium colli. Cleft palate. Bifid uvula. Micrognathia. Scoliosis/kyphosis. Cryptorchidism. Double uterus.

NATURAL HISTORY.

The extra eyelashes may cause irritative ocular problems and often require surgical removal. The lymphedema usually becomes evident between the ages of 5 and 20 years, especially at the time of adolescence and sometimes for the first time during pregnancy. The possibility of epidural cysts with secondary neurologic or other complications must always be considered in this disorder. Eyelash removal or surgery for the lymphedema is difficult to accomplish with good results, and hence, treatment is generally withheld unless grossly indicated.

ETIOLOGY.

Autosomal dominant inheritance with marked variability of expression. Diagnosis in sporadic cases is often difficult, since affected individuals might have only one of the characteristic features.

References

Falls, H. F., and Dertesz, E. D.: A new syndrome combining pterygium colli with developmental anomalies of the eyelids and lymphatics of the lower extremities. Trans. Am. Ophthalmol. Soc., 62:248, 1964.

Robinow, M., Johnson, G. F., and Verhagen, A. D.: Distichiasis-lymphedema. A hereditary syndrome of multiple congenital defects. Am. J. Dis. Child, 119:343, 1970.

Hoover, R. E., and Kelley, J. S.: Distichiasis and lymphedema: A hereditary syndrome with possible multiple defects—a report of a family. Trans. Ophthalmol. Soc., 69:293, 1971.

Holmes, L. B., Fields, J. P., and Zabriskiek, J. B.: Hereditary late onset lymphedema. Pediatrics, 61:575, 1978.

Schwartz, J. F., O'Brien, M. S., and Hoffman, J. C.: Hereditary spinal arachnoid cysts, distichiasis, and lymphedema. Ann. Neurol., 7:340, 1980.

Temple, I. K., and Collin, J. R. O.: Distichiasis-Lymphoedema syndrome: A family report. Clin. Dysmorphol., 3:139, 1994.

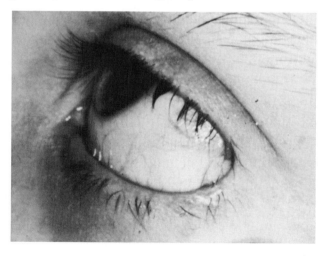

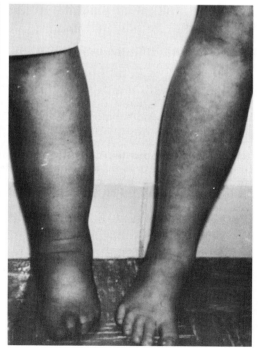

FIGURE 1. Distichiasis in the eye of this teen-age girl and lymphedema in her leg (*on right*) and more severely so in that of her affected mother (*on left*).

T

T. MISCELLANEOUS SEQUENCES

LATERALITY SEQUENCES

In addition to reversal of the sides, with partial to complete situs inversus, there can be bilateral left- or right-sidedness. The primary defect in both is a failure of normal asymmetry in morphogenesis. The basic problem would presumably be present prior to 30 days of development. The accompanying chart sets forth the differences as well as the similarities between the patterns due to predominantly left-sided bilaterality and due to right-sided bilaterality. Among other differences, the spleen dramatically reflects the variant laterality in the two. With left-sided bilaterality there is polysplenia (usually bilateral spleens plus rudimentary extra splenic tissue), and with right-sided bilaterality there is asplenia or a hypoplastic spleen. The defect in lateralization leading to the failure of normal asymmetry in morphogenesis is most likely etiologically heterogeneous. As such, although usually sporadic, autosomal dominant, autosomal recessive, and X-linked recessive inheritance have all been documented. A gene for X-linked laterality sequence has been mapped to Xq24-27.1.

BILATERAL LEFT-SIDEDNESS SEQUENCE (polysplenia syndrome). The sex incidence is about equal. The cardiac anomalies are usually not as severe as with bilateral right-sidedness.

BILATERAL RIGHT-SIDEDNESS SEQUENCE (asplenia syndrome, Ivemark syndrome, triad of spleen agenesis, defects of heart and vessels, and situs inversus). This is two to three times more common in males than in females. The complex cardiac anomalies, usually giving rise to cyanosis and early cardiac failure, are the major cause of early death. The possibility of gastrointestinal problems must also be considered, especially as related to the aberrant mesenteric attachments. Renal anomalies are also more frequent (25 per cent). Survivors have had an increased frequency of cutaneous, respiratory, and other infections, possibly related to the asplenia. Tests to detect asplenia include valuation of red blood cells for Howell-Jolly bodies and Heinz bodies.

OCCASIONAL ABNORMALITIES. Intestinal malrotation, biliary atresia, anomalous portal and hepatic vessels, intestinal obstruction, meningomyelocele, cerebellar hypoplasia, arrhinencephaly.

COMMENT. Both bilateral left-sidedness (polysplenia) and bilateral right-sidedness (asplenia) have been documented in different persons in the same family, indicating that the two conditions represent different manifestations of a primary defect in lateralization leading to failure of normal body asymmetry.

References

Freedom, R. M.: The asplenia syndrome. J. Pediatr., *81*: 1130, 1972.

Van Mierop, L. H. S., Gessner, I. H., and Schiebler, G. L.: Asplenia and polysplenia syndromes. Birth Defects, *8*:74, 1972.

Arnold, G. L., Bixler, D., and Gerod, D.: Probable autosomal recessive inheritance of polysplenia, situs inversus and cardiac defects in an Amish family. Am. J. Med. Genet., *16*:35, 1983.

Mathias, R. S., et al.: X-linked laterality sequence: Situs inversus, complex cardiac defects, splenic defects. Am. J. Med. Genet., *28*:111, 1987.

Casey, B., et al.: Mapping a gene for familial situs abnormalities to human chromosome Xq24-q27.1. Nat. Genet., *5*:403, 1993.

Mikkila, S. P., et al.: X-linked laterality sequence in a family with carrier manifestations. Am. J. Med. Genet., *49*:435, 1994.

Illustration on opposite page

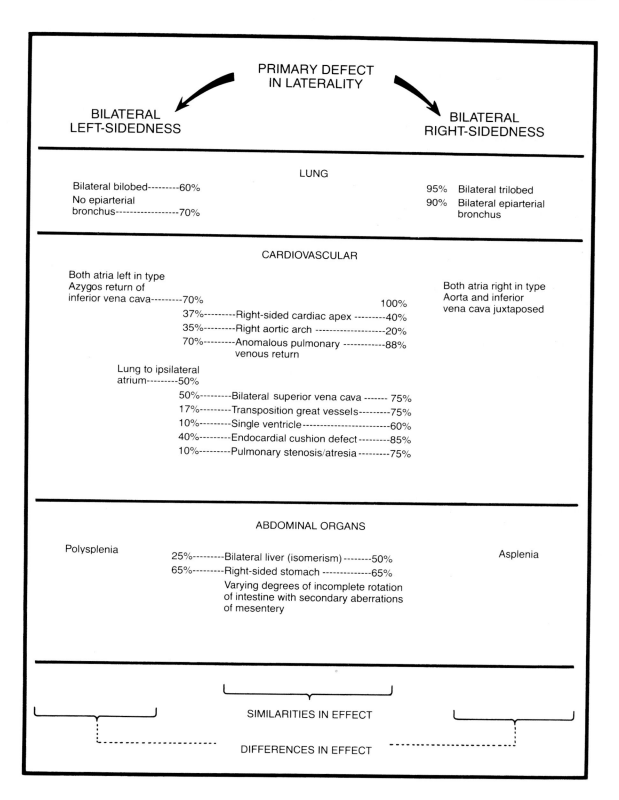

PRIMARY DEFECT
IN LATERALITY

BILATERAL
LEFT-SIDEDNESS

BILATERAL
RIGHT-SIDEDNESS

LUNG

Bilateral bilobed--------60%
No epiarterial
bronchus----------------70%

95%   Bilateral trilobed
90%   Bilateral epiarterial
        bronchus

CARDIOVASCULAR

Both atria left in type
Azygos return of
inferior vena cava--------70%
                                            100%
        37%--------Right-sided cardiac apex ---------40%
        35%--------Right aortic arch --------------------20%
        70%--------Anomalous pulmonary ------------88%
                        venous return
    Lung to ipsilateral
    atrium---------50%
        50%--------Bilateral superior vena cava ------- 75%
        17%--------Transposition great vessels---------75%
        10%--------Single ventricle------------------------60%
        40%--------Endocardial cushion defect---------85%
        10%--------Pulmonary stenosis/atresia---------75%

Both atria right in type
Aorta and inferior
vena cava juxtaposed

ABDOMINAL ORGANS

Polysplenia

        25%---------Bilateral liver (isomerism) --------50%
        65%---------Right-sided stomach -------------65%
        Varying degrees of incomplete rotation
        of intestine with secondary aberrations
        of mesentery

Asplenia

SIMILARITIES IN EFFECT

DIFFERENCES IN EFFECT

KARTAGENER SYNDROME

Situs Inversus, Sinusitis, Bronchiectasis

Described by Kartagener in 1933, this syndrome accounts for about one tenth of the cases of bronchiectasis and about one sixth of the cases of situs inversus. Kartagener syndrome is a subgroup of the immotile cilia syndrome.

ABNORMALITIES

Organ Orientation. Situs inversus, partial to complete, with gross defects in cardiac septation in 50 per cent; occasional asplenia. (See Laterality Sequences.)

Respiratory Tract. Absence of frontal sinus development. Lack of aeration of mastoids. Thick, tenacious mucus with problems of infection and stasis. Conductive deafness.

Other. Folliculitis. Nummular eczema. Pyoderma gangrenosum. Communicating hydrocephalus. Dull headaches. Endogenous depressions. Schizophrenia. Thyrotoxicosis.

NATURAL HISTORY. Provided the patient does not have a lethal cardiac anomaly, there is a variable age of onset and severity of chronic middle ear infection, rhinitis (sometimes with nasal polyps), sinusitis, pneumonia, chronic cough, and follicular bronchiectasis. *Haemophilus influenzae* and *Diplococcus pneumoniae* are the more common bacterial pathogens. Over 90 per cent of patients are symptomatic during childhood. The initial presentation of chronic rhinitis with wheezing and rales may falsely suggest an allergic problem. Middle ear problems frequently result in deafness. Partial lung resections may eventually be indicated for bronchiectasis. Occasional patients have had low IgA levels, but this does *not* appear to be the cause of this congenital defect in the function and integrity of the respiratory epithelium.

ETIOLOGY. Autosomal recessive inheritance implied. Abnormal cilia, the underlying cause of this disorder, lead to most of the clinical features. The ultrastructural abnormality is absence of ciliary dynein arms. Affected males are usually sterile because the sperm tail is a modified cilium. Affected females have decreased fertility.

References

Kartagener, M.: Zur Pathogenese der Bronkiektasien. Bronkiektasien bei situs viscerum inversus. Beitr. Klin. Tuberk., *83*:489, 1933.

Mayo, P.: Kartagener's syndrome. J. Thorac. Cardiovasc. Surg., *42*:39, 1961.

Holmes, L. B., Blennerhassett, J. B., and Austen, K. F.: A reappraisal of Kartagener's syndrome. Am. J. Med. Sci., *225*:13, 1968.

Hartline, J. V., and Zelkowitz, P. S.: Kartagener's syndrome in childhood. Am. J. Dis. Child., *121*:349, 1971.

Afzelius, A. B.: Kartagener's syndrome and abnormal cilia. N. Engl. J. Med., *297*:1011, 1977.

Jabourian, Z., et al.: Hydrocephalus in Kartagener's syndrome. Ear Nose Throat J., *65*:46, 1986.

Lunardi, P., et al.: Palinopsia: Unusual presenting symptom of a cerebral abscess in a man with Kartagener's syndrome. Clin. Neurol. Neurosurg., *93-4*:337, 1991.

Vazquez, J., et al.: Cutaneous manifestations in Kartagener's syndrome: Folliculitis, nummular eczema and pyoderma gangraenosum. Dermatology, *186*:269, 1993.

HOLOPROSENCEPHALY SEQUENCE

Arhinencephaly-Cebocephaly-Cyclopia: Primary Defect—In Prechordal Mesoderm

During the third week of fetal development, the prechordal mesoderm migrates forward into the area anterior to the notochord and is necessary for the development of the midface as well as having an inductive role in the morphogenesis of the forebrain. The consequences of prechordal mesoderm defect are varying degrees of deficit of midline facial development, especially the median nasal process (premaxilla), and incomplete morphogenesis of the forebrain. Cyclopia represents a severe deficit in early midline facial development, and the eyes become fused, the olfactory placodes consolidate into a single tube-like proboscis above the eye, and the ethmoid and other midline bony structures are missing. With cyclopia, there is failure in the cleavage of the prosencephalon, with grossly incomplete morphogenesis of the forebrain. Less severe deficits results in hypotelorism and varying degrees of inadequate midfacial and incomplete forebrain development that are more common than cyclopia and frequently include cleft lip and palate. The important clinical point is that incomplete midline facial development, such as hypotelorism or absence of the philtrum or nasal septum, suggests the possibility of a serious anomaly in brain development and function

Although the cause is unknown and the defects are isolated in the vast majority of cases, certain aneuploidy syndromes, particularly trisomies 13 and 18 as well as several structural chromosome aberrations including del (2) (p21), dup (3pter), del (7) (q36), del (13q), del (18p), and del (21) (q22.3) should be considered. In addition, there exists an autosomal dominant form of holoprosencephaly. Therefore, parents of an affected child should be checked for mild manifestations such as a single central incisor and absence of the nasal cartilage. In most families with autosomal dominant holoprosencephaly, the gene is located at 7q36 and is designated HPE3. This is the same gene that is deleted in some and rearranged in other sporadic cases with nonrandom chromosome anomalies involving 7q36. Finally, holoprosencephaly has been seen in the offspring of diabetic mothers and in the Meckel-Gruber syndrome. The prognosis for CNS function in individuals with this type of defect is very poor, and the author recommends serious consideration of limiting extraordinary medical assistance toward survival in patients in whom the forebrain is obviously severely affected.

References

Adelmann, H. B.: The problem of cyclopia. Part II. Q. Rev. Biol., 11:284, 1936.

DeMeyer, W., Zeman, W., and Palmer, C. G.: The face predicts the brain: Diagnostic significance of median facial anomalies for holoprosencephaly (arhinencephaly). Pediatrics, 34:256, 1964.

Cohen, M. M.: An update on the holoprosencephalic disorders. J. Pediatr., 101:865, 1982.

Siebert, J. R., Cohen, M. M., Sulik, K. K., Shaw, C. and Lemire, R. J.: Holoprosencephaly: An Overview and Atlas of Cases. New York, Wiley-Liss, 1990.

Gurrieri, F., et al.: Physical mapping of the holoprosencephaly critical region on chromosome 7q36. Nat. Genet., 3:247, 1993.

Muenke, M., et al.: Linkage of a human brain malformation, familial holoprosencephaly, to chromosome 7 and evidence for genetic heterogeneity. Proc. Natl. Acad. Sci. U. S. A., 91:8102, 1994.

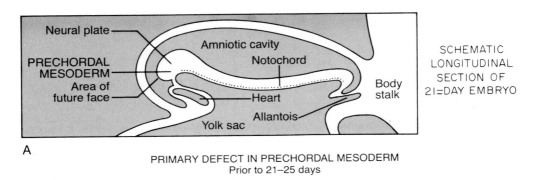

A

PRIMARY DEFECT IN PRECHORDAL MESODERM
Prior to 21–25 days

FIGURE 1. Holoprosencephaly sequence. *A*, Schematic longitudinal section of 21-day embryo.

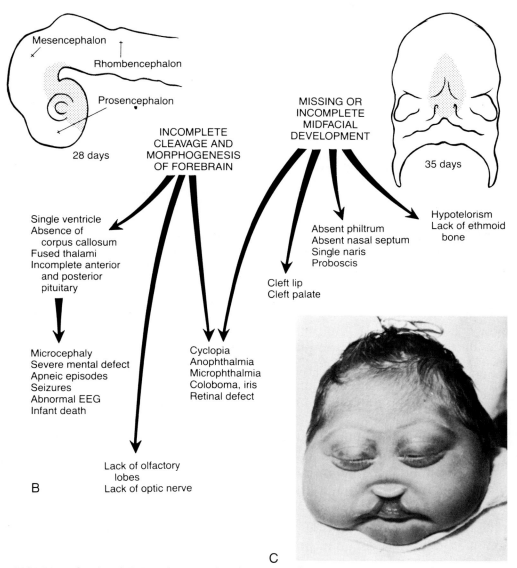

FIGURE 1. *Continued*. B, Developmental pathogenesis of the sequence. C, Affected individual.

MENINGOMYELOCELE, ANENCEPHALY, INIENCEPHALY SEQUENCES

Primary Defect—In Neural Tube Closure

The initiating malformation appears to be a defect in closure of the neural groove to form an intact neural tube, which is normally completely fused by 28 days. Anencephaly represents a defect in closure at the anterior portion of the neural groove. The secondary consequences are as follows: (1) The unfused forebrain develops partially and then tends to degenerate; (2) the calvarium is incompletely developed; and (3) the facial features and auricular development are secondarily altered to a variable degree, including cleft palate, and frequent abnormality of the cervical vertebrae.

Defects of closure at the mid or caudal neural groove can give rise to meningomyelocele and other secondary defects, as depicted. The early form of one such lesion is illustrated below.

Defects of closure in the cervical and upper thoracic region can culminate in the iniencephaly sequence, in which secondary features may include retroflexion of the upper spine with short neck and trunk, cervical and upper thoracic vertebral anomalies, defects of thoracic cage, anterior spina bifida, diaphragmatic defects with or without hernia, and hypoplasia of lung and/or heart. Recent evidence suggesting that there are four sites of anterior neural tube closure explains the variations observed in their location, recurrence risk, and etiology. Most commonly no mode of etiology is appreciated, and the recurrence risk is 1.9 per cent for parents who have had one affected child. Liberation of alpha-fetoprotein into the amniotic fluid from the anencephaly or meningomyelocele that is not skin covered allows for early amniocentesis detection, which may be augmented by sonography and/or radiography.

The U.S. Public Health Service has recommended that women of childbearing age should consume 0.4 mg of folic acid daily in order to reduce their risk of conceiving a child with a neural tube defect. For women who previously have had an affected infant, it has been recommended that 4.0 mg daily of folic acid should be consumed from 1 month prior to conception through 3 months of pregnancy.

References

Giroud, A.: Causes and morphogenesis of anencephaly. Ciba Foundation Symposium on Congenital Malformations, 1960, pp. 199–218.

Lemire, R. J., Shepard, T. H., and Alvord, E. C., Jr.: Caudal myeloschisis (lumbo-sacral spina bifida cystica) in a five millimeter (horizon XIV) human embryo. Anat. Rec., 152:9, 1965.

Lemire, R. J., Beckwith, J. B., and Shepard, T. H.: Iniencephaly and anencephaly with spinal retroflexion. Teratology, 6:27, 1972.

From the Centers for Disease Control and Prevention: Recommendations for use of folic acid to reduce number of spina bifida cases and other neural tube defects. J. A. M. A., 269:1233, 1993.

Van Allen, M. I., et al.: Evidence for multi-site closure of the neural tube in humans. Am. J. Med. Genet., 47:723, 1993.

Golden, J. A., and Chernoff, G. F.: Multiple sites of anterior neural tube closure in humans: Evidence from anterior neural tube defects (anencephaly). Pediatrics, 95:506, 1995.

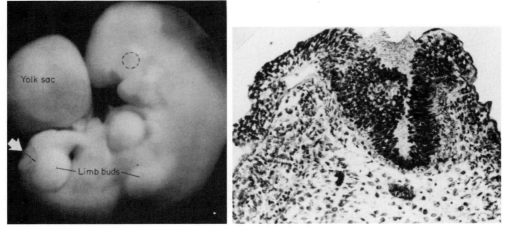

FIGURE 1. Meningomyelocele, anencephaly, iniencephaly sequences. Otherwise normal 28-day embryo with incomplete closure of the posterior neural groove (*arrow*), which shows aberrant growth of cells to the side in a transverse section (*right*). Had this embryo survived, it would presumably have developed a meningomyelocele. (From Lemire, R.: Anat. Rec., 152:9, 1965, with permission of John Wiley & Sons.)

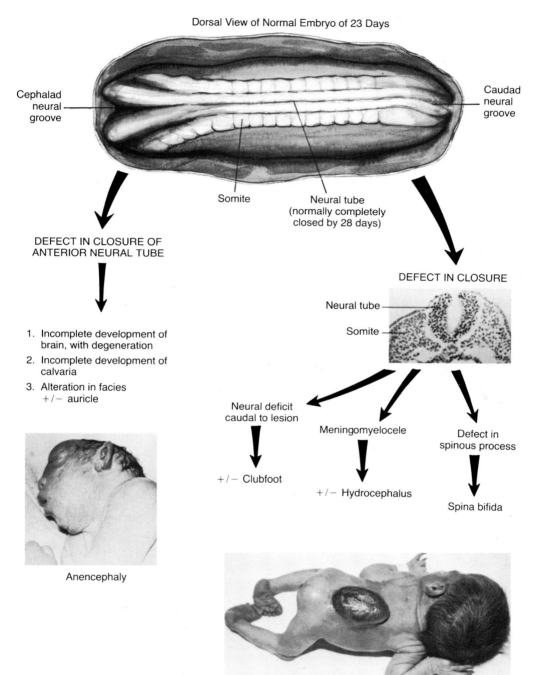

FIGURE 2. Developmental pathogenesis of anencephaly and meningomyelocele.

OCCULT SPINAL DYSRAPHISM SEQUENCE

(Tethered Cord Malformation Sequence)

Following closure of the neural groove at about 28 days, the cell mass caudal to the posterior neuropore tunnels downward and forms a canal in a process that gives rise to the most distal portions of the spinal cord—the filum terminale and conus medullaris. Failure of normal morphogenesis in this region leads to a spectrum of structural defects that cause orthopedic or urologic symptoms through tethering or compression of the sacral nerve roots, with restriction of the normal cephalic migration of the conus medullaris. Defects involve structures derived from both mesodermal and ectodermal tissue and include mesodermal hamartomata, sacral vertebral anomalies, hyperplasia of the filum terminale, and structural alterations of the distal cord itself. In most situations, there is a cutaneous marker at the presumed junction between the caudal cell mass and the posterior neuropore in the region of L2–L3. Markers consist of tufts of hair, skin tags, dimples, lipomata, and aplasia cutis congenita. Cutaneous markers such as a pit at the tip of the coccyx are extremely common and are not usually associated with a tethered cord.

The recognition of the surface manifestations of such a malformation sequence at birth should ideally lead to further evaluation and/or management. Roentgenograms of the spine may or may not show any abnormality. Ultrasound to document normal movement of the spinal cord with respiration followed by MRI in questionable cases is usually sufficient to document the defect. Early management will prevent neuromuscular lower limb and/or urologic problems such as retention, incontinence, and/or infection secondary to continued tractional tethering of the cord and nerve roots. If the physician waits for signs of such serious complications, the neurologic damage may not be reversible. A 4 per cent incidence of open neural tube defects has been documented in first-degree relatives of probands.

References

Anderson, F. M.: Occult spinal dysraphism: Diagnosis and management. J. Pediatr., 73:163, 1968.

Carter, C. O., Evans, K. A., and Till, K.: Spinal dysraphism: Genetic relation to neural tube malformations. J. Med. Genet., 13:343, 1976.

Tavafoghi, V., et al.: Cutaneous signs of spinal dysraphism. Arch. Dermatol., 114:573, 1978.

Higginbottom, M. C., et al.: Aplasia cutis congenita: Cutaneous marker of occult spinal dysraphism. J. Pediatr., 96:687, 1980.

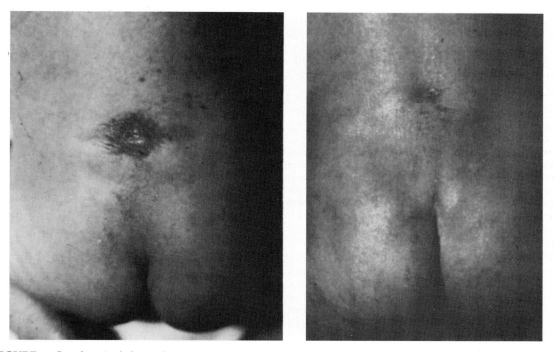

FIGURE 1. Occult spinal dysraphism sequence. Note the location of these lesions, which were the clues that resulted in surgical correction of tethered cord in early infancy. In addition to the flat hemangioma (*left*), the mound of connective tissue (*right*), and the localized absence of skin (*both*), surface anomalies may consist of lipomas, deep dimples, hair tufts, and skin tags. (From Higginbottom, M. C., et al.: J. Pediatr., *96:*687, 1980, with permission.)

SEPTO-OPTIC DYSPLASIA SEQUENCE

De Morsier recognized the association between the absence of the septum pellucidum and hypoplasia of the optic nerves and called it septo-optic dysplasia. The clinical spectrum of altered development and function arising from this defect has been reported by Hoyt and others to include hypopituitary dwarfism. The presumed developmental pathogenesis is depicted to the right.

ABNORMALITIES

Eyes. Hypoplastic optic nerves, chiasm, and infundibulum with pendular nystagmus and visual impairment, occasionally including field defects.

Endocrine. Low levels of growth hormone, thyroid-stimulating hormone, luteinizing hormone, follicle-stimulating hormone, and antidiuretic hormone.

Other. Agenesis of septum pellucidum in about half of cases. Schizencephaly.

OCCASIONAL ABNORMALITIES. Trophic hormone hypersecretion, including growth hormone, corticotropin, and prolactin. Sexual precocity. Hemiplegia. Spasticity. Athetosis. Epilepsy. Autism. Cranial nerve palsy. Mental retardation. Learning disabilities. Attention deficit disorders.

NATURAL HISTORY. Visual impairment, including partial to complete amblyopia, is frequent, and funduscopic evaluation discloses hypoplastic optic disks. Hypopituitarism of hypothalamic origin is a frequent feature and merits hormone replacement therapy. Affected newborns can develop hypoglycemia, apnea, hypotonia, or seizures. Kaplan found this sequence to be the most frequently recognized single defect in children with pituitary growth hormone deficiency. Most affected individuals are of normal intelligence, although mental deficiency does occur. Onset of puberty is variable.

Features of the septo-optic dysplasia sequence may occur as a part of a broader pattern of early brain defect, such as the holoprosencephaly type of defect, in which case the prognosis for brain function and survival is poor.

ETIOLOGY. Unknown. Though this defect is usually a sporadic occurrence, the author has evaluated one case in which the otherwise normal mother had unilateral amblyopia with a hypoplastic optic disk. In addition, two first cousins with hypopituitarism have been reported, one of whom had septo-optic dysplasia.

References

de Morsier, G.: Études sur les dysraphies crânioencéphaliques. III. Agénésie du septum lucidum avec malformation du tractus optique. La dysplasie septo-optique. Schweiz. Arch. Neurol. Neurochir. Psychiatr., 77:267, 1956.

Hoyt, W. F., et al.: Septo-optic dysplasia and pituitary dwarfism. Lancet, 1:893, 1970.

Kaplan, S., University of California School of Medicine, San Francisco; personal communication.

Brook, C. G. D., Sanders, M. D., and Hoare, R. D.: Septo-optic dysplasia. Br. Med. J., 3:811, 1972.

Haseman, C. A., et al.: Sexual precocity in association with septo-optic dysplasia and hypothalamic hypopituitarism. J. Pediatr., 92:748, 1978.

Blethen, S. L., and Weldon, V. V.: Hypopituitarism and septo-optic "dysplasia" in first cousins. Am. J. Med. Genet., 21:123, 1985.

Margalith, D., Tze, W. J., and Jan, J. E.: Congenital optic nerve hypoplasia with hypothalamic-pituitary dysplasia. Am. J. Dis. Child., 139:361, 1985.

Morgan, S. A., et al.: Absence of the septum pallucidum. Overlapping clinical syndromes. Arch. Neurol., 42:769, 1985.

Hanna, C. E., et al.: Puberty in the syndrome of septo-optic dysplasia. Am. J. Dis. Child., 143:186, 1989.

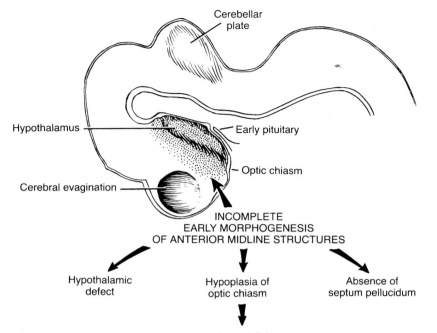

Cerebellar plate

Hypothalamus

Early pituitary

Optic chiasm

Cerebral evagination

INCOMPLETE
EARLY MORPHOGENESIS
OF ANTERIOR MIDLINE STRUCTURES

Hypothalamic defect

Hypoplasia of optic chiasm

Absence of septum pellucidum

Visual deficit pendular nystagmus

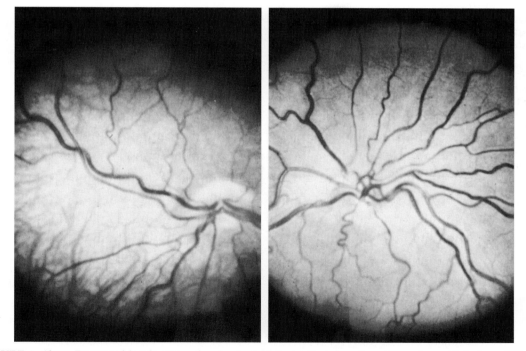

FIGURE 1. *Above,* Presumed localization of early single defect (*stippled area*) as shown in sagittal view of 38-day brain. *Below,* Photos of retinae of 4-year-old patient with the septo-optic dysplasia sequence who had reduced vision, pendular nystagmus, and growth deficiency secondary to pituitary growth hormone deficiency. Note the hypoplastic optic nerve heads and aberrant vascular arrangement.

ATHYROTIC HYPOTHYROIDISM SEQUENCE

(Hypothyroidism Sequence)

Primary Defect—In Development of Thyroid Gland

Athyrotic hypothyroidism is usually a sporadic occurrence in an otherwise normal child. Severe hypothyroidism does not give rise to growth deficiency until after birth. Postnatally, morphogenesis and function are grossly impaired as a metabolic consequence of the lack of thyroid hormone. Adequate thyroid hormone replacement therapy, at least ³/₄ grain of U.S.P. desiccated thyroid per day for the affected infant, will allow for a complete return to physical normality for age. However, the detrimental effect of the hypothyroid state on morphogenesis and function of the brain is irreparable. Therefore, the earlier a diagnosis is made and adequate thyroid hormone therapy instituted, the better the prognosis for mental function.

ABNORMALITIES. The following are some of the early signs that may allow for detection of the hypothyroid baby early in life.

General

Feeding problems	39%
Decreased activity	56%
Constipation	11%
Neonatal jaundice	50%
Prolonged gestation	

Cutaneous-Vascular

Cold to touch	33%
Dry skin	45%
Mottling	17%

Myxedema

Enlarged tongue	17%
Hoarse cry	39%
Periorbital edema	88%

Other

Umbilical hernia	58%
Enlarged anterior fontanel	71%
Enlarged posterior fontanel	65%
Cardiac defect	—

NATURAL HISTORY. When treatment is delayed until after 3 months, poor neurologic outcome is the rule. For those infants detected by neonatal screening and treated appropriately, growth and development have been demonstrated to be normal.

References

Wilkins, L.: The Diagnosis and Treatment of Endocrine Disorders in Childhood and Adolescence. Springfield, Ill., Charles C Thomas, 1965.

Smith, D. W., and Popich, G.: Large fontanels in congenital hypothyroidism. J. Pediatr., *80*:753, 1972.

Klein, A. H., et al.: Improved prognosis in congenital hypothyroidism treated before age three months. J. Pediatr., *81*:912, 1972.

Virtanen, M., et al.: Congenital hypothyroidism: Age at start of treatment versus outcome. Acta Paediatr. Scand., *72*:197, 1983.

New England Congenital Hypothyroidism Collaborative: Characteristics of infantile hypothyroidism discovered on neonatal screening. J. Pediatr., *104*: 539, 1984.

Thompson, G. N., et al.: Management and outcome of children with congenital hypothyroidism detected on neonatal screening in South Australia. Med. J. Aust., *145*:18, 1986.

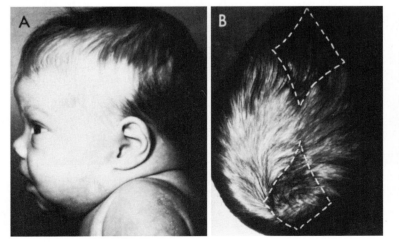

FIGURE 1. Evidence of osseous immaturity in a 3-month-old infant with athyrotic hypothyroidism. *A,* Immature facies with low nasal bridge. Note also the full subcutaneous tissues. *B,* Immaturity of osseous calvarium, with outer limits of large fontanels indicated. The bone age as determined from roentgenograms of the knee and foot was interpreted as being at about an 8-month fetal level.

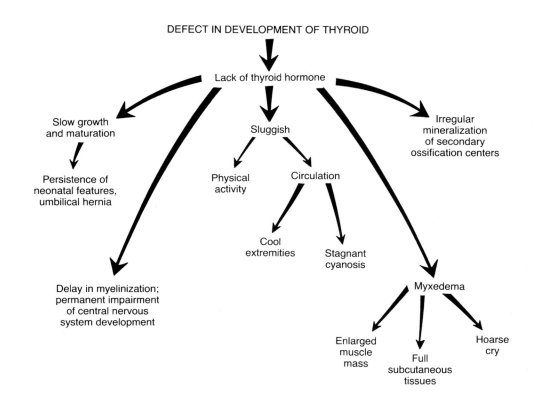

DEFECT IN DEVELOPMENT OF THYROID

Lack of thyroid hormone

Slow growth and maturation

Persistence of neonatal features, umbilical hernia

Sluggish

Physical activity

Circulation

Cool extremities

Stagnant cyanosis

Irregular mineralization of secondary ossification centers

Delay in myelinization; permanent impairment of central nervous system development

Myxedema

Enlarged muscle mass

Full subcutaneous tissues

Hoarse cry

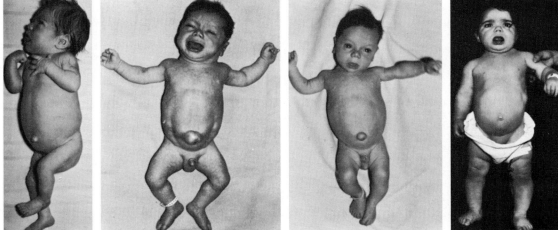

Age: 2 months
Height age: 1 month
Bone age: birth

Age: 9 months
Height age: 2 months
Bone age: birth

After 3 weeks of thyroid replacement

Age: 3 years, untreated
Height age: 12 months
Bone age: 3 months

FIGURE 2. *Above*, Developmental pathogenesis of athyrotic hypothyroidism. *Below*, Athyrotic patients.

DiGEORGE SEQUENCE

Primary Defect—Fourth Branchial Arch and
Derivatives of Third and Fourth Pharyngeal Pouches

This pattern of malformation was emphasized by DiGeorge and variably includes defects of development of the thymus, parathyroids, and great vessels. Conley et al. have observed 19 cases at necropsy. The illustration shows the presumed developmental pathogenesis.

ABNORMALITIES. Varying features from among the following:

Thymus. Hypoplasia to aplasia, with deficit of cellular immunity allowing for severe infectious disease.

Parathyroids. Hypoplasia to absence, allowing for severe hypocalcemia and seizures in early infancy.

Cardiovascular. Aortic arch anomalies, including right aortic arch, interrupted aorta, conotruncal anomalies such as truncus arteriosus and ventricular septal defect, patent ductus arteriosus, and tetralogy of Fallot.

Facial. (Specific to partial monosomy 22q: see below) Lateral displacement of inner canthi with short palpebral fissures, short philtrum, micrognathia, ear anomalies.

OCCASIONAL ABNORMALITIES. Mental deficiency of mild to moderate degree, esophageal atresia, choanal atresia, velopharyngeal insufficiency, imperforate anus, diaphragmatic hernia.

NATURAL HISTORY. There is a significant neonatal morbidity and mortality associated with the cardiac defects, sequelae of the immunodeficiency, and seizures relative to hypocalcemia. The natural history is dependent on the etiology of the DiGeorge sequence. For those children with partial monosomy of the long arm of chromosome 22, the natural history is the same as that of the Shprintzen syndrome.

ETIOLOGY. This pattern is etiologically heterogeneous. It has been associated with prenatal exposure to alcohol and Accutane, and a variety of chromosome abnormalities. The majority of cases, however, are a result of partial monosomy of the proximal long arm of chromosome 22 due to a microdeletion of 22q11.2 (usually detectable only on molecular or fluorescent in situ hybridization [FISH] analysis). For those individuals the parents should be evaluated for features of the Shprintzen syndrome including FISH analysis when the clinical features are suggestive.

References

Lobdell, D. H.: Congenital absence of the parathyroid glands. Arch. Pathol., 67:412, 1959.

Kretschmer, R., Say, B., Brown, D., and Rosen, F. S.: Congenital aplasia of the thymus gland (DiGeorge's syndrome). N. Engl. J. Med., 279:1295, 1968.

Freedom, R. M., Rosen, F. S., and Nadas, A. S.: Congenital cardiovascular disease and anomalies of the third and fourth pharyngeal pouch. Circulation, 46:165, 1972.

Conley, M. E., et al.: The spectrum of the DiGeorge syndrome. J. Pediatr., 94:883, 1979.

Greenberg, F., et al.: Familial DiGeorge syndrome and associated partial monosomy of chromosome 22. Hum. Genet., 65:317, 1984.

Stevens, C. A., et al.: DiGeorge anomaly and velocardiofacial syndrome. Pediatrics, 85:526, 1990.

Halford, S., et al.: Isolation of a gene expressed during early embryogenesis from the region of 22q11 commonly deleted in DiGeorge syndrome. Hum. Mol. Genet., 2:1577, 1993.

Halford, S., et al.: Isolation of a putative transcriptional regulator from the region of 22q11 deleted in DiGeorge syndrome, Shprintzen syndrome and familial heart disease. Hum. Mol. Genet., 2:2099, 1993.

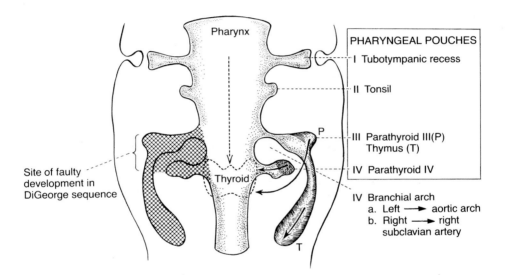

FIGURE 1. Schematic appearance of anterior foregut and its derivatives at around the fifth week of development, showing the presumed site of defect in the DiGeorge sequence.

KLIPPEL-FEIL SEQUENCE

*Short Neck With Low Hairline and Limited
Movement of Head: Primary Defect—
Early Development of Cervical Vertebrae*

In this malformation sequence, originally described by Klippel and Feil in 1912, the cervical vertebrae are usually fused, although hemivertebrae and other defects may also be found. There may also be secondary webbed neck, torticollis, and/or facial asymmetry. The frequency is about 1 in 42,000 births, and 65 per cent of patients are female. The sequence may be a part of a serious problem in early neural tube development, as is found in iniencephaly, cervical meningomyelocele, syringomyelia, or syringobulbia. Primary or secondary neurologic deficits may occur, such as paraplegia, hemiplegia, cranial or cervical nerve palsies, and synkinesia.

The following defects have occurred in a nonrandom association in patients with the Klippel-Feil sequence: deafness, either conductive or neural, noted in as many as 30 per cent; congenital heart defects, the most common being a ventricular septal defect; and mental deficiency, cleft palate, rib defects, the Sprengel anomaly, posterior fossa dermoid cysts, scoliosis, and renal abnormalities.

Lateral flexion-extension radiographs of the cervical spine should be performed on all patients to determine the motion of each open interspace. Clinically, flexion-extension is often maintained if a single functioning open interspace is maintained. Those with hypermobility of the upper cervical segment are at risk of developing neurologic impairment. They should be evaluated at least annually and should avoid violent activities. Affected individuals with hypermobility of the lower cervical segment are at increased risk for degenerative disk disease and should be treated symptomatically. Usually a sporadic occurrence of unknown etiology, this sequence has rarely been found in siblings. A close evaluation of the immediate family is indicated, since autosomal dominant inheritance with variable expression in affected individuals has been noted, although this is presumably rare.

References

Klippel, M., and Feil, A: Un cas d'absence des vertébres cervicales, avec cage thoracique remontant jusqu'à la base du crâne (cage thoracique cervicale) Mouv. Inconogr. Salpêt., 25:223, 1912.

Morrison, S. G., Perry, L. W., and Scott, L. P., III: Congenital brevicollis (Klippel-Feil syndrome) and cardiovascular anomalies. Am. J. Dis. Child., 115:614, 1968.

Palant, D. J., and Carter, B. L.: Klippel-Feil syndrome and deafness. Am. J. Dis. Child., 123:218, 1972.

Hensinger, R. W., Lang, J. E., and MacEwen, G. D.: Klippel-Feil syndrome. J. Bone Joint Surg., 56-A: 1246, 1974.

Dickey, W., et al.: Posterior fossa dermoid cysts and the Klippel-Feil syndrome. J. Neurol. Neurosurg. Psychiatry, 54:1016, 1991.

Pizzutillo, P. D., et al.: Risk factors in Klippel-Feil syndrome. Spine, 19:2110, 1994.

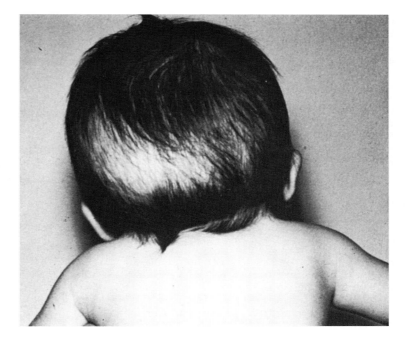

FIGURE 1. Infant with the Klippel-Feil sequence.

JUGULAR LYMPHATIC OBSTRUCTION SEQUENCE

The lymphatic channels in each upper quadrant drain into the jugular lymphatic sac, which, at about 40 days of development, opens into the jugular vein on that side. Failure of development of this communication results in stasis of the lymph fluid, which causes a host of consequences referred to as the jugular lymphatic obstruction sequence. The distended jugular lymph sac results in an excess of skin in the neck region with alteration in the zone of hair growth and the hair directional patterning plus elevation and sometimes protrusion of the lower auricle. The accumulating peripheral lymphedema causes full subcutaneous tissues with relative overgrowth of the overlying skin, prominent fingertip pads, and narrow hyperconvex nails, which are often deeply set at the base. The lack of lymphatic drainage results in an increased volume of fluid in the venous system, resulting in large veins. In addition there is a high incidence of flow-related cardiac defects such as hypoplastic left heart, aortic coarctation, and secundum atrial septal defect presumably related to mechanical distention of cardiac lymphatics at the ascending aorta as well as a variety of non–flow related cardiac defects.

This is apparently a lethal anomaly unless the communication between the jugular lymph sac and the jugular vein develops by mid to late fetal life. Once the link does occur, the distended jugular lymph sac collapses, leaving redundant overlying skin folds that are referred to as a pterygium colli. The drainage from the subcutaneous areas leaves relatively redundant skin, which is especially notable in the facies. The peripheral lymphedema may not have completely receded by birth, causing puffy hands and feet.

The jugular lymphatic obstruction sequence accounts for many of the features of the surviving individuals with the XO Turner syndrome and may be the predominant cause of the high early fetal lethality in this disorder. However, the sequence is a nonspecific defect and may occur in a number of disorders. When noted during the second trimester of pregnancy on ultrasound, a nuchal cystic hygroma is associated with a poor perinatal outcome, often due to a serious chromosomal error. When ascertained during the first trimester, the association with aneuploid remains. However, in the presence of a normal karyotype, prognosis is excellent.

The lymphatic channels in the lower quadrants drain into the iliac lymph sacs, which are analogous to the jugular lymph sacs. A lag in the communication with the venous system results in peripheral lymphedema in the lower limbs and sometimes the genital region. If the iliac lymph sacs are grossly distended, there may be distention of the abdomen. Decompression by communication with the venous system may yield a residuum of redundant abdominal skin that is one cause of the so-called prune belly.

References

Töndury, G., and Kubik, S.: Zur Ontogenese des lymphatischen systems. Handbuch der Allgemeinen Pathologie. Berlin, Springer-Verlag, 1975, pp. 2–38.

Van der Putte, S. C.: The development of the lymphatic system in man. Adv. Anat. Embryol., 51:1, 1975.

Van der Putte, S. C.: Lymphatic malformation in human fetuses. A study of fetuses with Turner's syndrome or status Bonnevie-Ullrich. Virchows Arch. (Pathol. Anat.), 376:233, 1977.

Trauffer, P. M. L., et al.: The natural history of euploid pregnancies with first-trimester cystic hygromas. Am. J. Obstet. Gynecol., 170:1279, 1994.

Berdahl, L. D., et al.: Web neck anomaly and its association with congenital heart disease. Am. J. Med. Genet., 56:304, 1995.

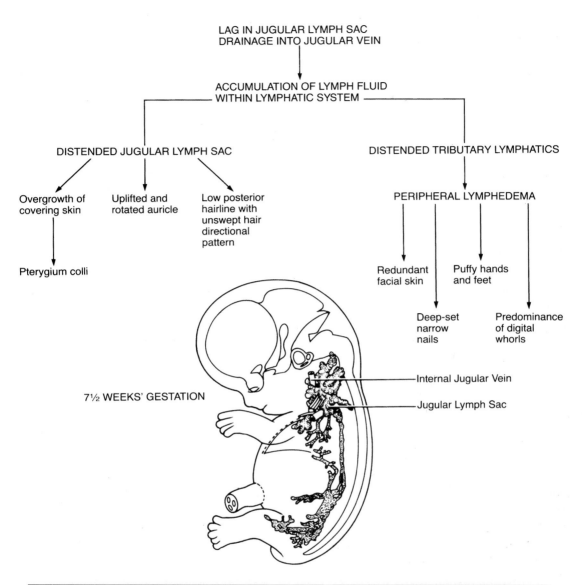

LAG IN JUGULAR LYMPH SAC
DRAINAGE INTO JUGULAR VEIN

ACCUMULATION OF LYMPH FLUID
WITHIN LYMPHATIC SYSTEM

DISTENDED JUGULAR LYMPH SAC

DISTENDED TRIBUTARY LYMPHATICS

Overgrowth of covering skin

Uplifted and rotated auricle

Low posterior hairline with unswept hair directional pattern

Pterygium colli

PERIPHERAL LYMPHEDEMA

Redundant facial skin

Puffy hands and feet

Deep-set narrow nails

Predominance of digital whorls

7½ WEEKS' GESTATION

Internal Jugular Vein

Jugular Lymph Sac

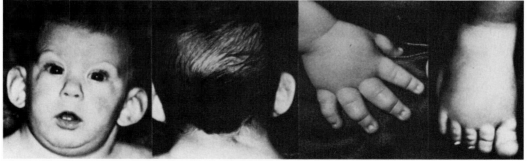

FIGURE 1. Presumed genesis of the jugular lymphatic obstruction sequence. The jugular lymph sac, shown here in a 7½-week embryo, normally opens into the jugular vein by about 40 days. Late communication may yield a number of residua engendered during the period of lymphatic obstruction.

EARLY URETHRAL OBSTRUCTION SEQUENCE

Early urethral obstruction is most commonly the consequence of urethral valve formation during the development of the prostatic urethra. Less commonly, it is due to urethral atresia, bladder neck obstruction, or distal urethral obstruction. With urine formation occurring, by 7 to 8 weeks of fetal life, there is a progressive back-up of urine flow, leading to the consequences shown in the flow diagram. The male-to-female ratio of 20:1 in this disorder is a result of the predominant malformations being in the development of the penile urethra. Cryptorchidism occurs secondary to the bulk of the distended bladder, preventing full descent of the testes. The back-pressure usually limits full renal morphogenesis and may result in dilatation of the renal tubules, which by histologic section examination may be interpreted as renal "cysts." Similarly, the hydrostatic pressure generated by distal obstruction most likely accounts for the hypoplastic prostate, seen in the majority of cases. The compressive mass of the bladder may limit full rotation of the colon and may even compress the iliac vessels to the point of causing partial defects or vascular disruption of the lower limb(s). The oligohydramnios will give rise to all the secondary phenomena of the oligohydramnios deformation sequence.

Severe early urethral obstruction is often lethal by mid to late fetal life unless the bladder ruptures and is thereby decompressed. The bladder rupture may occur through a patent urachus, an obstructing urethral "valve," or the wall of the bladder or ureter. Following decompression, the fetus will be left with a "prune belly."

Unfortunately, most of those who survive to term have incurred severe renal damage and are unable to live long after birth. Those who do survive may be assisted by urologic procedures to aid urinary drainage and control urinary tract infection. Respiration and bowel movements may be eased by wrapping the abdomen with a "belly binder." With advancing age, the hypoplastic abdominal musculature will usually improve in volume and strength to the point of being no serious problem.

The recurrence risk for the disorder is dependent on the specific cause of the urethral obstruction, and these data have not yet been determined. This defect most commonly occurs in an otherwise normal individual, but may be but one feature of a broader pattern of malformation, such as the VATER association. Early fetal diagnosis is possible, since sonography will show the distended bladder by 10 weeks from conception.

References

Stumme, E. G.: Ueber die symmetrischen kongenitalen Bauchmuskel defeckte und über die Kombination derselben mit anderen Bildunganomalien des Rumfes. Mitt. Grenzigebeite Med. Chir., 6:548, 1903.

Silverman, F. N., and Huang, N.: Congenital absence of the abdominal muscles. Am. J. Dis. Child., 80:91, 1950.

Lattimer, J. K.: Congenital deficiency of abdominal musculature and associated genitourinary anomalies. J. Urol., 79:343, 1958.

Pagon, R. A., Smith, D. W., and Shepard, T. H.: Urethral obstruction malformation complex: A cause of abdominal muscle deficiency and the "prune bell." J. Pediatr., 94:900, 1979.

Popek, E. J., et al.: Prostate development in prune belly syndrome. (PBS) and posterior urethral valves (PUV): Etiology of PBS lower urinary tract obstruction or primary mesenchymal defect? Pediatr. Pathol., 11:1, 1991.

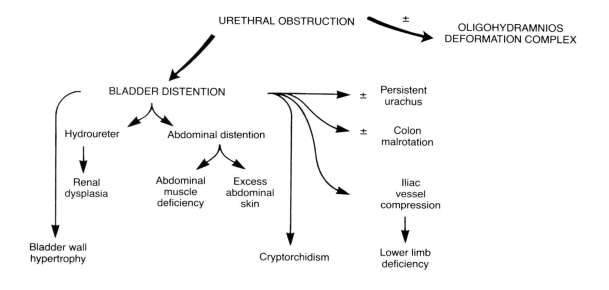

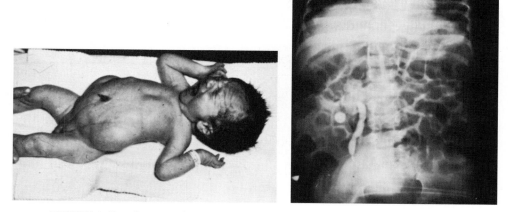

FIGURE 1. Developmental pathogenesis of early urethral obstruction sequence.

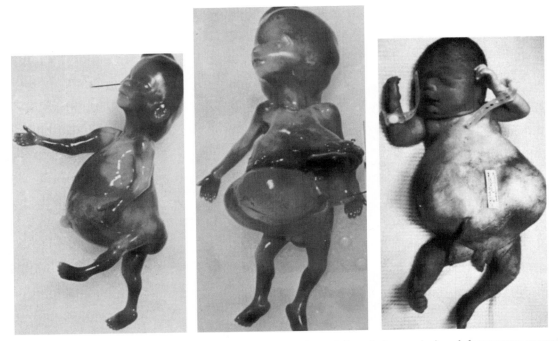

FIGURE 2. Early urethral obstruction sequence. *A* and *B*, A 10-week fetus before and after abdomen was opened, showing distended bladder due to urethral obstruction. (Courtesy of Dr. Thomas Shepard, University of Washington, Seattle, Wash.)

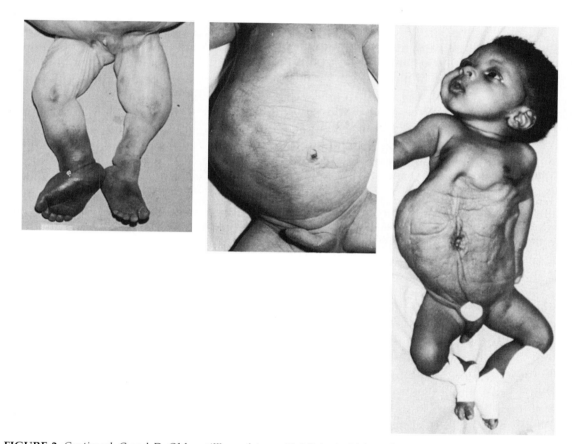

FIGURE 2. *Continued.* *C* and *D,* Older stillborn fetus with bilobed, thickened, massively distended bladder due to urethral obstruction. Vascular occlusion to legs resulted in ischemia and altered morphogenesis of the feet. (Courtesy of Cindy Dolan, Spokane, Wash.) *E* and *F,* Prenatal rupture of prostatic urethral obstruction decompressed the abdomen, leaving a "prune belly" as one residuum. (*F* Courtesy of Dr. Jaime L. Frias, University of South Florida, Tampa, Fla.)

EXSTROPHY OF BLADDER SEQUENCE

Primary Defect—In Infraumbilical Mesoderm

Normally the bladder portion of the cloaca and the overlying ectoderm are in direct contact (the cloacal membrane) until the infraumbilical mesenchyme migrates into the area at about the sixth to seventh week of fetal development, giving rise to the lower abdominal wall, genital tubercles, and pubic rami. A failure of the infraumbilical mesenchyme to invade the area allows for a breakdown in the cloacal membrane, in similar fashion to that which normally occurs at the oral, anal, and urogenital areas, where mesoderm does not intercede between ectoderm and endoderm. Thus the posterior bladder wall is exposed, in conjunction with defects in structures derived from the infraumbilical mesenchyme.

This malformation sequence is estimated to occur in approximately 1 in 30,000 births and is more likely to occur in the male than in the female. In most cases the defect can be closed within the first few days of life, genital function can be expected to be satisfactory, and urinary control will be achieved. Of 13 affected individuals greater than 17 years of age, 12 reported sexual experiences, 6 were married, 13 attended college, and 7 were employed. All were considered well-adjusted.

The recurrence risk for unaffected parents who have had a child with bladder exstrophy and/or epispadias is less than 1 per cent (1 in 275). For the offspring of a parent with bladder exstrophy or epispadias, recurrence risk is approximately 1 in 70 live-births.

References

Wyburn, G. M.: The development of the infraumbilical portion of the abdominal wall, with remarks on the aetiology of ectopia vesicae. J. Anat., 71:201, 1937.

Muecke, E. C.: The role of the cloacal membrane in exstrophy: The first successful experimental study. J. Urol., 92:659, 1964.

Shapiro, E., et al.: The inheritance of the exstrophy-epispadias complex. J. Urol., 132:308, 1984.

Jeffs, R. D.: Exstrophy, epispadias, and cloacal and urogenital sinus abnormalities. Pediatr. Clin. North Am., 34:1233, 1987.

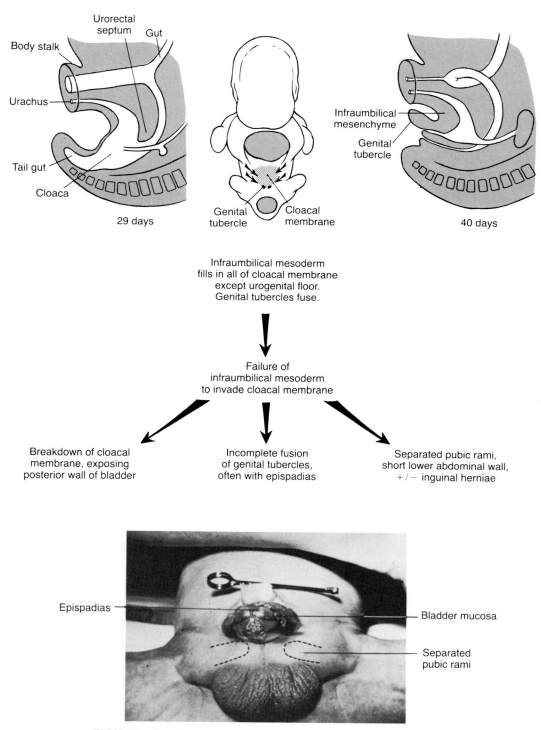

FIGURE 1. Developmental pathogenesis of exstrophy of bladder sequence.

EXSTROPHY OF CLOACA SEQUENCE

*Primary Defect—Early Mesoderm
That Will Contribute to Infraumbilical
Mesenchyme, Cloacal Septum, and Lumbosacral Vertebrae*

Occurring in approximately 1 in 400,000 births, the remarkable similarity among otherwise normal individuals with this bizarre type of defect suggests a similar mode of developmental pathology having its inception as a single localized defect—theoretically in the early development of the mesoderm, which will later contribute to the infraumbilical mesenchyme, cloacal septum, and caudal vertebrae. The consequences are (1) failure of cloacal septation, with the persistence of a common cloaca into which the ureters, ileum, and a rudimentary hindgut open; (2) complete breakdown of the cloacal membrane with exstrophy of the cloaca, failure of fusion of the genital tubercles and pubic rami, and often omphalocele; and (3) incomplete development of the lumbosacral vertebrae with herniation of a grossly dilated central canal of the spinal cord (hydromyelia), yielding a soft, cystic, skin-covered mass over the sacral area, sometimes asymmetric in its positioning. The rudimentary hindgut may contain two appendices, and there is no anal opening. The small intestine may be relatively short. Cryptorchidism is a usual finding in the male. Urinary tract anomalies including pelvic kidneys, renal agenesis, multicystic kidney, and ureteral duplication occur commonly. Affected females have unfused müllerian elements with completely bifid uterine horns and short, duplicated, or atretic vaginas. Most patients have a single umbilical artery, and anomalies of the lower limbs occasionally occur and include congenital hip dislocation, talipes equinovarus, and agenesis of a limb.

Excellent survival rates following surgical repair is now the rule. Since males have severe epispadias, which usually makes adequate reconstruction impossible, gender reassignment is recommended in most 46XY individuals. Although the "short bowel syndrome" is a significant problem in early years, the bowel usually adapts and nutritional status stabilizes. Urinary continence has been achieved in some patients. The chance of fecal continence is small. Reconstruction to create a vagina in teenage years must be anticipated.

References

Spencer, R.: Exstrophia splanchnica (exstrophy of the cloaca). Surgery, 57:751, 1965.

Beckwith, J. B.: The congenitally malformed. VII. Exstrophy of the bladder and cloacal exstrophy. Northwest Med., 65:407, 1966.

Jeffs, R. D.: Exstrophy, epispadius and cloacal and urogenital sinus abnormalities. Pediatr. Clin. North Am., 34:1233, 1987.

Hurwitz, R. S., et al.: Cloacal exstrophy: A report of 34 cases. J. Urol., 138:1060, 1987.

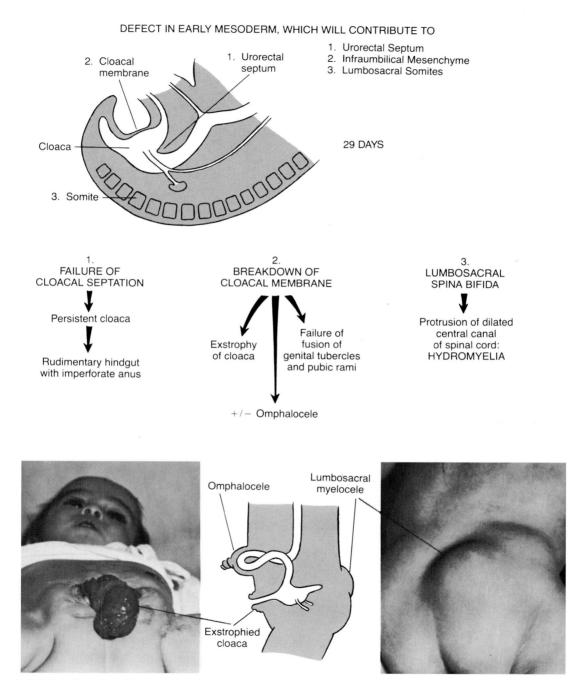

FIGURE 1. *Above*, Developmental pathogenesis of exstrophy of cloaca sequence. *Below, left*, infant with exstrophy of the cloaca (prolapsed intestine). Note separation of scrotal folds and genital tubercle.

URORECTAL SEPTUM MALFORMATION SEQUENCE

In 1987, Escobar et al. reported six patients with this disorder and reviewed a number of previously reported cases, many of which had been diagnosed as female pseudohermaphrodites. The vast majority of affected individuals have been females (46XX). The principal features in 46XX patients are the following: striking ambiguity of the external genitalia with a short phallus-like structure that lacks corpora cavernosa and absent urethra and vaginal openings; imperforate anus; bladder, vaginal and rectal fistulas; and müllerian duct defects.

It has been suggested that this pattern of malformation is due to two related events in the development of the urorectal septum. Normally, by the sixth week of development the urorectal septum divides the cloacal cavity into a urogenital sinus anteriorly and a rectum posteriorly and fuses with the cloacal membrane. At the same time that the urorectal septum approaches the cloacal membrane, the membrane breaks down, leaving an open urogenital sinus and rectum. Failure of the urorectal septum to divide the cloaca and/or approach the cloacal membrane leads in a cascading fashion to the urorectal septum malformation sequence.

Long-term survival of affected individuals is extremely rare. Virtually all patients are stillborn or die in the neonatal period secondary to respiratory complications of oligohydramnios or renal failure.

Recurrence risk for isolated cases of the urorectal septum malformation sequence is negligible. However, when it occurs as one feature in a multiple malformation syndrome, recurrence risk is for that disorder.

The reason that individuals with a 46XY karyotype are so infrequently affected is unknown.

References

Escobar, L. F., et al.: Urorectal septum malformation sequence: Report of six cases and embryological analysis. Am. J. Dis. Child., *141*:1021, 1987.

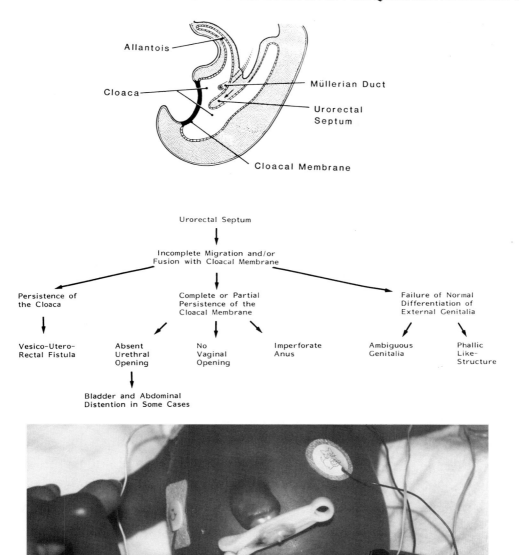

FIGURE 1. *Above*, Developmental pathogenesis of the urorectal septum malformation sequence. (From Escobar, L. F., et al.: Am. J. Dis. Child., *141*:1021, 1987, with permission. Copyright 1987, American Medical Association.) *Below*, 46XX individual with urorectal septum malformation sequence. Note the phallus-like structure, absent uretheral and vaginal opening, and imperforate anus.

OLIGOHYDRAMNIOS SEQUENCE

(Potter Syndrome)

Primary Defect—Development of Oligohydramnios

Renal agenesis, which must occur prior to 31 days of fetal development, will secondarily limit the amount of amniotic fluid and thereby result in further anomalies during prenatal life. The renal agenesis may be the only primary defect, or it may be one feature of a more extensive caudal axis anomaly. Other types of urinary tract defects such as polycystic kidneys or obstruction may also be responsible for oligohydramnios and its consequences. Another cause is chronic leakage of amniotic fluid from the time of midgestation. Regardless of the cause, the secondary effects of oligohydramnios are the same and would appear to be the result of compression of the fetus, as depicted below. The cause of death is respiratory insufficiency, with a lack of the late development of alveolar sacs. A similar lag in late development of the lung is observed with diaphragmatic hernia or asphyxiating thoracic dystrophy. In both of these latter situations, there is external compression of the developing lung; this is considered the most likely cause in oligohydramnios, as shown in the figure.

When the oligohydramnios is secondary to agenesis or dysgenesis of both kidneys or agenesis of one kidney and dysgenesis of the other, renal ultrasonographic evaluation of both parents and siblings of affected infants should be performed, since 9 per cent of first-degree relatives had asymptomatic renal malformations in a study by Roodhooft et al.

References

Potter, E. L.: Bilateral renal agenesis. J. Pediatr., 29:68, 1946.

Bain, A. D., and Scott, J. S.: Renal agenesis and severe urinary tract dysplasia. A review of 50 cases with particular reference to the associated anomalies. Br. Med. J., 1:841, 1960.

Thomas, I. T., and Smith, D. W.: Oligohydramnios, cause of the nonrenal features of Potter's syndrome, including pulmonary hypoplasia. J. Pediatr., 84:811, 1974.

Roodhooft, A. M., Birnholz, J. C., and Holmes, L. B.: Familial nature of congenital absence and severe dysgenesis of both kidneys. N. Engl. J. Med., 310: 1341, 1984.

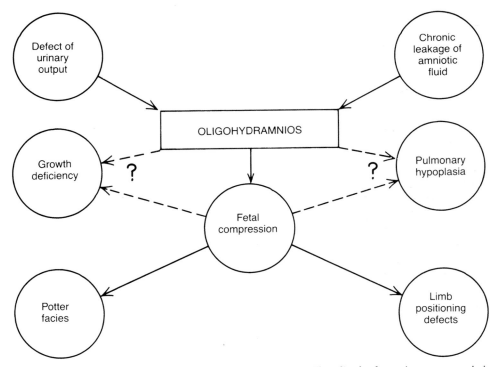

FIGURE 1. Depiction of the origin and effects of oligohydramnios. The oligohydramnios sequence is implied to be secondary to fetal compression.

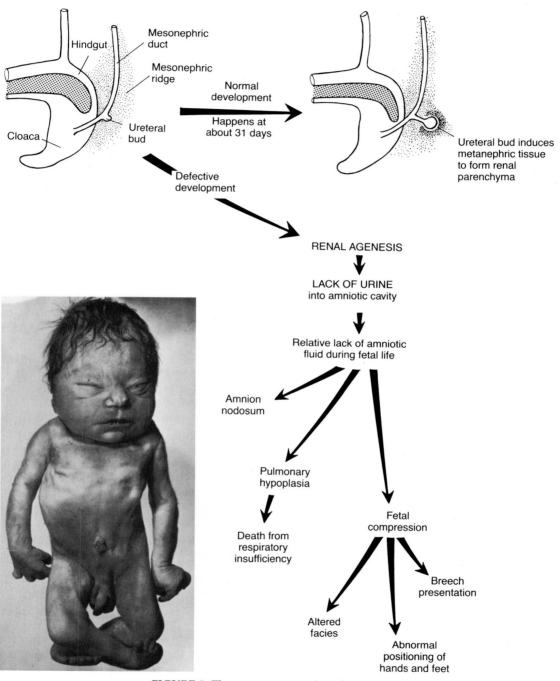

FIGURE 2. The consequences of renal agenesis.

SIRENOMELIA SEQUENCE

This defect has previously been thought to be the consequence of a wedge-shaped early deficit of the posterior axis caudal blastema, allowing for fusion of the early limb buds at their fibular margins with absence or incomplete development of the intervening caudal structures. However, Stevenson et al. have shown that sirenomelia and its commonly associated defects are produced by an alteration in early vascular development. Rather than blood returning to the placenta through the usual paired umbilical arteries arising from the iliac arteries, blood returns to the placenta through a single large vessel, a derivative of the vitelline artery complex, which arises from the aorta just below the diaphragm. The abdominal aorta distal to the origin of this major vessel is always subordinate and usually gives off no tributaries, especially renal or inferior mesenteric arteries, before it bifurcates into iliac arteries. This vascular alteration leads to a "vitelline artery steal" in which blood flow and thus nutrients are diverted from the caudal structures of the embryo to the placenta. Resultant defects include a single lower extremity with posterior alignment of knees and feet, arising from failure of the lower limb bud field to be cleaved into two lateral masses by an intervening allantois; absence of sacrum and other defects of vertebrae; imperforate anus and absence of rectum; absence of external and internal genitalia; renal agenesis; and absence of the bladder. Based on the variable alterations that could exist in blood flow, a variable spectrum of abnormalities occurs in structures dependent on the distal aorta for nutrients. Thus, as with other disruptive vascular defects, no two cases of sirenomelia are ever exactly the same.

References

Wolff, E.: Les bases de la tératogénèse expérimentale des vertèbres amniotes, d'après les résultats de méthodes directes. Arch. Anat. Histol. Embryol. (Strasb.), 22:1, 1936.

Stevenson, R. E., et al.: Vascular steal: The pathogenic mechanism producing sirenomelia and associated defects of the viscera and soft tissues. Pediatrics, 78: 451, 1986.

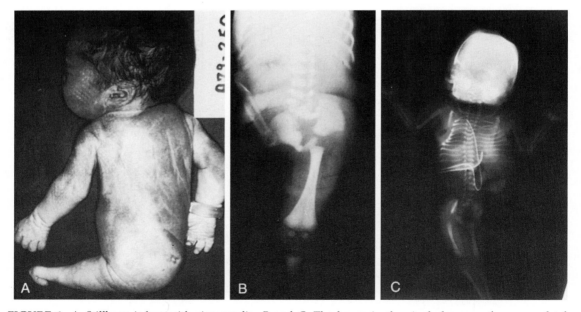

FIGURE 1. *A,* Stillborn infant with sirenomelia. *B* and *C,* The bones in the single leg vary from completely separate to a single broad femur with two distal ossification centers and a broad tibia with two ossification centers.

CAUDAL DYSPLASIA SEQUENCE
(Caudal Regression Syndrome)

This disorder has previously been grouped with sirenomelia, which was thought to represent its most severe form. Recent evidence suggests that the two are pathogenetically unrelated. Whereas sirenomelia and its associated defects are produced by an early vascular alteration leading to a "vitelline artery steal." The caudal dysplasia sequence is most likely heterogenous with respect to its etiology and developmental pathogenesis.

Structural defects of the caudal region observed in this pattern of malformation include the following to variable degrees: incomplete development of the sacrum and, to a lesser extent, the lumbar vertebrae; absence of the body of the sacrum leading to flattening of the buttocks, shortening of the intergluteal cleft, and dimpling of the buttocks; disruption of the distal spinal cord leading secondarily to neurologic impairment, varying from incontinence of urine and feces to complete neurologic loss; and extreme lack of growth in the caudal region resulting from decreased movement of the legs secondary to neurologic impairment. The most severely affected infants have flexion and abduction at the hips and popliteal webs secondary to lack of movement. Talipes equinovarus and calcaneovalgus deformities are common.

Occasional abnormalities include renal agenesis, imperforate anus, cleft lip, cleft palate, microcephaly, and meningomyelocele.

NATURAL HISTORY. In the most severely affected individuals, prognosis is poor. Urologic and orthopedic management is required in the vast majority of those who survive.

ETIOLOGY. Unknown. Sixteen per cent have occurred in offspring of diabetic mothers. Although usually sporadic, a few instances of affected siblings born to unaffected parents have been described.

References

Rusnak, S. L., and Driscoll, S. G.: Congenital spinal anomalies in infants of diabetic mothers. Pediatrics, 35:989, 1965.

Passarge, E., and Lenz, W.: syndrome of caudal regression in infants of diabetic mothers: Observations of further cases. Pediatrics, 37:672, 1966.

Gellis, S. S., and Feingold, M.: Picture of the month: Caudal dysplasia syndrome. Am. J. Dis. Child., 116: 407, 1968.

Price, D. L., Dooling, E. C., and Richardson, E. P.: Caudal dysplasia (caudal regression syndrome). Arch. Neurol., 23:212, 1970.

Finer, N. N., Bowen, P., and Dunbar, L. G.: Caudal regression anomalad (sacral agenesis in siblings). Clin. Genet., 13:353, 1978.

Stewart, J. M., and Stoll, S.: Familial caudal regression anomalad and maternal diabetes. J. Med. Genet., 16: 17, 1979.

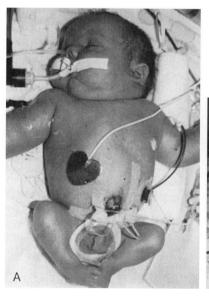

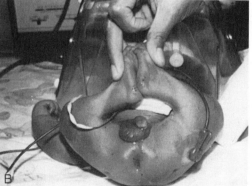

FIGURE 1. Caudal dysplasia sequence. *A,* Newborn male infant with a normal upper body and a short lower segment. *B,* Note the pterygia in the popliteal region, which are secondary to neurologically related flexion contractures at the knees.

AMNION RUPTURE SEQUENCE

Though the structural defects consequent to amnion rupture were reported by Portal in 1685, it was not until more recent times that the full spectrum of defects that can occur was delineated by Torpin as well as by others. Secondary to amnion rupture, small strands of amnion can encircle developing structures (usually the limbs) leading to annular constrictions, pseudosyndactyly, intrauterine amputations, and umbilical cord constriction. In addition to these disruptive defects, deformational defects can occur secondary to decreased fetal movement, the result of tethering of a limb by an amniotic band; or constraint, the result of decreased amniotic fluid. The decreased fetal activity may result in scoliosis and/or foot deformities. It may also cause edema, hemorrhage, and resorptive necrosis. As is the case with all disruptive defects, no two affected fetuses will have exactly the same features, and there is no single feature that consistently occurs. Examination of the placenta and membranes is diagnostic. Aberrant bands or strands of amnion are noted, and/or there may be the rolled-up remnants of the amnion at the placental base of the umbilical cord.

Incorrectly, thoraco- and/or abdominoschisis, exencephaly/encephalocele, and facial clefts usually associated with amnion adhesions and sometimes complicated by rupture of the amnion with amputation defects have been considered previously to be part of the amnion rupture sequence. This pattern of defects, now referred to as the limb–body wall complex, is due to a different pathogenetic mechanism.

NATURAL HISTORY AND MANAGEMENT. The natural history varies with the severity of the problem. Amnion constrictive bands and/or amputations of the limb in an otherwise normal child occurs most commonly. Occasionally, plastic surgery may be indicated, especially for the partially constrictive, deep residual groove that encircles a limb and is associated with partial limitation of vascular and/or lymphatic return from the distal limb. In such instances, a Z-plasty of the skin may be done to relieve the partial constriction. If there has been chronic amnion leakage, the neonate may show features of the oligohydramnios deformation sequence, including incomplete development of the lung, with respiratory insufficiency and development of hyaline membrane disease. Every attempt should be made to oxygenate and support such an infant, since with continued lung morphogenesis, the prognosis can be excellent. Because the result of amnion rupture is external compression and/or disruption, internal anomalies do not occur. Hence, the features evident by surface examination are usually the only abnormalities.

ETIOLOGY. The etiology has been, with rare exceptions, idiopathic. Those rare exceptions are known or presumed to be caused by trauma and include two examples of attempted early termination of pregnancy by using a coat hanger and one incident of a woman falling from a horse while pregnant. It has generally been a sporadic event in an otherwise normal family, and hence the recurrence risk is usually stated as being negligible. Although the disruptive defect resulting from amniotic bands may occur at any time during gestation, amnion rupture most likely occurs before 12 weeks' gestation. Prior to that time, the amnion and chorion are completely separate membranes and as such it has been suggested that the amnion is vulnerable to rupture.

References

Portal, P.: La Pratique des Accouchements. Paris, 1685.

Torpin, R.: Amniochorionic mesoblastic fibrous strings and amniotic bands: Associated constricting fetal malformations of fetal death. Am. J. Obstet. Gynecol., 91:65, 1965.

Torpin, R.: Fetal Malformations Caused by Amnion Rupture During Gestation. Springfield, Ill., Charles C Thomas, 1968.

Kalousek, D. K., and Bamforth, S.: Amnion rupture sequence in previable fetuses. Am. J. Med. Genet., 31:63, 1988.

Moerman, P., et al.: Constrictive amniotic bands, amniotic adhesions, and limb-body wall complex: Discrete disruption sequences with pathogenetic overlap. Am. J. Med. Genet., 42:470, 1992.

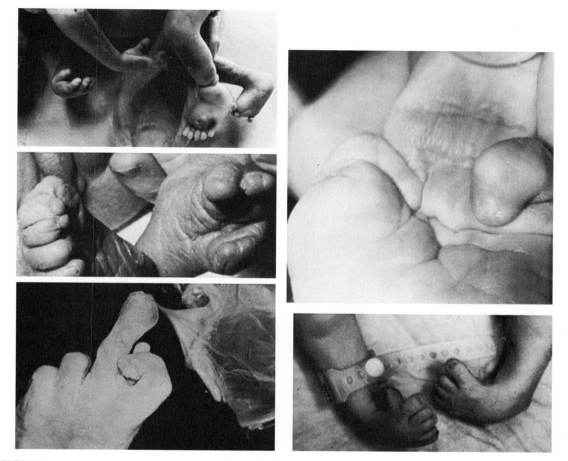

FIGURE 1. Amnion rupture sequence. Secondary limb problems include band-related constriction, band-related pseudosyndactyly (mid-left photo), compression or band-related deficiencies, and compression or band-related distortion. The lower left photo shows distortion with altered growth of a finger to which the amnion is still attached. Early compression may result in incomplete separation of the digits (syndactyly) or aberration in early finger rays with polydactyly, as shown in the photo to the right. (Courtesy of C. Dolan, Spokane, Wash.)

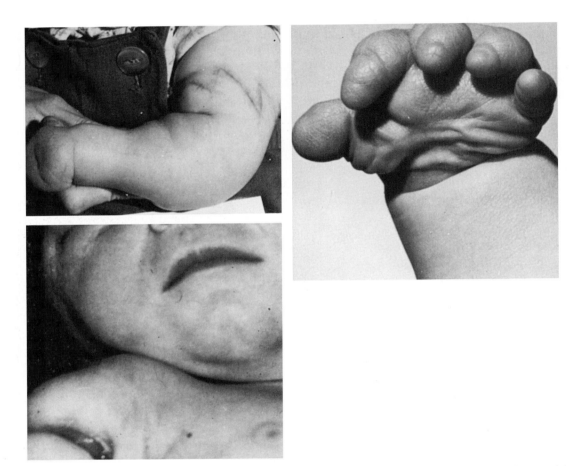

FIGURE 2. Amnion rupture sequence. A severe amnionic band constriction may result in hypoplasia and/or edema in the distal limb, as shown in the upper left and right photos. (Courtesy of Dr. Allan MacFarlane, Fairbanks, Alaska.) This infant had a multiple Z-plasty plastic surgical repair in order to improve partially the postnatal status of this amnionic band–induced limb deficiency. The neonate shown below had a severe band-induced constriction in the upper right arm.

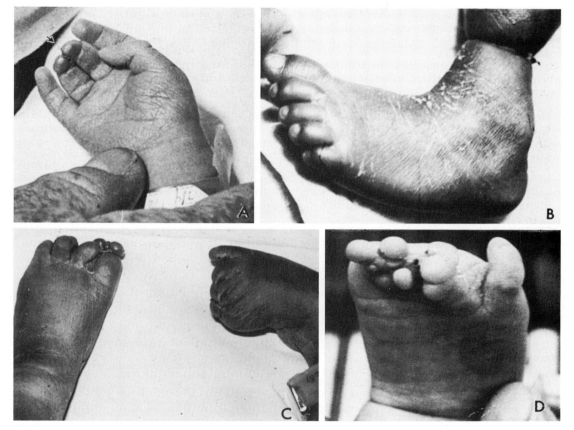

FIGURE 3. Amnion rupture sequence. Variable limb anomalies secondary to aberrant bands. *A*, The *arrow* denotes the broken band that caused the pseudosyndactyly. *B*, Band constricting the ankle. *C* and *D*, Pseudosyndactyly, amputation, and disruption of toe morphogenesis. (From Jones, K. L., et al.: J. Pediatr., *84*:90, 1974, with permission.)

LIMB–BODY WALL COMPLEX

The limb–body wall (LBW) complex consists of thoraco- and/or abdominoschisis and limb defects frequently associated with exencephaly/encephalocele and facial clefts. The vast majority of cases are spontaneously aborted; the remainder are stillborn.

The thoraco-abdominoschisis involves an anterolateral body wall defect with evisceration of thoracic and/or abdominal organs into a persistent extraembryonic coelom. The extraembryonic coelom, the space between the amnion and chorion, is obliterated normally by 60 days' gestation. Failure of the ventral body wall to fuse due to damage to part of the body wall or failure of normal ventral folding of the embryo leads to a persistence of the extraembryonic coelom. The amnion is continuous with the skin at the edge of the defect and the umbilical cord is short and partially devoid of its normal amniotic membrane covering. Limb defects similar to those seen in the amnion rupture sequence such as amputations secondary to ring constrictions and pseudosyndactyly occur occasionally. However, other limb defects such as single forearm and/or lower leg bones, ectrodactyly, radioulnar synostosis, and polydactyly (defects that cannot be explained on the basis of constriction or tethering by amniotic bands) occur more frequently. The encephaloceles are usually anterior, often multiple, and are occasionally attached to the amnion. The facial clefts do not conform to the usual lines of closure of the facial processes and are frequently associated with disruption of the frontonasal processes.

In addition, there is a high incidence of associated anomalies of the internal organs including the heart, lungs (lobation defects), diaphragm (absent), intestine (nonrotation, atresia, shortened), gallbladder, kidney (absent, hydronephrotic, dysplastic), and genitourinary tract (abnormal external genitalia or uterus, absent gonad, streak ovaries, bladder extrophy).

The developmental pathogenesis as well as the etiology of LBW complex is controversial. Incorrectly it has been included in the past as part of the spectrum of the amnion rupture sequence, a concept that is clearly untenable based on the observation that the amniotic membrane is intact in some cases.

Van Allen et al. have suggested that an early systemic alteration of embryonic blood supply between 4 and 6 weeks' gestation leads to disruptive vascular defects to the developing embryo including facial clefts, damage to the calvaria and/or brain resulting in neural tube–like defects, many of the limb reduction defects, and the internal visceral anomalies. Adhesion of the amnion to these necrotic areas could lead secondarily to amniotic adhesive bands. Failure of the ventral body wall to close due to vascular compromise could lead to persistence of the extraembryonic coelom. Features typical of the amnion band rupture sequence such as constriction bands are secondary to rupture of the amnion that is not adequately supported because the extraembryonic coelom has not been obliterated.

Others have suggested the LBW complex is secondary to early intrauterine constraint leading to the myriad of defects including the persistence of the extraembryonic coelom secondary to lack of ventral folding of the body wall.

It is most likely that the LBW complex is heterogeneous from the standpoint of etiology and developmental pathogenesis. However, recognition that the associated defects are disruptive in nature suggests that recurrence risk is negligible.

References

Graham, J. M., et al.: Limb reduction anomalies and early in-utero limb compression. J. Pediatr., 96;1052, 1980.

Miller, M. E., et al.: Compression-related defects from early amnion rupture: Evidence for mechanical teratogenesis. J. Pediatr., 98:292, 1981.

Van Allen, M. E., et al.: Limb-body wall complex: I. Pathogenesis. Am. J. Med. Genet., 28:529, 1987.

Van Allen, M. E., et al.: Limb-body wall complex II. Limb and spine defects. Am. J. Med. Genet., 28:549, 1987.

Luebke, H. J., et al.: Fetal disruptions: Assessment of frequency, heterogeneity, and embryologic mechanisms in a population referred to a community-based stillbirth assessment program. Am. J. Med. Genet., 36:56, 1990.

Moerman, P., et al.: Constrictive amniotic bands, amniotic adhesions, and limb-body wall complex: Discrete disruption sequences with pathogenetic overlap. Am. J. Med. Genet., 42:470, 1992.

Russo, R., et al.: Limb body wall complex: A critical review and a nosological proposal. Am. J. Med. Genet., 47:893, 1993.

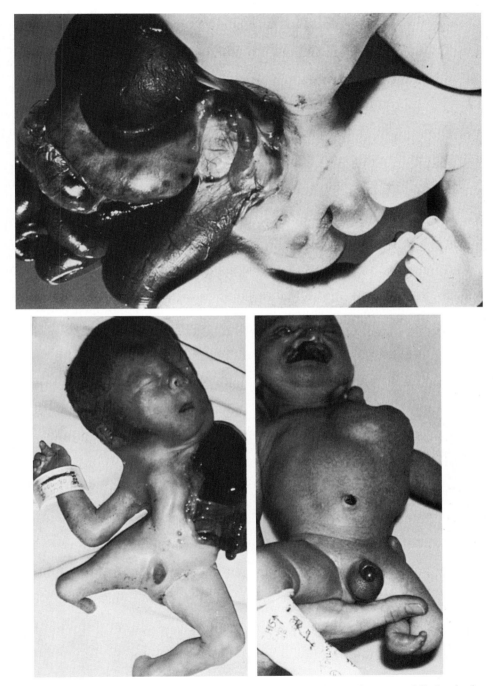

FIGURE 1. Limb–body wall complex. Affected fetuses with multiple involvement of limbs, body wall, and craniofacies. The body wall defect may occasionally be skin covered, as is the case in the lower right photo.

U

U. SPECTRA OF DEFECTS

OCULO-AURICULO-VERTEBRAL SPECTRUM

(First and Second Branchial Arch Syndrome, Facio-Auriculo-Vertebral Spectrum, Hemifacial Microsomia, Goldenhar Syndrome)

The predominant defects in this nonrandom association of anomalies represent problems in morphogenesis of the first and second branchial arches, sometimes accompanied by vertebral anomalies and/or ocular anomalies. The occurrence of epibulbar dermoid with this pattern of anomaly, especially when accompanied by vertebral anomaly, was designated as the Goldenhar syndrome, and the predominantly unilateral occurrence was designated as hemifacial microsomia. However, the occurrence of various combinations and gradations of this pattern of anomalies, both unilateral and bilateral, with or without epibulbar dermoid, and with or without vertebral anomaly, has suggested that hemifacial microsomia and the Goldenhar syndrome may simply represent gradations in severity of a similar error in morphogenesis. The frequency of occurrence is estimated to be 1 in 3000 to 1 in 5000, and there is a slight (3:2) male predominance.

ABNORMALITIES. Variable combinations of the following, tending to be *asymmetric* and 70 per cent unilateral.

Facial. Hypoplasia of malar, maxillary, and/or mandibular region, especially ramus and condyle of mandible and temporomandibular joint. Lateral cleft-like extension of corner of mouth (macrostomia). Hypoplasia of facial musculature. Hypoplasia of depressor anguli oris.

Ear. Microtia, accessory preauricular tags and/or pits, most commonly in a line from the tragus to the corner of the mouth. Middle ear anomaly with variable deafness.

Oral. Diminished to absent parotid secretion. Anomalies in function or structure of tongue. Malfunction of soft palate.

Vertebral. Hemivertebrae or hypoplasia of vertebrae, most commonly cervical but may also be thoracic or lumbar.

OCCASIONAL ABNORMALITIES

Eye. Epibulbar dermoid, lipodermoid, notch in upper lid, strabismus, microphthalmia.

Ear. Inner ear defect with deafness.

Oral. Cleft lip, cleft palate.

Cardiac. Ventricular septal defect, patent ductus arteriosus, tetralogy of Fallot, and coarctation of aorta, in decreasing order.

Genitourinary. Ectopic and/or fused kidneys, renal agenesis, vesicoureteral reflux, ureteropelvic junction obstruction, ureteral duplication, and multicystic dysplastic kidney.

Other. Mental deficiency (I.Q. below 85 in 13 per cent). Branchial cleft remnants in anterior-lateral neck, laryngeal anomaly, hypoplasia to aplasia of lung. Hydrocephalus. Arnold-Chiari malformation. Occipital encephalocele. Agenesis of corpus callosum. Calcification of falx cerebri. Hypoplasia of septum pellucidum, intracranial dermoid cyst. Lipoma in corpus callosum. Radial and/or rib anomalies. Prenatal growth deficiency. Low scalp hairline.

NATURAL HISTORY. Cosmetic surgery is strongly indicated. Most of these patients are of normal intelligence. Mental deficiency is more common in association with microphthalmia. Deafness should be tested for at an early age.

ETIOLOGY. Unknown. Usually sporadic. Estimated recurrence in first-degree relatives is about 2 per cent, although minor features of this disorder may be more commonly noted in relatives. When unilateral it tends to be right-sided. Summitt has reported one family with dominant inheritance of varying degrees of this pattern of anomalies, indicating heterogeneity of cause.

References

Goldenhar, M.: Associations malformatives de l'oeil et de l'oreille. J. Genet. Hum., 1:243, 1952.

Summitt, R. L.: Familial Goldenhar syndrome. Birth Defects, 5:106, 1969.

Pashayan, H., Pinsky, L., and Fraser, F. D.: Hemifacial microsomia-oculo-auriculo-vertebral dysplasia. A patient with overlapping features. J. Med. Genet., 7:185, 1970.

Baum, J. L., and Feingold, M.: Ocular aspects of Goldenhar's syndrome. Am. J. Ophthalmol., 75:250, 1973.

Rollnick, B. R., et al.: Oculoauriculovertebral dysplasia and variants. Phenotypic characteristics of 294 patients. Am. J. Med. Genet., 26:631, 1987.

Cohen, M. M., Jr., et al.: Oculoauriculovertebral spectrum: An updated critique. Cleft Palate J., 26:276, 1989.

Kumar, A., et al.: Pattern of cardiac malformation in oculoauriculovertebral spectrum. Am. J. Med. Genet., 46:423, 1993.

Ritchey, M. L., et al.: Urologic manifestations of Goldenhar syndrome. Urology, 43:88, 1994.

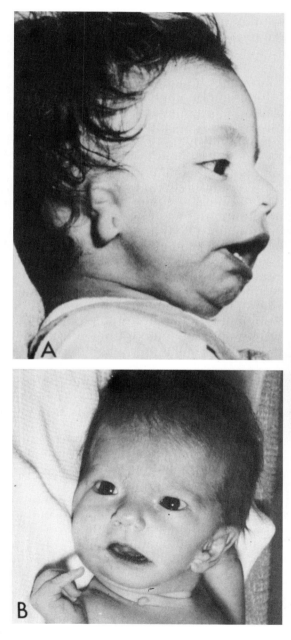

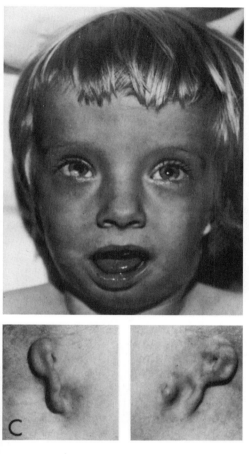

FIGURE 1. Oculo-auriculo-vertebral spectrum. *A*, Right-sided "hemifacial microsomia." Note the macrostomia and micrognathia. *B*, Asymmetric bilateral involvement, with left-sided facial weakness. Note the skin tag, which contained cartilage, in the anterior left neck. There were slight epibulbar dermoids, and there was transposition of the great vessels of the heart. *C*. A 2⁶/₁₂-year-old A laryngeal cyst was excised when the patient was 4 months of age. She has a 40- to 50-dB hearing deficit by air conduction but normal reception by bone conduction. Note the epibulbar lipodermoids.

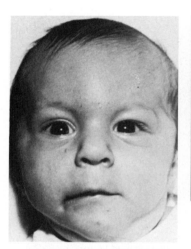

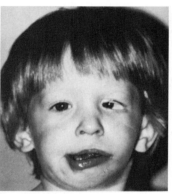

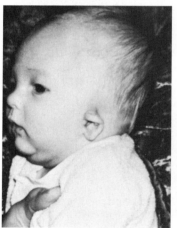

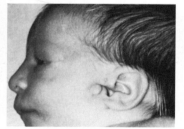

FIGURE 2. Oculo-auriculo-vertebral spectrum. Variation in severity of effects on the eye region, corners of the mouth, nasal region, mandible, and auricular region.

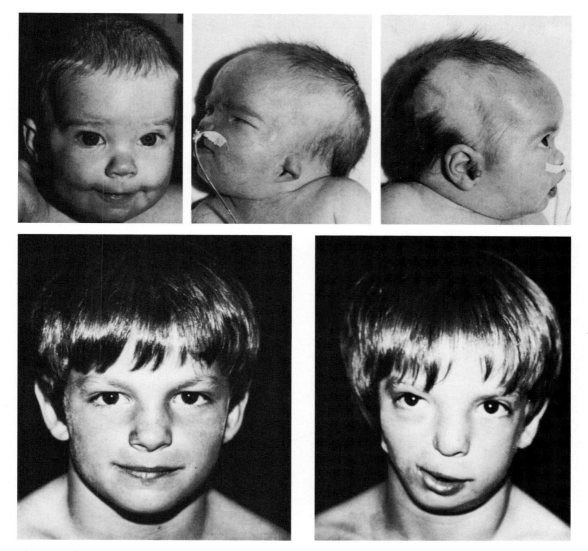

FIGURE 3. Oculo-auriculo-vertebral spectrum. This pattern of defect appears to be more common in monozygotic (MZ) twins and usually affects only one of them. These two sets of MZ twins not only illustrate this but provide an excellent illustration (*left*) on how the individual on the right would have appeared if this problem in facial morphogenesis had not occurred. (*Above*, courtesy of Dr. Uta Burck, Institut für Humangenetik, Universität Hamburg; *below*, courtesy of Dr. Jaime Frias, University of South Florida, Tampa, Fla.)

OROMANDIBULAR-LIMB HYPOGENESIS SPECTRUM

(Hypoglossia-Hypodactyly Syndrome, Aglossia-Adactyly Syndrome, Glossopalatine Ankylosis Syndrome, Facial-Limb Disruptive Spectrum)

Limb Deficiency, Hypoglossia, Micrognathia

In 1932, Rosenthal described aglossia and associated malformations. More recently, Kaplan et al. have emphasized a "community" or spectrum of disorders and have suggested some common elements in modes of developmental pathology.

ABNORMALITIES. Various combinations from among the following features:

Craniofacial. Small mouth, micrognathia, hypoglossia, variable clefting or aberrant attachments of tongue; mandibular hypodontia; cleft palate; cranial nerve palsies including Moebius sequence; broad nose; telecanthus; lower eyelid defect; facial asymmetry.

Limbs. Hypoplasia of varying degrees, to point of adactyly. Syndactyly.

Other. Brain defect, especially of cranial nerve nuclei, causing Moebius sequence. Splenogonadal fusion.

NATURAL HISTORY. Early feeding and speech difficulties may occur. Orthopedic and/or plastic surgery may be indicated for the limb problems. Intelligence and stature are generally normal. Serious problems with hyperthermia can occur in children with four-limb amputation.

ETIOLOGY. Unknown, usually sporadic. The hypothesis that the abnormalities are the disruptive consequence of hemorrhagic lesions has experimental backing from the studies of Poswillo. The presumed vascular problem is more likely to occur in distal regions, such as the distal limbs, tongue, and occasionally parts of the brain. Chorionic villus sampling, particularly when performed between 56 and 66 days of gestation, has been associated with this disorder giving further credence to a disruptive vascular hypothesis.

References

Rosenthal, R.: Aglossia congenita. A report of the condition combined with other congenital malformations. Am. J. Dis. Child., 44:383, 1932.

Poswillo, D.: The pathogenesis of the first and second branchial arch syndrome. Oral Surg., 35:302, 1973.

Kaplan, P., Cummings, C., and Fraser, F. C.: A "community" of face-limb malformation syndromes. J. Pediatr., 89:241, 1976.

Pauli, R. M., and Greenlaw, A.: Limb deficiency and splenogonadal fusion. Am. J. Med. Genet., 13:81, 1982.

Lipson, A. H., and Webster, W. S.: Transverse limb deficiency, oro-mandibular limb hypogenesis sequences, and chorionic villus biopsy. Human and animal experimental evidence for a uterine vascular pathogenesis. Am. J. Med. Genet., 47:1141, 1993.

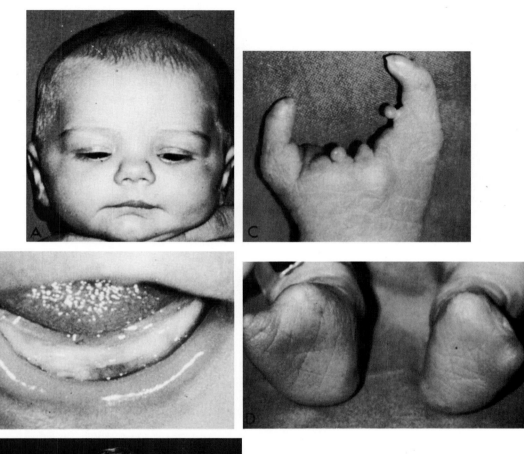

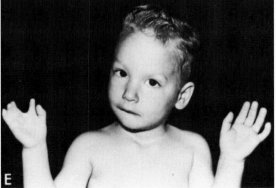

FIGURE 1. Oromandibular-limb hypogenesis spectrum. *A* to *D*, Young infant showing small mandible and crease below the lower lip; small tongue, protruded to its fullest, and hypoplastic alveolar ridge; and limb reduction defects. (*C, D,* From Hall, B. D.: Birth Defects, 7(7):233, 1971, with permission of the copyright holder, March of Dimes Birth Defects Foundation.) *E,* A 3-year-old male showing lower lip indentation and asymmetric hand anomalies.

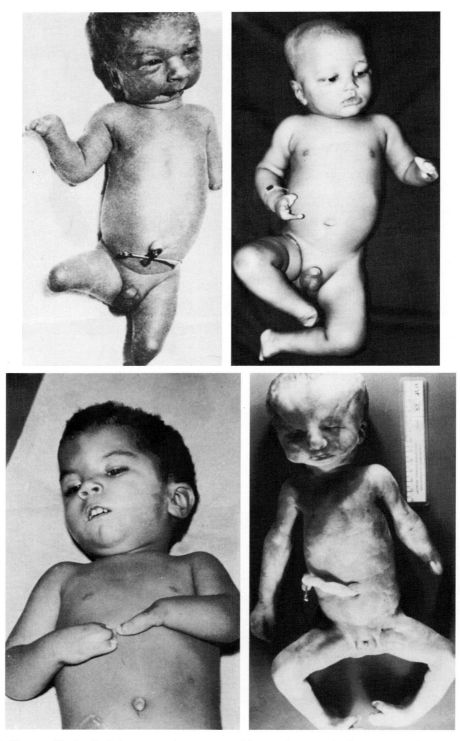

FIGURE 2. Oromandibular-limb hypogenesis spectrum. No one instance is the same as the next. There are varying degrees of limb deficiency, hypoglossia, and/or micrognathia.

CONGENITAL MICROGASTRIA–LIMB REDUCTION COMPLEX

Microgastria, Limb Defects, Splenic Abnormalities

Robert described the first patient with this disorder in 1842. Subsequently, nine additional cases have been described.

ABNORMALITIES

Gastrointestinal. Microgastria. Intestinal malrotation.

Limb. Varying degrees of radial and ulnar hypoplasia, bilateral in 40 per cent of cases. Isolated absence of thumbs (20 per cent). Terminal transverse defects of humerus (10 per cent). Phocomelia (10 per cent). Oligodactyly.

Spleen. Abnormalities in 70 per cent including asplenia, hyposplenia, and/or splenogonadal fusion.

Other. Renal anomalies in 40 per cent including pelvic kidney in two cases, and unilateral renal agenesis and bilateral cystic dysplasia in one patient each. Cardiac defects in 20 per cent (secundum atrial septal defect and type I truncus arteriosus). Central nervous system defects in 20 per cent (arrhinencephaly, fused thalami, polymicrogyria, and agenesis of corpus callosum).

OCCASIONAL ABNORMALITIES. Congenital megacolon, abnormal lung lobation, anophthalmia and porencephalic cyst, cryptorchidism, bicornuate uterus, horseshoe kidney, and absent gallbladder.

NATURAL HISTORY. Microgastria usually presents with gastroesophageal reflux and failure to thrive. Surgical intervention to create a gastric reservoir improves the ability of patients to tolerate normal feeding volumes.

ETIOLOGY. Unknown. All ten cases of this disorder have represented sporadic events in otherwise normal families.

References

Robert, H. L. F.: Hummungsbildung des magens, mangel der milz und des netzes. Arch. Anat. Physiol. Wissenschaftliche Med., *57*, 1942.

Lueder, G. T., et al.: Congenital microgastria and hypoplastic upper limb anomalies. Am. J. Med. Genet., 32:368, 1989.

Meinecke, P., et al.: Microgastria-hypoplastic upper limb association: A severe expression including microphthalmia, single nostril and arrhinencephaly. Clin. Dysmorphol., *1*:43, 1992.

Cunniff, C., et al.: Congenital microgastria and limb reduction defects. Pediatrics, *91*: 1192, 1993.

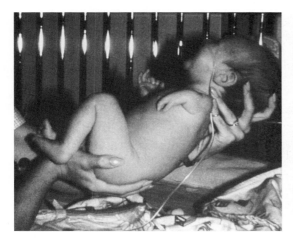

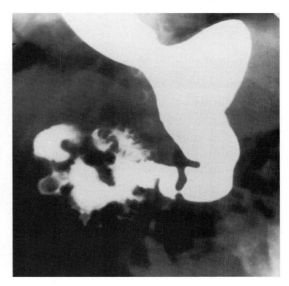

FIGURE 1. Note the limb reduction anomaly and, on the barium-contrast roentgenogram, microgastria and intestinal malrotation.

STERNAL MALFORMATION–VASCULAR DYSPLASIA SPECTRUM

In 1985, Hersh et al. described two patients with this disorder and summarized the findings in 13 previously reported cases. The principal features include cleft of the sternum that is covered with atrophic skin; a median abdominal raphe extending from the sternal defect to the umbilicus; and cutaneous craniofacial hemangiomata.

In 13 of the cases, the hemangiomata were localized to cutaneous structures, while in one the upper respiratory tract was involved and in another there were multiple hemangiomata in the mucosa of the small bowel, mesentery, and pancreas. The sternal defect varies from a complete cleft to a partial cleft involving the upper one third of the sternum.

Occasional abnormalities have included absent pericardium anteriorly, unilateral cleft lip, micrognathia, and glossoptosis.

A significant morbidity is related to respiratory compromise, gastrointestinal bleeding, and infection, as rapid expansion of the vascular lesion leads to tissue hypoxia and necrosis.

All reported cases of this disorder have been sporadic events in otherwise normal families with the exception of a male with asternia and a facial hemangioma who had a sister with isolated asternia. The etiology of this condition is unknown.

References

Hersh, J. H., et al.: Sternal malformation–vascular dysplasia association. Am. J. Med. Genet., *21*:177, 1985.

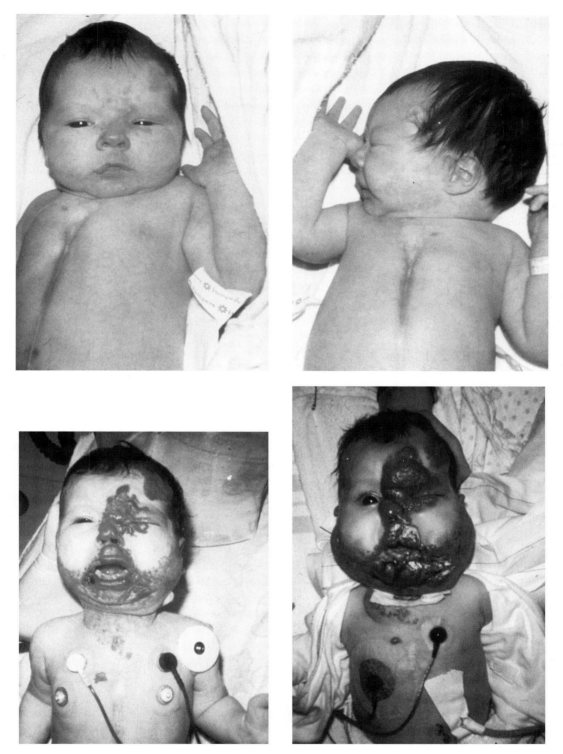

FIGURE 1. Affected child in newborn period, at 6 weeks, and at 4 months. Note the capillary hemangiomata over the face and the cleft of the upper one third of the sternum, which is covered with atrophic skin. (From Hersh, J. H.: Am. J. Med. Genet., 21:177, 1985, with permission from Wiley-Liss, a division of John Wiley & Sons.)

MONOZYGOTIC (MZ) TWINNING AND STRUCTURAL DEFECTS—GENERAL

Monozygotic (MZ) twinning occurs in about 1 in 200 births and, as such, represents the most common aberration of morphogenesis noted in the human. The frequency of MZ twin conceptuses is probably appreciably higher than 1 in 200. Livingston and Poland found a threefold excess of MZ twins among spontaneous abortuses versus live-born twins, with the ratio of MZ to DZ (dizygotic) being 17:1 in the abortuses versus 0.8:1 in the live-born twins. Most of these MZ aborted twins had structural defects and may represent the early lethal effect of the types of structural defects that have been noted to occur with excess frequency in MZ twins.

Structural defects occur two to three times more commonly in live-born MZ twins than in DZ twins or singletons. The origin and nature of these defects are summarized in Table 1–2, and the first three categories are individually set forth in the following subsections. The fourth category of deformation due to in utero crowding, which is not increased in MZ versus DZ twins, is set forth in *Smith's Recognizable Patterns of Human Deformation* and will not be detailed here.

MZ twinning may occur soon after conception, and this type may even have separate placentas with dichorionic-diamnionic membranes. The development of two embryonic centers in the blastocyst by 4 to 5 days of gestation yields twins with monochorionic-diamnionic membranes, the most common type of MZ twinning.

The final potential timing for the induction of MZ twinning is by 15 to 16 days of development, with the formation of more than one Hensen node and primitive streak in the embryonic plate. This will result in monochorionic-monoamnionic twins, who account for about 4 per cent of MZ twins.

In addition to the problems that were alluded to concerning MZ twins, there appears to be an increased likelihood of fetal death in one or more of MZ twins who develop in a monoamnionic sac, at least partially because of cord entanglements leading to vascular problems. There is also an overall excess of perinatal mortality in MZ twins. The primary cause is prematurity, but the excess of structural defects also contributes to this high mortality.

The value and importance of examining the placenta for the condition of the membranes, vascular interconnections between the twins, and evidence of a deceased twin should be obvious.

The etiologies for MZ twining are largely unknown. A single-gene, dominant type of inheritance has been implicated in an occasional family. Experimental studies have implied environmental factors, such as late fertilization of the ovum in the rabbit and vincristine administration in the rat.

Table continued on opposite page

TABLE 1–2. ORIGIN AND TYPES OF STRUCTURAL DEFECTS IN MZ TWINS

Origin	Types of Defects
A. ? The same causative factor that gave rise to MZ twinning	Early malformations or malformation sequences
B. Incomplete twinning	Conjoined twins
C. Consequence of vascular placental shunts	
1. Artery-artery	Disruptions, including acardiac and amorphous twins
2. Artery-vein	Twin-twin transfusion, causing unequal size, unequal hematocrit, and/or other problems
3. Death of one twin with thromboplastin embolic release to co-twin	
D. Constraint in fetal life	Deformations due to uterine constraint

A.   MZ TWINS AND EARLY MALFORMATIONS

The excess of early types of malformation among MZ twins may be the consequence of the same etiology that gave rise to the MZ twinning aberration of morphogenesis. For example, Stockard was able to produce both MZ twinning *and* early malformation such as cyclopia by early environmental insults (alterations of oxygen level and temperature) to the developing Atlantic minnow (*Fundulus*). The findings of Schinzel et al. are in keeping with this hypothesis. They found that the malformations in MZ twins were predominantly early defects, presumably engendered at the same time as the MZ twinning. The incidence of associated early malformations was greatest in the monochorionic-monoamnionic cases, which would usually have been induced at the time of embryonic plate development and hence would theoretically be more likely to have associated early malformations. The early types of defects that have been considered to be of excess frequency in MZ twins are as follows:

1.   Sacrococcygeal teratoma.
2.   Sirenomelia (see page 634).
3.   The VATER association (see page 664).
4.   Exstrophy of the cloaca malformation sequence (see page 628).
5.   Holoprosencephaly malformation sequence (see page 605).
6.   Anencephaly (see page 608).

About 5 to 20 per cent of such cases are concordant; thus, the majority are nonconcordant. When one twin has the more severe degree of a malformation sequence, the other twin may show lesser degrees of the same type of initiating defect.

These early defects are individually presented in this text. Most are early lethals and cause spontaneous abortion. This is probably a partial explanation of the excess of MZ twins among spontaneous abortuses.

Recurrence risk counseling should involve the total problem, namely, the MZ twinning plus the associated malformation sequence. To our knowledge, this risk is of low to negligible magnitude, although the specific etiologies for this type of problem are unknown.

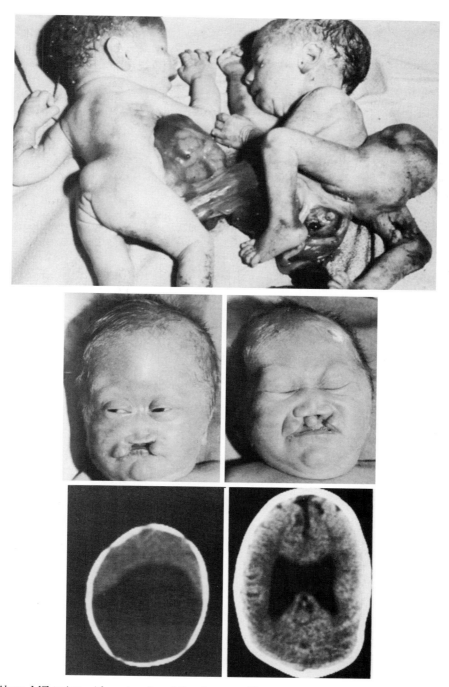

FIGURE 1. *Above*, MZ twins with exstrophy of the cloaca malformation sequence. Note that the severity of the individual components of this malformation sequence, such as the skin-covered myelocele, varies from one twin to the other. *Middle* and *below*, Holoprosencephaly malformation sequence of varying severity in MZ twins (8 days), with CAT scans showing single ventricle (died at 18 days) and more normal ventricular development on the right. (*Middle* and *bottom* photos courtesy of Dr. Uta Burck, Institut für Humangenetik, Universität Hamburg.)

B. Conjoined Twins

Conjoined twins may be viewed as examples of incomplete twinning and occur in about 1 per cent of MZ twins. Although it is feasible that two closely placed embryonic centers in the 4- to 5-day-old blastocyst could result in conjoined twins, it seems more likely that they originate at the primitive streak stage of the embryonic plate (15 to 17 days). Current experimental techniques in animals have not been successful in producing conjoined twins.

The most common type of conjoined twins is termed thoracopagus, in which the twins are joined at the thorax. Juncture at the head, buttocks, and less commonly, other anatomic sites also occurs. Partial to complete duplication of only the upper or lower body parts may also take place.

As with MZ twins in general, there is a higher incidence of early malformations in conjoined twins. Disregarding the incidence of anomalies related to the sites of juncture, there is a 10 to 20 per cent occurrence of major early defects. As with separate MZ twins, the malformations in conjoined twins are often not concordant. The high frequency of associated malformations in conjoined twins may relate to the timing of the defect, which is presumed to be at the embryonic plate–primitive streak stage of development.

The likelihood of particular types of early malformation occurring in certain kinds of conjoined twins is increased very nonrandomly. For example, the dicephalic conjoined twin frequently has anencephaly, most commonly affecting only one of the heads. Whether this relates to differences in early blood flow to the respective heads remains to be determined. The recurrence risk for conjoined twins appears to be negligible.

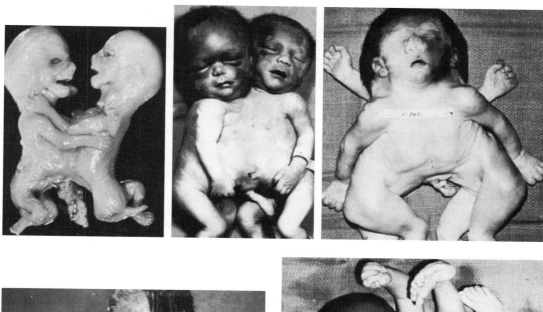

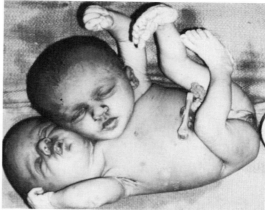

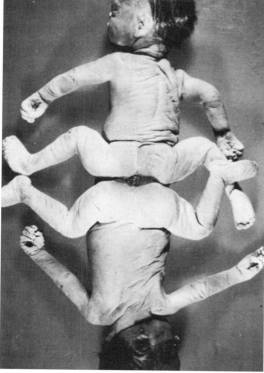

FIGURE 2. *Upper*, Varying degrees of conjoined twins attached at the chest (thoracopagus), which is the most common type. *Lower left*, Joined at the buttocks. *Lower right*, Two heads (dicephaly), sometimes having anencephaly on one side. (*Upper left*, courtesy of Dr. Allan Ebbin; others, courtesy of Dr. Bruce Beckwith and Dr. Thomas Shepard.)

C. PLACENTAL VASCULAR SHUNTS IN MZ TWINS—GENERAL

Benirschke has indicated that the great majority of monochorionic (single placenta) twins have a conjoined placenta with vascular interconnections. These develop on a chance basis and are usually evident on the fetal surface of the placenta where the major vessels course between the fetuses and the major cotyledons. The magnitude of intertwin vascular shunts may be judged by the caliber of the connecting vessels, which relates to the amount of flow they have carried. Much of the early in utero mortality and excess of structural defects in MZ twins may well relate to the secondary consequences of these vascular connections between the twins. Some of the types of shunts and their adverse effects on one or both of the MZ twins are set forth subsequently.

C–1. ARTERY-ARTERY TWIN DISRUPTION SEQUENCE

Benirschke emphasized the dire consequences that could result from a sizable artery-artery placental shunt, usually accompanied by a vein-vein shunt. The tendency will be for the arterial pressure of one twin to overpower that of the other, usually early in morphogenesis. The "defeated" recipient then has reverse flow from the co-twin. This sends "used" arterial blood from the donor into the iliac vessels of the recipient, perfusing the lower part of the body more than the upper part. The results are a host of disruptions, with deterioration of previously existing tissues as well as incomplete morphogenesis (malformation) of tissues that are in the process of formation. The variably missing tissues include the head, heart, upper limbs, lungs, pancreas, and upper intestine. Rudiments of early disrupted tissues may be found in the residuum. The extent of disruption may be even broader, leaving as the residuum an "amorphous" twin. There is every gradation, from amorphia to acardia to less severe degrees of disruption, with no one case being identical to another. Examples of some of the gradations of severity are shown in the accompanying figure.

The donor twin may have an excessive cardiac load resulting in cardiomegaly and even cardiac decompensation, with secondary liver dysfunction, hypoalbuminemia, and edema. Sometimes this may progress to the level of hydrops.

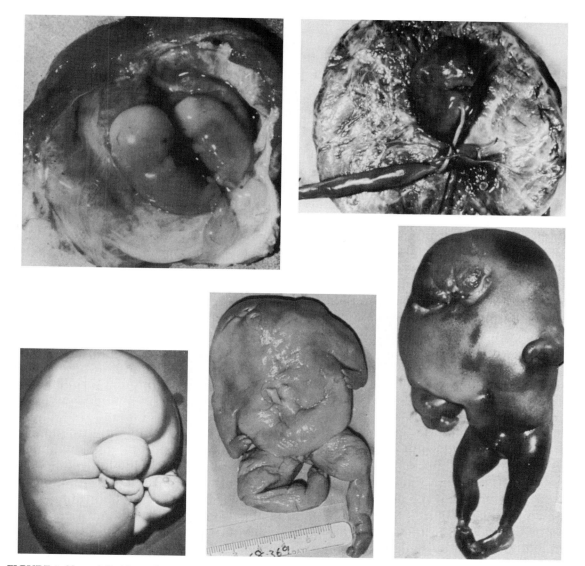

FIGURE 3. *Upper left,* Aborted twin embryo in situ. Note the growth deficiency, especially in the head and upper limbs of the twin to the right. This may well represent the early stage of artery-artery disruptive transfusion from the twin on the left to the one on the right, the early genesis of the acardiac situation. (Courtesy of Dr. Lewis Holmes, Massachusetts General Hospital, Boston, Mass.) *Upper right,* amorphous acardiac, partially embedded in the placenta and not detected by the delivering physician. Note the twisted cord (held up by the probe) that partially occluded vascular flow for both the acardiac fetus and the surviving fetus. (Courtesy of Dr. Mason Barr, Jr., University of Michigan Medical School, Ann Arbor, Mich.) *Lower,* Gradations of severity, from amorphous twin to acephalic, with upper limb deficiency due to artery-artery shunt and reverse circulation from co-twin. (Courtesy of Dr. Thomas Shepard, University of Washington School of Medicine, Seattle, Wash.)

C-2. ARTERY-VEIN TWIN TRANSFUSION SEQUENCE

Artery-vein transfusion may result in problems such as those summarized in Table 1–3. The excessive volume in the recipient twin not only tends to lead to increased growth and an enlarged heart but also causes increased kidney size and excess urine output, with resultant polyhydramnios. The high hematocrit may constitute a serious risk of vascular problems and merits early postnatal management. The donor twin, being hypovolemic, tends to have diminished renal blood flow, smaller kidneys, and oligohydramnios (when the twins are diamnionic). There may even be evidence of transient renal insufficiency in the smaller twin during the first days after birth, as the kidneys have been hypofunctional since before birth.

Tan et al. have found that 18 per cent of MZ twins are discrepant in size and hematocrit at birth; hence, this is not a rare occurrence. Treatment may be warranted soon after birth to provide each affected twin with a more normal hematocrit.

TABLE 1–3. PROBLEMS SECONDARY TO ARTERIOVENOUS TWIN-TWIN TRANSFUSION

Feature	Donor Twin	Recipient Twin
Growth	Smaller size	Larger size
Hematocrit	Low	High
Blood volume	Hypovolemia	Hypervolemia
Renal blood flow and renal size	Diminished	Increased
Amnionic fluid	Oligohydramnios	Polyhydramnios
Heart size	Diminished	Increased

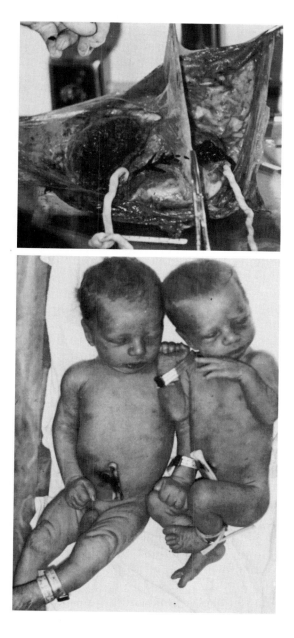

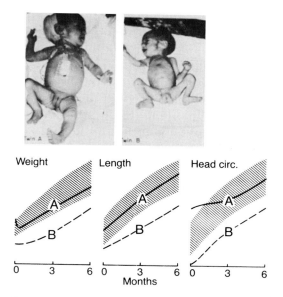

FIGURE 4. *Left,* Discrepant size of MZ twins as the result of an arteriovenous shunt in the monochorionic-diamnionic placenta. The direction of the flow is shown by the *arrows,* from the anemic transfuser at the right to the plethoric, overgrown recipient at the left. The hypovolemic smaller twin had transient evidence of renal insufficiency in the first days after birth. *Above,* Marked discrepancy in size at birth. Note the rapid initial drop in the hypervolemic recipient's (*twin A*) weight after birth. She was given a shunt for "hydrocephalus"; however, in the opinion of the author, this represented large head size secondary to hypervolemia. The smaller donor twin (*twin B*) had evidence of transient renal insufficiency soon after birth, which resolved. She continued to grow at a slow rate. Postnatal growth in the smaller twin has varied from full catch-up to no catch-up and may be dependent on the in utero age of onset of the growth deficiency; the earlier the growth deficiency, the less likely it will be for catch-up growth to occur. The larger *twin B* developed a proencephalic cyst presumably secondary to the plethora, and a vascular problem as a consequence. No aggressive therapy had been pursued relative to the plethora.

C–3. COMPLICATIONS IN AN MZ TWIN FROM THE IN UTERO DEATH OF THE CO-TWIN

Benirschke first implicated death of an MZ co-twin (stillborn or fetus papyraceus) as a potential cause for problems in the surviving twin as a consequence of thromboplastin gaining access to the survivor's circulation and causing disseminated intravascular coagulation. The other possibility is that emboli from the deceased co-twin enter the circulation of the survivor. Either mechanism can give rise to areas of ischemia and disruption, with subsequent loss of tissue. Some of the defects occurring in the co-twin of the deceased MZ twin are the following:

1. Disseminated intravascular coagulation.
2. Aplasia cutis.
3. Porencephalic cyst to hydranencephaly.
4. Limb amputation.
5. Intestinal atresia.
6. Gastroschisis.

Melnick has concluded from the Collaborative Perinatal Project (50,000 deliveries) that about 3 per cent of near-term MZ twins have a deceased co-twin, and about one third of the survivors, or 1 per cent of MZ twin births, have severe brain defects as a consequence of the foregoing mechanisms. The surviving infants with porencephalic cysts and/or hydranencephaly are usually severely mentally deficient with microcephaly, spastic diplegia, and seizures.

References

General

Stockard, C. R.: Developmental rate and structural expression: An experimental study of twins, "double monsters," and single deformities and the interaction among embryonic organs during their origin and development. Am. J. Anat., 28:115, 1921.
Benirschke, K.: Twin placenta in perinatal mortality. N.Y. State J. Med., 61:1499, 1961.
Benirschke, K., and Driscoll, S. G.: The placenta in multiple pregnancy. Handbuch Pathol. Histol., 7: 187, 1967.
Bomsel-Helmreich, O.: Delayed ovulation and monozygotic twinning in the rabbit. Acta Genet. Med. Gemellol., 23:19, 1974.
Myrianthopoulos, N. C.: Congenital malformations in twins. Acta Genet. Med. Gemellol., 24:331, 1976.
Harvey, M. A. S., Huntley, R. M., and Smith, D. W.: Familial monozygotic twinning. J. Pediatr., 90:246, 1977.
Kaufman, M. H., and O'Shea, K. S.: Induction of monozygotic twinning in the mouse. Nature, 276: 707, 1978.
Schinzel, A. A. G. L., Smith, D. W., and Miller, J. R.: Monozygotic twinning and structural defects. J. Pediatr., 95:921, 1979.

Livingston, J. E., and Poland, B. J.: A study of spontaneously aborted twins. Teratology, 21:139, 1980.

Early Malformations in MZ Twins

Stockard, C. R.: Developmental rate and structural expression: An experimental study of twins, "double monsters," and single deformities and the interaction among embryonic organs during their origin and development. Am. J. Anat., 28:115, 1921.
Gross, R. E., Clatworthy, H. W., and Mecker, J. A.: Sacrococcygeal teratomas in infants and children. Surg. Gynecol. Obstet., 92:341, 1951.
Davies, J., Chazen, E., and Nance, W. E.: Symmelia in one of monozygotic twins. Teratology, 4:367, 1976.
Mohr, H. P.: Misibilundugen bei Zwillingen. Ergeb. Inn. Med. Kinderheilkd., 33:1, 1972.
Smith, D. W., Bartlett, C., and Harrah, L. M.: Monozygotic twinning and the Duhamel anomalad (imperforate anus to sirenomelia): A nonrandom association between two aberrations in morphogenesis. Birth Defects, 12:53, 1976.
Schinzel, A. A. G. L., Smith, D. W., and Miller, J. R.: Monozygotic twinning and structural defects. J. Pediatr., 95:921, 1979.
Livingston, J. E., and Poland, B. J.: A study of spontaneously aborted twins. Teratology, 21:139, 1980.

Conjoined Twins

Riccardi, V. M., and Bergmann, C. A.: Anencephaly with incomplete twinning (diprosopus). Teratology, 16:137, 1977.
Schinzel, A. A. G. L., Smith, D. W., and Miller, J. R.: Monozygotic twinning and structural defects. J. Pediatr., 95:921, 1979.

Vascular Shunts Between MZ Twins

Confalonieri, C.: Gravidanza gemellare monocoriale biamniotica con feto papiraceo ed atresia inestinale congenita nell'altro feto. Riv. Ost. Ginec. Prat., 33: 199, 1951.
Naeye, R. L.: Human intrauterine parabiotic syndrome and its complications. N. Engl. J. Med., 268: 804, 1963.
Hague, I. U., and Glassauer, F. E.: Hydranencephaly in twins. N.Y. State J. Med., 69:1210, 1969.
Moore, C. M., McAdams, A. J., and Sutherland, J.: Intrauterine disseminated intravascular coagulation: A syndrome of multiple pregnancy with a dead twin fetus. J. Pediatr., 74:523, 1969.
Saier, F., Burden, L., and Cavanagh, D.: Fetus papyraceus. An unusual case with congenital anomaly of the surviving fetus. Obstet. Gynecol., 45:271, 1975.
Balvour, R. P.: Fetus papyraceus. Obstet. Gynecol., 47: 507, 1976.
Weiss, D. B., Aboulafia, Y., and Isackson, M.: Gastroschisis and fetus papyraceus in double ovum twins. Harefuah, 91:392, 1976.
Benirschke, K., and Harper, V.: The acardiac anomaly. Teratology, 15:311, 1977.

Mannino, F. L., Jones, K. L., and Benirschke, K.: Congenital skin defects and fetus papyraceus. J. Pediatr., 91:599, 1977.

Melnick, M.: Brain damage in survivor after death of monozygotic co-twin. Lancet, 2:1287, 1977.

Schinzel, A. A. G. L., Smith, D. W., and Miller, J. R.: Monozygotic twinning and structural defects. J. Pediatr., 95:921, 1979.

Tan, K. L., et al.: The twin transfusion syndrome. Clin. Pediatr., 18:111, 1979.

Jones, K. L., and Benirschke, K.: The developmental pathogenesis of structural defects: The contribution of monozygotic twins. Semin. Perinatol., 7:239, 1983.

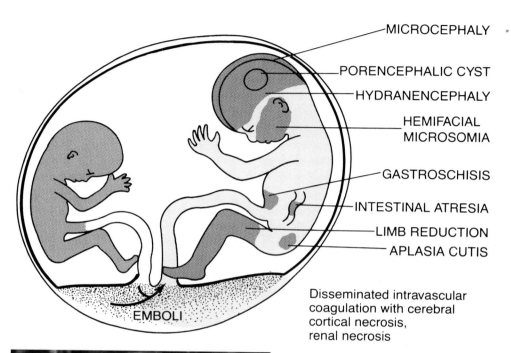

MICROCEPHALY

PORENCEPHALIC CYST

HYDRANENCEPHALY

HEMIFACIAL MICROSOMIA

GASTROSCHISIS

INTESTINAL ATRESIA

LIMB REDUCTION

APLASIA CUTIS

EMBOLI

Disseminated intravascular coagulation with cerebral cortical necrosis, renal necrosis

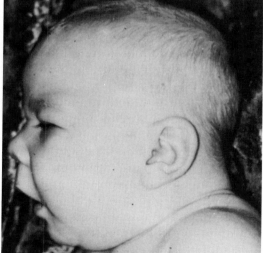

FIGURE 5. *Above*, Impact of death of MZ twin on co-twin can include the release of thromboplastin and/or emboli, which may cause vascular disruptive defects in the surviving co-twin. *Below*, A 5-month-old infant, with severe microcephaly, hypertonic diplegia, seizures, and developmental deficiency, who had hydranencephaly. At birth, there was a macerated 30-cm co-twin of the same sex whose death was considered to be the cause of the disruptive brain problem in the surviving twin. The recurrence risk was judged to be negligible.

V

V. MISCELLANEOUS ASSOCIATIONS

VATER ASSOCIATION

A nonrandom association of vertebral defects, imperforate anus, and esophageal atresia with tracheoesophageal (T-E) fistula has long been appreciated. Say and Gerald noted the association of imperforate anus, vertebral defects, and polydactyly, and Say et al. extended the latter to include polyoligodactyly. The spectrum was broadened by Quan and Smith to include *ver*tebral defects, *a*nal atresia, *T-E* fistula with esophageal atresia, and *r*adial and *r*enal dysplasia, and the acronym VATER association was utilized to designate this complex. Cardiac defects and a single umbilical artery as well as prenatal growth deficiency were also nonrandom features of this pattern of anomalies, and these were emphasized by Temtamy and Miller, who utilized the acronym VATERS association, with the *V* standing for both vertebral defects and ventricular septal defect and the *S* designating single umbilical artery. The general spectrum of the pattern in a total of 34 cases is presented below, as summarized by Temtamy and Miller.

ABNORMALITIES. Thirty-four cases with three or more VATER association defects.

Vertebral anomalies	70%
Ventricular septal defects and other cardiac defects	53%
Anal atresia with or without fistula	80%
T-E fistula with esophageal atresia	70%
Radial dysplasia, including thumb or radial hypoplasia, preaxial polydactyly, syndactyly	65%
Renal anomaly	53%
Single umbilical artery	35%

OTHER LESS FREQUENT DEFECTS. Prenatal growth deficiency, postnatal growth deficiency, laryngeal stenosis, ear anomaly, large fontanels, defect of lower limb (23 per cent), rib anomaly, defects of external genitalia, spinal dysraphia with tethered cord.

NATURAL HISTORY. Though many of these patients may fail to thrive and have slow developmental progress in early infancy related to their defects, the majority of them have normal brain function and thus merit vigorous attempts toward rehabilitation, surgical and otherwise.

ETIOLOGY. This pattern of malformation has generally been a sporadic occurrence in an otherwise normal family. The etiology is unknown. It has been more frequently seen in the offspring of diabetic mothers.

COMMENT. This spectrum of anomalies may occur as a part of a broader pattern, such as the trisomy 18 or del(13q) syndromes, in which case the prognosis is not favorable. It is also important to appreciate that cases with radial dysplasia and cardiac defect may be mistakenly designated as the Holt-Oram syndrome. In addition, a distinct, genetically determined disorder referred to as VATER with hydrocephalus has been reported. Both autosomal and X-linked recessive inheritance have been documented for that disorder. The hydrocephalus is due to aqueductal stenosis. Although a poor prognosis is the rule, survival with a relatively good outcome has been noted in some cases.

References

Say, B., and Gerald, P. S.: A new polydactyly, imperforate anus, vertebral anomalies syndrome. Lancet, 2:688, 1968.

Say, D., et al.: A new syndrome of dysmorphogenesis-imperforate anus associated with poly-oligodactyly and skeletal (mainly vertebral) anomalies. Acta Paediatr. Scand., 60:197, 1971.

Silver, W., et al.: The Holt-Oram syndrome with previously undescribed associated anomalies. Am. J. Dis. Child., 124:911, 1972.

Quan, L., and Smith, D. W.: The VATER association, Vertebral defects, Anal atresia, T-E fistula with esophageal atresia, Radial and Renal dysplasia: A spectrum of associated defects. J. Pediatr., 82:104, 1973.

Temtamy, S. A., and Miller, J. D.: Extending the scope of the VATER association: Definition of a VATER syndrome. J. Pediatr., 85:345, 1974.

Evans, J. A., et al.: VACTERL with hydrocephalus: Further delineation of the syndrome(s). Am. J. Med. Genet., 34:177, 1989.

Wang, H., et al.: VACTERL with hydrocephalus: Spontaneous chromosome breakage and rearrangement in a family showing apparent sex-linked recessive inheritance. Am. J. Med. Genet., 47:114, 1993.

James, H. E., et al.: Distal spinal cord pathology in the VATER association. J. Pediatr. Surg., 29:1501, 1994.

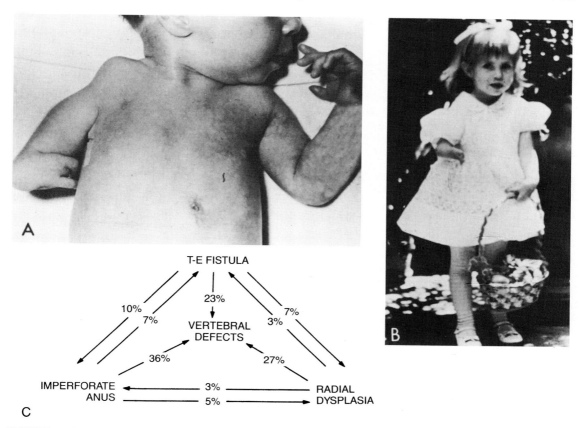

FIGURE 1. *A*, Young infant with vertebral anomalies, anal atresia, esophageal atresia with T-E fistula, radial aplasia on the right, and thumb hypoplasia on the left. *B*, Same patient at 2 years of age, with normal intelligence. *C*, Relative frequencies of some of the other VATER association defects when the patient is ascertained by virtue of having one of the defects. (From Quan, L., and Smith, D. W.: J. Pediatr., *82*:104, 1973, with permission.)

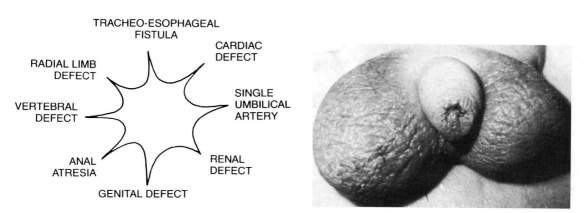

FIGURE 2. *Left*, Expanded VATER association of defects, including genital anomaly (*right*).

MURCS ASSOCIATION

Müllerian Duct, Renal and Cervical Vertebral Defects

The MURCS association, as described in 30 patients by Duncan et al. in 1979, consists of a nonrandom association of *m*üllerian duct aplasia, *r*enal aplasia, and *c*ervicothoracic *s*omite dysplasia.

ABNORMALITIES

Growth. Small stature.

Skeletal. Cervicothoracic vertebral defects, especially from C5–T1 (80 per cent), sometimes to the extent of being termed the Klippel-Feil malformation sequence.

Genitourinary. Absence of proximal two thirds of vagina and absence to hypoplasia of uterus (96 per cent, but there is an ascertainment bias for this defect; sometimes referred to as the Rokitansky malformation sequence). Renal agenesis and/or ectopy (88 per cent).

OCCASIONAL ABNORMALITIES. Moderate frequency of rib anomalies, upper limb defects, and Sprengel scapular anomaly. Infrequent features include deafness, cerebellar cyst, external ear defects, facial asymmetry, cleft lip and palate, micrognathia, gastrointestinal defects, and defects of laterality.

NATURAL HISTORY. Most patients are ascertained because of primary amenorrhea or infertility associated with normal secondary sexual characteristics. Rarely, the MURCS association may be diagnosed in the course of an investigation for a renal malformation or because of multiple malformations. Small stature is frequent, with adult stature usually being less than 152 cm.

ETIOLOGY. The etiology is not known, and it is usually a sporadic disorder in an otherwise normal family.

COMMENT. The Rokitansky malformation sequence, one of the defects that makes up the MURCS association, is characterized by an incomplete to atretic vagina and a rudimentary to bicornuate uterus. The fallopian tubes and ovaries are usually nearly normal with normal secondary sexual characteristics, except for a lack of menstruation. The lower vagina, which is derived from an outpouching from the urogenital sinus, is usually present as a blindly ending pouch. The cause is unknown. Although most cases are sporadic, about 4 per cent of cases have been familial, with affected female siblings.

The Rokitansky malformation sequence may be a part of a broader pattern of malformation such as the MURCS association. In addition, Winter et al. reported four sisters; three had vaginal atresia, all had unilateral or bilateral renal agenesis, and the two survivors had conductive deafness.

References

Rokitansky, K.: Über sog. Verdoppelung des Uterus. Med. Jahrb. des Osterreich. Staates., *26*:39, 1838.

Byran, A. L., et al.: One hundred cases of congenital absence of the vagina. Surg. Gynecol. Obstet., *88*:79, 1949.

Winter, J. S. D., et al.: A familial syndrome of renal, genital, and middle ear anomalies. J. Pediatr., 72:88, 1968.

Duncan, P. A.: Embryologic pathogenesis of renal agenesis associated with cervical vertebral anomalies (Klippel-Feil phenotype). Birth Defects, *13*(3D): 91, 1977.

Duncan, P. A., et al.: The MURCS association: Müllerian duct aplasia, renal aplasia, and cervicothoracic somite dysplasia. J. Pediatr., *95*:399, 1979.

Greene, R. A., et al.: MURCS association with additional congenital anomalies. Hum. Pathol., *17*:88, 1986.

Mahajan, P., et al.: MURCS association—a review of 7 cases. J. Postgrad. Med., *38*:109, 1992.

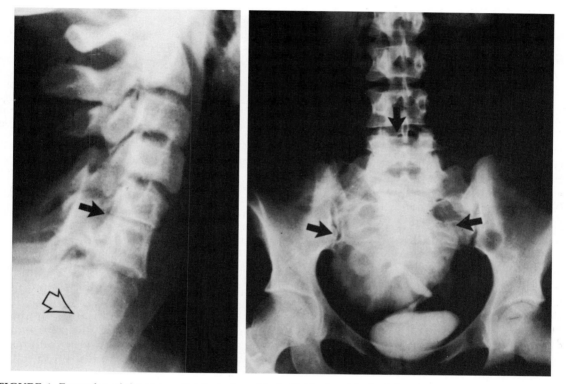

FIGURE 1. Examples of the types of defects found in individuals with the MURCS association include partial to complete cervical vertebral fusion (*left, arrows*) and ectopic pelvic single large kidney in intravenous pyelogram (*right, arrows*).

CHARGE ASSOCIATION

This association was first summarized by Hall, and many similar anomalies have been observed in patients ascertained for ocular coloboma. The spectrum was broadened by Pagon et al. to include *c*oloboma, *h*eart disease, *a*tresia choanae, *r*etarded growth and development and/or CNS anomalies, *g*enital anomalies and/or hypogonadism, and *e*ar anomalies and/or deafness. This latter report utilized the acronym CHARGE association, reported 21 new cases, and summarized the findings in 41 previously reported cases.

ABNORMALITIES. Sixty-two cases with four or more of the seven major CHARGE association defects.

Colobomatous malformation sequence (ranging from isolated iris coloboma without visual impairment to clinical anophthalmos; retinal coloboma most common) 80%

Heart defect (tetralogy of Fallot, patent ductus arteriosus, double-outlet right ventricle with an atrioventricular canal, ventricular septal defect, atrial septal defect, right-sided aortic arch) —

Atresia choanae (membranous and/or bony) 58%

Growth deficiency (usually postnatal) 87%

Mental deficiency (ranging from mild to profound with several patients at autopsy demonstrating arhinencephaly variants and several adults demonstrating hypogonadotropic hypogonadism reminiscent of Kallmann syndrome) 94%

Genital hypoplasia (in males) 75%

Ear anomalies and/or deafness (ranging from small ears without malformation of the pinna to cup-shaped, lop ears; either sensorineural or mixed sensorineural and conductive deafness, ranging from mild to profound) 88%

OTHER FINDINGS. Micrognathia, including Robin malformation sequence; cleft lip; cleft palate; multiple cranial nerve abnormalities; facial palsy; feeding difficulties resulting from poor suck and velopharyngeal incompetence; DiGeorge sequence; renal anomalies; omphalocele; tracheoesophageal fistula; rib anomalies; ptosis; ocular hypertelorism; microcephaly; anal atresia and/or stenosis; growth hormone deficiency.

NATURAL HISTORY. In some instances, the severity of these defects has been such that death has occurred during the perinatal period, the result of either respiratory insufficiency, intractable hypocalcemia, or congenital heart disease. Though prenatal growth deficiency has been present in some cases, most patients have been the appropriate size for gestational age, with linear growth shifting down to or below the third percentile during the first 6 months of life which in some cases has been due to growth hormone deficiency. Most patients have shown some degree of mental deficiency and/or CNS defects, and visual or auditory handicaps may further compromise cognitive function. Multiple cranial nerve abnormalities may be more common than previously appreciated and may be responsible for the facial palsy, feeding difficulties, and sensorineural hearing loss.

The CHARGE association shows some phenotypic overlap with the VATER association and also shares some phenotypic features with recognized chromosomal syndromes such as trisomy 13, trisomy 18, del(4p) syndrome, and cat-eye syndrome. In addition, choanal atresia can be one feature of a variety of monogenic disorders, such as Apert syndrome, Crouzon syndrome, Saethre-Chotzen syndrome, or Treacher Collins syndrome. The nature of the associated defects is sufficient to distinguish the CHARGE association from these latter conditions.

ETIOLOGY. Unknown. Many of the anomalies present in the CHARGE association may derive from altered morphogenesis during the second month of gestation. The choanae are formed between days 35 and 38 of gestation, when the bucconasal membrane ruptures as the epithelia lining the oral and nasal cavities come into contact with each other. Colobomata result from failure of the fetal fissure to close during the fifth week of gestation. Cardiac septation begins with the appearance of the septum primum from the midline of a common atrium at about day 32, proceeds through fusion of the midatrioventricular canal at approximately day 38, and is reasonably complete by day 45, when the outflow tracts, valves, and membranous ventricular septum have been formed.

Holoprosencephaly variants may reflect altered morphogenesis during the fourth to fifth weeks of gestation and may result in hypogonadotropic hypogonadism, growth deficiency, and mental retardation. External ear morphogensis occurs during the sixth week of gestation, shortly after the cochlea begins to form on day 36 (its full length being established by 75 days of gestation). Thus, the defects seen in the CHARGE association might be attributed to ar-

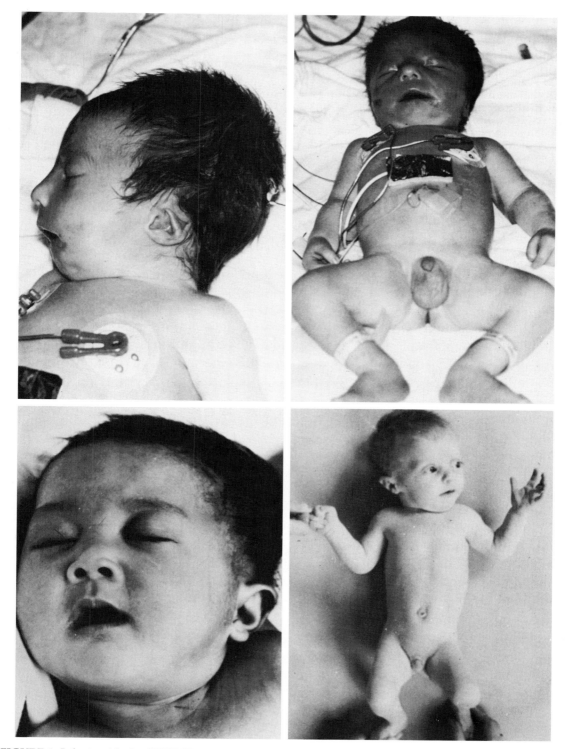

FIGURE 1. Infants with the CHARGE association. The above infant had choanal atresia, aberrant auricles, micrognathia, a short neck with low hairline, a cardiac defect, hypertonicity, seizures, and a micropenis. (The lower two infants, courtesy of Dr. Bryan Hall, University of Kentucky, Lexington, Ky.)

rested development between days 35 and 45 following conception. The causes for such arrested development are probably heterogeneous. There have been instances in which familial recurrence of some of the associated anomalies has suggested a possible genetic etiology, but reduced reproductive fitness has made this possibility difficult to evaluate. The normal parents of an affected child appear to have a low but not negligible recurrence risk.

References

Hall, B. D.: Choanal atresia and associated multiple anomalies. J. Pediatr., *95*:395, 1979.

Hittner, H. M., et al.: Colobomatous microphthalmia, heart disease, hearing loss, and mental retardation —a syndrome. J. Pediatr. Ophthalmol. Strabismus, *16*:122, 1979.

Pagon, R. A., et al.: Coloboma, congenital heart disease, and choanal atresia with multiple anomalies. CHARGE association. J. Pediatr., *99*:1981.

August, J. P., et al.: Hypopituitarism and the CHARGE association. J. Pediatr., *103*:424, 1983.

Davenport, S. L. H., et al.: The spectrum of clinical features in CHARGE association. Clin. Genet., *29*: 298, 1986.

Byerly, K. A., and Pauli, R. M.: Cranial nerve abnormalities in CHARGE association. Am. J. Med. Genet., *45*:751, 1993.

Derenoncourt, A., et al.: CHARGE association and growth hormone deficiency. Clin. Res., *42*:51A, 1994.

ALPHABETICAL LISTING OF SYNDROMES

671

2

Approaches to Categorical Problems of growth deficiency, mental deficiency, arthrogryposis, ambiguous external genitalia

Many patients with specific patterns of malformation may initially be evaluated by the clinician because of a categorical problem such as growth deficiency or mental deficiency. The physician is challenged to arrive at a specific overall diagnosis that will be of value in the management of and prognosis and counsel for that particular patient and family. This chapter sets forth approaches toward a specific diagnosis for several of the more common or more difficult categorical types of problems. It is designed to provide an overall diagnostic point of view, placing the patterns of malformation in relevant perspective to other types of disorders in which such a problem may occur.

Each categorical problem is considered from the standpoint of normal morphogenesis, mechanisms by which abnormal morphogenesis may occur, and the clinical manner of proceeding toward a specific overall diagnosis. These approaches are designed to be rational for the particular problem and germane for the specific patient.

APPROACH TO GROWTH DEFICIENCY

Normal Growth

Assuming proper skeletal organization and ossification, adult stature and the age at which it is achieved are the respective consequences of the following phenomena:

1. *Mitotic* Rate and thereby rate of increasing cell number, especially in the epiphyses.
2. *Maturational* rate of the skeletal system toward final epiphyseal ossification, which can be assessed as "bone age."

677

Both of these processes are influenced by many genes (polygenic). Some of these genes are apparently located on the sex chromosomes. For example, the XY male tends to be taller than the XX female, even in childhood, and the XYY individual is generally taller than the XY male. The XX female matures more rapidly and at a more consistent rate than the XY male and thus reaches the advent of adolescence and final height attainment at an earlier chronologic age than the male. The genetically determined potential for stature and pace of maturation are dependent upon an adequate supply of certain nutrients, vitamins, hormones, and oxygen to the skeletal cells. The dramatic trend toward increasing size and pace of maturation during the past 100 years is most likely related to better nutrition and relatively less chronic disease during childhood.

Causes of Growth Deficiency

Growth deficiency, although a valuable clinical sign, is a highly nonspecific one. Five general categories of growth deficiency are presented subsequently, each having somewhat different overall characteristics in terms of growth pattern, mode of evaluation toward a specific diagnosis, prognosis for eventual stature, and/or management. The first two categories are variants of normal growth, and the other three represent abnormalities in the growth process. This classification, with the exception of prenatal infectious disease, is summarized in Table 2–1.

Variants of Normal

Familial Short Stature. Familial short stature is characterized by an otherwise normal small child who is maturing at a normal rate, as indicated by "bone age," with a family history of small stature in otherwise normal close relatives. Such individuals are usually within normal limits for size at birth, have a consistently slow pace of linear growth during childhood, reach adolescence at a usual age, and are relatively short in final stature.

Familial Slow Maturation. Familial slow maturation is characterized by a slowly maturing child who is short for chronologic

TABLE 2–1. CLASSIFICATION OF GROWTH DEFICIENCY

	Normal Variants	
Features	*Familial Short Stature*	*Familial Slow Maturation*
Onset of growth deficiency	Postnatal	Postnatal (early childhood)
Rate of maturation	Normal	Slow
Family history	Short stature	Slow maturation
Final stature	Short	Normal limits
Therapy to increase eventual stature	None	None

	Abnormals*	
Features	*Primary Skeletal Growth Deficiency*	*Secondary Growth Deficiency*
Onset of growth deficiency	Usually prenatal	Usually postnatal
Rate of maturation	Variable, usually normal	Usually retarded
Associated anomalies	Frequent	Unusual, except when causative anomaly
Malproportionment	Frequent	Unusual, except for rickets
General modes of etiology	Chromosomal abnormalities	Environmental
	Mutant gene syndromes, including the osteochondrodysplasias	Defect in nonskeletal organ, including endocrine
	Syndromes of unknown etiology	Metabolic disorders
		Chronic infectious disease
Therapy to increase eventual stature	None at present	Specific treatment can result in "catch-up" growth

*Prenatal infectious disease and fetal alcohol syndrome are not included.

age but not for maturational age (bone age), with a family history of slow maturation. The latter is indicated by late advent of adolescence and final height attainment in one or more close relatives. Such individuals are usually within normal limits for size at birth, with slowing in the pace of growth and maturation becoming evident during late infancy or early childhood. They have a late onset of normal adolescence and usually achieve a final height within the normal range, but at a late chronologic age.

Abnormal Growth

Aside from the rare and rather obvious situation of sexual precocity leading to rapid growth and accelerated maturation with an early and relatively short final height attainment, the other growth deficiency disorders can be grouped into three general categories.

Primary Skeletal Growth Deficiency. The implication for this category is that of a primary intracellular problem that affects the growth of the skeletal system. The growth deficiency is usually of prenatal onset and is often accompanied by malproportionment or defects in skeletal molding. The same problem that affects cellular growth and morphogenesis in the skeleton may have affected other tissues as well. Thus the patient often presents with a *pattern* of multiple malformations, the recognition of which may allow for a concise overall diagnosis.

Postnatal growth generally proceeds at a consistently slow pace. Although the anomalous skeletal development may lead to difficulty in the interpretation of "bone age," maturation usually advances at a near-normal rate, and adolescence is achieved at a usual age. As yet, there is no known therapy for increasing the eventual stature of persons with any one of the disorders within this category. The prognosis of stature can best be inferred with knowledge of the final height attainment of other patients with the same disorder. Many of the problems of malformation presented in this text have primary growth deficiency as one feature. These include chromosomal abnormality syndromes, osteochondrodysplasias and many other mutant gene syndromes, plus a number of syndromes of unknown

etiology. For a few of them, such as the Hurler syndrome, the Hunter syndrome, and X-linked spondyloepiphyseal dysplasia, the growth deficiency does not become manifest until months or years after birth.

Secondary Skeletal Growth Deficiency. The implication for this category is that the skeletal cells are normal. The growth deficiency is *secondary* to a problem outside the skeletal system that limits its capacity for growth. The problem may exist in the delivery of nutrients, hormones, or oxygen to the skeletal cells or in the maintenance of extracellular homeostasis. Specific types of secondary growth deficiency disorders are listed in Table 2–2. It is unusual for these types of problems to give rise to growth deficiency during fetal life,* and hence the onset of growth deficiency is usually *postnatal.* As illustrated in Figure 2–1, defects in the development and function of the brain, pituitary, thyroid, heart, lungs, liver, intestines, or kidneys seldom have a serious effect on prenatal growth but can cause postnatal growth deficiency. Since the growth problem is of postnatal onset, there usually are no associated malformations, except for an anomaly that may be responsible for the growth deficiency. Furthermore, the skeletal system is normally proportioned and modeled, except in the case of rickets.

Skeletal maturation is usually retarded to about the same extent as linear growth, with the exception of primary hypothyroidism, in which case osseous maturation is usually relatively more retarded than is linear growth.

When the cause of the secondary growth deficiency is recognized and rectified, one may witness the amazing phenomenon of catch-up growth, an acceleration of growth and maturation toward expectancy for chronologic age. This phenomenon dramatically emphasizes the fact that there is no primary growth problem within the skeletal system. The extent of catch-up growth varies in accordance with the age of onset, duration, and nature of the growth problem—plus the adequacy of therapy.

---

*Mild degrees of prenatal secondary growth deficiency may occur with maternal toxemia, malnutrition, or heavy cigarette smoking, and prenatal onset of serious persisting growth deficiency may occur in the offspring of women with chronic alcoholism.

TABLE 2–2. SECONDARY GROWTH DEFICIENCY

Problem	Reason for Growth Deficiency	Diagnostic Studies

Nutritional
  a. Inadequate intake
  b. Partial intestinal obstruction
  c. Malabsorption
	Nutritional deficiency	Response to adequate intake
		GI radiographic studies
		Absorption, GI enzyme studies

Deprivation syndrome	Neglect, abuse, nutritional	Response to environmental change Home and family investigation
Mental deficiency, usually severe	Unknown	Exclude other causes of mental deficiency

Cardiac defect
  a. Large left to right shunt
  b. Cyanotic type
	?Rapid circulation time
	?Hypoxia, sluggish circulation
		Cardiac evaluation

Respiratory insufficiency	?Hypoxia	Usually obvious
Renal dysfunction	Acidosis Polyuria with dehydration Rickets	Urine pH, serum electrolytes, CO_2, urine concentrating ability Serum calcium, phosphorus
Pituitary growth hormone deficiency	?Diminished lipolysis and amino acid transport to cell	Stimulated serum growth hormone values
Hypothyroidism	Deficit in energy metabolism	Serum thyroxine or protein-bound iodine
Chronic serious infectious disease (not upper-respiratory)	Unknown	

Metabolic disorders such as hypercalcemia, hypophosphatemic rickets, hypokalemia, galactosemia, glycogen storage disease, salt-losing congenital adrenal hyperplasia

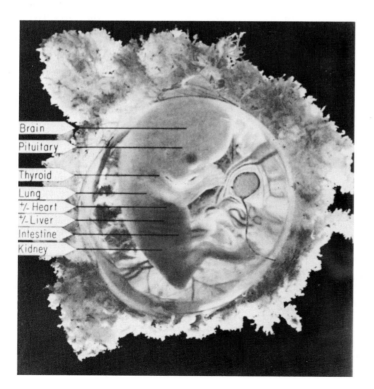

FIGURE 2–1. Serious problems in development and function of the listed tissues usually do not have an adverse effect on prenatal growth, whereas each problem can be the cause of serious postnatal secondary growth deficiency.

Prenatal Infectious Disease. Certain prenatally acquired infectious diseases such as toxoplasmosis, cytomegalic inclusion disease, and rubella may give rise to a chronic disease that can adversely affect growth, presumably by direct involvement of the skeletal system. The onset of growth deficiency is prenatal. Such babies often demonstrate other signs of prenatal infectious disease such as hepatosplenomegaly, brain dysfunction and, in the case of rubella, the patient may have cataracts and cardiac and/or auditory defects. There is inadequate knowledge about the eventual growth pattern in such babies, although the growth rate may improve after 1 to 2 years of age.

Clinical Approach to Growth Deficiency

Emphasis should be placed on the following:

1. Family history relative to stature and maturational rate.
2. History of patient's growth, plotted on normal grids. Of particular importance is the *age of onset* of growth deficiency and the *rate* of growth. Compare with normals for the mean parental stature when possible.
3. A complete physical evaluation should include height, weight, head circumference, and facial anomalies. Check closely for evidence of malproportionment, including asymmetry. Measure span and upper-to-lower segment ratio when indicated.
4. Based on the findings, most patients can be separated into one of the following three categories:
   a. Normal for genetic background. No further studies indicated.
   b. Prenatal onset of growth deficiency. Strive to recognize a specific overall syndrome among the primary growth deficiency disorders presented in this text. Also consider prenatal infectious disease, the fetal alcohol syndrome, and the fetal hydantoin syndrome.
   c. Postnatal onset of growth deficiency. Generally, obtain a bone age

determination (roentgenographs of knee and foot prior to 3 months, usually just hand and wrist thereafter). Consider such secondary growth deficiency disorders as those set forth in Table 2–2 plus the few primary skeletal growth deficiency syndromes that have a postnatal onset of growth deficiency.

APPROACH TO MENTAL DEFICIENCY

Since knowledge about the development of the central nervous system (CNS) and the causes of mental deficiency is rather incomplete, the following section should be interpreted as being preliminary and tentative.

Normal Development of CNS[5]

At 18 days of fetal development, the thickened neural plate becomes a neural groove, the margins of which join to form the neural tube, which is completely closed by 28 days. Rapid growth takes place anteriorly with formation of the primitive brain vesicles: the prosencephalon (forebrain), mesencephalon (midbrain), and rhombencephalon (hindbrain). By 23 days, the optic outpouchings are occurring from the prosencephalon, and by 33 days, its lateral outpouchings (i.e., the early cerebral hemispheres) are evident. Major brain morphogenesis continues for many months; the cerebellum does not begin its major period of morphogenesis until 4 to 5 fetal months. Within the cerebral hemispheres, the inner layer of neuroepithelial cells differentiates to become neuroblasts, which migrate outward in successive waves to form the cortical mantle layers. By 10 weeks, the cerebral cortex is quite thin, with only one outer cortical layer in contrast with the relatively large size of the lateral ventricles, as shown in Figure 2–2. Cell numbers are increasing rapidly, with a major addition of neurons at approximately 4 to 5 fetal months. New cells are being added well into postnatal life, as indicated in Figure 2–3. Although most of the neurons are present at birth, a major addition of glial cells occurs during

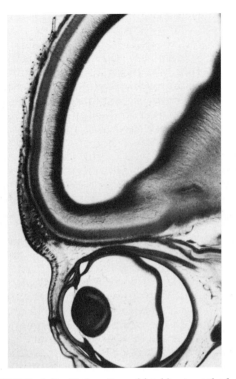

FIGURE 2–2. Sagittal section of fetal brain at the level of the eye at 10 weeks of development. Note the single cortical zone of the cerebral cortex and the relatively large ventricular space. (From Smith, D. W., and Gong, B. T.: Teratology, 9:17, 1974, with permission of John Wiley & Sons.)

the first 6 postnatal months. Most of the myelinization process, the responsibility of glial cells, occurs during the first year. The "wiring" of the axon networks, so integral to advancing and integrated function, is also occurring; however, less is known about critical periods for these interconnections between neurons. The functional consequences of this rapid brain growth and integration of neurons are reflected in the orderly progression of advancing performance during this time. Brain growth is almost complete by 2 years, with the organ reaching about 80 per cent of its adult size by this age.

Approach to Problems in Which Mental Deficiency is a Feature

Clinical Subcategorization of Mental Deficiency Relative to Diagnostic Studies

The majority of children with milder degrees of mental deficiency, having intelligence quotients (I.Q.s) in the range of 50 to 70, come from mentally dull and/or socioeconomically deprived parents, related to polygenic and/or environmental factors.[7] This group also includes some XXY boys; and an occasional XXX girl; some children with malformation syndromes; some chil-

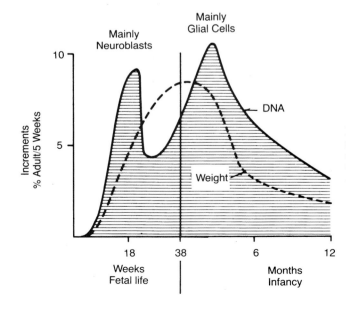

FIGURE 2–3. Rate of brain growth in terms of new cells (DNA) and weight during the most critical period of brain morphogenesis. (Adapted from Dobbin, J.: Am. J. Dis. Child., 120:411, 1970, with permission.)

dren with the fragile X syndrome and the fetal alcohol syndrome; and some patients with inborn errors of metabolism, milder defects of CNS development, or residual CNS insults. Among the more severely mentally deficient patients, with I.Q.s below 50, it is possible to arrive at a precise overall diagnosis in between 58 and 71 per cent of patients.[8] Though the following categorical breakdown of mental deficiency is especially relevant for severely affected patients, it is applicable for all degrees of mental deficiency.

This general subcategorization was designed to be of clinical value to aid in the rational diagnostic evaluation of a given patient with mental deficiency. It is based on findings derived from an appropriate family history, prenatal and birth history, postnatal history, and physical examination, with the latter including a careful search for associated major and minor malformations. It is the author's contention that, having obtained such information, there is no single laboratory study that is indicated for all patients with evidence of mental deficiency. Rather, the next phase of the diagnostic evaluation should be individualized in accordance with the findings from the history and physical examination. It is important to emphasize that laboratory tests are primarily of value in this group of patients for confirming clinical suspicions and that only rarely will a "shot-gun approach" utilizing routine laboratory tests yield an unexpected diagnosis.[9] This subcategorization is predominantly based on the apparent *age of onset of the problem*. Table 2–3 summarizes the subgroups and the types of diagnostic laboratory studies that might merit consideration of each subgroup. These are elaborated upon in the following text.

Category I: Prenatal Problem in Morphogenesis of the Brain. This group is the largest one, making up 44 per cent of 1224 seriously mentally deficient patients evaluated by Kaveggia et al.,[10] approximately the same percentage in two similarly conducted studies,[8,11] and 53 per cent of a less severely mentally deficient group reported by Smith and Simons.[12] Between 15 and 33 per cent of this subcategory of patients were considered to have a single primary defect in brain morphogenesis, such as primary microcephaly, hydrocephalus, hydranencephaly, a defect of neural tube closure, or other types of cerebral dysmorphogenesis. The others had multiple major and/or mi-

TABLE 2–3. CATEGORIZATION OF MENTAL DEFICIENCY*

		Category	Subgroups		Studies to Consider
I	44%	Prenatal onset of problem in morphogenesis	Single defect of brain	14%	Consider CAT scan
			Multiple defect, including brain		
			Chromosomal	12%	Chromosome studies
			Unknown	6%	
			Known syndrome, not chromosomal	6%	
II	?3%	Perinatal insult to brain	Trauma		
			Metabolic		
			Infectious		
			Other		
III	?12%	Postnatal onset of problem	Environmental		
			Metabolic disorders, including known inborn errors	4%	Indicated metabolic study
			Infectious		
			Other		
IV	41%	Undecided age of onset of problem			Consider metabolic studies, chromosome study
	?Very small %	Disorders that might present *clinically* in several of the above categories	Prenatal infectious disease		Appropriate culture and/or antibody studies
			Hypothyroidism, congenital		PBI or T_4

*The percentage figures were obtained from Kaveggia et al.[10] and represent the approximate percentage of each category and subgroup from the *total* of 1224 seriously mentally deficient patients in their study.

nor malformations of non-CNS structures, and by inference, the mental deficiency was also considered to be the consequence of a defect in early morphogenesis of the brain. This latter discrimination is often dependent upon a cautious total physical examination with the purpose of detecting minor as well as major anomalies. For example, Smith and Bostian[13] evaluated 50 consecutive patients with idiopathic mental deficiency and found that 42 per cent of them had three or more extra-CNS major and/or minor anomalies of prenatal onset versus none with three or more associated anomalies in 100 concomitantly examined control children without mental deficiency. Within Kaveggia et al.'s[10] multiple defect subcategory, 41 per cent of patients had a chromosomal abnormality, mostly the Down syndrome, 18 per cent had known syndromes of nonchromosomal etiology, and 41 per cent had patterns of malformation of unknown etiology.

Category II: Perinatal Insult to Brain. This group includes kernicterus, severe neonatal hypoglycemia, intracerebral hemorrhage, perinatal hypoxia, and meningitis and sepsis—all more common in the prematurely born infant. Caution should be exerted before assuming that problems of birth and perinatal adaptation are the *primary* cause of mental deficiency in patients who have evidence of *prenatal* onset of a problem in morphogenesis. Such patients, especially those who have a severe defect of early brain development and those with prenatal onset of growth deficiency, are more likely to have problems in neonatal adaptation.

Category III: Postnatal Onset of Problem in Brain Function. These patients generally appear normal as newborns. After a variable period of time, during which they have normal appearance and function, there is a slowing and/or deterioration in developmental progress and performance. This group includes environmental insults such as trauma, meningitis, encephalitis, hypernatremia, water intoxication, severe hypoglycemia, severe hypoxemia, and lead encephalopathy plus certain enzymatic defects of amino acid, carbohydrate, uric acid, mucopolysaccharide, and brain lipid metabolism. Though some of these latter inborn errors of metabolism may have a prenatal onset, only a few of them, such as the Leroy I-cell syndrome or generalized gangliosidosis,

have gross clinical manifestations by the time of birth. Thus the *clinical* implication is usually that of a postnatal onset of the problem. Kaveggia et al.[10] found that 4.3 per cent of 1224 seriously mentally deficient patients had established inborn errors of metabolism, of which one third had phenylketonuria.

Category IV: Undecided Age of Onset of the Problem in Brain Function. These are the patients who show no obvious evidence of a prenatal problem in morphogenesis, have no established history of a gross insult to the brain in the perinatal period, and who have been rather consistently slow in postnatal developmental progress of CNS dysfunction, such as spasticity, hypotonia, seizures, and/or aberrant behavior. This is the second largest group, making up 41 per cent of the series studied by Kaveggia et al.[10]

Disorders That May Present Clinically in Several of the Four Categories

1. *Prenatal infectious disease.* The patient with mental deficiency as a consequence of prenatally acquired infectious disease such as rubella, cytomegalic inclusion disease, or toxoplasmosis may have obvious historical and physical indications of prenatal onset of the disorder, may have had serious problems in perinatal adaptation, or may have had no obvious problems until a later age. Thus, their clinical presentation may be in any one of the above categories.

2. *Congenital hypothyroidism.* Early detection of congenital hypothryoidism, with thyroid hormone replacement, is critical in preventing or at least limiting the adverse effect of hypothyroidism on early brain development.[14] Signs of prenatal onset of osseous immaturity, such as unusually large fontanels[15] and facial immaturity with a short nose, are usually present at birth, and perinatal problems not uncommonly include persisting indirect bilirubinemia, lethargy, and/or poor feeding. Unfortunately, congenital hypothyroidism is seldom detected on the basis of these early signs and symptoms. Most commonly, it is not suspected until postnatal onset of slow growth, sluggish activity, myx-

edema, and lag of developmental progression become evident. Patients with partial degrees of congenital hypothyroidism may not show signs of myxedema and may have a very subtle postnatal onset of slowness in growth, maturation, and developmental progress, with borderline sluggishness in activity. Thus the clinician could interpret the patients as belonging in any of the above categories, although they obviously belong in category I (prenatal onset).

3. *Fragile X syndrome.* Although affected individuals sometimes have a characteristic clinical phenotype in association with mental deficiency, the phenotype is often extremely subtle, particularly in females. Thus, their clinical presentation may be in any one of the above categories. Recommendations for diagnostic and carrier testing have been set forth that imply that virtually all mentally retarded individuals should be tested.[16] It has been the author's practice to perform fragile X testing on undiagnosed mentally retarded individuals of either sex if they satisfy the following criteria: (1) They have characteristic physical or behavioral features of fragile X syndrome in the absence of minor or major malformations never seen in the disorder or (2) they have a normal physical examination but have male or female relatives with undiagnosed mental retardation or with fragile X syndrome.

Diagnostic Studies in Patients With Mental Deficiency—Their Rational Usage

1. Studies that may resolve the diagnosis.
    a. *Chromosome studies.* Indications for chromosome studies are largely limited to appropriate patients in category I who have multiple malformations and to those in category IV (undecided) when the clinical findings do not *exclude* the possibility of XXY or XXX.
    b. *Molecular analysis.* At this time, indications for DNA testing are limited to patients for whom there is a high suspicion of a specific diagnosis such as fragile X syndrome.
    c. *Studies for inborn errors of metabolism.* Patients with mental deficiency due to an inborn error of metabolic function, most commonly the consequence of a recessively inherited enzyme defect, often have one or more additional clues besides mental deficiency alone. Some of these are set forth in Table 2–4. These patients usually fit into category III. They appear normal at birth and then at variable postnatal ages develop diffuse nonlateralizing evidence of CNS deficit or deterioration of function. A history of intermittent lapses of consciousness, inanition, unexplained hypoglycemia, or recurrent acidosis should each be potential clues toward an inborn error of metabolism. For example, acidosis may be a feature of lactic acidemia, and intermittent loss of consciousness may occur in the severe form of maple syrup urine disease or in hyperammonemia.
    d. *Studies for prenatal infectious disease.* Patients with mental deficiency as the result of congenital rubella, cytomegalic inclusion disease, or toxoplasmosis usually also have one or more of the following features: microcephaly, chorioretinitis, prenatal onset growth deficiency, hepatosplenomegaly, neonatal petechiae, jaundice, and/or deafness. Patients with congenital rubella may also have cataract, cardiac defect, and other anomalies. Those mentally deficient patients who have one or more of these additional findings and whose total findings do not *exclude* the possibility of the disorder being due to prenatal infectious disease should be considered for one or more of the following studies: direct culture of the infectious agent (in early infancy), specific fluorescent IgM antibody determination, and complement-fixation antibody determination.
    e. *Thyroid studies.* A protein-bound iodine (PBI) or serum thyroxine determination is merited for the mentally deficient patient who has

TABLE 2–4. EXAMPLES OF FEATURES IN ADDITION TO MENTAL DEFICIENCY THAT OFTEN OCCUR POSTNATALLY IN CERTAIN INBORN ERRORS OF METABOLISM

Disorder	Features
Phenylketonuria, classic; autosomal recessive	Light pigmentation, eczema (33%); poor coordination, seizures (25%), autistic behavior
Sanfilippo syndrome (MPS III); autosomal recessive	Developmental lag after 1 year with deterioration toward restless behavior, clumsiness by age 6–7 yr; development of coarse facies and hair by 2–3 yr; gum hypertropy, mild limitation in finger extension
Hurler syndrome (MPS I); autosomal recessive	Developmental lag after 6–10 mo, with deterioration and growth deficiency, coarse facies, stiff joints, gibbus, hepatosplenomegaly, cloudy corneas, rhinitis
Hunter syndrome (MPS II), severe type; X-linked recessive	Developmental lag after 6–12 mo, with growth deficiency, coarse facies, stiff joints, hepatosplenomegaly; no gibbus or cloudy corneas
Galactosemia, severe type; autosomal recessive	Development in early infancy (on cow's milk feeding) of lethargy, hypotonia, heptomegaly, icterus, hypoglycemia, cataract, with failure to thrive
Lesch-Nyhan syndrome; X-linked recessive	Development after 6–8 mo of spasticity, choreoathetosis, self-mutilation, autistic behavior, growth deficiency; tophi in late childhood
Homocystinuria; autosomal recessive	Mild arachnodactyly, pectus, genu valgus, pes cavus, mild limitation of finger extension; downward lens dislocation, usually by age 10 yr; wide facial pores, malar flush; thrombotic phenomena, contributing to CNS problems
Argininosuccinicaciduria; autosomal recessive	Onset in first 1–2 yr of growth deficiency, mild hepatomegaly, skin lesions, dry brittle hair with trichorrhexis nodosa, seizures

evidence of osseous immaturity, slow postnatal growth, sluggish physical activity, and myxedematous fullness in the tissues. Thyroid studies are *not* indicated in the patient with mental deficiency and short stature who does not show any other clinical indication of having hypothyroidism.

2. Ancillary studies that may assist in the diagnosis.

  a. *Computed axial tomography (CAT) scan* may occasionally be indicated in a category I patient with a primary defect in brain morphogenesis in an effort to delineate the nature and extent of the brain malformation more fully. This may be of particular relevance for hydrocephalus. For other defects, the study may provide a better perspective toward prognosis as well as genetic counseling.

  b. *Skull roentgenograms* merit consideration in a patient with clinical signs of craniosynostosis, evidence of increased intracranial pressure, cutaneous signs of tuberous sclerosis or Sturge-Weber malformation sequence, or evidence of prenatal infectious disease, especially toxoplasmosis. Otherwise, there is seldom any clinically relevant information to be derived from this study.

  c. *Long-bone roentgenograms* may be indicated by clinical findings such as skeletal abnormalities. Bone age determination may be indicated in patients with decelerating growth, especially those in whom the overall findings are compatible with hypothyroidism, and in patients with excessive rate of growth, but it is of little practical value in patients with prenatal onset of growth deficiency.

  d. *Electroencephalograms* may be warranted in patients with a history of seizures or suspected seizure-equivalent.

  e. *Fasting blood glucose* level merits consideration in patients with a history suggestive of hypoglycemic signs and symptoms but is not necessarily indicated for all patients with seizures.

f. *Other serum chemistries*, blood studies, and urinalysis should be performed only as prompted by findings other than mental deficiency in the history or examination.

APPROACH TO ARTHROGRYPOSIS

(Prenatal Onset of Joint Contractures)

Normal Development of Joints

Joint development begins secondarily within the early mesenchymal condensations of the precartilaginous bone at about $5^1/_2$ weeks. By 7 weeks, many joint spaces exist, and by 8 weeks, there is movement of the limbs. Figure 2–4 shows the early development. Motion is essential for the normal development of the joints and their contiguous structures.

Problems That Can Cause Congenital Joint Contractures

Joint contractures can be secondary to factors intrinsic to the developing fetus such as early-onset neurologic, muscle, and/or joint problems or to factors extrinsic to the developing fetus such as fetal crowding and constraint (Fig. 2–5).

1. *Neurologic abnormality* has been the most common cause of arthrogryposis in the experience of the author. The neurologic disorders that may be responsible for the secondary arthrogryposis include meningomyelocele; anterior motor horn cell deficiency; prenatal spasticity; and certain gross brain defects such as anencephaly, hydranencephaly, and holoprosencephaly.
2. *Muscle problems* such as muscle agenesis, rare fetal myopathies, and occasionally myotonic dystrophy.
3. *Joint and contiguous tissue problems* such as synostosis, lack of joint development, aberrant fixation of joints as in dia-

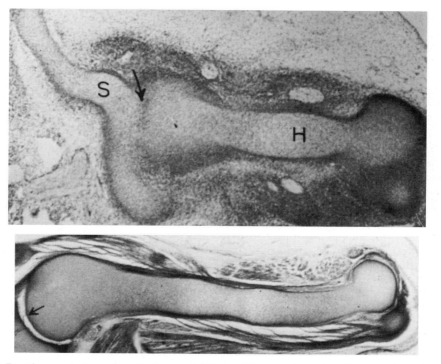

FIGURE 2–4. Development of scapulo (S) -humoral (H) shoulder joint (*arrow*) at 38 days of development (*above*) and at about 47 days (*below*). Note that joint morphogenesis occurs secondarily. By the time the joint is formed, functional muscle has differentiated.

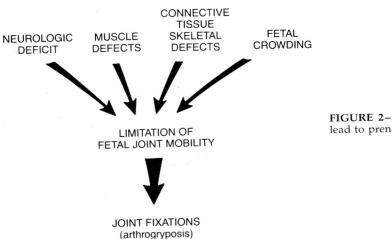

FIGURE 2–5. The types of problems that can lead to prenatal joint contractures.

strophic dysplasia, aberrant laxity of joints with dislocations as in the Larsen syndrome, and aberrant soft tissue fixations as in the popliteal pterygium syndrome.

4. *Fetal crowding and constraint* as with multiple births or with oligohydramnios in disorders such as renal agenesis or early persisting leakage of amniotic fluid.

Methods of Evaluation

1. *History.* The history relative to arthrogryposis should include information on the onset and character of fetal movements (often diminished), mode of delivery (often breech), and amniotic fluid (oligohydramnios may give rise to fetal crowding while polyhydramnios secondary to decreased fetal swallowing is sometimes seen in situations associated with neurologic abnormalities).

2. *Total pattern of anomalies.* Non–joint-related anomalies may indicate that the arthrogryposis is part of a multiple defect syndrome such as the trisomy 18 syndrome.

3. *Joint and skeletal evaluation.* Physical and radiologic assessment of joints and skeletal system is indicated. Determine whether the joint fixation is a result of an anatomic anomaly, such as lack of development of a joint or synostosis, or a deficit in functional movement with

no primary structural cause. Always check for scoliosis and for hip dislocation.

4. *Evaluation of hand and foot creases.* The palmar and finger creases and the sole creases represent the planes of early flexional function and are evident by 11 to 12 weeks of fetal age. Absent or abnormal creases are secondary to aberrant form or function in the early hand or foot development. They also provide a historical record of the flexional planes of function that have existed and thus facilitate decisions relative to rehabilitation of existing function.

5. *Search for dimples.* When close fetal contact between bone and overlying skin has occurred, there may be failure in the development of subcutaneous and adipose tissue at that locale, thereby causing a dimple. The finding of aberrant dimples implies an early fetal onset of the problem, resulting in aberrant cutaneous-osseous approximation, as shown in Fig. 2–6.

6. *Cautious neurologic and muscle assessment.* Attempts to determine whether there is a primary neurologic or muscle problem can be most difficult, since deficit in either one can lead to aberrant function of the other. Electromyographic (EMG) studies occasionally may be of value. In the great majority of patients with arthrogryposis who have abnormal study results, the evidence points toward neuropathy and

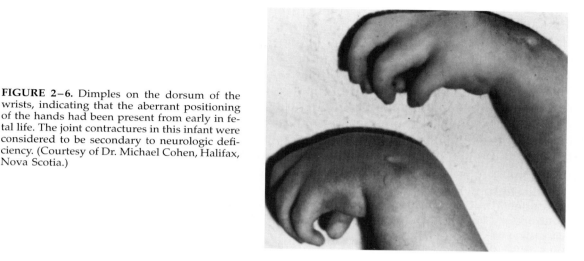

FIGURE 2–6. Dimples on the dorsum of the wrists, indicating that the aberrant positioning of the hands had been present from early in fetal life. The joint contractures in this infant were considered to be secondary to neurologic deficiency. (Courtesy of Dr. Michael Cohen, Halifax, Nova Scotia.)

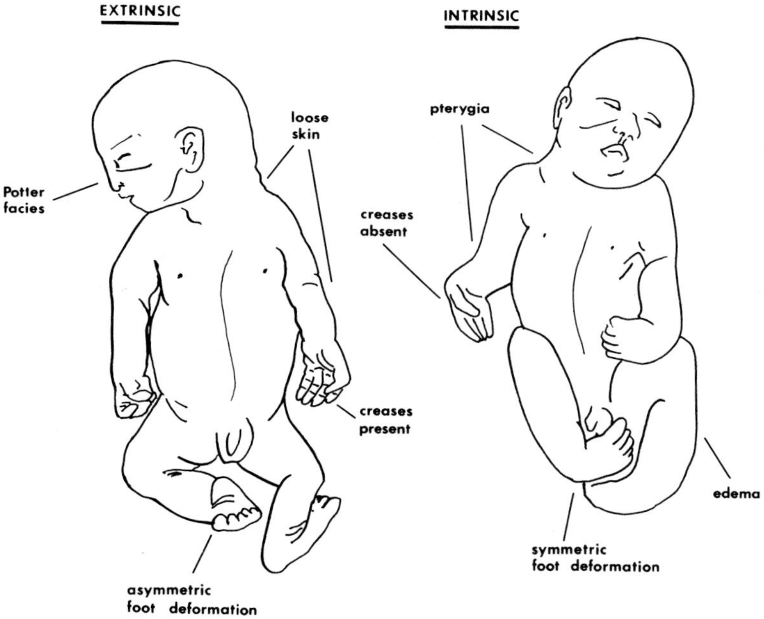

FIGURE 2–7. Differentiation between intrinsically and extrinsically derived deformational defects.

rarely to a myopathy. Muscle biopsy may only occasionally be of value, since it is difficult to determine whether muscle hypoplasia and/or fibrosis is a primary or secondary phenomenon.

7. *Distinction between joint contractures caused by a problem intrinsic to the fetus versus those due to intrauterine constraint* (Fig. 2–7). Intrinsically derived contractures are symmetric and polyhydram-nios is often present. The skin is taunt and pterygia cross the joints. Flexion creases are lacking. By contrast, the infant with extrinsically derived contractures has positional limb anomalies, large ears, and loose skin. Flexion creases are normal or often exaggerated. Distinction between these two categories is important for the family, since children with extrinsically derived

constraint-related arthrogryposis have an excellent prognosis and a low recurrence risk, while both recurrence risk and prognosis are dependent on the etiology of the joint contractures when they are intrinsically derived.

Comment and Management

When a particular diagnosis can be delineated, the management should be specific for that disorder. There remain a number of patients with multiple congenital joint contractures for whom no specific diagnosis can presently be clearly determined. Based on a study of over 350 patients with congenital contractures of joints, Dr. Judith Hall, University of British Columbia, Vancouver, has made the most significant contribution to our understanding of this problem as well as to an approach to its etiology.[19,20]

APPROACH TO AMBIGUOUS (PARTIALLY MASCULINIZED) EXTERNAL GENITALIA

Normal Development

Genes on the Y chromosome determine testicular differentiation of the gonad, which at about 8 weeks' gestation begins producing testosterone, actively causing masculinization of the external genitalia, with fusion of the labioscrotal folds to form a scrotum, enlargement of the phallus, and fusion of the labia minora folds into a penile urethra, as shown in Figure 2–8. The testes descend into the scrotum by 7 to 8 fetal months.

Methods of Evaluation

In evaluation of the child with ambiguous genitalia, the focus should be to establish an etiologic diagnosis as rapidly as possible so that sex of rearing can be assigned confidently and so that the metabolic complications of some of the potential diagnosis can be treated promptly.

With respect to sex of rearing, the vast majority of affected children can be raised in concordance with their genetic sex. The exceptions are XY infants with severe perineal malformations who have insufficient tissue to allow reconstruction of a phallus (e.g., exstrophy of the cloaca) and those XY individuals who have inadequate masculinization on the basis of androgen insensitivity.

The approach outlined in Figure 2–9 is predicated on determining if the infant is an XY individual who is incompletely masculinized or an XX individual who is virilized. Central to the diagnosis is determination of genetic sex usually by peripheral blood chromosomes. Fluorescent in situ hybridization (FISH) or molecular analysis for uniquely Y sequences may be helpful adjuncts to diagnosis but are not usually part of the initial evaluation.

A complete physical examination is extremely helpful in determining genetic sex. The presence of associated nongenital anomalies rules out the various types of congenital adrenal hyperplasia and usually indicates that the affected child has either a defect in the mesodermal primordia that form the external genitalia or incomplete masculinization from inadequate follicle-stimulating hormone (FSH) and/or luteinizing hormone (LH) production, inadequate production of cholesterol precursor for steroid hormone synthesis, or a genital malformation as part of an overall pattern of malformation, some of which are due to a chromosome abnormality. The majority of multiply malformed infants with ambiguous genitalia are XY. The only pattern of malformation that is likely to present confusion is the XX infant with the urorectal septum malformation sequence (see Chapter 1). These infants are readily identified by the lack of defined structures on the perineum (e.g., imperforate anus, no labioscrotal folds, an ill-defined phallus with or without a single perineal opening).

The algorithm in Figure 2–9 outlines the approach to the child with ambiguous external genitalia who has associated nongenital anomalies versus the child with ambiguous external genitalia who lacks associated nongenital anomalies.

Ambiguous External Genitalia with Associated Nongenital Anomalies. For infants with the urorectal septum malformation se-

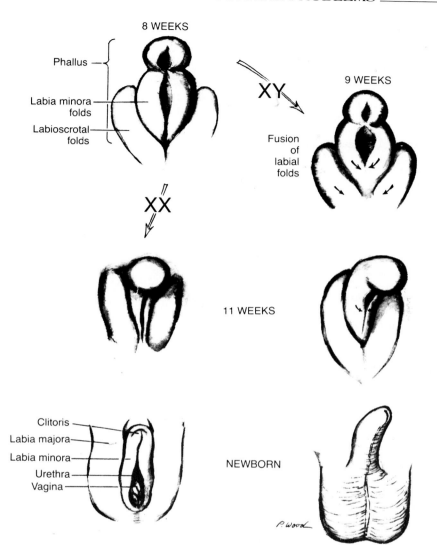

FIGURE 2–8. Normal morphogenesis of external genitalia. The normal male development is induced by testosterone derived from the fetal testicle. (Illustrations adapted from photos supplied by Dr. Jan Jirásek, Prague, Czech Republic.)

quence or ectopically positioned genital parts, search should be made for defects in other mesodermally derived structures. For infants with incomplete masculinization manifest by hypospadias and/or a shawl scrotum, evaluation of serum cholesterol and 7-dehydrocholesterol to rule out Smith-Lemli-Opitz syndrome should be performed and other multiple malformation syndromes associated with ambiguous external genitalia should be considered. For infants with ambiguity that reflects micro-

penis and cryptorchidism, the hypothalamic axis and brain need to be evaluated. It is important to recognize, however, that most patients who present with a normally structured micropenis and/or cryptorchidism lack associated nongenital anomalies.

Ambiguous External Genitalia Without Associated Nongenital Anomalies. For this group of infants, determination of the following features of the genital anatomy can often provide strong evidence for genetic sex while chromosomes are pending.

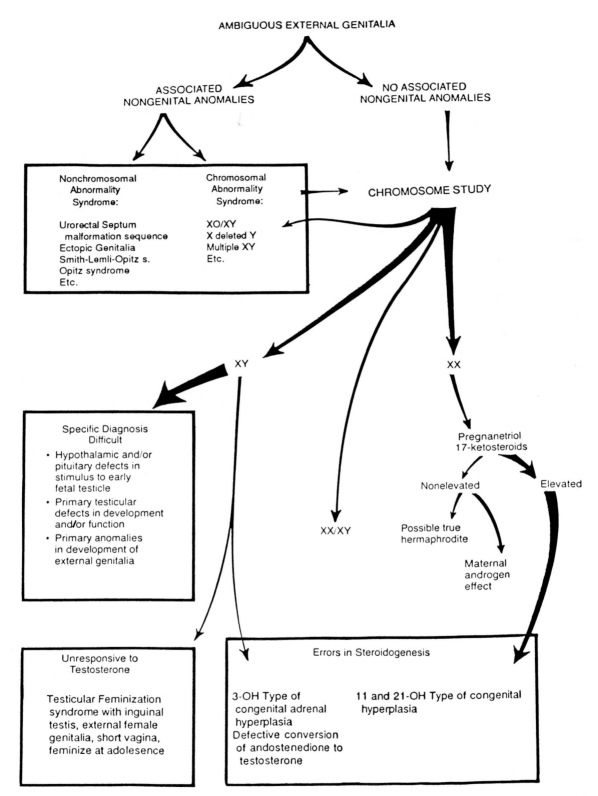

FIGURE 2–9. Approach toward arriving at a specific overall diagnosis in the patient who has ambiguous external genitalia.

Gonads. If no gonads are found in the scrotal area, place a finger over the inguinal canal to prevent the ascent of any inguinal gonad and palpate the inguinal areas carefully, ideally with three fingers. If one or more gonads are found, it is highly unlikely that the patient is a partially masculinized female, since inguinal or lower gonads are usually testes. Only in the situation of inguinal hernia may one find an ovary in the inguinal area.

Phallus. If it is a relatively thin phallus, the patient is unlikely to be a female with congenital adrenal hyperplasia, since she would be under "active" androgen stimulation with increased caliber to the phallus. If there is a single opening at the base of the phallus and also a small "pit" on the glans, the former represents the urethral opening and the latter is of no significance.

Urogenital sinus or urethra; vagina. When there is only a single opening at the base of the phallus, insert a relatively stiff catheter or sterile probe into it. Direct the catheter tip downward in the direction of the anal opening. If it goes in that direction easily and can be palpated beneath the perineal skin, there is probably a urogenital sinus with both urethral and vaginal orifices, as in the female with congenital adrenal hyperplasia. If it is "penile" urethra, the catheter will usually go cephalad and cannot be easily palpated in the perineal area. Inject radiopaque material into the single opening under pressure and obtain a lateral roentgenogram to demonstrate whether there is a vaginal pouch. If a vaginal opening is evident, insert a catheter into it and determine its depth.

Uterus. Do a cautious rectal examination with the little finger, feeling for a uterine body. When removing the finger in the neonate, stroke the anterior rectal area outward. If there is a vagina, this maneuver will often result in the extrusion of vagina mucus from the single urogenital opening. The majority of diagnoses that cause inadequate virilization of the external genitalia in an XY individual do not interfere with production of müllerian inhibiting factor. Thus on rectal exam no cervix or uterus should be palpable. In addition, pelvic ultrasound should not demonstrate müllerian derivatives.

XX individuals who are masculinized. These infants either have been exposed to exogenous androgen or have defects in adrenal steroid biosynthesis that cause them to produce endogenous androgen. The former may be identified on questioning the mother. A 17-OH-progesterone level is the most useful screen for the latter, as it will be elevated in the most common inborn error (21-hydroxylase deficiency).

XY individuals who are inadequately masculinized. These infants fall into one of three categories: (1) Those with globally inadequate androgen production either on a central (hypothalamic) or peripheral (testis) basis; (2) those with inborn errors of testosterone biosynthesis; or (3) those with androgen resistance. Since testosterone levels in the first month of life in XY individuals are usually near adult levels, measurement of FSH, LH, testosterone and its precursors can usually separate infants in category 1 (low testosterone) from categories 2 (low testosterone), elevated precursors) and 3 (normal to high testosterone). Defining the etiology of inadequate androgen production frequently involves assessment of the gonad itself. Separating patients in categories 2 and 3 may require more specific assay of genital skin fibroblasts, although category 3 patients frequently have a history of maternal female relatives with infertility.

Using this approach, it is usually possible to reach a diagnosis with a minimum of laboratory tests and a high degree of diagnostic certainty.

References

Growth Deficiency

1. Faulkner, F., ed.: Human Development. Philadelphia, W. B. Saunders Co., 1966.
2. Gardner, L. I., ed.: Endocrine and Genetic Diseases of Childhood and Adolescence, 2nd ed. Philadelphia, W. B. Saunders Co., 1975.
3. Garn, S. M., and Rohmann, C. G.: Interaction of nutrition and genetics in the timing of growth and development. Pediatr. Clin. North Am., 13: 353, 1966.
4. Tanner, J. M., Goldstein, H., and Whitehouse, R. H.: Standards for children's height at ages two to nine years allowing for height of parents. Arch. Dis. Child., 45:755, 1970.
5. Smith, D. W.: Growth and Its Disorders. Basics and Standards, Approach and Classifications,

Growth Deficiency Disorders, Growth Excess Disorders, Obesity. Philadelphia, W. B. Saunders Co., 1977.

Mental Deficiency

6. O'Rahilly, R., and Gardner, E.: The timing and sequence of events in the development of human nervous system during the embryonic period proper. Z. Anat. Entwicklungsgesch., 34:1, 1971.
7. Drillen, C. M., Jameson, S., and Wilkinson, E. M.: Studies in mental handicap, Part I: Prevalence and distribution by clinical type and severity of defect. Arch. Dis. Child., 41:528, 1966.
8. Pai, G. S.: Diagnostic approach to the etiology of mental retardation. Indian Pediatr., 31:879, 1994.
9. Jaffe, M., et al.: Diagnostic approach to the etiology of mental retardation. Isr. J. Med. Sci., 20:136, 1984.
10. Kaveggia, E. G., et al.: Diagnostic genetic studies on 1,224 patients with severe mental retardation. Proceedings of the Third Congress of the International Association for Scientific Study of Mental Deficiency. Held at The Hague, Holland, September 4–12, 1973.
11. Hunter, A. G. W., et al.: A study of institutionalized mentally retarded patients in Manitoba. I. Classification and preventability. Dev. Med. Child. Neurol., 22:145, 1980.
12. Smith, D. W., and Simons, F. E. R.: Rational diagnostic evaluation of the child with mental deficiency. Am. J. Dis. Child., 129:1285, 1975.
13. Smith, D. W., and Bostian, K. D.: Congenital anomalies associated with idiopathic mental retardation. J. Pediatr., 65:189 1964.

14. Smith, D. W., Blizzard R. M., and Wilkins, L.: The mental prognosis in hypothyroidism in infancy and childhood: A review of 128 cases. Pediatrics, 19:1011, 1957.
15. Smith, D. W., and Popich, G.: Large fontanels in congenital hypothyroidism: A potential clue toward earlier recognition. J. Pediatr., 80:753, 1972.
16. Park, V., et al.: Policy Statement: American College of Medical Genetics. Fragile X syndrome: Diagnostic and carrier testing. Am. J. Med. Genet., 53:380, 1994.

Arthrogryposis

17. Fisher, R. L., et al.: Arthrogryposis multiplexed congenita, a clinical investigation. J. Pediatr., 76:255, 1970.
18. Jones, M. C.: Intrinsic versus extrinsically derived deformational defects: A clinical approach. Semin. Perinatol., 7:237, 1983.
19. Hall, J. G., Reed, S. D., and Greene, D.: The distal arthrogryposes: Delineation of new entities—review and nosologic discussion. Am. J. Med. Genet., 11:185, 1982.
20. Hall, J. G., Reed, S. D., and Driscoll, E. P.: Part I. Amyoplasia: A common sporadic condition with congenital contractures. Am. J. Med. Genet., 15:571, 1983.

Ambiguous External Genitalia

21. Summitt, R. L.: Differential diagnosis of genital ambiguity in the newborn. Clin. Obstet. Gynecol., 15:112, 1972.
22. Guthrie, R. D., Smith, D. W., and Graham, C. B.: Testosterone treatment for the micropenis during early childhood. J. Pediatr., 83:247, 1973.

3
Morphogenesis and Dysmorphogenesis

Knowledge of normal morphogenesis may assist in the interpretation of structural defects, and the study of structural defects may assist in the understanding of normal morphogenesis. Each anomaly must have a logical mode of development and cause. When interpreting a structural defect, the clinician is looking back to an early stage in development with which he or she has often had little acquaintance. This chapter sets forth some of the phenomena of morphogenesis and the normal stages in early human development, followed by the types of abnormal morphogenesis and the relative timing of particular malformations.

NORMAL MORPHOGENESIS

Phenomena of Morphogenesis

The genetic information that guides the morphogenesis and function of an individual is all contained within the zygote. After the first few cell divisions, differentiation begins to take place, presumably through activation or inactivation of particular genes, allowing cells to assume diverse roles. The entire process is programmed in a timely and sequential order with little allowance for error, especially in early morphogenesis.

Although little is known about the fundamental processes that control morphogenesis, it is worthwhile to mention some of the normal phenomena that occur and to give examples of each.

Cell Migration

The proper migration of cells to a predestined location is critical in the develop-

ment of many structures. For example, the germ cells move from the yolk sac endoderm to the urogenital ridge, where they interact with other cells to form the gonad.

Control Over Mitotic Rate

The size of particular structures, as well as their form, is to a large extent the consequence of control over the rates of cell division.

Interaction Between Adjacent Tissues

The optic cup induces the morphogenesis of the lens from the overlying ectoderm, the ureteric bud gives rise to the development of the kidney from the adjacent metanephric tissue, the notochord is essential for normal development of the overlying neural tissue, and the prechordal mesoderm is important for the normal morphogenesis of the overlying forebrain. These are but a few examples of the many interactions that are essential features in morphogenesis.

Adhesive Association of Like Cells

In the development of a structure such as long bone, the early cells tend to aggregate closely in condensations, a membrane comes to surround them, and only later do they resemble cartilage cells. The association of like cells is dramatically demonstrated by admixing trypsinized liver and kidney cells in vitro and observing them reaggregate with their own kind.

Controlled Cell Death

Controlled cell death plays a role in normal morphogenesis. Examples include death of tissue between the digits resulting in separation of the fingers and recanalization of the duodenum. The dead cellular debris is engulfed by large macrophages, leaving no trace of the tissue.

Hormonal Influence Over Morphogenesis

Androgen effect is one example of a hormonal influence over morphogenesis—in this case, that of the external genitalia. Normally, the individual with a Y chromosome has testosterone from the fetal testicle that induces enlargement of the phallus, closure of the labia minoral folds to form a penile urethra, and fusion of the labioscrotal folds to form a scrotum. Prior to 8 week's gestation, the genitalia appear female in type and will remain so unless androgenic hormone is present.

Mechanical Forces

Mechanical forces play a major role in morphogenesis. The size, growth, and form of the brain and its early derivatives, for example, have a major function in the formation of the calvarium and upper face. The alignment of collagen fibrils and bone trabeculae relates directly to the direction of forces exerted on these tissues. The role of mechanical factors in development is covered in the text *Smith's Recognizable Patterns of Human Deformation*.

Normal Stages in Morphogenesis

The general steps in normal morphogenesis as set forth here are illustrated in Figures 3–1 to 3–16. The first week is a period of cell division without much enlargement, the conceptus being dependent on the cytoplasm of the ova for most of its metabolic needs. By 7 to 8 days, the zona pellucida is gone, and the outlying trophoblast cells invade the endometrium and form the early placenta that must function both to nourish the parasitic embryo and to maintain the pregnancy via its endocrine function. During this time, a relatively small inner cell mass has become a bilaminar disk of ectoderm and endoderm, each with its own fluid-filled cavity, the amniotic sac and yolk sac, respectively. By the end of the second week, a small mound, a primitive node, has developed in the ectoderm, and behind it a primitive streak forms. The embryo now has an axis to which further morphogenesis will relate. Cells migrate forward from the node between the ectoderm and endoderm to form an elastic cord, the notochord, which temporarily provides axial support for the embryo as well as influencing the adjacent morphogenesis. Ectodermal cells migrate through the node and the primitive streak to specific areas between the ectoderm and endoderm, becoming the mesoderm. One of the early mesodermal derivatives is a circulatory system; during the

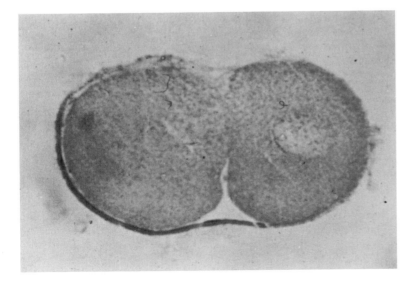

FIGURE 3–1. Two-cell specimen, within zona pellucida. (From the Department of Embryology, Carnegie Institution of Washington, D.C., Baltimore.)

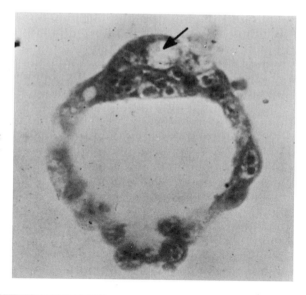

FIGURE 3–2. A 4- to 5-day blastocyst. The embryonic cell mass (*top*). (From the Department of Embryology, Carnegie Institution of Washington, D.C., Baltimore.)

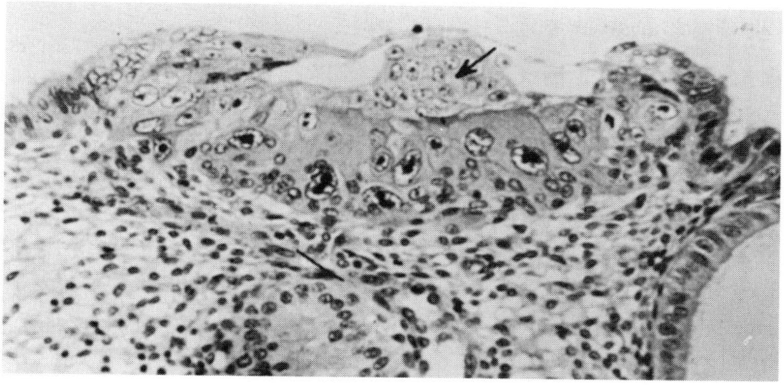

FIGURE 3–3. *Seven days.* The major part of the conceptus, the cytotrophoblast, has invaded the endometrium, and the embryo (*arrow*) is differentiating into two diverse cell layers, the ectoderm and endoderm. The amniotic cavity is beginning. (From the Department of Embryology, Carnegie Institution of Washington, D.C., Baltimore.)

FIGURE 3–4. *Fourteen to 16 days.* The thicker ectoderm (*arrow*) has its continuous amniotic sac, whereas the underlying endoderm has its yolk sac. Major changes will now begin to take place.

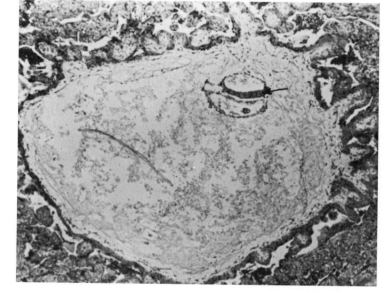

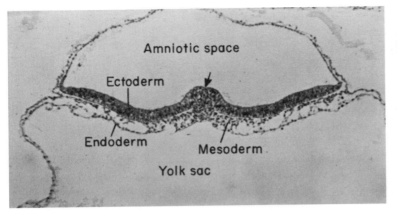

FIGURE 3–5. *Seventeen to 18 days.* Mesoblast cells migrate from the ectoderm through the node (the hillock marked by the *arrow*) and the primitive streak to specific locations between the ectoderm and endoderm, there constituting the highly versatile mesoderm. Anterior to the node the notochordal process develops, providing axial support and influencing subsequent development such as that of the overlying neural plate.

FIGURE 3–6. *Twenty-one to 23 days.* The midaxial ectoderm has thickened and formed the neural groove *arrow*, partially influenced by the underlying notochordal plate (N). Lateral to it, the mesoblast has now segmented into somites (S), intermediate mesoderm (IM), and somatopleure and splanchnopleure as intervening steps toward further differentiation. Vascular channels are developing in situ from mesoderm, blood cells are being produced in the yolk sac wall, and the early heart is beating. Henceforth, development is extremely rapid, with major changes each day.

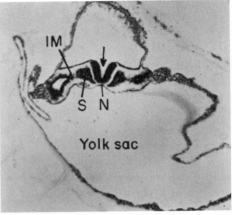

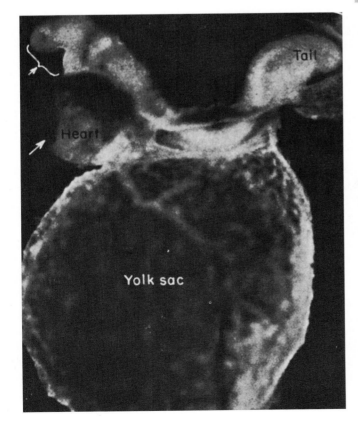

FIGURE 3–7. *Twenty-four days.* The fore part of the embryo is growing rapidly, especially the anterior neural plate. The cardiac tube, under the developing face (*arrow*), is functional. (From the Department of Embryology, Carnegie Institution of Washington, D.C., Baltimore.)

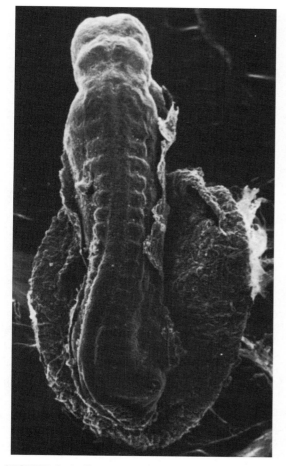

FIGURE 3–8. Scanning EM photograph of human embryo of about 23 to 25 days' gestation, with the amnion largely stripped away. This dorsal view beautifully shows the developing brain (anterior) and spinal cord just after neural tube formation and the orderly bilateral segmentation of the somites. (Courtesy of Dr. Jan E. Jirásek, Prague, Czech Republic.)

third week, the heart begins to develop, vascular channels form in situ, and blood cells are produced in the yolk sac. By the end of the third week, the heart is pumping, a neural groove has formed anterior to the node, the para-axial mesoderm has begun to be segmented into somites, the anterior and posterior regions of the embryo have begun to curl under, and the foregut and hindgut pouches become distinct. The stage is now set for the period of major organogenesis, which is best considered in relation to individual structures.

Early morphogenesis is set forth in the accompanying figures. As noted in the il-

lustrations found on the inside front cover and inside back cover of this book, each stage of development represents a synchronous syndrome of characteristics.

ABNORMAL MORPHOGENESIS

As mentioned in the introduction, there are four general types of developmental pathology leading to structural defects. The first type is malformation, which is poor formation of the tissue. The second is deformation due to altered mechanical forces on a normal tissue. Deformation may be secondary to extrinsic forces, such as uterine constraint on a normal fetus, or to intrinsic forces related to a more primary malformation. The third type of pathology is disruption, which is a result of the breakdown of a previously normal tissue. An example of the latter is porencephalic cyst of vascular causation. The fourth mechanism of abnormal morphogenesis is dysplasia, in which there is a lack of normal organization of cells into tissue. Hamartomata are examples of this latter mechanism. These anomalies represent an organizational defect leading to an abnormal admixture of tissues, often with a tumor-like excess of one or more tissues. Some have malignant potential. Examples of hamartomata are hemangiomata, melanomata, fibromata, lipomata, adenomata, and some strange admixtures that defy traditional classification.

Extrinsic deformation is set forth in a separate text, *Smith's Recognizable Patterns of Human Deformation*. A few disruption patterns of anomaly are considered in this book, as well as some dysplasias, with the major emphasis being on patterns of malformation, including malformation sequences. However, it is very important for the reader to appreciate that many of the anomalies in a given malformation sequence or syndrome are actually deformations that are engendered by the altered mechanical forces resulting from the more primary malformation. For example, most minor anomalies represent deformations, often secondary to a malformation.

Malformations may be broken down into a number of subcategories in terms of the nature of the poor formation.

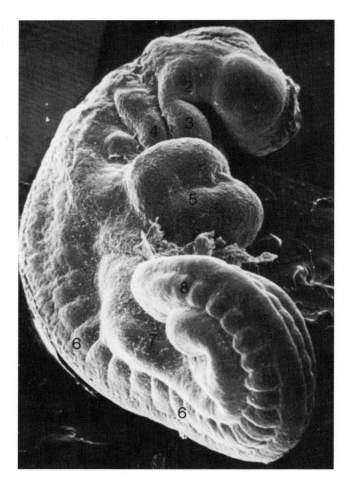

FIGURE 3–9. Scanning EM photograph of a 28- to 30-day human embryo with the amnion removed, showing the following features: *1,* early optic vesicle outpouching; *2,* maxillary swelling; *3,* mandibular swelling; *4,* hyoid swelling; *5,* heart; *6,* somites, with adjacent spinal cord; *7,* early rudiments of upper limb bud; and *8,* the tail. (Courtesy of Dr. J. E. Jirásek, Prague, Czech Republic.)

FIGURE 3–10. *Twenty-eight to 30 days.* The optic cup has begun to invaginate. Between it and the mandibular process is the area of the future mouth, where the buccopharyngeal membrane, with no intervening mesoderm, has broken down. Within the recess of the mandibular (M) and hyoid (H) processes, the future external auditory meatus will develop (*arrow*), and dorsal to it the otic vesicle (O) forms the inner ear. The relatively huge heart must pump blood in the yolk sac and developing placenta as well as to the embryo proper. Foregut outpouchings and evaginations will now begin to form various glands and the lung and liver primordia. Foregut and hindgut are now clearly delineated from the yolk sac. The somites, which will differentiate into myotomes (musculature), dermatomes (subcutaneous tissue), and sclerotomes (vertebrae), are evident on into the tail bud.

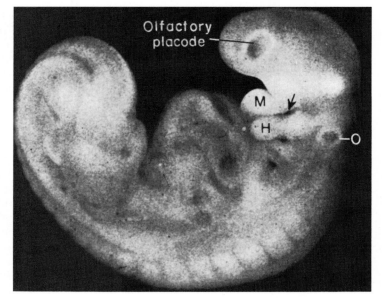

FIGURE 3–11. *About 30 to 31 days.* The brain is rapidly growing and its early cleavage into bilateral future cerebral hemispheres is evident in the telencephalic outpouching of the forebrain (FB). To the right of this is the developing eye with the optic cup (*arrow*) and the early invagination of the future lens from surface ectoderm. From the somatopleura the limb swellings (L) have developed. The loose mesenchyme of the limb bud, interacting with the thickened ectodermal cells at its tip, carries all the potential for the full development of the limb. The liver is now functional and will be a source of blood cells. The mesonephric ducts, formed in the mesonephric ridges, communicate to the cloaca, which is beginning to become septated, and the yolk sac is regressing.

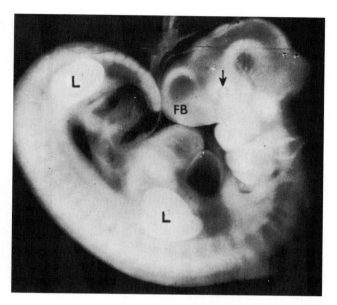

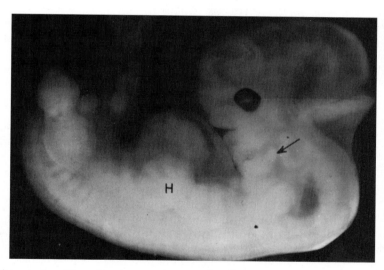

FIGURE 3–12. *Thirty-six days.* The retina is now pigmented, still incompletely closed at its inferomedial margin. Closure of the retinal fissure is nearly complete. The auricular hillocks are forming the early auricle (*arrow*) from the adjacent borders of the mandibular and hyoid swellings. The hand plate (H) has formed with condensation of mesenchyme into the five finger rays. The lower limb lags behind the upper limb in its development. The ventricular septum is partitioning the heart. The ureteral bud from the mesonephric duct has induced a kidney from the mesonephric ridge, which is also forming gonad and adrenal. Cloacal septation is nearly complete; the infraumbilical mesenchyme has filled in all the cloacal membrane except the urogenital area; and the genital tubercles are fused, whereas the labioscrotal swellings are unfused. The gut is elongating, and a loop of it may be seen projecting out into the body stalk.

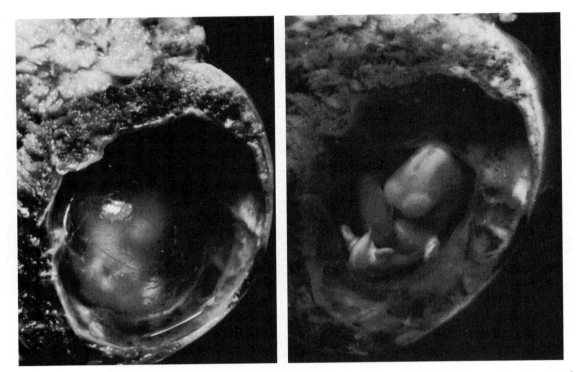

FIGURE 3–13. *Forty-two days.* In situ embryo (*left*) with the amnion removed (*right*) to show the phenomenal extent of early brain development with formation of the cerebral hemispheres, large heart, still "paddle-like" limbs, and the regressing tail. (Courtesy of Dr. Jan E. Jirásek, Prague, Czech Republic.)

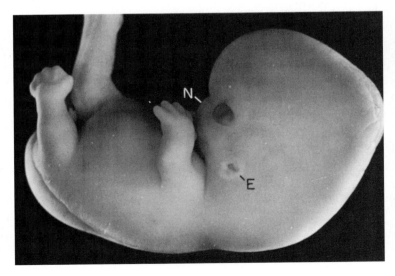

FIGURE 3–14. *Forty-five days.* The nose (N) is relatively flat, and the external ear (E) is gradually shifting in relative position as it continues to grow and develop. A neck area is now evident, the anterior body wall has formed, and the thorax and abdomen are separated by the septum transversum (diaphragm). The fingers are now partially separated, and the elbow is evident. The major period of cardiac morphogenesis and septation is complete. The urogenital membrane has now broken down, yielding a urethral opening. The phallus and lateral labioscrotal folds are the same for both sexes at this age.

FIGURE 3–15. *A 10-week male.* The eyelids have developed and fused, not to reopen until 4 to 5 months. Muscles are developed and functional, normal morphogenesis of joints is dependent on movement, and primary ossification is occurring in the centers of developing bones. In the male, the testicle has produced androgen and masculinized the external genitalia, with enlargement of the genital tubercle, fusion of the labioscrotal folds into a scrotum, and closure of the labia minoral folds to form a penile urethra, these structures being unchanged in the female. The testicle does not descend into the scrotum until 8 or 9 months.

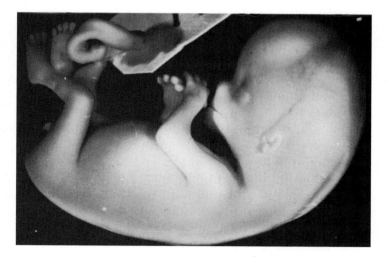

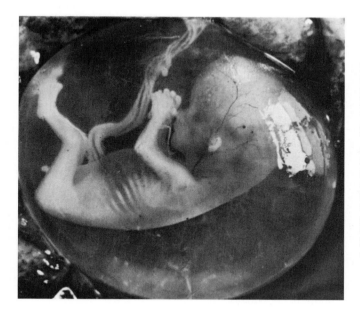

FIGURE 3–16. A 3½-*month male.* The fetus is settling down for the latter two thirds of prenatal life. The morphogenesis of the lung, largely solid at this point in development, will not have progressed to the capacity for aerobic exchange for another 3 to 4 months. The skin is increasing in thickness, and its accessory structures are differentiating. The form of the palmar surface of the hand and foot, especially the character of the prominent apical and other pads, will influence the patterning of parallel dermal ridges that form transversely to the relative lines of growth stress on the palms and soles between 16 and 19 weeks. Subcutaneous tissue is thin, and adipose tissue does not develop until 7 to 8 months.

TABLE 3-1. RELATIVE TIMING AND DEVELOPMENTAL PATHOLOGY OF CERTAIN MALFORMATIONS

Tissues	Malformation	Defect In	Causes Prior To	Comment
Central nervous system	Anencephaly	Closure of anterior neural tube	26 days	Subsequent degeneration of forebrain
	Meningomyelocele	Closure in a portion of the posterior neural tube	28 days	80% lumbosacral
Face	Cleft lip	Closure of lip	36 days	42% associated with cleft palate
	Cleft maxillary palate	Fusion of maxillary palatal shelves	10 weeks	
	Branchial sinus and/or cyst	Resolution of branchial cleft	8 weeks	Preauricular and along the line anterior to sternocleidomastoid
Gut	Esophageal atresia plus tracheoesophageal fistula	Lateral septation of foregut into trachea and foregut	30 days	
	Rectal atresia with fistula	Lateral septation of cloaca into rectum and urogenital sinus	6 weeks	
	Duodenal stresia	Recanalization of duodenum	7 to 8 weeks	Associated incomplete or aberrant mesenteric attachments
	Malrotation of gut	Rotation of intestinal loop so that cecum lies to the right	10 weeks	
	Omphalocele	Return of midgut from yolk sac to abdomen	10 weeks	
	Meckel diverticulum	Obliteration of vitelline duct	10 weeks	May contain gastric and/or pancreatic tissue
	Diaphragmatic hernia	Closure of pleuroperitoneal canal	6 weeks	
Genitourinary system	Exstrophy of bladder	Migration of infraumbilical mesenchyme	30 days	Associated müllerian and wolffian duct defects
	Bicornuate uterus	Fusion of lower portion of müllerian ducts	10 weeks	
	Hypospadias	Fusion of urethral folds (labia minora)	12 weeks	
	Cryptorchidism	Descent of testical into scrotum	7 to 9 months	
Heart	Transposition of great vessels	Directional development of bulbus cordis septum	34 days	
	Ventricular septal defect	Closure of ventricular septum	6 weeks	
	Patent ductus arteriosus	Closure of ductus arteriosus	9 to 10 months	
Limb	Aplasia of radius	Genesis of radial bone	38 days	Often accompanied by other defects of radial side of distal limb
	Syndactyly, severe	Separation of digital rays	6 weeks	
Complex	Cyclopia, holoprosencephaly	Prechordal mesoderm development	23 days	Secondary defects of midface and forebrain

Types of Malformation

Incomplete Morphogenesis

These are anomalies that represent incomplete stages in the development of a structure; they include the following subcategories, with one example listed for each:

Lack of development: renal agenesis secondary to failure of ureter formation.

Hypoplasia: micrognathia.

Incomplete separation: syndactyly (cutaneous).

Incomplete closure: cleft palate.

Incomplete septation: ventricular septal defect.

Incomplete migration of mesoderm: exstrophy of bladder.

Incomplete rotation: malrotation of the gut.

Incomplete resolution of early form: Meckel diverticulum.

Persistence of earlier location: cryptorchidism.

Aberrant Form

An occasional anomaly may be interpreted as an aberrant form that never exists in any stage of normal morphogenesis. An example is the pelvic spur in the nail-patella syndrome. Such an anomaly may be more specific for a particular clinical syndrome entity than anomalies of incomplete morphogenesis.

Accessory Tissue

Accessory tissue such as polydactyly, preauricular skin tags, and accessory spleens may be presumed to have been initiated at approximately the same time as the normal tissue, developing into finger rays, auricular hillocks of His, and spleen, respectively.

Functional Defects

Function is a necessary feature in joint development, and hence joint contractures such as clubfoot may be caused by functional deficit in the use of the lower limb resulting from a more primary malformation.

RELATIVE TIMING OF MALFORMATIONS

Malformations resulting from incomplete morphogenesis usually have their origin *prior* to the time when normal development would have proceeded beyond the form represented by the malformation. This type of developmental timing should not be construed as indicating that something happened *at* a particular time; all one can say is that a problem existed *prior* to a particular time. Serious errors in early morphogenesis seldom allow for survival; hence, only a few malformation problems are seen that can be said to have occurred prior to 23 days. The cyclopia-cebocephaly type of defect appears to be the consequence of a defect in the prechordal mesoderm, and presumably developed prior to 23 days. Aside from this example, the vast majority of serious malformations represent errors that occur after 3 weeks of development.

Table 3–1 sets forth the relative timing as well as the presumed developmental error for some of the malformations that appear to represent incomplete stages in morphogenesis.

References

Ebert, J. D., and Sussex, I.: Interacting Systems in Development. New York, Holt, Rinehart & Winston, 1970.

Graham, J. M.: Smith's Recognizable Patterns of Human Deformation, 2nd ed. Philadelphia, W. B. Saunders Co., 1988.

Gilbert, S. F.: Developmental Biology, 4th ed., Sunderland, Mass., Sinauer Associates, 1994.

Hamilton, W. J., Boyd, J. D., and Mossman, H. W.: Human Embryology, Baltimore, Williams & Wilkins Co., 1962.

Millen, J. W.: Timing of human congenital malformations. Dev. Med. Child. Neurol., 5:343, 1963.

Moore, K. L., and Persaud, T. V. N.: The Developing Human: Clinically Oriented Embryology, 5th ed. Philadelphia, W. B. Saunders Co., 1993.

Moore, K. L., Persaud, T. V. N., and Shiota, K.: Color Atlas of Human Embryology. Philadelphia, W. B. Saunders Co., 1994.

O'Rahilly, R., and Muller, F.: Human Embryology and Teratology. New York, Wiley-Liss, 1992.

Sadler, T. W.: Langman's Medical Embryology, 6th ed. Baltimore, Williams & Wilkins Co., 1990.

Nilsson, L., Ingelman-Sundberg, A., and Wirsen, C.: A Child is Born. New York, Dell Books, 1986.

Streeter, G. L.: Developmental Horizons in Human Embryos; Age Groups XI to XXIII. Washington, D.C., Carnegie Institute of Washington, 1951.

Willis, R. A.: The Borderland of Embryology and Pathology. Washington, Butterworth, 1962.

4

Genetics, Genetic Counseling, and Prevention

The basic process of morphogenesis is genetically controlled. However, the ability of an individual to reach his or her genetic potential with respect to structure, growth, and/or cognitive development is impacted by environmental factors in both prenatal and postnatal life. Review of the etiologies of those structural abnormalities and syndromes for which an etiology is known indicates that the majority of malformations and syndromes appear to be genetically determined. The purpose of this chapter is to outline the most prevalent mechanisms through which genetic abnormalities impact morphogenesis, to suggest genetic counseling strategies for each, and to discuss approaches to prevention.

The structure and function of a human being is determined by roughly 100,000 genes, which come in pairs. The great majority of these genes are distributed in the 46 chromosomes that are found in the nucleus of the cell. A few genes reside in the cytoplasm inside the mitochondria, the energy-producing apparatus of the cell. Genetic abnormalities may be grossly divided into those that affect gene dosage (chromosomal abnormalities), those that involve changes in the actual genes themselves (single-gene disorders), and those that create a susceptibility to developmental errors that is then modified by factors in the environment (multifactorial inheritance). The frequency with which each of these genetic mechanisms contributes to malformation and disease depends upon the time in development at which inquiry is made. For example, roughly half of all first-trimester miscarriages are a consequence of chromosomal abnormalities, whereas only 6 of 1000 live-born infants are similarly affected. Figure 4–1 provides a perspective as to the frequency with which each mechanism contributes to birth defects and/or human disease over the lifetime of a population. Each of these problems is considered separately as it relates to malformation, especially multiple defect syndromes. Recommended genetic counseling is presented at the end of each section.

GENETIC IMBALANCE DUE TO GROSS CHROMOSOMAL ABNORMALITIES

The 46 normal chromosomes consist of 22 homologous pairs of autosomes plus an XX pair of sex chromosomes in the female or an XY pair in the male. Normal development is not only dependent on the gene content of these chromosomes but on the gene balance as well. An altered number of chromosomes most commonly arises because of fault in chromosome distribution at cell division. During the gametic meiotic reduction division (Fig. 4–2), one of each pair of autosomes and one of the sex chromosomes are distributed randomly to each daughter cell, whereas during mitosis (Fig. 4–3) each replicated chromosome is separated longitudinally at the centromere such

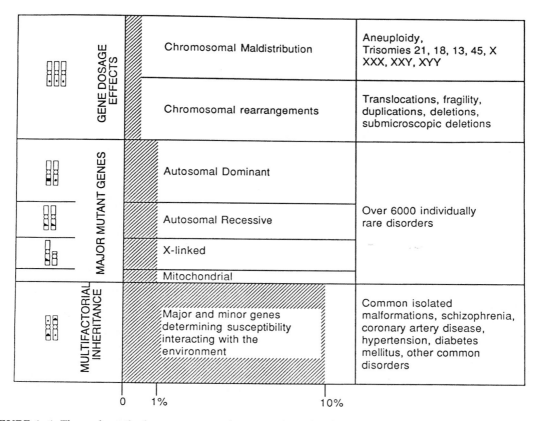

		Chromosomal Maldistribution	Aneuploidy, Trisomies 21, 18, 13, 45, X XXX, XXY, XYY
GENE DOSAGE EFFECTS		Chromosomal rearrangements	Translocations, fragility, duplications, deletions, submicroscopic deletions
MAJOR MUTANT GENES		Autosomal Dominant	Over 6000 individually rare disorders
		Autosomal Recessive	
		X-linked	
		Mitochondrial	
MULTIFACTORIAL INHERITANCE		Major and minor genes determining susceptibility interacting with the environment	Common isolated malformations, schizophrenia, coronary artery disease, hypertension, diabetes mellitus, other common disorders

0   1%   10%

FIGURE 4–1. The scale at the base represents the percentage of individuals born who do have, or will have, a problem in life secondary to a genetic difference. The three categories of genetic aberration are depicted to the left. The *dots* within the chromosomes represent "normal" genes, the *bar* represents a dominant mutant gene, the *hash-bar* represents a recessive mutant gene, and the *triangles* denote major and minor genes that confer susceptibility to a given process.

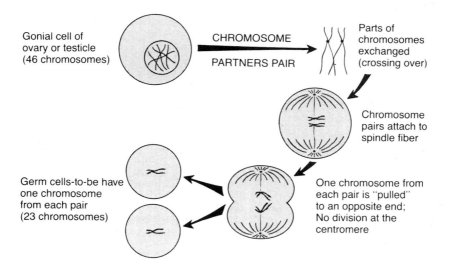

Gonial cell of ovary or testicle (46 chromosomes)

CHROMOSOME PARTNERS PAIR

Parts of chromosomes exchanged (crossing over)

Chromosome pairs attach to spindle fiber

Germ cells-to-be have one chromosome from each pair (23 chromosomes)

One chromosome from each pair is "pulled" to an opposite end; No division at the centromere

FIGURE 4–2. Meiotic reduction division in development of gametes (sex cells). One pair of chromosomes is followed through the cycle.

that each daughter cell receives an identical complement of genetic material.

Figure 4–4 shows the natural appearance of the stained chromosomes at early, middle, and later stages of mitosis. It would obviously be difficult to count these chromosomes or to distinguish their individual structure from such preparations. In order to obtain adequate preparations for the study of chromosome number and morphology, the cultured cells are treated with an agent that blocks the spindle formation and thus leads to the accumulation of cells at the metaphase of mitosis. These cells are then exposed to a hypotonic solution that spreads the unattached chromosomes, allowing for such preparations as that shown in Figure 4–5. Various techniques, such as trypsin treatment and Giemsa staining, can be employed to allow for the identification of individual chromosomes. The development of synchronized culture techniques that allow evaluation of chromosomes in prophase and prometaphase have greatly enhanced the ability to detect subtle abnormalities and have expanded our understanding of the impact of chromosomal rearrangement on morphogenesis. A chromosome analysis using this technique is a high-resolution analysis (Fig. 4–6).

Figure 4–7 illustrates some of the mechanisms that can lead to genetic imbalance (too many or too few copies of normal genes) as a consequence of chromosomal rearrangement and maldistribution. Such abnormalities occur in at least 4 per cent of recognized pregnancies. Most of these imbalances have such an adverse effect on morphogenesis that the conceptus does not survive. Figure 4–8 summarizes the frequency and types of chromosomal abnormalities found in newborns and spontaneous abortuses. About 50 per cent of the latter have a chromosome abnormality compared to 0.5 per cent of live-born babies. The nature of the abnormalities detected in live-born infants differs from those seen in abortuses, with sex chromosomal aneuploidies and trisomy 21 (Down syndrome) accounting for most of the anomalies observed because these are least likely to have an early lethal effect. It has been estimated that only about 1 in 500 45,X conceptuses survives to term compared to 4 per cent of trisomy 18 and 13, and 20 per cent of trisomy 21 conceptuses. There are some data to suggest that survival is impacted by the presence of a normal as well as an aneuploid cell line (mosaicism).

Although little is known about the etiology of faulty chromosomal distribution, one recognized factor is older maternal age. This applies especially to the autosomal trisomy syndromes and, to a lesser extent,

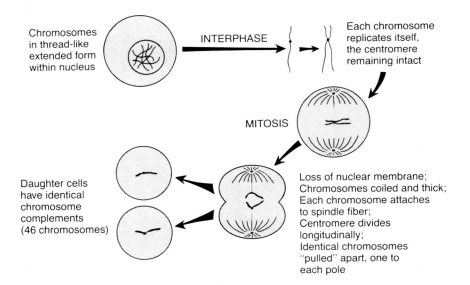

FIGURE 4–3. Normal mitotic cell division. One chromosome is followed through the cycle.

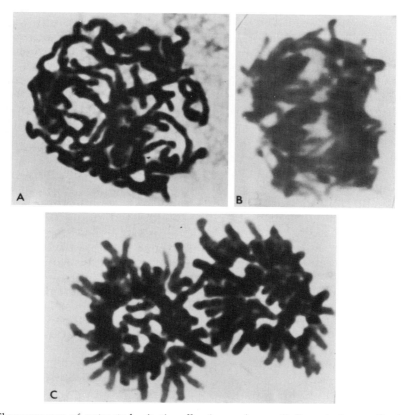

FIGURE 4–4. Chromosomes of untreated mitotic cells: *A*, prophase cell; *B*, metaphase cell with chromosomes attached to the spindle fibers and beginning to separate; *C*, anaphase cell with identical chromosomal complements having been "pulled apart" toward the development of two daughter cells.

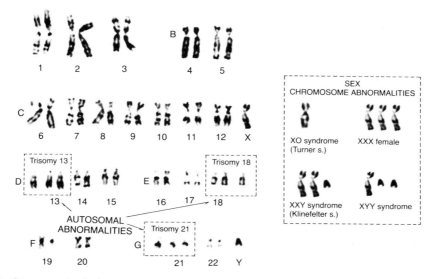

FIGURE 4–5. Giemsa-stained chromosomes arranged into a karyotype by letter grouping and number designation on the basis of length of the chromosome, position of the centromere, and banding patterns. The most common types of aneuploidy are shown within the boxes.

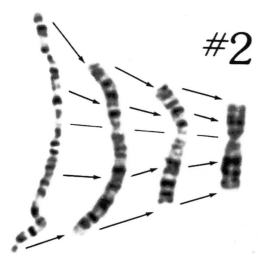

FIGURE 4–6. Giemsa-stained chromosome number 2 harvested at different points in the cell cycle. The prometaphase appearance is on the left, while the metaphase is on the right. Note the dramatic increase in detail visible in the prometaphase chromosome. (Courtesy of Dr. James T. Mascarello, Children's Hospital, San Diego, Calif.)

some of the sex chromosome aneuploidies. Figure 4–9 shows the progressive increase in the frequency of live-born infants with the Down syndrome during the later period of a woman's reproductive life. The frequency of aneuploidy detected by amniocentesis at 14 to 16 weeks' gestation is appreciably higher because some of the aneuploid conceptuses detected at this early stage in gestation would normally abort spontaneously or die in utero later in pregnancy.

The timing of the error in chromosome distribution can seldom be stated with assurance from a routine karyotype, although molecular techniques, as will be discussed below, have permitted detailed investigation of this issue in certain aneuploidy states. Numerical errors may result from altered chromosomal segregation in the cells that will give rise to the germ cells (gonadal mosaicism), or in either the first or second division of meiosis leading to an abnormal chromosome number in the egg or sperm (nondisjunction), or during the first division of the newly formed zygote. Errors in the assortment of chromosomes may also occur later in embryogenesis, giving rise to mosaic individuals who have two populations of cells from the standpoint of chromosome number. Mosaicism also develops when a trisomic conceptus "self-corrects" and loses one copy of the trisomic chromosome in early cell division, thus establishing a normal along with the aneuploid cell line. Individuals who are mosaic for a condition show every gradation of the phenotype associated with that chromosomal abnormality, from a pattern indistinguishable from complete aneuploidy to near normal appearance and function. In general, the degree of mosaicism present in the peripheral blood is not, in and of itself, that helpful in predicting prognosis. Detection of mosaicism may require the sampling of more than one tissue such as assessment of cultured fibroblasts from a skin biopsy.

New molecular techniques that allow identification of the parent of origin of individual chromosomes have shed some light on the source of the extra or deleted chromosome and the stage of cell division during which accidents leading to aneuploidy occur. In conceptuses and live-born individuals with 45,X, the chromosome that is deleted is usually paternal in origin.[1] This is consistent with the observation that maternal age is not related to a 45,X karyotype in the fetus. By contrast, the extra chromosome in trisomy 21 is of maternal origin in 95 per cent of cases.[2] Most of the maternal errors involve nondisjunction in meiosis I.[3] Of the paternally derived chromosomes, most represent errors in meiosis II. Similarly, the extra X chromosome in 47,XXX females is usually maternally derived. In 47,XXY the source of the extra chromosome appears to be equally divided.[4] In those cases of 47,XXY and XXX with a maternally derived extra chromosome, increasing maternal age correlated with errors in the first meiotic cell division but not with errors in meiosis II or in postzygotic events. The etiology of nondisjunction is unknown. Although relatively little is known about the frequency of aneuploidy in normal human oocytes, between 1 and 5 per cent of sperm from chromosomally normal men are aneuploid.

In addition to errors in chromosome number, genetic imbalance can result from chromosomal rearrangement (Fig. 4–7). A break in one chromosome may result in loss

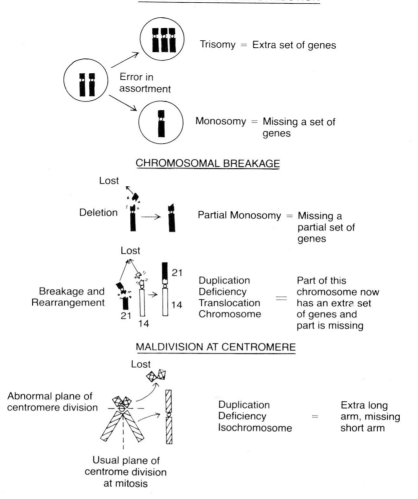

FIGURE 4–7. Types of chromosomal abnormalities leading to genetic imbalance.

of information (deletion). If more than one chromosome breaks, rearrangement of the resulting pieces may take place creating a translocation. An individual can have a translocation between chromosomes with no evident problem as long as he or she has a balanced set of genes. However, as illustrated in Figure 4–10, a balanced carrier of a translocation has a significant risk of producing unbalanced germ cells during the meiotic reduction division, meiosis I. Should a germ cell receive the translocation chromosome as well as the normal 21 chromosome from the same parent, the resulting zygote would be trisomic for most of chromosome 21. Such individuals generally

have Down syndrome. About 4 per cent of patients with Down syndrome have 46 chromosomes, with the extra set being attached to another chromosome. Similarly, a small proportion of patients with the trisomy 18 or trisomy 13 syndromes have the extra set of genes attached as part of a translocation chromosome.

Less commonly, a pattern of malformation will result from a deletion of chromosomal material in which the missing piece is so small that routine chromosome analysis cannot detect the abnormality. Such conditions are referred to as microdeletion syndromes to denote the fact that the phenotype is a consequence of imbalance in

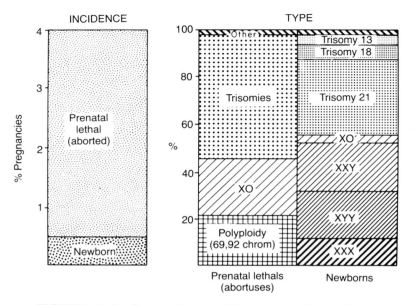

FIGURE 4–8. Incidence and types of chromosomal abnormalities.

dosage of several genes that lie next to each other along a chromosome.

The major reason for doing chromosome studies on individuals with autosomal trisomy syndromes, beyond confirmation of the clinical diagnosis, is to determine whether the patient has a translocation chromosome rather than the more usual complete trisomy. If a translocation is identified, then both parents should be studied to determine whether either of them is a balanced translocation carrier with a con-

sequent increased risk of having affected offspring. Fortunately, only about one third of the patients with partial translocation trisomy will be found to have a carrier parent, because most of them represent fresh occurrences for which there is a negligible recurrence risk.

Surveys of the incidence of chromosomal abnormalities in newborns have documented that roughly 1 in 520 normal individuals has a balanced structural chromosomal rearrangement, whereas 1 in 1700 newborns has an unbalanced rearrangement. Systematic surveys of undiagnosed children with mental retardation and multiple structural defects have documented an 8 per cent incidence of chromosome abnormalities.[5] With the use of high-resolution chromosome analysis, subtle abnormalities, which would have escaped detection on a routine study, will be identified in an additional 1.1 per cent of patients evaluated for similar indications.[6]

In clinical situations in which a specific disorder is known to be associated with a characteristic but subtle cytogenetic abnormality (microdeletion syndrome), a focused chromosome analysis may be recommended to address the question. High-resolution methodology is imperative for this type of evaluation. An alternative

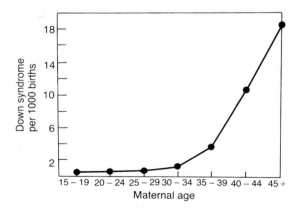

FIGURE 4–9. Increasing incidence of the Down syndrome during the latter period of a woman's reproductive period. (From Smith, D. W.: Am. J. Obstet. Gynecol., *90*:1055, 1964, with permission.)

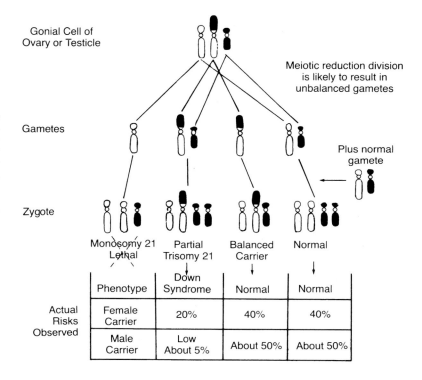

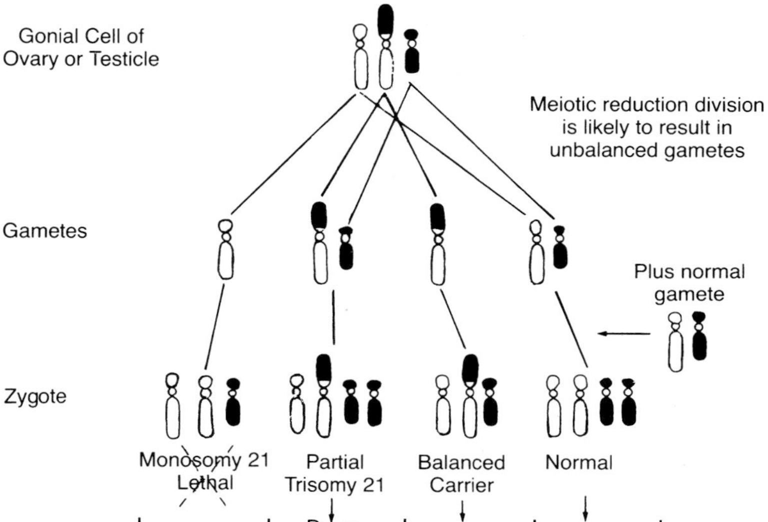
Gonial Cell of
Ovary or Testicle
Meiotic reduction division
is likely to result in
unbalanced gametes
Gametes
Plus normal
gamete
Zygote
Monosomy 21
Lethal
Partial
Trisomy 21
Balanced
Carrier
Normal

	Phenotype	Down Syndrome	Normal	Normal
Actual Risks Observed	Female Carrier	20%	40%	40%
	Male Carrier	Low About 5%	About 50%	About 50%

FIGURE 4–10. Potential inheritance from balanced translocation carrier using a 21/14 translocation as an example. Only chromosomes 21 and 14 are depicted. The translocation could be constitutional (in all the cells in the body) or a fresh occurrence in the gonial cell (gonadal mosaicism). The cartoon illustrates the theoretical risk for balanced and unbalanced offspring. The table beneath lists the actual observed risks by sex of the carrier parent. For many rare translocations this type of empiric information is not available. The example documents how difficult it is to predict the actual outcome in the offspring of translocation carriers.

laboratory approach that has proved quite useful in this situation is fluorescent in situ hybridization (FISH). In this technique, a molecular probe of DNA, complementary to the sequence to be identified, is synthesized and tagged with a fluorescent marker. When applied to cultured cells, the probe hybridizes with its complementary sequence and a fluorescent signal can be detected. The technique allows ready identification of the number of copies of the sequence in question in a given cell (Fig.

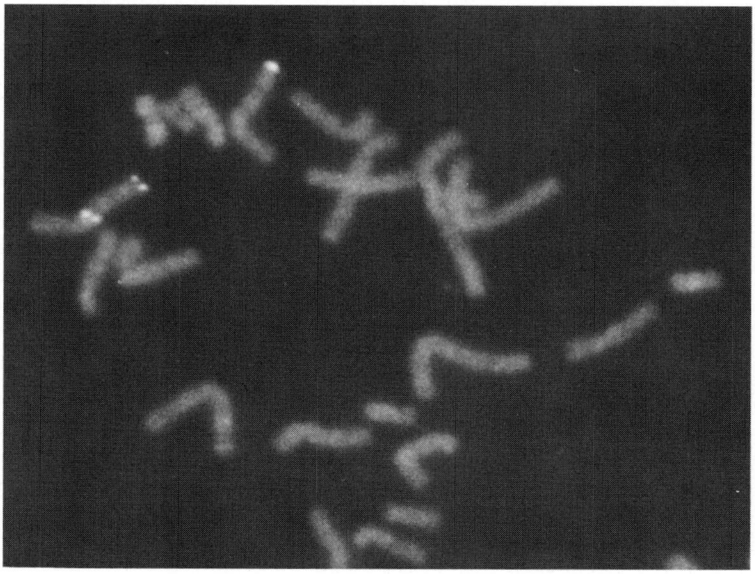

FIGURE 4–11. FISH analysis for elastin locus in a patient with Williams syndrome. Two fluorescent probes are used. One hybridizes with the telomere of chromosome 7 allowing ready identification of both chromosomes. The second probe identifies the elastin locus. In this patient only one signal is visible, consistent with a submicroscopic deletion in the other chromosome. (Courtesy of Dr. James T. Mascarello, Children's Hospital, San Diego, Calif.)

4–11). Focused analysis has proved useful in the diagnosis of Prader-Willi syndrome, 11p13 deletion causing aniridia and Wilms tumor, and in some cases of del(4p) syndrome. FISH probes are available for the diagnosis of Prader-Willi syndrome, DiGeorge sequence/velocardiofacial syndrome, and Williams syndrome, among others. Both techniques are most useful when there is a high index of clinical suspicion.

Another type of chromosomal abnormality that can lead to genetic imbalance is maldivision or breakage at the centromere during mitosis, leading to the formation of an isochromosome (Fig. 4–7). The cell receiving the isochromosome has an extra dose of the long arm of the parent chromosome and is missing the set of genes on the short arm. Occasionally, autosomal trisomy syndromes may be found to have an isochromosome of the long arm (21, 13, or 18) accounting for the imbalance. Also, isochromosome X accounts for roughly 10 per cent of the cases of Turner syndrome in liveborn female infants.

GENETIC COUNSELING FOR CHROMOSOMAL ABNORMALITIES

Autosomal Trisomy Syndromes

Chromosomal studies are warranted on all individuals suspected of having an autosomal trisomy syndrome in order to determine whether full trisomy (47 chromosomes) or an unbalanced translocation is involved. If a full trisomy is identified, the risk for recurrence is roughly 1 per cent. For older mothers, the risk is based upon the maternal age at delivery in the subsequent pregnancy. Parental karyotypes are suggested *only* if a second child in the same sibship has an identical trisomy. In this rare circumstance, mosaicism in one of the parents may be detected in as many as 38 per cent of families if a diligent search is made. The presence of a second- or third-degree relative with a similar trisomy can be accounted for by chance alone and does not appear to increase the risk for recurrence.[7]

Should an unbalanced translocation be identified, both parents must be evaluated to determine if either one is a balanced translocation carrier, a finding in about one third of cases. The recurrence risk for chromosomally normal parents is very small (probably less than 1 per cent) and reflects the unlikely possibility of gonadal mosaicism that cannot be identified by peripheral blood karyotype. The recurrence risk for a carrier parent is obviously greater, but is often less than the theoretical possibilities might indicate (Fig. 4–10).

Informing parents that their child has an autosomal trisomy is best accomplished in as straightforward yet compassionate a manner as possible. Knowledge of the natural history of the specific trisomy should serve as a guideline for anticipatory guidance; however, it is best to approach the child as an individual with respect to such issues as survival (in trisomy 18 and 13) and intellectual potential (in trisomy 21). The karyotype does not predict either of these issues with complete accuracy. There is no substitute for clinical correlation and longitudinal follow-up.

Other Chromosomal Disorders

45,X Syndrome

Suspicion of Turner syndrome should lead to a chromosome study. Although a wide variety of chromosomal rearrangements are known to produce the phenotype (including X/XX mosaicism, X,iso X, or X, deleted X) the recurrence risk for these arrangements is low to negligible.

Any Case With a Deletion, Duplication, or Unbalanced Translocation

In this situation, chromosome studies should be done on both parents to rule out a rearrangement such as a pericentric inversion or balanced translocation that could predispose to recurrence of the abnormality. If parental karyotypes are normal, as is the case in the majority of families, the recurrence risk is low. If a parental rearrangement is identified, the theoretical risk for recurrence is increased. For some of the more common rearrangements, empiric risk figures are available in the literature. The actual risks often do not coincide with the theoretical risk as has been previously reviewed (Fig. 4–10).

Microdeletion Syndromes

Although microdeletion syndromes are chromosomal abnormalities because the problem that produces the phenotype is genetic imbalance rather than genetic mutation and because the abnormality is identified using cytogenetic methodology, from a counseling standpoint the conditions behave like dominantly inherited mendelian disorders. The majority of cases represent de novo events that carry a negligible risk for recurrence. Evaluation of parents using FISH analysis or focused high-resolution cytogenetics may be recommended, since vertical transmission of microdeletion syndromes is reported. However, the overwhelming majority of parents who are identified to have deletions also express the phenotype to some degree. Recurrence risk for these individuals is 50 per cent for each subsequent pregnancy.

GENETIC IMBALANCE DUE TO SINGLE-GENE DISORDERS

Genes located on the X chromosome are referred to as X-linked genes and those on the autosomes as autosomal genes. Man is a diploid organism with two sets of chromosomes, one set being derived from each parent. Each pair of chromosomes will have comparable gene determinants located at the same position on each chromosome pair. The pair of genes may be referred to as *alleles*, or partners, which normally work together. Thus with the exception of the genes of the X and Y chromosomes in the male, each genetic determinant is present in two doses, one from each parent. A mutant gene indicates a changed gene. A major mutant gene is herein defined as a genetic determinant that has changed in such a way that it can give rise to an abnormal characteristic. If a mutant gene in single dose produces an abnormal characteristic despite the presence of a normal allele (partner), it is referred to as dominant because it causes abnormality even when counterbalanced by a normal gene partner. A mutant gene that causes an abnormal characteristic when present in double dosage (or single dosage

without a normal partner, as for an X-linked mutant gene in the male) is referred to as recessive. These principles, set forth diagrammatically in Figure 4–12, reflect mendelian laws of inheritance, which equate the presence of an altered gene or pair of genes with a phenotype or trait. As more is learned about the molecular biology of mutant genes, the distinction between dominant and recessive genes becomes blurred. In general, however, mutations in genes that code for structural proteins, in which an abnormal product is made, tend to function in a dominant fashion, since the abnormal product often has the capacity to interfere with the function of the product of the normal partner. The various forms of osteogenesis imperfecta are good examples of dominant mutations. Since collagen is a triple helical molecule, mutations that give rise to one abnormal procollagen molecule will impact the final assembly process. Recessive mutations often serve to reduce the quantity of product made by half; however, many biologic systems are forgiving of quantitative decrease in enzyme function, hence the silence of recessive mutations when present in single copy. Hurler syndrome is an example. Half of the normal amount of activity of alpha-iduronidase has no effect on the individual with the altered gene; however, the enzyme deficiency resulting from a double dose of the altered gene produces a severe phenotype.

Expression is a term used to indicate the extent of abnormality that is due to a genetic aberration. The expression may be stated as severe, usual, mild, or no expression, the latter being synonymous with lack of penetrance in an individual who has the genetic aberration. Individuals with the same genetic aberration frequently show variance in expression, especially with respect to structural defects.

Traditionally, the mutant gene disorders have been categorized into those due to genes located on the autosomes—autosomal dominant and autosomal recessive—and disorders due to genes on the X chromosome—X-linked dominant and X-linked recessive.

Autosomal Dominant Disorders

Autosomal dominant disorders show a wide variation in expression among af-

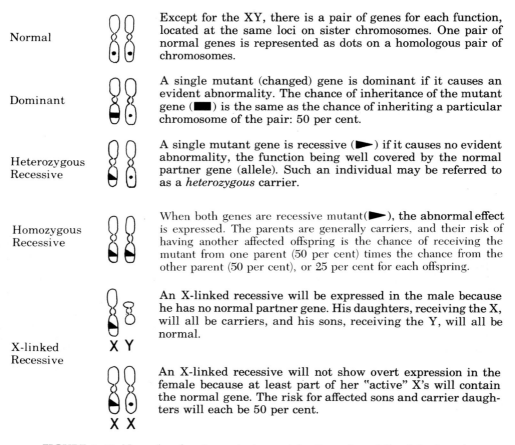

Normal

Except for the XY, there is a pair of genes for each function, located at the same loci on sister chromosomes. One pair of normal genes is represented as dots on a homologous pair of chromosomes.

Dominant

A single mutant (changed) gene is dominant if it causes an evident abnormality. The chance of inheritance of the mutant gene (■) is the same as the chance of inheriting a particular chromosome of the pair: 50 per cent.

Heterozygous Recessive

A single mutant gene is recessive (►) if it causes no evident abnormality, the function being well covered by the normal partner gene (allele). Such an individual may be referred to as a *heterozygous* carrier.

Homozygous Recessive

When both genes are recessive mutant(►), the abnormal effect is expressed. The parents are generally carriers, and their risk of having another affected offspring is the chance of receiving the mutant from one parent (50 per cent) times the chance from the other parent (50 per cent), or 25 per cent for each offspring.

X-linked Recessive

An X-linked recessive will be expressed in the male because he has no normal partner gene. His daughters, receiving the X, will all be carriers, and his sons, receiving the Y, will all be normal.

An X-linked recessive will not show overt expression in the female because at least part of her "active" X's will contain the normal gene. The risk for affected sons and carrier daughters will each be 50 per cent.

FIGURE 4–12. Normal and major mutant gene inheritance (mendelian inheritance).

fected individuals, presumably because of differences in the normal allele (partner) of the mutant gene as well as other differences in the genetic and environmental background of the affected individual. Figure 4–13 demonstrates the variation in expression for an autosomal dominant disorder, ectrodactyly. The risk of the single mutant gene being passed to a given offspring is 50 per cent, yet the risk of a severe defect of hand development is less than 50 per cent because of variation in expression. To utilize the example of Waardenburg syndrome, the risk of inheritance of the mutant gene from an affected individual is 50 per cent, yet only about 20 per cent of affected individuals have deafness, the most disturbing expression of the mutant gene. Hence, the risk of deafness in offspring of a parent with the Waardenburg syndrome is the risk of receiving the mutant gene (50 per cent) times the likelihood of expression for deafness in the disorder (20 per cent), or 10 per cent.

This dichotomy between the risk of receiving the gene and the risk of a particular expression of the disorder must be utilized in counseling, especially for autosomal dominant conditions. A significant proportion of autosomal dominant patterns of malformation appear to represent fresh gene mutations in the individuals who express the condition. In reproductive counseling for the family, it is important to try to distinguish between lack of expression in the parent due to variability and fresh gene mutation in the child. Knowledge of both the natural history and the clinical variability of the disorder is extremely helpful in these determinations. Fresh gene mutation is more likely at older paternal age, as has been shown for at least 12 autosomal dominant multiple malformation syndromes.[8]

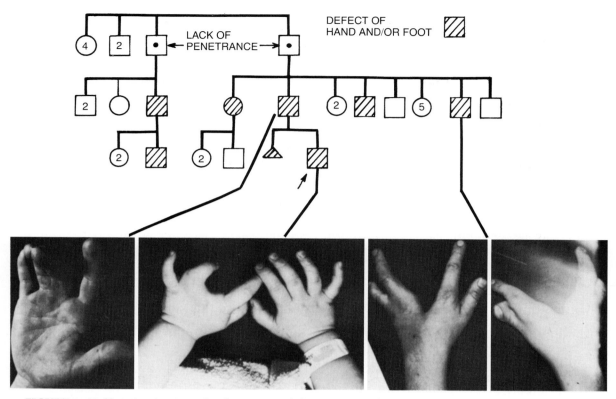

FIGURE 4–13. Variation in expression for autosomal dominant ectrodactyly among various related individuals. Note also the *intraindividual* asymmetry of expression in the propositus (*arrow*). (From Smith, D. W.: J. Pediatr., *69*:1150, 1966, with permission.)

Hence, paternal age should always be noted in the evaluation of disorders that may be the consequence of a single mutant gene.

Autosomal Recessive Disorders

Autosomal recessive disorders generally have less variation in expression than do dominant syndromes. The inheritance is from clinically normal parents who both have the same, or an allelic, recessive mutant gene in single dose. The likelihood of this occurring is enhanced if the parents are related. Hence, the possibility of consanguinity should always be addressed in disorders known to be autosomal recessive as well as when evaluating patterns of malformation of unknown cause.

X-Linked Disorders

Mutations on the X chromosome may be dominant or recessive in nature. Dominant mutations produce obvious clinical effects in XX females and either severe or lethal effects in the XY male who has no normal gene to lessen the impact of the mutation. By contrast, X-linked recessive mutations usually have minimal to no impact on the XX (carrier) female, whereas XY males demonstrate a phenotype.

Parent-of-Origin Effects

Although it has been assumed that genes inherited from mother and father are equally weighted in terms of expression and effect, observations in a variety of clinical settings have led to the appreciation that this is not invariably the case. Triploid conceptuses, who have an entire extra complement of genes, provide graphic illustration of this point.[9] When triploidy is produced by one maternal and two paternal sets of chromosomes, the pregnancy consists of a large hydatidiform placenta with a proportionate fetus. If two maternal and one paternal set of chromosomes is responsible, the fetus is disproportionately growth retarded and the placenta is usually extremely small, confirming observations in mouse embryos that paternal genes contribute to placental development, whereas maternal genes tend to define the embryo.

Genomic *imprinting* is a phenomenon first described in mice whereby certain genes are marked differently during male versus female germ cell formation such that apparently identical genes possess dissimilar function depending upon whether they are passed from the mother or the father. Imprinting commonly serves to "turn off" a gene or reduce its expression. Current understanding suggests that imprinting involves methylation analagous to the process of X-inactivation in normal females. Imprinting has been shown to play a role in a number of human syndromes including Prader-Willi syndrome, Angelman syndrome, and Beckwith syndrome. Prader-Willi syndrome occurs if the paternal copy of genes in the q11 region of chromosome 15 are missing through deletion of that region or disomy as discussed below. The inference from this observation is that the maternally inherited genes at this locus are normally imprinted or turned off. Absence for whatever reason of the paternally derived copies produces the phenotype. In Beckwith syndrome, a variety of different abnormalities involving chromosome 11p appear to be capable of producing the phenotype. Investigation of the homologous region on mouse chromosome 17 has documented the presence of the gene for insulin-like growth factor II (IGF II) (only the paternal copy is expressed) and the gene for the receptor for IGF II (only the maternal copy is expressed). Presumably, the phenotype may result from disturbed imprinting of either or both of these loci.[10]

Uniparental *disomy* is a term that indicates that both members of a chromosome pair or both alleles of a gene pair come from the same parent. This situation usually occurs when an embryo, initially trisomic for a certain chromosome, "self-corrects" by eliminating one of the extra chromosomes. In one third of such cases, the remaining two chromosomes will have the same parent of origin, resulting in uniparental di-

somy for the genes on that chromosome. The impact of uniparental disomy on morphogenesis is just beginning to be understood. Uniparental disomy for chromosome 16 has been documented in several growth-retarded fetuses in whom mosaicism for trisomy 16 was confined to the placenta.[11] Moreover, uniparental disomy may account for some of the phenotypic effects observed in individuals with apparently balanced Robertsonian translocations involving chromosome 14.[12] The implication is that certain chromosomes contain genes that are either paternally or maternally imprinted. Two copies from one parent would disturb the gene balance required for normal development. Uniparental disomy from correction of a trisomic conceptus is one mechanism that is known to produce Prader-Willi syndrome.

Unstable DNA Mutations

Throughout the human genome there are a number of sites in which short triplet repeated sequences of nucleotides normally occur. Although the purpose of these triplet repeats is not always known, the number of repeats at a given site is usually transmitted in a stable fashion from one generation to the next. An unstable DNA mutation occurs when the number of copies of a repeated sequence becomes increased. Expansion in the number of repeats at a locus may produce disease directly or it may create what has been termed a premutation. The latter indicates that the expanded sequence has no clinical effects on the individual; however, the sequence is likely to be unstable during meiosis (germ cell formation), resulting in offspring with clinical abnormalities. Although unstable DNA mutations usually expand further during meiosis, contraction of unstable sequences is documented. Unstable DNA mutations account for some observations that seem to defy the laws of single-gene inheritance such as anticipation (a condition getting worse in successive generations) and unaffected transmitting males in X-linked recessive disorders.[13] Parent-of-origin effects are common in unstable mutations, with some expanding only when transmitted through the mother and others showing paternal effects. The fragile X syndrome and Steinert myotonic dystrophy are examples of conditions that result from unstable DNA mutations.

Mitochondrial Mutations

The DNA of the normal mitochondrion is a circular molecule that contains 37 genes encoding 22 types of transfer RNA, two types of ribosomal RNA, and 13 structural proteins which are all subunits of the respiratory chain complexes involved in oxidative phosphorylation. Any given cell may contain from a hundred to several thousand mitochondria. Since the mitochondria are the energy-producing apparatus of the cell, most mitochondrial disorders described to date present postnatally with visual loss, progressive myopathy, seizures, encephalopathy, and/or diabetes presumably as a consequence of insufficient energy production in a critical tissue. The effects of mitochondrial mutation appear to worsen over time.[14] The impact of these abnormalities on morphogenesis is unknown.

GENETIC COUNSELING FOR SINGLE-GENE DISORDERS

For single-gene disorders it is a good general rule to consult the literature directly before counseling families or affected individuals regarding the availability of testing as it pertains to carrier detection, presymptomatic diagnosis, and prenatal diagnosis, since the nature of the work-up that is required to address many of these questions changes dramatically as the level of the understanding of the genetic abnormality becomes more refined.

Autosomal Dominant Disorders

The parents and siblings of the affected individual should be examined to determine whether any of them show any features of the disorder in question. The nature of the "examination" to exclude the effects of an altered gene varies by disorder from simple assessment of parental stature in achondroplasia to cutaneous examination plus eye evaluation plus cranial and renal imaging in tuberous sclerosis. If neither parent shows any features of the condition, it is appropriate to counsel the family that the condition in the child likely represents a fresh gene mutation (gene change in one of the germ cells that went to make the baby) for which the risk for recurrence is negligible. More distant relatives need have no concern of having affected children.

The risk for an *affected* individual having an affected child is 50 per cent for each offspring. This number represents the risk for vertical transmission of the altered gene; however, it does not predict the severity of the affect in offspring who inherit the mutation. Knowledge of the frequency of various features in affected individuals is helpful in outlining not only the risk for transmission but also the likelihood of particular complications.

In the uncommon circumstance in which a dominant condition is the result of an unstable mutation in DNA, the likelihood of anticipation (increasing severity in subsequent generations) should be addressed if the affected parent is the sex in which expansion of the unstable sequence is known to occur. For example, congenital myotonic dystrophy occurs only when the altered gene is transmitted through the mother.

Explanation of how the phenotype relates to the effects of the single altered gene is often helpful in outlining the natural history of the condition and need for follow-up of certain specific issues.

Autosomal Recessive Disorders

Inheritance is from clinically normal parents who both have the same, or an allelic, recessive mutant gene in single dose. The risk is obviously enhanced if the parents are related. The possibility of consanguinity should always be addressed in disorders known to be autosomal recessive and when evaluating patterns of malformation of unknown cause. Autosomal recessive disorders generally have less variation in expression than autosomal dominant conditions. This is likely because homozygosity for recessive mutations (both copies of the gene are mutated) leads to absence of gene function, which is consistent from child to child within the same sibship.

Recurrence risk from the same parentage is 25 per cent for each subsequent pregnancy. The risk of any relative having an affected child may be calculated by multiplying their risk of being a heterozygote (carrier) times the risk of marrying a heterozygote (the general carrier frequency for that gene in the population) times one fourth (the chance of two heterozygotes) having an affected offspring).

In counseling parents of individuals with recessive disorders it is helpful to emphasize that most people have several altered genes that cause no problem because each is balanced by a normal partner. They happen to have one altered gene in common. The normal children of carrier parents have a two out of three chance of being carriers as well. However, their risk of randomly marrying another carrier is low, thus their risk for affected offspring is low.

X-Linked Recessive Disorders

The X-linked genes in the XY male are present in but a single dose with no partner gene. Hence, a single copy of a mutant gene on the X chromosome will express a full recessive disorder. The chance of an XX female having a pair of such X-linked recessive genes and expressing the same disorder as the XY male is very small. The following generalizations apply to this pattern of inheritance: with rare exception, only males are affected; transmission is through unaffected or mildly affected (carrier) females; male-to-male transmission does not occur.

X-linked disorders in the male often represent fresh gene mutation. These disorders present a problem in striving to determine in which generation the gene mutation arose, for it could be in the patient alone or in the mother or even further back in the family, having been silently passed through carrier females. For some X-linked disorders, such as hypohidrotic ectodermal dysplasia, this dilemma can be resolved by demonstrating the presence or absence of mild (carrier) expression in the females in question. Older paternal age has been noted to be a factor in fresh X-linked mutation; however, the older age effect is seen in the father of the mother (maternal grandfather) of the first affected XY male rather than the boy's father from whom he does not receive his X.[15]

For unstable X-linked mutations, such as those that account for the fragile X syndrome, counseling needs to incorporate knowledge of parent-of-origin effects. Unstable X-linked mutations tend to expand when passed through the mother, accounting for a more severe phenotype in offspring of carrier women who inherit the altered gene.

If the mother is not a carrier, the risk for recurrence is low. If the mother is a carrier, she has a 50 per cent risk that any future male will be affected. Normal sons cannot transmit the disorder. All sons of affected males are normal. All daughters of affected males are usually clinically normal carriers.

In general, all daughters of carrier mothers will be clinically normal, although 50 per cent will carry the altered gene and have themselves a risk for vertical transmission. The major exception is the case of unstable DNA mutation in which daughters of carrier mothers who inherit an expanded mutation often show clinical effects.

X-Linked Dominant Inheritance

X-linked dominant disorders show expression in the XX female, usually with more severe, often lethal, effects in the XY male. This type of inheritance is most commonly confused with autosomal dominant inheritance from which it may be discriminated in the following ways: males are more severely affected than females, although affected males are underrepresented in large kindreds, reflecting the male lethality of X-linked dominant conditions; male-to-male transmission is not observed; instead, affected males have normal sons and all of their daughters are affected.

Affected females have a 50 per cent risk for affected daughters. Although the risk that an XY fetus will inherit the gene is also 50 per cent, the probability of a live-born affected male is usually significantly less because of the selection pressure against affected XY conceptuses. Males born to affected women are usually normal. The affected males represent early miscarriages.

Mothers of females with X-linked dominant conditions should be examined closely for evidence of clinical effect. If the mother is normal, fresh gene mutation in the offspring is likely and the risk for recurrence is negligible. If not, counseling is the same as for affected females above.

Mitochondrial Inheritance

Since mitochondria are exclusively maternally inherited, males with disorders due to mitochondrial mutations have no risk for affected offspring. Females, on the other hand, have a risk that approaches 100 per cent, since the human egg is the source of all of the mitochondria for the offspring. Most affected women have both normal and abnormal mitochondria, thus any given egg will have both types in different proportions. Random distribution of mitochondria in dividing cells in the early embryo creates different proportions of abnormal to normal mitochondria in different tissues. A clinical phenotype occurs only when a threshold of abnormal to normal mitochondria is exceeded in a critical tissue. Thus all offspring of affected women may be assumed to have inherited some abnormal mitochondria; however, not all will manifest disease. Clinically unaffected daughters of affected women also have a risk for vertical transmission, since lack of clinical disease does not preclude the possibility that some of the daughter's mitochondria might harbor the mutation.

MULTIFACTORIAL INHERITANCE

In the mid 1960s a model was advanced to explain the findings emerging from a variety of epidemiologic studies, which suggested that a broad number of common malformations including cleft lip and palate, isolated cleft palate, neural tube defects, club foot, and pyloric stenosis among others tended to cluster in families although the pattern of inheritance did not conform to the laws of gene transmission as set forth by Mendel.[16,17] The model involved the concept of genetic liability or susceptibility to a given characteristic, governed by many different genes, and a threshold, determined by both genetic and environmental factors. Individuals lying beyond the threshold exhibited the phenotype, whereas those who did not were phenotypically normal. The model converted the normal distribution of a morphogenetic process within a population into an "all-or-none" expression of a structural defect. As initially proposed, the many genes contributing to susceptibility were given equal weight. The multifactorial/threshold model makes several predictions which in large measure, are in accord with the clinical and epidemiologic observations regarding given malformations:

1. *Familial clustering is observed.* As stated above, clustering is observed among family groups. In addition, many common malformations have different birth frequencies in different populations. Since numerous subtle genetic differences are presumed to account for some of the normal variation observed among ethnic groups, it is hypothesized that some of these differences may confer susceptibility for certain developmental problems. Thus, the model would predict variation in the prevalence of certain malformations by ethnic groups, a finding that is well documented in population surveys.

2. *The risk for first-degree relatives (parents, siblings, and offspring) approximates the square root of the population risk.* Table 4–1 lists the frequency of recurrence of the same defect in offspring of normal parents who have had one affected child. For the majority of defects, the risk is 2 to 5 per cent, which is 20 to 40 times the frequency of the problem in the general population. The figures in Table 4–1 are derived from direct observations in clinical populations and correlate well with the numbers predicted by the model.

3. *Second-degree relatives (uncles, aunts, half-siblings) have a sharply lower risk than first-degree relatives.* This characteristic differentiates multifactorial inheritance from autosomal dominant inheritance in which the risk drops only by half with each degree of relational distance from the affected individual and from autosomal recessive inheritance in which the major risk is for full siblings.

4. *The greater the number of affected family members, the greater the risk for recurrence.* This pattern of recurrence of multifactorial traits is in contrast to both dominant and recessive inheritance in which the risk for future offspring remains unchanged despite recurrences.

TABLE 4–1. RECURRENCE RISKS FOR SOME DEFECTS[16,17]

Defect	Recurrence Risk For		
	Normal Parents of One Affected Child	Future Males	Future Females
Cleft lip with or without cleft palate	4–5%*		
Cleft palate alone	2–6%		
Cardiac defect (common type)	3–4%		
Pyloric stenosis	3%	4%	2.4%
Hirschsprung anomaly	3–5%		
Clubfoot	2–8%		
Dislocation of hip	3–4%	0.5%	6.3%
Neural tube defects—anencephaly, meningomyelocele	3–5%		
Scoliosis	10–15%		

*Range of recurrence risks observed.

5. *Consanguinity increases the risk.* This concept relates to the fact that inbreeding increases the number of "susceptibility genes," thus making a developmental problem more likely.

6. *The more severe the malformation the greater the risk for recurrence.* This presumes that the severity of the malformation reflects a greater adverse genetic influence, thereby increasing the risk from the same parentage. Certainly with cleft lip and palate, data support the hypothesis, since the risk for recurrence in subsequent children when an offspring has a severe bilateral cleft lip and palate is 5.7 per cent as contrasted with a 2.5 per cent recurrence risk when the offspring has a less severe degree of defect.[16]

7. *The risk for recurrence will be increased for relatives of the least affected sex, if sex differences are noted.* The sex difference between the XX and XY genetic background has an appreciable effect on the occurrence of many malformations (Fig. 4–14). Some of the sex differences in malformation occurrence may be explained as the direct effects of structural genital differences, such as hypospadias in the male. Similarly, the marked male predominance of the urethral obstruction sequence may be explained by the fact that the most common site of urethral obstruction is the prostatic urethra.[18] The humoral impact of testosterone, which makes connective tissue tougher in the male, may explain the preponderance of dislocation of the hip, related to connective tissue laxity, in the female. Also, testosterone, which is produced by the male during

the first few postnatal months, may enhance the likelihood of muscle hypertrophy and thereby increase the tendency to develop hypertrophic pyloric stenosis.[18] The sex differences related to the incidence of other structural defects would appear to imply that genes on the X and/or Y chromosome may increase the likelihood of particular anomalies developing during morphogenesis.

One indirect manner in which the genetic background of XX versus XY may influence the frequency of structural defects at birth is simply the growth rate in utero. Thus, with the exception of anomalies related to joint laxity, most late uterine constraint-induced deformations are more common in the male, who is normally growing faster in the last trimester of gestation than the female.[19]

The hypothesis reasons that if it takes more genetic factors to give rise to an anomaly in the female, then the affected female should pass on more of these genetic factors to her offspring, who would have a higher frequency of the anomaly than

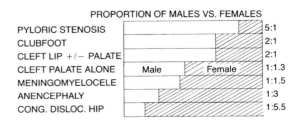

PROPORTION OF MALES VS. FEMALES

PYLORIC STENOSIS		5:1
CLUBFOOT		2:1
CLEFT LIP +/– PALATE		2:1
CLEFT PALATE ALONE	Male / Female	1:1.3
MENINGOMYELOCELE		1:1.5
ANENCEPHALY		1:3
CONG. DISLOC. HIP		1:5.5

FIGURE 4–14. Relative sex incidence of single common malformations.

would offspring of affected males. Observational studies in pyloric stenosis documenting a 24 per cent risk of transmission from affected mothers compared to 6 per cent from affected fathers bear this out.

8. *Concordance in twins.* If both twins have a defect, they are concordant for the anomaly. If one twin has the defect and the other does not, they are discordant. The frequency of concordance and discordance in monozygotic and dizygotic twins has been used to argue both for environmental and for single-gene causation of common malformations. For most of these defects, the incidence of concordance in dizygotic twins is similar to that of siblings born of separate pregnancies, arguing against both a single-gene etiology and a major environmental influence.

In the last several years, numerous investigators have reanalyzed specific, previously published data sets with respect to a variety of alternative hypotheses, most of which assume the impact of a single major gene on susceptibility. For cleft lip with or without cleft palate, the observed distributions and family clustering is best explained by a single major "susceptibility" locus in the majority of populations.[20,21] Molecular methodology is allowing investigators to explore linkage between a specific phenotype and a variety of "candidate genes" chosen because the mechanism of action of the gene in experimental animal models suggested a possible connection. For cleft lip with or without cleft palate, linkage has been demonstrated between the phenotype and the transforming growth factor alpha locus[22] and the retinoic acid receptor.[23]

Despite the accumulating evidence that suggests that the multifactorial model is probably not the best construct for explaining what constitutes genetic susceptibility to a given malformation, the empiric data obtained from the observational studies used to construct the model remain the basis for genetic counseling of families.

That environmental influences play a role in the determination of common malformations is born out by many studies such as those of anencephaly and meningomyelocele that document that social class is a variable that impacts birth frequency.[24] Birth order influences have also been noted, with congenital dislocation of the hip and pyloric stenosis being more likely to occur in first-born children.[16] One obvious environmental factor is fetal in utero constraint leading to deformation. Such constraint is more common in the first-born who is the first to distend the uterus and the abdominal wall.[19] Environmental factors such as this probably explain the greater frequency of dislocation of the hip as well as most other deformations in the first-born.

Studies in experimental animals have dramatically illustrated the profound influence that genetic background may have on the likelihood of a given environmental teratogen causing malformation. For example, Fraser[25] could regularly produce cleft palate in mouse embryos of the A/Jax strain by giving the mothers a high dose of cortisone during early gestation, whereas the same treatment in a different strain led to only 17 per cent affected offspring. In humans, genetic susceptibility to hydantoin-induced teratogenesis appears to correlate with the genetically determined activity levels of epoxide hydrolase, one of the enzymes necessary for the metabolism of hydantoin.[26] Expression of the phenotype requires both genetic susceptibility and drug exposure.

The search for environmental factors that allow for expression of a single malformation obviously should continue. However, just as the genetic differences that contribute to susceptibility are multiple and difficult to characterize, so environmental factors are likely to be multiple and subtle in character. The total factors combine to approach the threshold for a particular error in morphogenesis, a threshold predominantly set by the genetic makeup of the individual.

GENETIC COUNSELING FOR DEFECTS THAT ARE A RESULT OF MULTIFACTORIAL INHERITANCE

For many common single defects, empiric risk figures relative to recurrence of the problem in a subsequent pregnancy are available.[27] The risk is 3 to 5 per cent or less for most of the common single defects, with the exception of scoliosis (Table 4–1). The risk figures may be slightly increased when the defect in the affected individual is severe in degree, and decreased when the anomaly is mild in degree. If the sex of the child impacts the condition (such as in pyloric stenosis and hip dislocation), sex-specific risks for recurrence may be appropriate. If two offspring are affected, the risk for the next child is two to three times greater, or approximately 10 to 15 per cent. Since recurrence risk figures address the risk for first-degree relatives, the risk that an affected individual will have affected offspring is similar in magnitude to that of the sibling risk (or 3 to 5 per cent). As the factors that influence both genetic and environmental susceptibility to multifactorial traits become elucidated, it is expected that more precise counseling will be possible.

The multifactorial model is useful in explaining common malformations to parents, as it dictates that the genetic factors which contribute come from both sides of the family. It is helpful to explain the developmental pathology of the defects so that parents can appreciate that there was only a single localized problem in the early development of their child. A discussion that the localized problem in development must have occurred prior to a particular time in gestation may be helpful in dispelling any concerns over later gestational events that are likely to have had no impact on the occurrence on the particular malformation. The prognosis of multifactorial traits is dependent upon the amenability of the specific malformation to surgical intervention or, in the case of constraint-related problems, to postural intervention. The prognosis is poor for certain neural tube defects, but may be quite good for cardiac malformations and other defects in which advances in therapy have improved both morbidity and mortality.

PRENATAL DIAGNOSIS

Technologic advancement as well as progress in the understanding of the etiology and pathogenesis of many disorders have made the possibility for prenatal diagnosis an increasing reality for many families. For a very few conditions, fetal therapy may be available; however, most prenatal diagnosis is offered to allow parents options for managing their reproductive risk. The following are some of the techniques for early fetal evaluation along with indications for their application.

Screening Approaches for the General Pregnant Population

Chromosomal Abnormalities

Because the risk for many chromosomal aneuploidy states increases with advancing maternal age, a variety of approaches have been developed to assess fetal karyotypes in older mothers. The most accurate way to address this issue is with direct assessment of the fetal chromosomes, which requires a sample of fetal cells. The traditional method by which this is done is *amniocentesis* at 15 to 18 weeks of pregnancy. Although highly accurate,[28] the procedure carries a roughly 1 in 200 risk for miscarriage, which is a deterrent to some couples. *Chorionic villus sampling* (CVS) affords the advantage of earlier diagnosis, as the procedure is done at 11 to 12 weeks of pregnancy. The test carries an increased risk for miscarriage even correcting for the earlier gestational age at which testing is done. In addition, mosaicism in the sampled placental cells is documented in about 1 per cent of cases, causing counseling dilemmas. Noninvasive serum screening using alpha-fetoprotein determination (AFP testing) or triple markers (AFP, HCG, and estriol) analysis is a useful way to modify the age-related risk for Down syndrome to determine which women in the population are at high enough risk that more invasive testing should be offered.[29] The application of triple marker screening in women over 35 is the subject of considerable debate at the present time, since not all abnormalities for which older women are at risk will be detected by this approach.[30]

Single-Gene Disorders

Carrier screening is available for a number of single-gene disorders that are inherited in an autosomal recessive fashion and that have a high prevalence in certain populations. Examples include Tay-Sachs disease, sickle cell anemia, and cystic fibrosis. For most of the conditions in this book, approaches for carrier screening in the general population have not been developed.

Multifactorial Conditions

The only multifactorial conditions for which population screening is specifically available are the neural tube closure defects. Elevation of alpha-fetoprotein both in the amniotic fluid and in maternal serum (*MSAFP*) has been associated with the presence of an open defect in the fetus. Serum screening in conjunction with thorough *ultrasound evaluation* should detect over 90 per cent of affected pregnancies.

Ultrasonography is also a potential screening tool for a number of other malformations; however, variations in equipment and operator experience make this an imperfect technique as it is currently practiced.[31]

Prenatal Diagnostic Approaches for Specific Disorders

Chromosomal Abnormalities

Amniocentesis or CVS should be offered in the following situations:

1. Previous child with trisomy 21.
2. Parental balanced translocation.
3. Affected parent with a microdeletion syndrome.
4. Any de novo abnormality in which the parents, although chromosomally normal, are interested, since this is the only way to exclude recurrence from gonadal mosaicism.

Single-Gene Disorders

Prenatal testing for single-gene disorders is more difficult because the approach that is used for any given condition depends upon, among other things, the level of understanding of the molecular basis of the disorder in question. Testing can be done at the level of the gene (DNA), the message (RNA), the product (biochemical analysis), or the phenotype produced (gross morphology). Even in situations in which the gene that causes a specific condition is known, direct analysis of the gene is not always the easiest, least costly, and most reliable approach to prenatal testing. The rapidity with which changes occur in this arena dictates that the literature be reviewed at the time prenatal diagnosis is requested. Information available in textbooks will be out of date for some conditions at the time of publication.

1. For conditions in which the specific gene mutation is known, prenatal diagnosis is often possible using amniocentesis or CVS to collect fetal cells for direct mutation analysis. If a common mutation accounts for the majority of the cases (such as achondroplasia) the approach can be relatively straightforward. By contrast, in conditions such as Marfan syndrome in which multiple different mutations within the same gene produce the same phenotype, prenatal diagnosis using direct DNA analysis is possible only if the family's specific mutation is known.

2. For disorders in which the location of the gene is known, linkage analysis may be useful. This technique dictates that DNA samples be obtained on multiple family members and often requires a confirmed diagnosis in more than one family member. Nonpaternity is occasionally discovered in the course of this type of investigation.

3. Biochemical studies may be diagnostic in conditions in which the approach is based upon analysis of gene product. Some tests are performed on amniotic fluid directly. Other studies demand cultured fetal cells for enzyme analysis requiring amniocentesis or CVS.

4. For X-linked conditions in which neither direct DNA analysis nor linkage are available, prenatal sex determination may be an option. However, 50 per cent of the male offspring of carrier women would be expected to be normal.

5. For conditions in which the diagnosis is made on the clinical phenotype, prenatal diagnosis is dependent upon the ability of ultrasound to visualize specific features of the condition such as severe limb shortening in some of the skeletal dysplasias.

Multifactorial Conditions

For conditions that have neither a chromosomal or genetic marker, prenatal diagnosis is entirely dependent upon the amenability of the specific structural defects to ultrasound imaging. For example, holoprosencephaly is readily visualized with level II imaging, whereas isolated cleft palate is not at the time of this writing. (Level II scanning is defined by the sophistication of the equipment and the experience of the operator.) It is important that clinicians be aware of the limitations of ultrasound. Studies from experienced tertiary care centers have documented that ultrasound misses up to 37 per cent of second defects in scans in which a primary abnormality is identified.[32] This is not to downplay the usefulness of ultrasound imaging, but rather to foster realistic expectations among families and physicians.

References

1. Hassold, T., Pettay, D., Robinson, A., and Uchida, I.: Molecular studies of parental origin and mosaicism in 45,X conceptuses. Hum. Genet. *89*: 647, 1992.
2. Antonarakis, S. E., and the Down Syndrome Collaborative Group: Parental origin of the extra chromosome in trisomy 21 using DNA polymorphism analysis. N. Engl. J. Med., *324*:872, 1991.
3. Antonarakis, S. E., et al.: The meiotic stage of nondisjunction in trisomy 21: Determination by using DNA polymorphisms. Am. J. Hum. Genet., *50*:544, 1992.
4. MacDonald, M., Hassold, T., Harvey, J., Wang, L. H., Morton, M. E., and Jacobs, P.: The origin of 47,XXY and 47,XXX aneuploidy: Heterogeneous mechanisms and role of aberrant recombination. Hum. Mol. Genet., *3*:1365, 1994.
5. Summitt, R.: Cytogenetics in mentally retarded children with anomalies: A controlled study. J. Pediatr., *74*:58, 1969.
6. Mascarello, J. T., and Hubbard, V.: Routine use of methods for improved G-band resolution in a population of patients with malformations and developmental delay. Am. J. Med. Genet., *38*:37, 1991.
7. Pangalos, C. G., et al.: DNA polymorphism analysis in families with recurrence of free trisomy 21. Am. J. Hum. Genet., *51*:1015, 1992.
8. Jones, K. L., et al.: Older paternal age and fresh gene mutation. J. Pediatr., *86*:84, 1975.
9. McFadden, D. E., and Kalousek, D. K.: Two different phenotypes of fetuses with chromosomal triploidy: Correlation with parental origin of the extra haploid set. Am. J. Med. Genet., *38*:535, 1991.
10. Wilson, G. N., Hall, J. G., and de la Cruz, F.: Genomic imprinting: Summary of an NICHD conference. Am. J. Med. Genet., *46*:675, 1993.
11. Kalousek, D. K., Langlois, S., Barrett, I., et al.: Uniparental disomy for chromosome 16 in humans. Am. J. Hum. Genet., *52*:8, 1993.
12. Donnai, D.: Robertsonian translocations: Clues to imprinting. Am. J. Med. Genet., *46*:681, 1993.
13. Caskey, C. T., Pizzuti, A., et al.: Triplet repeat mutations in human disease. Science, *256*:784, 1991.
14. Wallace, D. C.: Mitochondrial genetics: A paradigm for aging and degenerative diseases? Science, *256*:628, 1992.
15. Herrmann, J.: Ein Einfluss des zeugungsalters auf die Mutationen zu Hamophilie A. Humangenetik, *3*:1, 1966.
16. Carter, C. O.: The inheritance of common congenital malformations. Progr. Med. Genet., *4*:59, 1965.
17. Smith, D. W., and Aase, J. M.: Polygenic inheritance of certain common malformations. J. Pediatr., *76*:653, 1970.
18. Arenas, F., and Smith, D. W.: Sex liability to single structural defects. Am. J. Dis. Child., *132*:970, 1978.
19. Graham, J. M.: Smith's Recognizable Patterns of Human Deformation, 2nd ed. Philadelphia, W. B. Saunders Co., 1988.
20. Chung, C. S., Bixler, D., Watanabe, T., et al.: Segregation analysis of cleft lip with or without cleft palate: A comparison of Danish and Japanese data. Am. J. Hum. Genet., *39*:603, 1986.
21. Marazita, M. L., Hu, D. N., Spence, M. A., et al.: Cleft lip with or without cleft palate in Shanghai, China: Evidence for an autosomal major locus. Am. J. Hum. Genet., *51*:648, 1992.
22. Ardinger, H. H., Buetow, K. H., Bell, G. I., et al.: Association of genetic variation of the transforming growth factor alpha gene with cleft lip and palate. Am. J. Hum. Genet., *45*:348, 1989.
23. Chenevix-Trench, G., Jones, K., Green, A. C., et al.: Cleft lip with or without cleft palate: Associations with transforming growth factor alpha and retinoic acid receptor loci. Am. J. Hum. Genet., *51*:1377, 1992.
24. Edwards, J. H.: Congenital malformations of the central nervous system in Scotland. Br. J. Prev. Soc. Med., *12*:115, 1958.
25. Fraser, F. C.: The use of teratogens in the analysis of abnormal developmental mechanisms. First International Conference on Congenital Malformations. Philadelphia, J. B. Lippincott Co., 1961.
26. Buehler, B. A., Delimont, D., van Waes, M., et al.: Prenatal prediction of risk of the fetal hydantoin syndrome. N. Engl. J. Med., *322*:1567, 1990.
27. Harper, P.: Practical Genetic Counseling, 4th ed. Oxford, Butterworth-Heinemann, Ltd., 1993.
28. Golbus, M. S., Loughman, W. D., Epstein, C. J., et al.: Prenatal genetic diagnosis in 3000 amniocenteses. N. Engl. J. Med., *300*:157, 1979.
29. Haddow, J. E., Palomai, G. E., Knight, G. J., et al.: Prenatal screening for Down's syndrome with use of maternal serum markers. N. Engl. J. Med., *327*:588, 1992.
30. Haddow, J. E., Palomake, G. E., Knight, G. J., et al.: Reducing the need for amniocentesis in women 35 years of age or older with serum markers for screening. N. Engl. J. Med., *330*:1114, 1994.
31. Ewigman, B. G., Crane, J. P., Frigoletto, F. E., et al.: Effect of prenatal ultrasound screening on perinatal outcome. N. Engl. J. Med., *329*:821, 1993.
32. Manchester, K. D., Pretorius, D. H., Avery, C., et al.: Accuracy of ultrasound diagnoses in pregnancies complicated by suspected fetal anomalies. Prenat. Diagn., *8*:109, 1988.

5

Minor Anomalies
as clues to more serious problems and toward the recognition of malformation syndromes

Minor anomalies are herein defined as unusual morphologic features that are of no serious medical or cosmetic consequence to the patient. The value of their recognition is that they may serve as indicators of altered morphogenesis in a general sense or may constitute valuable clues in the diagnosis of a specific pattern of malformation. Those wanting a more detailed discussion of this subject or those desiring information on a minor malformation not addressed in this chapter are referred to the elegant text by Jon M. Aase, *Diagnostic Dysmorphology*, New York, Plenum Medical Book Co., 1990.

Regarding the general occurrence of minor anomalies detectable by surface examination (except for dermatoglyphics), Marden et al.[1] found that 14 per cent of newborn babies had a single minor anomaly. This was of little concern because the frequency of major defects in this group was not appreciably increased. However, only 0.8 per cent of the babies had two minor defects, and in this subgroup, the frequency of a major defect was five times that of the general group. Of special importance were the findings in babies with three or more minor anomalies. This was found in only 0.5 per cent of babies (20), and 90 per cent of them had one or more major defects as well, as depicted in Figure 5–1.

In two additional studies, Mehes et al.[2] and Leppig et al.[3] demonstrated that 26 per

cent and 19.6 per cent of newborn infants with three or more minor anomalies, respectively, had a major malformation, a much lower incidence than documented in the study by Marden et al. and most likely related to differences in study design. Based on these studies, it is concluded that any infant with three or more minor anomalies should be evaluated for a major malformation, many of which are occult.

These minor external anomalies are most common in areas of complex and variable features, such as the face, auricles, hands, and feet. Before ascribing significance to a given minor anomaly in a patient, it is important to note whether it is found in other family members. Almost any minor defect may occasionally be found as a usual feature in a particular family, as noted in Figure 5–2.

The following figures illustrate certain minor anomalies and allude to their developmental origin and relevance (Figs. 5–3 to 5–8). Many, if not most, minor anomalies represent deformations due to altered mechanical forces affecting the development of otherwise normal tissue. The reason for the deformation may be purely external uterine constraint. Thus, most minor anomalies of external ear formation at birth are constraint-induced. However, the minor deformational anomaly may be the result of a

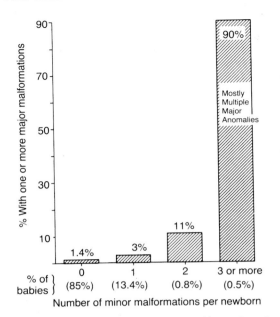

FIGURE 5–1. Frequency of major malformations in relation to the number of minor anomalies detected in a given newborn baby. (From Marden, P. M., Smith, D. W., and McDonald, M. J.: J. Pediatr., *64*:357, 1964, with permission.)

more primary malformation, and this is the presumed reason for the association between minor anomalies and major malformations. Also depicted, for the purpose of perspective, are some minor variants found in newborn babies with sufficient frequency that they should not be classed as anomalies (Fig. 5–9).

CALVARIUM

The presence of unusually *large fontanels* (see standards in Chapter 6) may be a nonspecific indicator of a general lag in osseous maturation.[4] It may, for example, lead to the detection of congenital hypothyroidism in the newborn or young infant, as shown in Figure 5–10.[5] The finding of a large posterior fontanel is especially helpful in this regard, since the posterior fontanel is normally fingertip size or smaller in 97 per cent of full-term neonates. Large fontanels may also be a feature in certain skeletal dysplasias and can, of course, be a sign of increased intracranial pressure.

DERMAL RIDGE PATTERNS (DERMATOGLYPHICS)

The parallel dermal ridges on the palms and soles form between the 13th and 19th fetal weeks. Their patterning appears to be dependent on the surface contours at the time, and the parallel dermal ridges tend to develop transversely to the planes of growth stress.[8] Curvilinear arrangements occur when there was a surface mound, for example, over the fetal pads that are prominently present during early fetal life on the

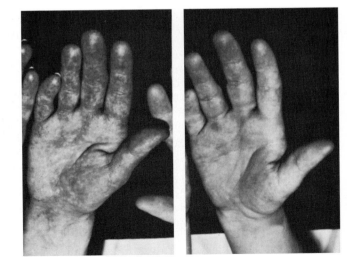

FIGURE 5–2. An otherwise normal mother (*left*) and daughter with clinodactyly of the fifth finger. A family history should be obtained before ascribing significance to a given minor anomaly.

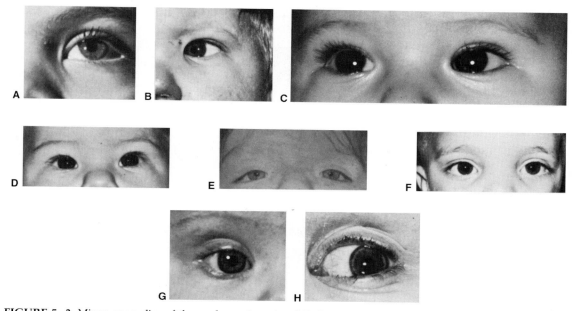

FIGURE 5–3. Minor anomalies of the ocular region. *A* and *B, Inner epicanthal folds* appear to represent redundant folds of skin, secondary to either low nasal bridge (most common) or excess skin, as in cutis laxa. Minor folds are frequent in early infancy, and as the nasal bridge becomes more prominent, they are obliterated. *C,* A unilateral epicanthal fold is indicative of torticollis. (From Jones, M. C.: J. Pediatr., *108*:707, 1986 with permission.) *D* and *E,* Telecanthus is the consequence of lateral displacement of the inner canthi, which partially obscures the medial portion of the eye and gives a false impression of strabismus and of hyperterlorism. *Slanting of the palpebral fissures* seems to be secondary to the early growth rate of the brain above the eye versus that of the facial area below the eye. For example, the patient with up-slanting (*D*) had mild microcephaly with a narrow frontal area, resulting in the up-slant; the patient with down-slanting (*E*) had maxillary hypoplasia, resulting in the down-slant. Mild degrees of up-slant were noted in 4 per cent of 500 normal children. *F, Ocular hypertelorism* refers to widely spaced eyes. A low nasal bridge will often give rise to a visual impression of ocular hypertelorism. This should always be determined by measurement. Measurement of inner canthal distance, coupled with the visual distinction of whether telecanthus is present, is usually sufficient. *G* and *H, Brushfield spots* are speckled rings about two thirds of the distance to the periphery of the iris. There is relative lack of patterning beyond the ring. These spots are found in 20 per cent of normal newborn babies, but they are found in 80 per cent of babies with Down syndrome.

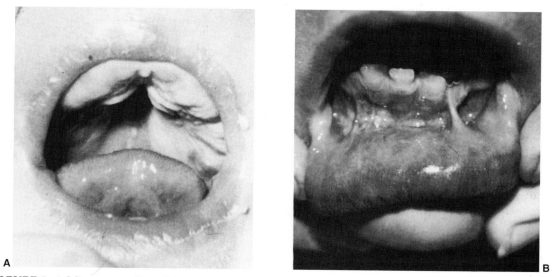

FIGURE 5–4. Minor anomalies of the oral region. *A, Prominent later palatal ridges* may be secondary to a deficit of tongue thrust into the hard palate, allowing for relative overgrowth of the lateral palatal ridges. Such a ridge may be a feature in a variety of disorders, especially those with hypotonia and with serious neurologic deficits related to sucking. As such, it can be a useful sign of a long-term deficit in function. *B, Aberrant frenula.*

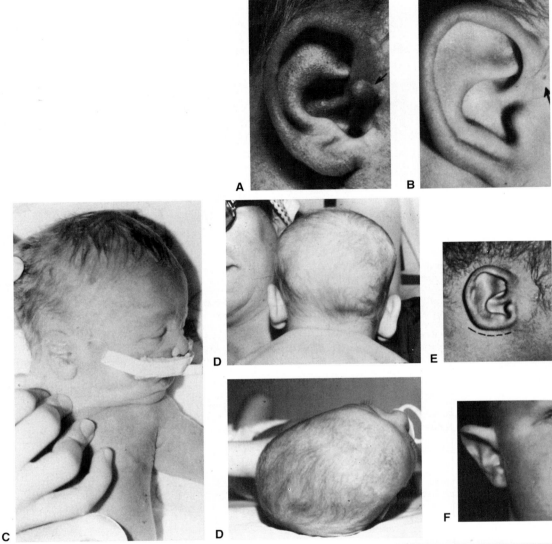

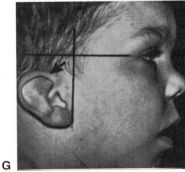

FIGURE 5–5. Minor anomalies of the auricular region. *A,* *Preauricular tags,* which often contain a core cartilage, appear to represent accessory hillock of His, the hillocks that normally develop in the recess of the mandibular and hyoid arches and coalesce to form the auricle. *B, Preauricular pits* may be familial, are twice as common in females as in males, and are more common in blacks than in whites. *C,* Large ears are often due to intrauterine constraint as in this child with oligohydramnios. Asymmetric ear size can be secondary to torticollis as in *D.* The child's head was positioned constantly on his right side, leading to plagiocephaly and enlargement of the right ear. *E, Lack of lobulus. F, Protruding ear* is usually due to lack of development or function of the posterior auricular ear muscle.[16] *G, Low-set ears*: This designation is made when the helix meets the cranium *arrow* at a level below that of a horizontal plane which may be an extension of a line through both inner canthi. This latter plane may relate to the lateral vertical axis of the head. *Ears slanted*: When the angle of the slope of the auricle exceeds 15 degrees from the perpendicular. Note: The findings of low placement and slanted auricle often go together and usually represent a lag in morphogenesis, since the auricle is normally in that position in early fetal life. It is important to appreciate that deformation of the head secondary to in utero constraint may temporarily distort the usual landmarks.[14]

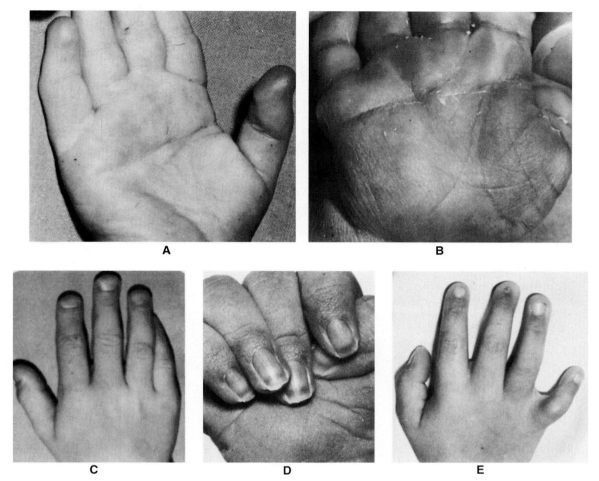

FIGURE 5–6. Minor anomalies of the hands. *A* and *B*, Creases represent the planes of folding (flexion) of the thickened volar skin of the hand. As such, they are simply deep wrinkles. The finger creases relate to flexion at the phalangeal joints, and if there has been no flexion, there is no crease.[7] Hypoplasia of the middle phalanx may result in only one plane of flexion on that finger (*A*). The thenar crease is the consequence of oppositional flexion of the thumb. Hence, if there is no oppositional flexion, there will be no crease. The slanting upper palmar crease reflects the palmar plane of folding related to the slope of the third, fourth, and fifth metacarpolphalangeal joints. The midpalmar crease is the plane of skin folding between upper palmar crease and the thenar crease. Any alteration in the slope of the third, fourth, and fifth metacarpolphalangeal planes of flexion, or relative shortness of the palm, may give rise to but a single midpalmar plane of flexion and thereby the *simian crease* (*A*). The latter is found unilaterally in about 4 per cent of normal infants and bilaterally in 1 per cent. Davies[6] found the incidence to be 3.7 per cent in newborn babies and noted that the simian crease is twice as common in males as in females. All degrees are found between normal and *simian crease*, including the *bridged palmar crease* (*B*). The creases are evident by 11 to 12 weeks of fetal life; hence, any gross alteration in crease patterning is usually indicative of an *abnormality in form and/or function of the hand prior to 11 fetal weeks.*[7] Clinodactyly (*curved finger*) (*A*) is most common in the fifth finger and is the consequence of hypoplasia of the middle phalanx, normally the last digital bone to develop. Up to 8 degrees of inturning of the fifth finger is within normal limits. Regardless of which digits are affected (fingers or toes), there is usually incurvature toward the area between the second and third digits. Partial *cutaneous syndactyly* (*A*) represents an incomplete separation of the fingers and most commonly occurs between the third and fourth fingers and between the second and third toes. *C* to *E*, The *nails* generally reflect the size and shape of the underlying distal phalanx. Hence, the *short, broad nail* (*C*), the *narrow hyperconvex nail* (*D*), and the *hypoplastic nail* (*E*) reflect dimensions of the underlying respective phalanges. *Asymmetric length* (*E*) of fingers is usually the result of hypoplasia of one or more fingers. *Camptodactyly* (*E*) most commonly affects the fifth, fourth, and third digits in decreasing order of frequency. It is presumably the consequence of relative shortness in the length of the flexor tendons with respect to the growth of the hand.

Illustration continued on following page

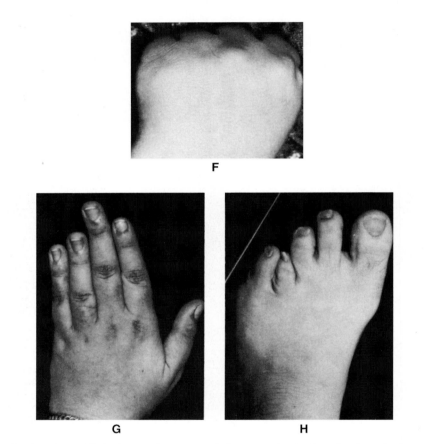

FIGURE 5–6. *Continued F* to *H, Malproportionment* or disharmony in the length of particular segments of the hand is not uncommon. The most common is a short middle phalanx of the fifth finger with clinodactyly. Another is relative shortness of the fourth and/or fifth metacarpal or metatarsal bone (*H*). This is best appreciated in the hand by having the patient make a fist and observing the position of the knuckles as shown in *F*. The altered alignment of these metacarpophalangeal joints may result in an altered palmar crease, especially the simian crease. It may also yield the impression of partial syndactyly between the third, fourth, and fifth fingers. Such relative shortness of the fourth and fifth metacarpals *may develop* postnatally by there being earlier than usual fusion of the respective metacarpoepiphyseal plates. When this happens, it tends to occur in the center of the epiphyseal plate first, yielding the radiographic appearance of a "coned-down" epiphysis. This is a nonspecific anomaly that may occur by itself or as one feature of a number of syndromes.

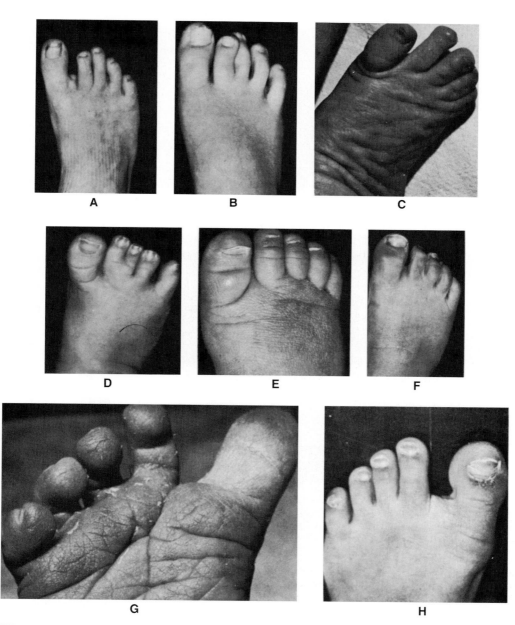

FIGURE 5–7. Minor anomalies of the feet. *A*, Asymmetric length of toes. *B*, Clinodactyly of second toe with overlapping. *C*, Short first metatarsal with dorsiflexion of hallux. *D*, Syndactyly (most commonly between digits 2 and 3). *E*, Hypoplasia of nails (in a 2⁶/₁₂-year-old). *F*, Short, broad toenail. *G*, Deep crease between hallux and second toe. *H*, Wide gap between hallux and second toe.

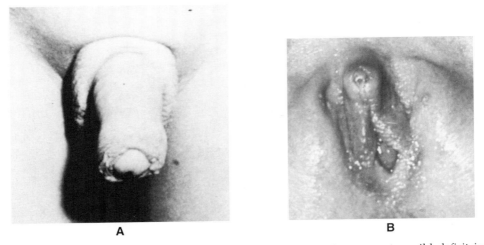

FIGURE 5–8. Minor anomalies of genitalia. *A, Shawl scrotum* appears to represent a mild deficit in the full migration of the labial-scrotal folds and as such may be accompanied by other signs of incomplete masculinization of the external genitalia. This photo shows a patient with the Aarskog syndrome. *B, Hypoplasia of the labia majora* may give rise to the false visual impression of a large clitoris, as in this patient with the trisomy 18 syndrome.

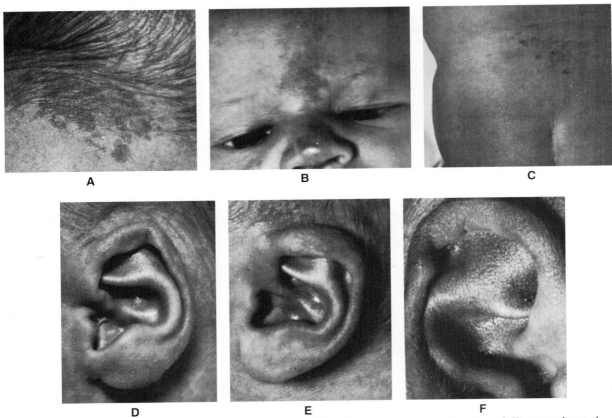

FIGURE 5–9. Minor variants in the newborn that should *not* be classed as anomalies. *A* to *C,* Fine nonelevated pink to red capillary hemangiomata at nape of neck (*A*), over central forehead and eyelids (*B*), and in lumbosacral area (*C*). *D* and *E,* Incompletely outfolded scapha helix. *F,* Darwinian tubercle.

Illustration continued on opposite page

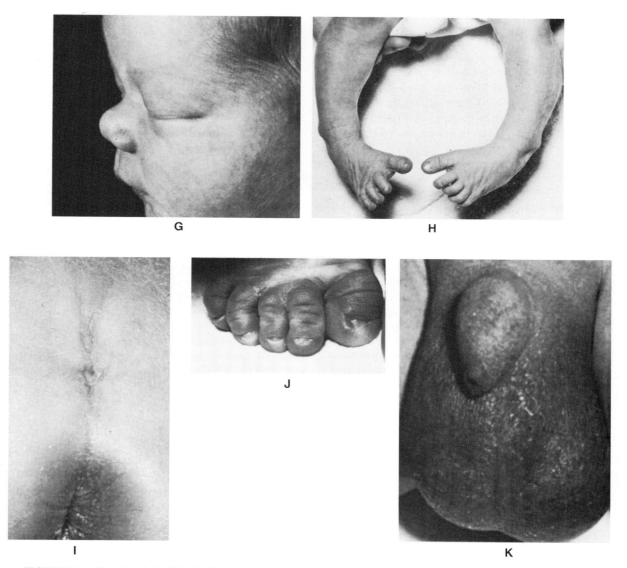

FIGURE 5–9. *Continued. G*, "Saddle" nose, mildly upturned nares. *H*, Mild to moderate inbowing of lower leg, with tibial torsion. *I*, Sacral dimple, not deep. *J*, Mild syndactyly of second and third toes; also, toenail hypoplasia in newborn. *K*, Hydrocele of testicle.

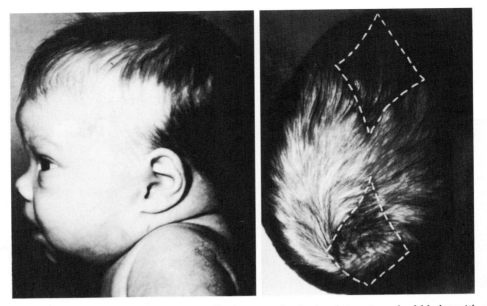

FIGURE 5–10. Unusually large fontanels, especially the posterior fontanel, in a 6-week-old baby with athyrotic hypothyrodism. The fetal onset of retarded osseous maturation is also evident in the immature facial bone development. (From Smith, D. W., and Popich, G.: J. Pediatr., *80*:753, 1972, with permission.)

fingertips, on the palm between each pair of fingers, and occasionally in the hypothenar area. Indirect evidence suggests that a high fetal fingertip pad tends to give rise to a whorl pattern, a low pad yields an arch pattern, and an intermediate pad produces a loop, as illustrated in Figure 5–11*B*. The dermal ridge patterning thereby provides an indelible historical record that indicates the form of the early fetal hand (or foot). Mild to severe alterations in hand morphology occur in a variety of syndromes, and hence it is not surprising that dermatoglyphic alterations have been noted in numerous dysmorphic syndromes. These alterations have seldom been pathognomonic for a particular condition. Rather, they simply provide additional data that, viewed in relation to the total pattern of malformation, may enhance the clinician's capacity to arrive at a specific overall diagnosis. Dermal ridge patterning may be evaluated utilizing a seven-power illuminated magnifying device such as an otoscope or a stamp collector's flashlight, which has a wider field of vision. Permanent records may be obtained by a variety of techniques.[9–11] There are two general categories of dermatoglyphic alterations: an *aberrant pattern* and

unusual frequency and/or *distribution of a particular pattern on the fingertips.*

Aberrant Patterning

Distal Axial Palmar Triradius (Fig. 5–11*A*). Triradii occur at the junction of three sets of converging ridges. There are usually no triradii between the base of the palm and the interdigital areas of the upper palm. However, patterning in the hypothenar area often gives rise to a distal axial triradius located, by definition, greater than 35 per cent of the distance from the wrist crease to the crease at the base of the third finger. This alteration, found in about 4 per cent of whites, is a frequent feature in a number of patterns of malformation.

Open Field in Hallucal Area (Arch Tibial) (Fig. 5–11*A*). Open field simply means that there is a relative lack of complexity in patterning and thereby implies a low surface contour in the that area at the time ridges developed. The hallucal area of the sole usually has a loop or whorl pattern, and a lack of such a pattern is unusual in the normal individual but is found in about 50 per cent of patients with the Down syn-

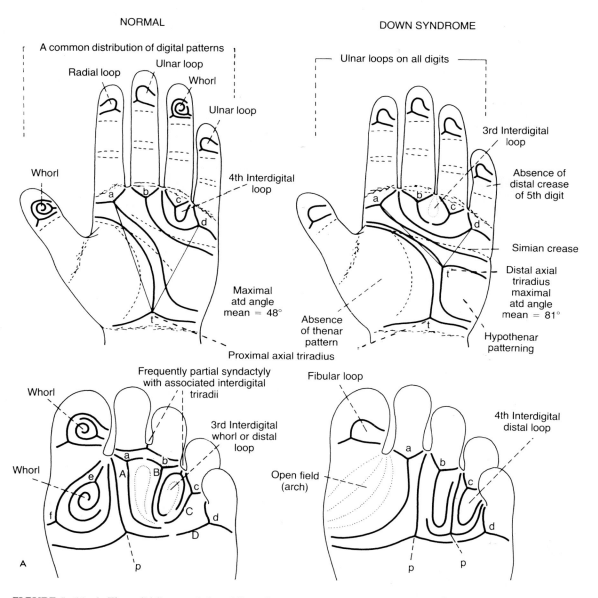

NORMAL

A common distribution of digital patterns

Radial loop

Ulnar loop

Whorl

Ulnar loop

Whorl

4th Interdigital
loop

Maximal
atd angle
mean = 48°

Absence
of thenar
pattern

Proximal axial triradius

Whorl

Frequently partial syndactyly
with associated interdigital
triradii

3rd Interdigital
whorl or distal
loop

Whorl

DOWN SYNDROME

Ulnar loops on all digits

3rd Interdigital
loop

Absence of
distal crease
of 5th digit

Simian crease

Distal axial
triradius
maximal
atd angle
mean = 81°

Hypothenar
patterning

Fibular loop

4th Interdigital
distal loop

Open field
(arch)

A

FIGURE 5–11. *A,* The *solid lines* and *dotted lines* denote the dermal ridge configurations, and the *dashes* within the palm represent the creases. (Courtesy of Dr. M. Bat-Miriam; prepared by Mr. R. Lee of the Kennedy-Galton Center near St. Albans, England.)

Illustration continued on following page

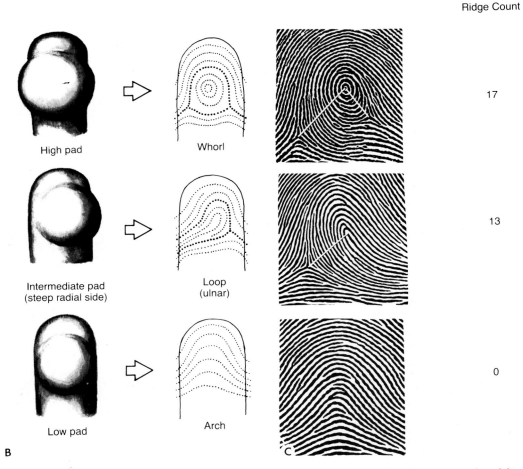

Ridge Count

High pad → Whorl — 17

Intermediate pad (steep radial side) → Loop (ulnar) — 13

Low pad → Arch — 0

B

C

FIGURE 5–11. *Continued B,* Presumed relationship between fetal fingertip pads at 16 to 19 weeks of fetal life and the fingertip dermal ridge pattern, which develops at that time. *C,* Technique for dermal ridge counting: A line is drawn between the center of the pattern and the more distal triradius, and the number or ridges that touch this line is the fingertip ridge count. The sum of the ten fingertip ridge counts is the total ridge count; this average is 144 in the male and 127 in the female. (From Holt, S.: Br. Med. Bull. *17:*247, 1961, with permission.)

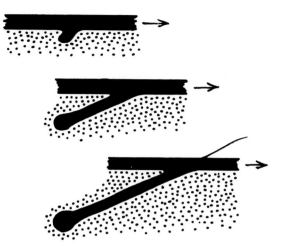

FIGURE 5–12. Hair follicles over the scalp begin their downgrowth into the loose underlying mesenchyme at 10 fetal weeks. The slope of each hair follicle and thereby the hair directional patterning is determined by the direction of growth stretch (*arrows*) exerted on the surface skin by the development of underlying tissues. For the scalp hair, the patterning relates to the growth in size and form of the underlying brain during the period of 10 to 16 weeks. By 18 weeks, when hairs are extruded onto the surface, their patterning is set. (From Smith, D. W., and Gong, B. T.: Teratology, *9*:17, 1974, with permission of John Wiley & Sons.)

drome and as an occasional feature in other syndromes.

Lack of Ridges. The failure of development of ridges in an area, most commonly the hypothenar region of the palm, is an occasional but nonspecific feature in the de Lange syndrome.

Other Patterns. There are a number of other unusual patterns, especially in the upper palmar, hypothenar, and thenar areas, which may be of clinical significance, but these are so rarely of value in an individual case that they will not be discussed.

Unusual Frequency or Distribution of Patterns on the Fingertips

A quantitation of the overall extent of patterning on the ten fingertips may be achieved by obtaining fingerprints and recording the total fingertip ridge count, as illustrated in Figure 5–11C

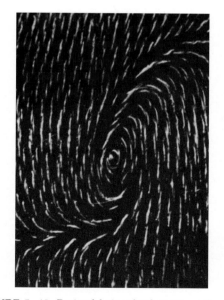

FIGURE 5–13. Parietal hair whorl at 18 weeks. This appears to be the fixed focal point from which the skin is being stretched by the dome-like outgrowth of the brain between 10 and 16 weeks. (From Smith, D. W., and Gong, B. T.: Teratology, *9*:17, 1974, with permission of John Wiley & Sons.)

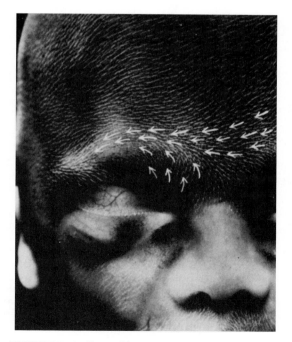

FIGURE 5–14. Frontal hair stream at 18 weeks, arcing laterally from the ocular punctum to meet with the downsweeping parietal hair stream. The frontal hair stream has been influenced by the growth of the underlying upper facial structures and the forebrain. (From Smith, D. W., and Gong, G. T.: Teratology, *9*:17, 1974, with permission of John Wiley & Sons.)

High Frequency of Low Arch Configurations. It is unusual to find a normal person with more than six of ten fingertips having a low arch configuration; however, this is a frequent feature in the trisomy 18 syndrome and the XXXXY syndrome, presumably reflecting hypoplasia of the fetal fingertip pads in these disorders. High frequency of low arches is nonspecific, being an occasional finding in certain other syndromes and in about 0.9 per cent of normal individuals.

High Frequency of Whorl Patterning. It is unusual to find nine or more fingertip whorls in an individual (3 per cent in normal persons). Excessive patterning, presumably reflecting prominent fetal pads, is more likely to be found in the XO syndrome, the Smith-Lemli-Opitz syndrome, occasionally in other patterns of malformation, and in some normal individuals.

Unusual Distribution, Especially of Radial Loop Patterns. Loops opening to the radial side of the hand are unusual on the fourth and fifth fingers. Radial loop patterns on these fingers are more common in people with Down syndrome (12.4 per cent)

than in individuals who are normal (1.5 per cent).

HAIR: ORIGIN AND RELEVANCE OF ABERRANT SCALP AND UPPER FACIAL HAIR PATTERNING AND GROWTH

The origin and relevance of hair directional patterning and aberrant hair growth[12] will be considered individually.

Hair Directional Patterning

Normal Development and Relevance. The origin of the sloping angulation of each hair follicle, which determines the surface hair directional patterning, is derived from the direction of stretch on the surface skin during the time the hair follicle is growing down from it into the loose underlying mesenchyme, as shown in Figure 5–12. Over the scalp and upper face, this directional patterning reflects the plane of growth stretch on the surface skin that was exerted by the growth of underlying struc-

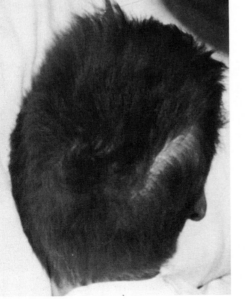
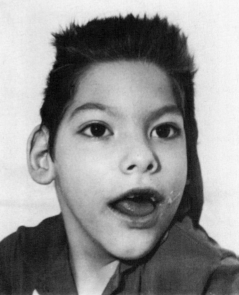

FIGURE 5–15. Hair patterning in a patient with primary microcephaly. The posterior scalp shows a lack of concise whorl, and the anterior scalp shows a marked frontal upsweep. These findings are interpreted as being the consequence of a deficit in growth of the brain prior to and during the period of hair follicle development and thus imply an early defect in morphogenesis of the brain, prior to 10 to 16 weeks. (From Smith, D. W., and Gong, B. T.: Teratology, 9:17, 1974, with permission of John Wiley & Sons.)

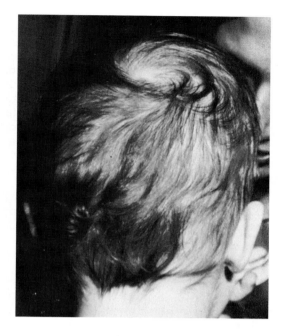

FIGURE 5–16. Posterior scalp hair of the type more commonly found in mild microcephaly, in this instance, the Down syndrome. The parietal whorl tends to be more central and posterior than usual, being over the former position of the posterior fontanel. This is considered secondary to the brain having been smaller and more symmetric than usual at 10 to 16 weeks, the time when the hair follicles develop. (From Smith, D. W., and Gong, B. T.: Teratology, 9:17, 1974, with permission of John Wiley & Sons.)

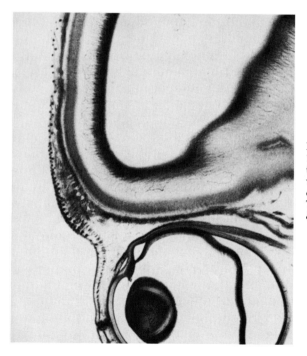

FIGURE 5–17. Sagittal section of forebrain area of a 10-week fetus, showing the early stage of cerebral cortical development and the lack of any organized calvarium at the time the hair follicles are beginning their downgrowth. (From Smith, D. W., and Gong, B. T.: Teratology, 9:17, 1974, with permission of John Wiley & Sons.)

FIGURE 5–18. Aberrant mid eyebrow patterning, which implies an aberration in growth and/or form of underlying facial structures by 10 to 16 fetal weeks. This patient has the Waardenburg syndrome, in which aberrant mid upper facial development is a usual feature.

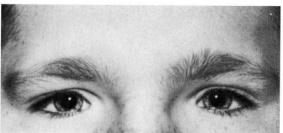

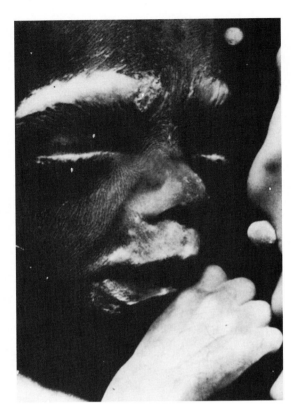

FIGURE 5–19. Hair growth on the face at 18 weeks, shortly after the hairs have been extruded onto the surface skin. (From Nilsson, L., Ingelman-Sundberg, A., and Wirsen, C.: A Child is Born. New York, Delacorte Press, 1966, with permission.)

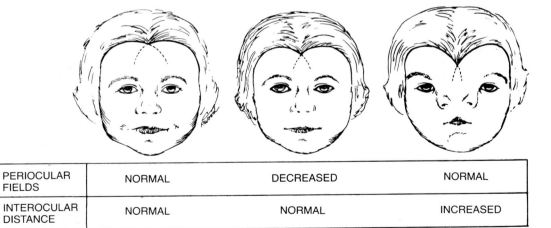

PERIOCULAR FIELDS	NORMAL	DECREASED	NORMAL
INTEROCULAR DISTANCE	NORMAL	NORMAL	INCREASED

FIGURE 5–20. If the eyes are widely spaced, or the area of periocular hair growth suppression is smaller than usual, the bilateral zones of periocular hair growth suppression may overlap at a lower point than usual, allowing for the presence of a widow's peak. The drawing on the right is of a patient with the frontonasal dysplasia anomaly. (From Smith, D. W., and Cohen, M. M., Jr.: Lancet, 2:1127, 1973, with permission.)

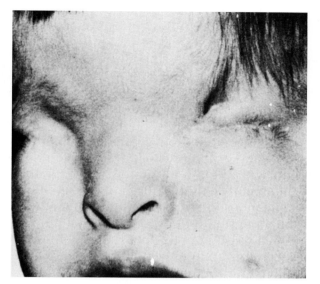

FIGURE 5–21. Aberrant growth of hair in lateral forehead area, related to the cryptophthalmos anomaly. (From Bergsma, D., McKusick, V. A. (eds.): National Foundation—Birth Defects. Baltimore, Williams & Wilkins Co., 1973, p. 27, with permission.)

tures during the period of hair follicle downgrowth, which takes place from 10 to 16 weeks of fetal life. Thus the parietal hair whorl, or crown, is interpreted as representing the focal point from which the posterior scalp skin was under growth tension exerted by the dome-like outgrowth of the early brain during this fetal period (Fig. 5–13). Its location is normally several centimeters anterior to the position of the posterior fontanel. Fifty-six per cent of single parietal hair whorls are located to the right of the midline; 30 per cent are left-sided, and 14 per cent are midline in location. Five per cent of normal individuals have bilateral parietal hair whorls. From the posterior whorl, the parietal hair stream flares out progressively, sweeping anteriorly to the forehead. Over the frontal region, the growth of the forebrain and the upper face

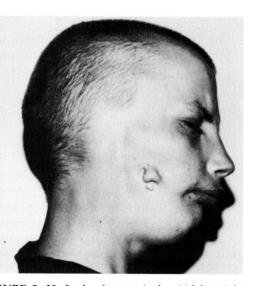

FIGURE 5–22. Lack of preauricular (sideburn) hair growth in relation to a deficit of auricular development. (Courtesy of Dr. Michael Cohen, Halifax, Nova Scotia.)

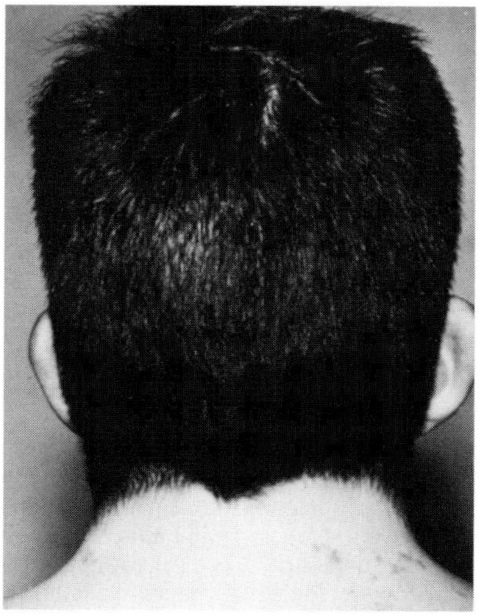

FIGURE 5–23. Low posterior hairline, usually related to either a short or webbed neck.

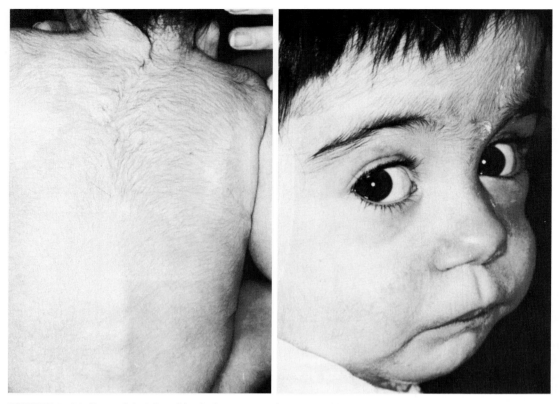

FIGURE 5-24. General facial and body hirsutism, often normal but sometimes related to failure to thrive.

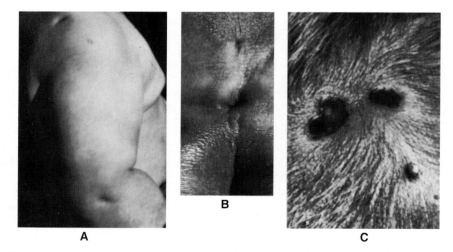

A

B

C

FIGURE 5-25. Unusual *dimples* (*A* and *B*) may occur at a location where there has been a closer than usual proximity between the skin and underlying bony structures during fetal life, resulting in deficient development of subcutaneous tissue at that locus. Such dimples may be secondary either to a deficit in early subcutaneous tissue or to an aberrant bony promontory. They tend to occur at the elbows, knees, over the acromion promontories, and over the lower sacrum, as shown above. In the latter location, they often have subsidiary creases and pits and should be distinguished from a pilonidal sinus. *C, Punched-out scalp lesions* are most commonly found toward the midline in the posterior parietal scalp area. The skin is usually totally lacking, but the crater becomes covered with scar tissue postnatally. The developmental pathology for these lesions is unknown.

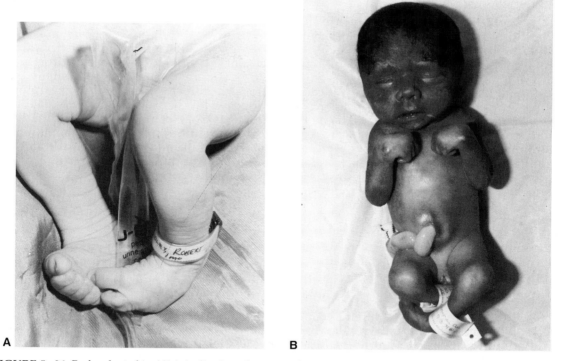

FIGURE 5–26. Redundant skin (*A*) is indicative of tangential traction produced by external constraint. Compare the redundant skin in *A* to the tight, thin skin over the joints in *B*, which is indicative of early onset lack of mobility secondary to neurologic impairment.

results in bilateral frontal hair streams that emanate from the fixed points of the ocular puncta and tend to arc outward in a lateral direction, thereby affecting eyebrow hair directional patterning (Fig. 5–14). The anterior parietal hair stream normally converges with the upsweeping frontal hair stream on the forehead, resulting in a variety of forehead hair patterning, such as converging whorls and quadriradial patterns. If the frontal hair stream meets the parietal hair stream above the forehead, there may be an anterior upsweep of the scalp hair, known as a "cowlick." Mild to moderate lateral upsweep or central upsweep of the scalp hair occurs in 5 per cent of normal individuals.

Defects of the calvarium, such as primary craniosynostosis, have not been noted to affect hair patterning, since the calvarium is not yet developed at the time of hair follicle downgrowth.

Relevance and Nature of Aberrant Scalp and Upper Facial Hair Directional Patterning. Abnormal size and/or shape of the brain and upper facial area during the 10-

to 16-week fetal period can apparently result in aberrant hair patterning. Severe microcephaly may lead to a lack of a parietal hair whorl (25 per cent) and/or a frontal upsweep of the scalp hair (70 per cent), as shown in Figure 5–15. The latter feature appears to relate to the individual who has a narrow and smaller frontal area of the brain.

The parietal whorl is more likely to be midline and posteriorly located in patients with microcephaly, as shown in Figure 5–16. In a variety of other gross defects of early brain development, the hair directional patterning may be secondarily altered. In each case, the aberrant scalp hair patterning reflects the altered shape and/or growth of the early fetal brain. Gross aberrations of hair patterning often imply a serious degree of mental deficient, since the brain is at such an early stage of development at 10 to 16 weeks (Fig. 5–17). Abnormal eyebrow patterning, such as the unusual outflaring of the medial eyebrows of the patient shown in Figure 5–18, implies that there was abnormal shape and/or growth in the upper midface prior to or during the period of hair follicle downgrowth, which occurs from 10 to 16 weeks of fetal development.

Hair Growth Patterns

Normal Development and Relevance. At 18 fetal weeks, when hair first emerges, it grows on the entire face and scalp, as noted in Figure 5–19. Later, the eyebrows and scalp hair predominate, and the growth of hair over the remainder of the face is apparently suppressed. Studies imply that there is a periocular zone of hair growth suppression.

Nature and Relevance of Aberrant Facial Hair Growth Patterns. The V-shaped midline, downward projection of the scalp hair, known as the "widow's peak," is considered to represent an upper forehead intersection of the bilateral fields of periocular hair growth suppression.[13] This may occur because the fields are widely spaced, as in ocular hypertelorism, or because the ocular fields of hair growth suppression are smaller with a low scalp hairline and low position of intersection, as illustrated in Figure 5–20. In the presence of cryptophthalmos, there may be an abnormal projection of scalp-like hair growth toward the ocular area (Fig. 5–21). The auricle appears to influence hair growth in the region anterior to the ear. With absence of the auricle, there is usually absence of hair growth in the sideburn area (Fig. 5–22) anterior to the ear. When there is a rudimentary ear, such as is often found in Treacher Collins syndrome, there may be an aberrant tongue of hair growth projecting onto the cheek area.

Usually, a short neck or webbed neck may be associated with the secondary feature of a low posterior hairline, especially at the lateral borders, as shown in Figure 5–23.

Whether the facial body hirsutism (Fig. 5–24) found in patients with the de Lange syndrome and in a variety of failure to thrive growth deficiency disorders represents a more generalized failure of normal growth suppression in these conditions remains to be determined.

OTHER CUTANEOUS ANOMALIES

Cutaneous features such as unusual dimples and punched-out scalp lesions are shown in Figure 5–25. The skin normally grows in response to the growth of the structure which it invests. Tangential traction on the skin produced by external constraint can lead to redundant skin (Fig. 5–26).[17] Differentiation between talipes equinovarus due to intrauterine constraint as opposed to a neurologic problem that limits joint mobility can sometimes be made by observing the skin, which in the latter situation is taut and thin secondary to early onset lack of movement in a fetus that has had ample space to move.

References

1. Marden, P. M., Smith, D. W., and McDonald, M. J.: Congenital anomalies in the newborn infant, including minor variations. J. Pediatr., *64*:357, 1964.
2. Mehes, K., et al.: Minor malformation in the neonate. Helv. Pediatr. Acta, *28*:477, 1973.
3. Leppig, K. A., et al.: Predictive value of minor anomalies. Association with major malformations. J. Pediatr., *110*:530, 1987.
4. Popich, G. A., and Smith, D. W.: Fontanels: Range of normal size. J. Pediatr., *80*:479, 1972.
5. Smith, D. W., and Popich, G. A.: Large fontanels in congenital hypothyroidism: A potential clue toward earlier recognition. J. Pediatr., *80*:753, 1972.
6. Davies, P.: Sex and the single transverse crease in newborn singletons. Dev. Med. Child Neurol., *8*:729, 1966.
7. Popich, G. A., and Smith, D. W.: The genesis and significance of digital and palmar hand creases: Preliminary report. J. Pediatr., *77*:1917, 1970.
8. Mulvihill, J., and Smith, D. W.: Genesis of dermal ridge patterning. J. Pediatr., *75*:1969.
9. Ford-Walker, N.: Inkless methods of finger, palm and sole printing. J. Pediatr., *50*:27, 1957.
10. Uchida, I. A., and Soltan, H. C.: Evaluation of dermatoglyphics in medical genetics. Pediatr. Clin. North. Am., *10*:409, 1963.
11. Aase, J. M., and Lyons, R. B.: Technique for recording dermatoglyphics. Lancet, *1*:32, 1971.
12. Smith, D. W., and Gong, B. T.: Scalp hair patterning as a clue to early fetal brain development. J. Pediatr., *83*:374, 1973 and Teratology, *9*:17, 1974.
13. Smith, D. W., and Cohen, M. M., Jr.: Widow's peak scalp anomaly, origin and relevance to ocular hypertelorism. Lancet, *2*:1127, 1973.
14. Graham, J. M.: Recognizable Patterns of Human Deformation, 2nd ed. Philadelphia, W. B. Saunders Co., 1988.
15. Jones, M. C.: Unilateral epicanthal folds: Diagnostic significance. J. Pediatr., *108*:702, 1986.
16. Smith, D. W., and Takashima, H.: Protruding auricle, a neuromuscular sign. Lancet, *1*:747, 1978.
17. Aase, J. M.: Structural defects as a consequence of late intrauterine constraint: Craniotabes, loose skin and asymmetric ear size. Semin. Perinatol., *7*:237, 1983.

6

Normal Standards

The following compilation of normal measurements is set forth as an aid in determining whether or not a given feature is abnormal. Such data may be especially useful when the visual impression is potentially misleading For example, when the nasal bridge is low-set, the visual impression may falsely suggest ocular hypertelorism, and when the patient is obese, the hands may *appear* to be small. Besides comparing patient measurements with these normal cross-sectional population standards, it may be important to contrast the findings of the patient with those of his parents and/or siblings in an attempt to determine whether or not a given feature is unusual for that particular family.

These measurements have been predominantly obtained from whites and hence may not be accurate for other racial groups. Separate data are presented for males and females, except for features that do not show significant differences between the sexes. For paired structures, the measurements are given for the right side. Many of the charts were kindly supplied by Dr. Murray Feingold from his Boston study of normal measurements. For normal measurements of structures not included in this chapter, the reader is referred to the excellent reference by Hall et al., *Handbook of Normal Physical Measurements*, New York, Oxford University Press, 1989.

STANDARDS FOR HEIGHT AND WEIGHT*

The growth charts for young children (Figs. 6–1 to 6–4) were developed by J. M.

Tanner and R. H. Whitehouse at the University of London Institute of Child Health. The data on means and standard deviations (Tables 6–1 and 6–2) relate to the four growth charts for young children. The subsequent four charts, which concern growth from birth through adolescence (Figs. 6–5 to 6–8), are from Tanner et al.[1]

Notes on Use

1. *Weight* is preferably taken in the nude; otherwise, the estimated weight of clothing is subtracted before plotting.

2. When a child is born earlier than 40 weeks' gestation preterm, the birth weight is plotted at the appropriate number of weeks on the chart. Subsequent weights are plotted in relation to this "conception age"; thus for a child born at 32 weeks, the 8-weeks-after-birth weight is plotted at B (birth) on the scale, the 12-week weight at 4 weeks after B, and so on. Length is plotted in the same manner.

3. *Supine length* (up to age 2.0 years) should be taken with the infant lying on a measuring table constructed for this purpose. One person holds the infant's head so that he looks straight upward (the lower borders of the eye sockets and the external auditory meati should be in the same vertical plane) and pulls very gently to bring the top of the head into contact with the fixed measuring board. A second person, the measurer, presses the infant's knees down into contact with the board, and, also pulling gently to stretch the infant out, holds the infant's feet, with the toes pointing directly upward. He brings the movable

*Obtainable from Creaseys Ltd., Print Division, Bull Plain, Hertford, England.

747

footboard to rest firmly against the infant's heels and reads the measurement to the last completed 0.1 cm.

4. *Standing height* should be taken without shoes, the child standing with heels and back in contact with an upright wall or preferably a stadiometer made for this purpose.[†] His head is held so that he looks straight forward, with the lower borders of the eye sockets on the same horizontal plane as the external auditory meati (i.e., head not with nose tipped upwards). A right-angled block (preferably counterweighted) is slid down the wall until its bottom surface touches the child's head, and a scale fixed to the wall is read. During this measurement, the child should be told to stretch his neck to be as tall as possible, though care must be taken to prevent his heels from coming off the ground. The measurer should apply gentle but firm upward pressure under the mastoid processes to help the child stretch. In this way, the variation in height from morning to evening is minimized. Standing height should be recorded to the last completed 0.1 cm.

5. The sources of the standards on young children are (a) weight from 32 to 40 weeks'

gestation, Tanner-Thomson standards (published by Creaseys, 1970 and in Arch. Dis. Child., *45*:566, 1970) from Aberdeen data; (b) length from 32 to 40 weeks estimated from West European and North American data, not available for England; and (c) weight and length after 40-week birth, same sources as Tanner-Whitehouse 0- to 18-year-old standards (published by Creaseys, 1966 and detailed in Arch. Dis. Child., *41*:454, 613, 1966.)

OTHER STANDARDS

The reader will find charts showing normal measurements for head circumference, chest, hand, foot, inner and outer canthal distances, palpebral fissure, length, fontanel, ear, penis, and testis (Figs. 6–9 to 6–21) after the growth charts.

Reference

1. Tanner, J. M., Whitehouse, R. H., and Takaishi, M.: Standards from birth to maturity for height, weight, height velocity, and weight velocity. Arch. Dis. Child., *41*:613, 1966.

[†]Obtainable from Holtain Ltd., Crymmych, Pembrokeshire, England.

LINEAR GROWTH
MALES, FIRST 5 YEARS

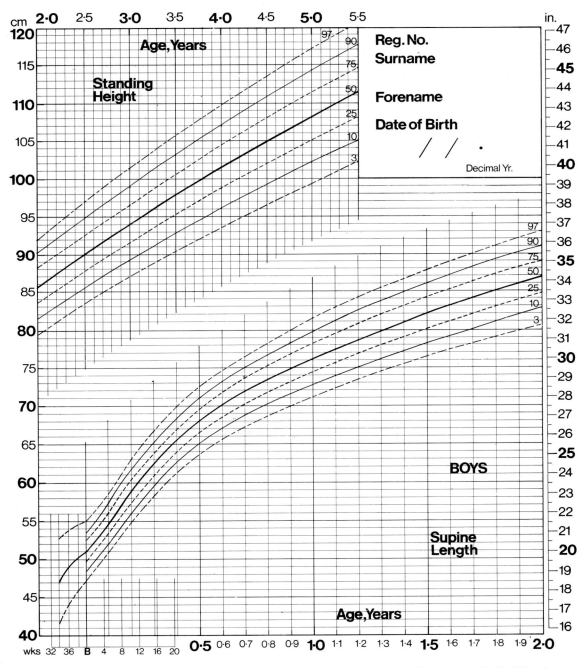

FIGURE 6–1. Linear growth, males, first 5 years. (Chart prepared by J. M. Tanner and R. H. Whitehouse, University of London Institute of Child Health, for the Hospital for Sick Children, Great Ormond Street, London, W. C.I. Printed by Creaseys of Hertford, Ltd. No. Ref SHWB28. For information on sources used to develop standards, see text, item 5.)

WEIGHT GROWTH
MALES, FIRST 5 YEARS

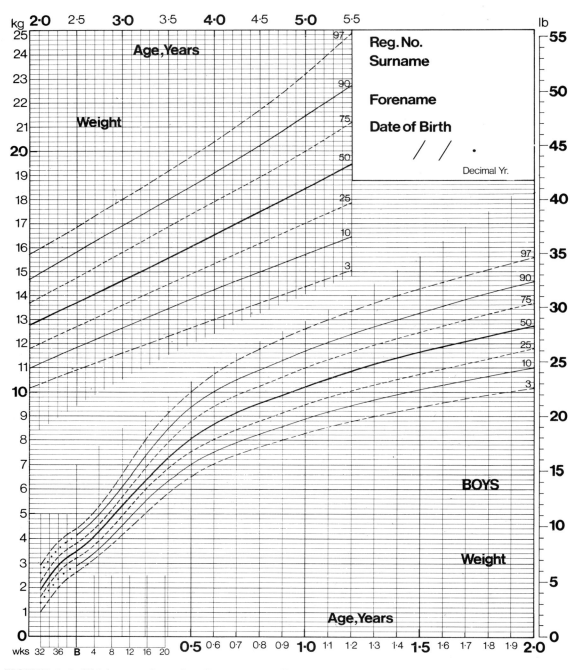

FIGURE 6–2. Weight growth, males, first 5 years. (Chart prepared by J. M. Tanner and R. H. Whitehouse, University of London Institute of Child Health, for the Hospital for Sick Children, Great Ormond Street, London, W. C.I. Printed by Creaseys of Hertford, Ltd. No. Ref SHWB28. For information on sources used to develop standards, see text, item 5.)

LINEAR GROWTH
FEMALES, FIRST 5 YEARS

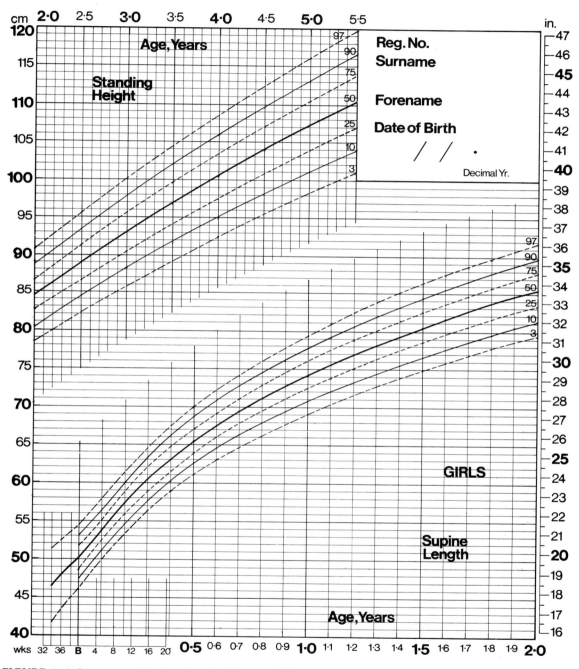

FIGURE 6–3. Linear growth, females, first 5 years. (Chart prepared by J. M. Tanner and R. H. Whitehouse, University of London Institute of Child Health, for the Hospital for Sick Children, Great Ormond Street, London, W. C.I. Printed by Creaseys of Hertford, Ltd. No. Ref SHWB28. For information on sources used to develop standards, see text, item 5.)

WEIGHT GROWTH
FEMALES, FIRST 5 YEARS

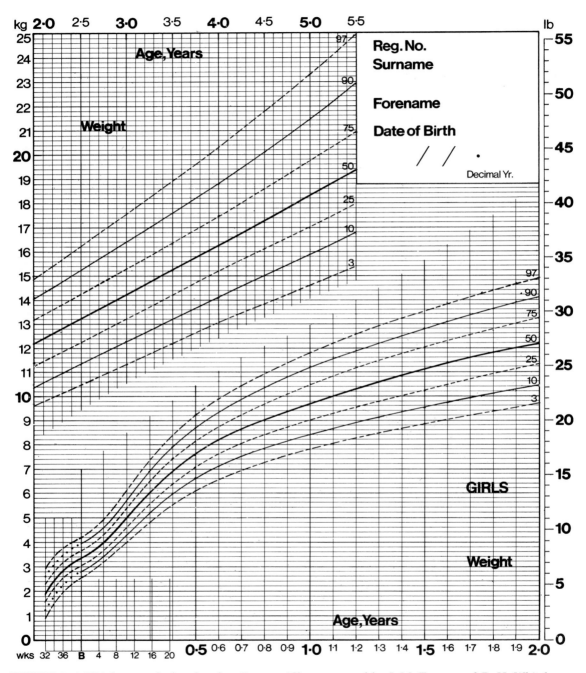

FIGURE 6–4. Weight growth, females, first 5 years. (Chart prepared by J. M. Tanner and R. H. Whitehouse, University of London Institute of Child Health, for the Hospital for Sick Children, Great Ormond Street, London, W. C. I. Printed by Creaseys of Hertford, Ltd. No. Ref SHWB28. For information on sources used to develop standards, see text, item 5.)

TABLE 6–1. MEANS AND STANDARD DEVIATIONS—MALES*

Weight		Head Circumference		Length Velocity	Height Velocity	Weight Velocity		Triceps Skinfold		Subscapular Skinfold	
Mean	SD	Mean	SD	(Mean)	(SD)	Mean	SD	Mean	SD	Mean	SD
3.50	0.53	36.00	1.97	47.00	3.00	8.93	1.80	175.0	12.56	172.0	14.8
5.93	0.66	40.20	1.70	36.00	2.63	9.85	2.38	193.0	12.10	182.0	14.8
7.90	0.80	43.65	1.60	24.00	2.34	6.80	1.61	201.0	12.00	184.8	15.0
9.20	1.15	45.60	1.60	16.25	2.15	4.30	1.22	202.0	12.50	184.0	15.2
10.20	1.01	46.65	1.60	13.40	1.98	3.33	0.93	201.0	12.70	182.0	15.8
11.60	1.17	48.10	1.49	10.50	1.75	2.44	0.71	198.3	12.90	173.0	15.6
12.70	1.33	49.03	1.49	8.90/9.00	1.48/1.64	2.10	0.63	195.8	13.10	168.0	15.2
14.70	1.61	50.37	1.41	7.88	1.34	1.96	0.69	191.0	10.40	162.0	15.5
16.60	1.90	51.12	1.36	7.00	1.12	1.90	0.77	187.0	13.50	158.3	16.2
18.50	2.17	51.60	1.33	6.48	1.03	1.92	0.85	183.5	13.90	155.2	16.6
20.50	2.44	51.88	1.33	6.09	0.91	2.07	0.94	181.4	14.70	153.4	16.8
22.60	2.75	52.12	1.33	5.79	0.87	2.31	1.02	180.3	15.60	153.0	17.5
25.00	3.12	52.29	1.33	5.55	0.77	2.47	1.14	180.0	17.00	153.8	18.3
27.50	5.98	52.43	1.36	5.35	0.76	2.67	0.88	180.8	18.70	155.5	19.9
30.30	7.04	52.70	1.49	5.16	0.70	2.87	1.60	182.4	20.70	158.0	23.4
33.30	7.78	53.10	1.46	5.01	0.68	3.08	1.70	184.4	22.40	162.0	26.0
36.50	8.48	53.60	1.54	4.98	0.79	3.50	1.75	186.0	23.00	165.8	26.5
40.70	8.47	54.10	1.54	6.55	1.03	5.13	1.78	184.4	23.70	187.0	25.2
48.40	9.42	54.59	1.54	9.45	1.20	9.06	1.95	181.0	23.50	186.0	23.1
56.30	9.52	54.85	1.49	5.86	1.13	5.68	1.89	178.4	23.20	188.0	20.7
60.20	9.63	55.00	1.46	2.65	0.91	2.60	1.00	178.8	23.40	179.6	18.7
62.10	9.60			1.00	0.50			182.0	21.70	185.7	17.8
63.00	9.69			0.05	0.40			185.7	21.50	190.4	17.5
								188.8	21.20	192.3	17.5

*Adapted from data in Forfar, J. O., and Arneil, G. C.: Textbook of Pediatrics, 2nd edition. Edinburgh, Scotland, Churchill Livingstone, 1978; and from Tanner, J. M., and Whitehouse, R. H.: Personal communication.

TABLE 6–2. MEANS AND STANDARD DEVIATIONS—FEMALES*

Weight		Head Circumference		Length Velocity	Height Velocity	Weight Velocity		Triceps Skinfold		Subscapular Skinfold	
Mean	SD	Mean	SD	(Mean)	(SD)	Mean	SD	Mean	SD	Mean	SD
3.40	0.57	34.00	1.60	41.00	3.00	7.42	1.91	175.7	10.9	173.2	12.3
5.56	0.64	39.60	1.52	32.00	2.63	9.25	2.69	189.7	10.5	183.0	12.9
7.39	0.80	42.60	1.44	22.50	2.34	6.60	1.55	196.3	11.9	186.0	14.1
8.72	0.90	44.62	1.44	16.45	2.15	4.29	1.32	198.8	12.9	184.8	14.4
9.70	1.01	45.45	1.41	14.70	1.98	3.37	0.99	199.5	13.6	182.0	14.0
11.10	1.12	46.90	1.38	11.20	1.75	2.44	0.72	199.4	13.8	177.3	14.4
12.20	1.33	47.90	1.37	9.15/9.30	1.43/1.64	2.08	0.57	198.7	13.7	173.8	14.8
14.30	1.54	49.33	1.25	7.90	1.34	2.00	0.73	196.8	13.6	169.0	16.3
16.30	1.69	50.20	1.28	7.03	1.15	2.00	0.78	194.7	13.4	166.0	17.5
18.30	2.65	50.80	1.28	6.48	1.09	2.05	1.10	192.5	13.9	163.4	18.5
20.40	3.39	51.20	1.28	6.09	0.95	2.17	1.22	190.7	14.7	162.0	19.1
22.60	4.23	51.50	1.28	5.82	0.87	2.30	1.34	190.0	16.1	162.1	20.7
25.10	5.24	51.70	1.28	5.55	0.80	2.54	1.38	191.7	17.6	164.2	23.2
27.70	6.34	51.90	1.28	5.47	0.78	2.81	0.96	194.6	18.7	167.8	25.5
30.70	7.72	52.15	1.30	5.47	0.83	3.16	1.56	197.0	19.4	172.2	27.7
34.20	8.68	52.65	1.33	6.50	1.01	4.05	1.65	198.7	19.8	178.0	28.0
39.60	9.52	53.20	1.33	8.33	1.10	7.43	1.42	199.8	20.1	184.0	26.5
47.80	9.79	53.62	1.28	5.50	1.05	7.25	1.40	201.5	19.9	188.3	24.7
53.00	9.79	53.97	1.20	2.36	0.84	3.55	1.30	205.3	19.2	193.0	22.6
55.20	9.79	54.18	1.14	0.60	0.52	1.48	1.41	209.8	18.2	198.7	19.9
56.00	9.79	54.27	1.14	0.20	0.52	0.22	1.11	213.4	17.4	201.5	19.0
56.40	9.79			0.00	0.50			215.0	16.6	202.8	18.3
56.60	9.79			0.00	0.40			215.5	16.4	203.0	18.7
								215.5	16.4	203.0	18.7

*Adapted from data in Forfar, J. O., and Arneil, G. D.: Textbook of Paediatrics, 2nd edition. Edinburgh, Scotland, Churchill Livingstone, 1978; and from Tanner, J. M., and Whitehouse, R. H.: Personal communication.

LINEAR GROWTH
MALES

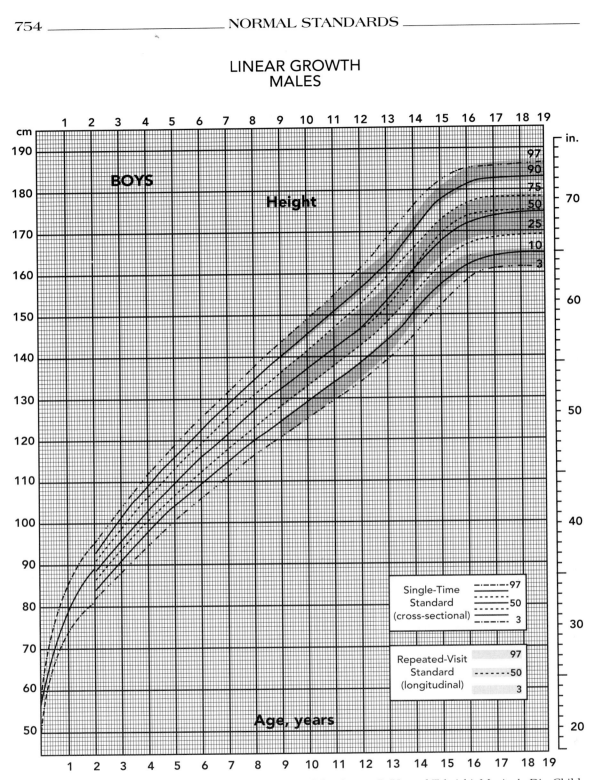

FIGURE 6–5. Linear growth, males. (From Tanner, J. M., Whitehouse, R. H., and Takaishi, M.: Arch. Dis. Child., *41*:613, 1966, with permission.)

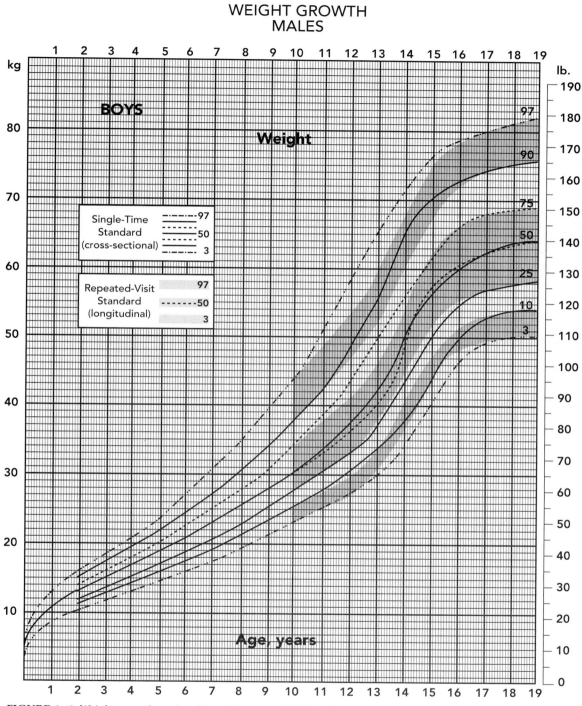

FIGURE 6–6. Weight growth, males. (From Tanner, J. M., Whitehouse, R. H., and Takaishi, M.: Arch. Dis. Child., *41*:613, 1966, with permission.)

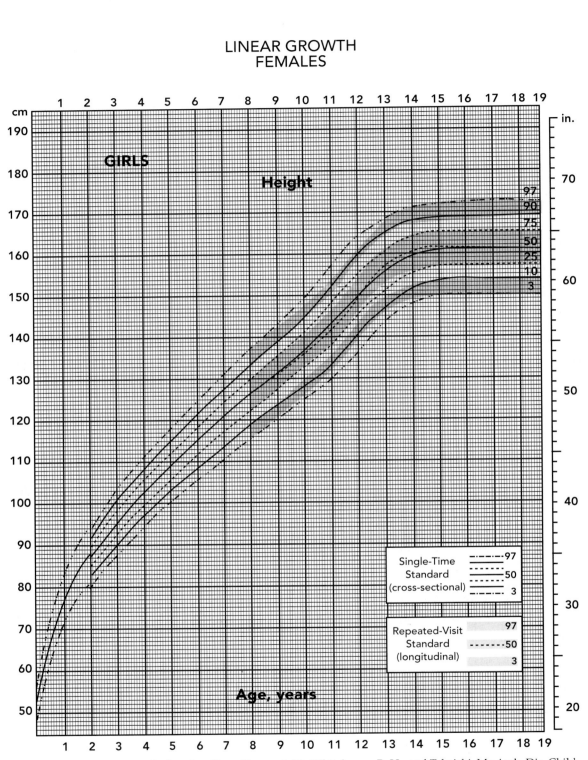

FIGURE 6–7. Linear growth, females. (From Tanner, J. M., Whitehouse, R. H., and Takaishi, M.: Arch. Dis. Child., *41*:613, 1966, with permission.)

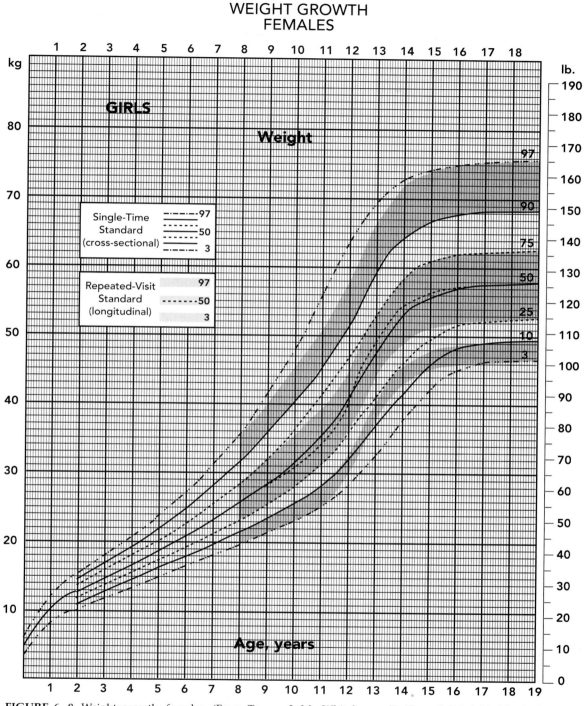

FIGURE 6–8. Weight growth, females. (From Tanner, J. M., Whitehouse, R. H., and Takaishi, M.: Arch. Dis. Child., *41*:613, 1966, with permission.)

HEAD CIRCUMFERENCES

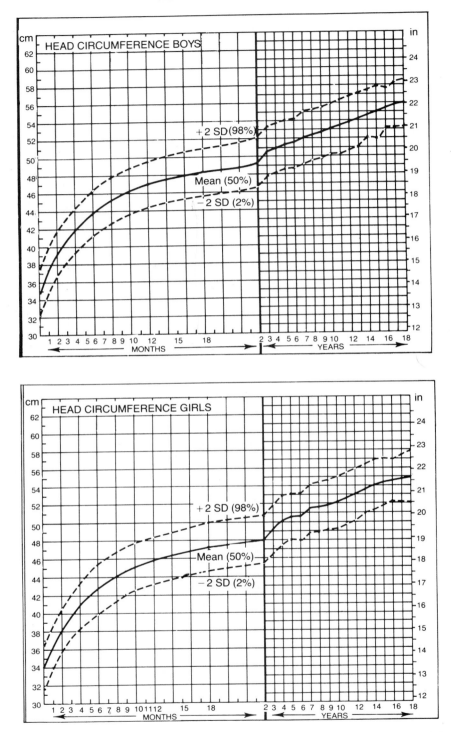

FIGURE 6–9. Head circumferences. (From Nellhaus, G.: Pediatrics, *41*:106, 1968. University of Colorado Medical Center Printing Services.)

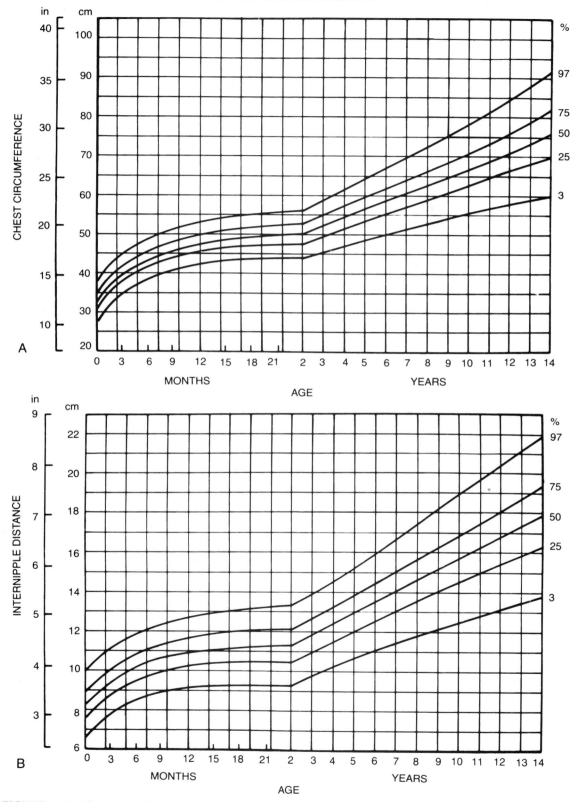

FIGURE 6–10. Chest circumference (*A*) and internipple distance (*B*). (From Feingold, M., and Bossert, W. H.: Birth Defects, *10*[Suppl. 13]: 1974. With permission of the copyright holder, March of Dimes Birth Defects Foundation.)

HAND MEASUREMENTS

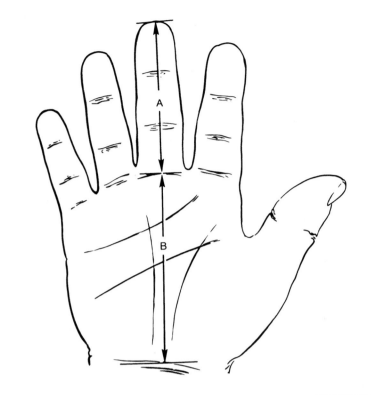

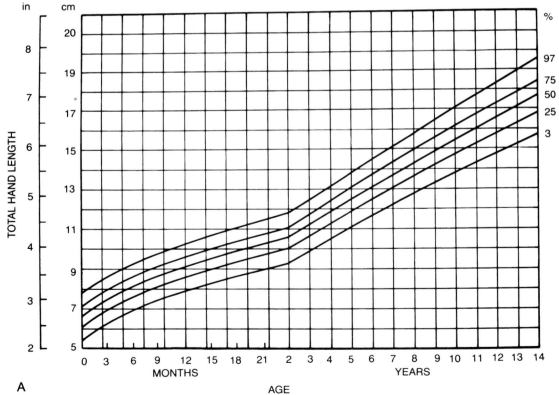

FIGURE 6–11. Hand length (*A*), middle finger length (*B*), and palm length (*C*). (From Feingold, M., and Bossert, W. H.: Birth Defects, *10*[Suppl. 13]: 1974. With permission of the copyright holder, March of Dimes Birth Defects Foundation.)

Illustration continued on opposite page

HAND MEASUREMENTS

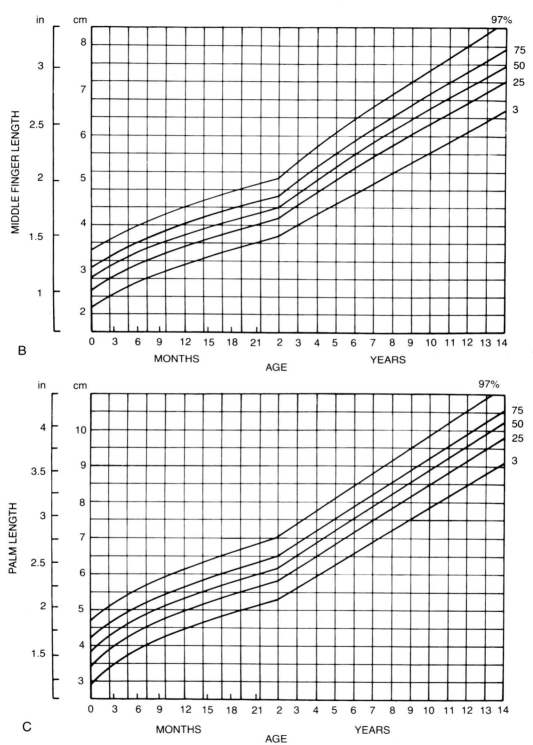

HAND MEASUREMENTS

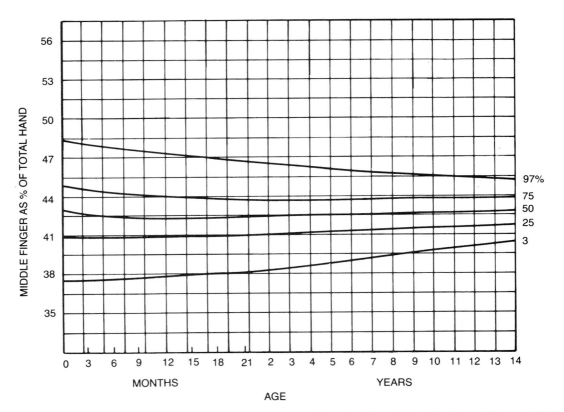

FIGURE 6–12. Proportion (per cent) of middle finger to hand length. (From Feingold, M., and Bossert, W. H.: Birth Defects, *10*[Suppl. 13]: 1974. With permission of the copyright holder, March of Dimes Birth Defects Foundation.)

FOOT LENGTH

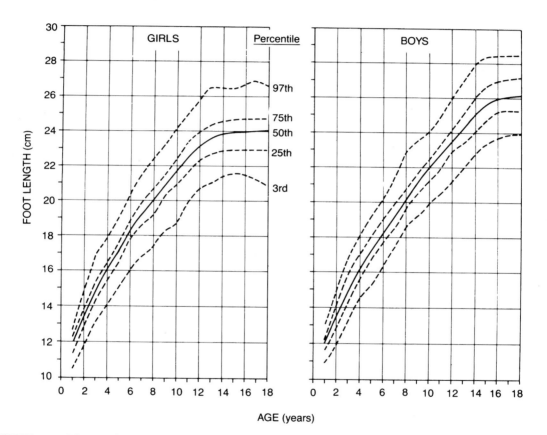

FIGURE 6–13. Mean and percentile values for foot length. Note: The adolescent growth spurt of the foot usually begins prior to the general linear growth spurt and ends before final height attainment. Thus, the foot growth spurt is a good early indicator of adolescence. (Adapted from Blais, M. M., Green, W. T., and Anderson, M.: J. Bone Joint Surg., *38-A*:998, 1956, with permission.)

FACIAL MEASUREMENTS

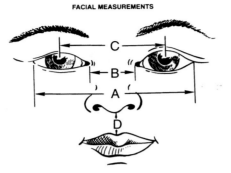

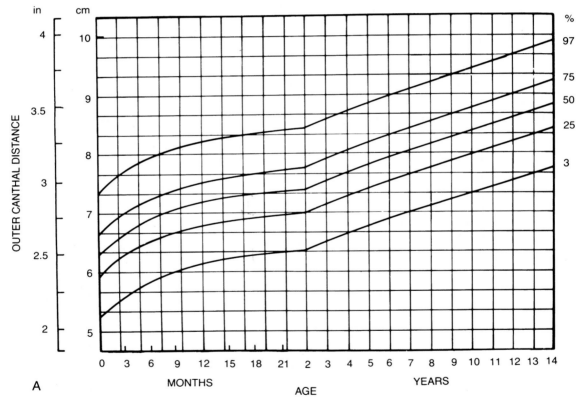

A

FIGURE 6–14. Outer canthal (*A*), inner canthal (*B*), and interpupillary (*C*) measurements. (From Feingold, M., and Bossert, W. H.: Birth Defects, *10*[Suppl. 13]: 1974. With permission of the copyright holder, March of Dimes Birth Defects Foundation.)

Illustration continued on facing page

FACIAL MEASUREMENTS

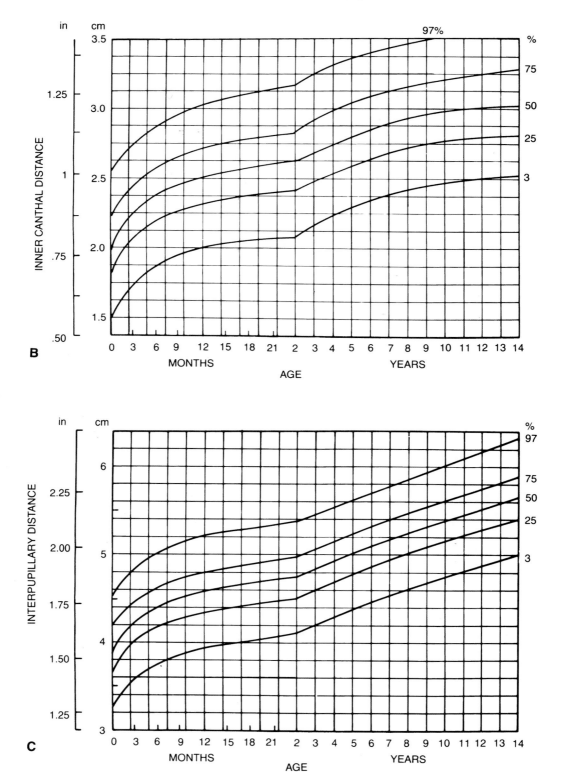

EYE MEASUREMENTS

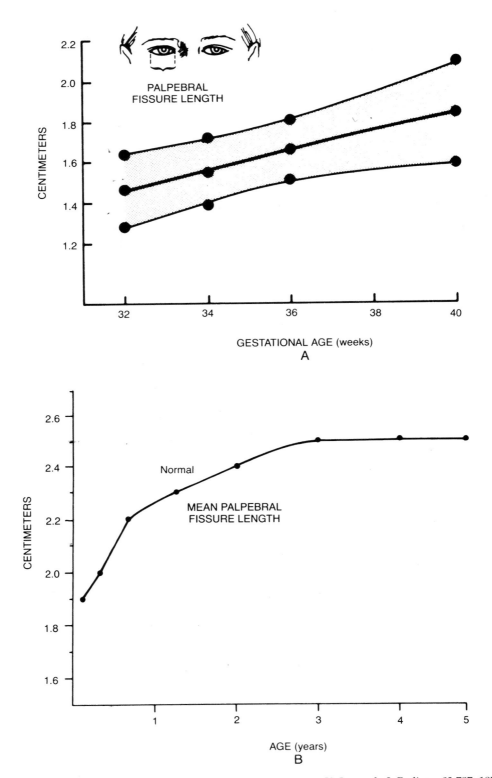

FIGURE 6–15. *A*, Palpebral fissure length, 32–40 weeks. (From Jones, K. L., et al.: J. Pediatr., *92*:787, 1978, with permission.) *B*, Palpebral fissure length, from inner to outer canthus, 1 to 5 years. (Data from Chouke, K. S.: Am. J. Phys. Antropol., *13*:255, 1929.)

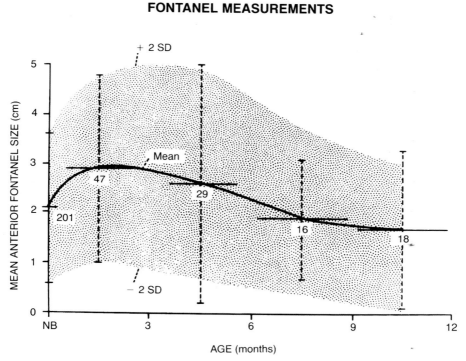

FONTANEL MEASUREMENTS

FIGURE 6–16. Mean anterior fontanel measurement (length plus width divided by 2) during the first year. The numbers below the mean line indicate the number of normal infants measured at each age. Note: The posterior fontanel was fingertip size or smaller in dimension in 97 per cent of newborn infants. (From Popich, G., and Smith, D. W.: J. Pediatr., *80*:749, 1972, with permission.)

EAR LENGTH

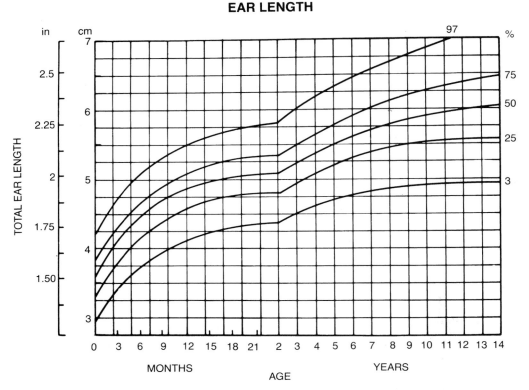

FIGURE 6–17. Maximum ear length. (From Feingold, M., and Bossert, W. H.: Birth Defects, *10*[Suppl. 13]: 1974. With permission of the copyright holder, March of Dimes Birth Defects Foundation.)

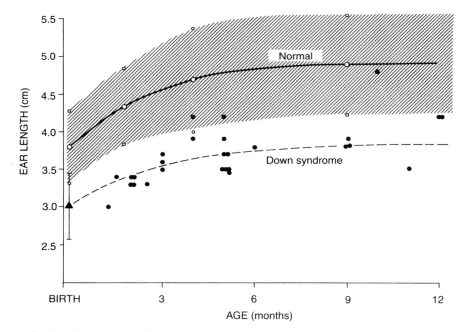

FIGURE 6–18. Ear length in normals during the first year, showing mean 2 standard deviations in hatched area, as contrasted with ear length in the Down syndrome, showing mean and 2 standard deviations for 26 affected newborns and individual values (*black dots*) during the first year. (From Aase, J. M., et al.: J. Pediatr., *82*:845, 1973, with permission.)

PENILE LENGTH

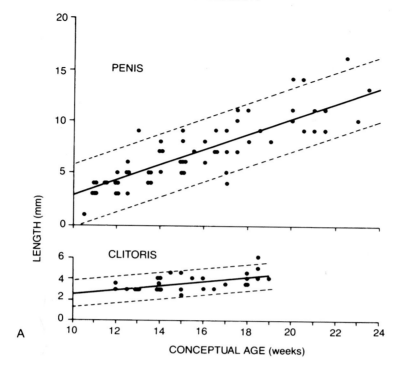

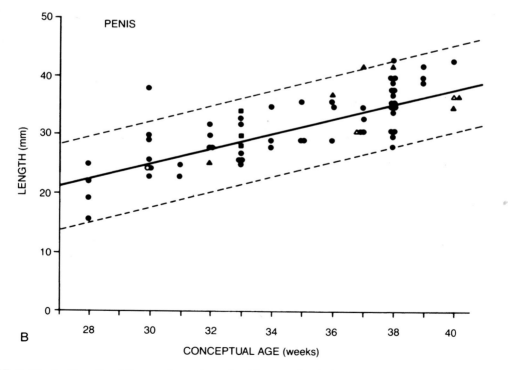

FIGURE 6–19. *A,* Growth of the penis contrasted with growth of the clitoris from formalin-fixed fetuses. *B,* Penile stretched length (from public bone to tip of glans) in the newborn. The mean full-term length is 3.5 cm with a 2–standard deviation range, from 2.8 to 4.2 cm. The *solid line* approximates the mean values, and the *broken lines* the 2–standard deviation values. (From Feldman, K. W., and Smith, D. W.: J. Pediatr., *86:*395, 1975, with permission.)

PENILE AND TESTICULAR GROWTH

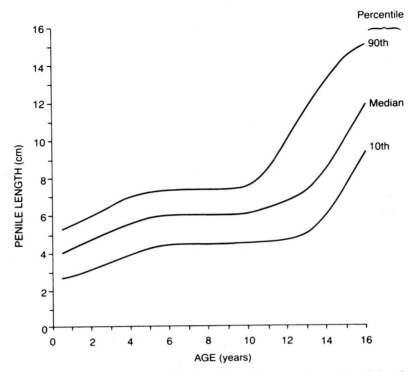

FIGURE 6–20. Penile growth in stretched length (from the pubic ramus to the tip of the glans) from infancy into adolescence. (From Schonfeld, W. A.: Am. J. Dis. Child., *65*:535, 1943, with permission.)

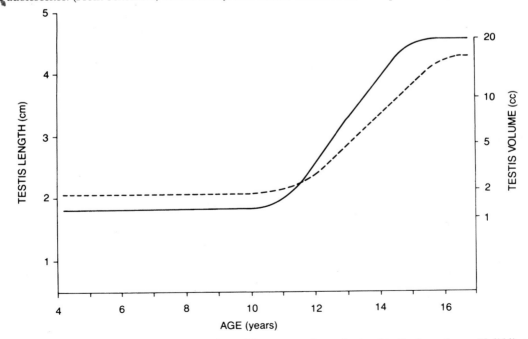

FIGURE 6–21. Testicular growth in length, adapted from normal standards of testicular volume. (*Solid line* from data of A. Prader, Zurich; *broken line* from data of Laron, A., and Zilka, E.: J. Clin. Endocrinol. Metab., *29*:1409, 1969.)

APPENDIX:
Pattern of Malformation Differential Diagnosis by Anomalies

The following lists were developed from the syndromes delineated in Chapter One. Listed for each anomaly are the syndromes in which this defect is a frequent feature, as well as those syndromes in which it is an occasional feature. Characteristics such as mental or growth deficiency are not considered because they are frequent features in a large number of disorders.

The anomalies are set forth under the following headings:

1. Central Nervous System Dysfunction other than Mental Deficiency
2. Deafness
3. Brain: Major Anomalies
4. Cranium
5. Scalp and Facial Hair Patterning
6. Facies
7. Ocular Region
8. Eye
9. Nose
10. Maxilla and Mandible
11. Oral Region and Mouth
12. Teeth
13. External Ears
14. Neck, Thorax, and Vertebrae
15. Limbs
16. Limbs: Nails, Creases, Dermatoglyphics
17. Limbs: Joints
18. Skin and Hair
19. Cardiac
20. Abdominal
21. Renal
22. Genital
23. Endocrine and Metabolic
24. Immune Deficiency
25. Hematology-Oncology
26. Unusual Growth Patterns

1. CENTRAL NERVOUS SYSTEM DYSFUNCTION OTHER THAN MENTAL DEFICIENCY

Hypotonicity

Frequent in

Occasional in

Hypertonicity

Frequent in

Occasional in

Ataxia

Frequent in

Occasional in

Seizures

Frequent in

2. DEAFNESS

Frequent in

Occasional in

3. BRAIN: MAJOR ANOMALIES

Anencephaly/Meningomyelocele

Occasional in

Encephalocele

Frequent in

Occasional in

Hydrocephalus

Frequent in

Occasional in

Microcephaly

Frequent in

Frontal Bossing or Prominent Central Forehead

5. SCALP AND FACIAL HAIR PATTERNING

Anterior Upsweep, Scalp

Posterior Midline Scalp Defects

6. FACIES

"Flat" Facies

Occasional in

Slanted Palpebral Fissures

Frequent in

Occasional in

Shallow Orbital Ridges

Frequent in

Occasional in

Prominent Supraorbital Ridges

Frequent in

Prominent Eyes

Frequent in

Occasional in

Periorbital Fullness of Subcutaneous Tissue

Frequent in

Eyebrows Extending to Midline (Synophrys)

Frequent in

Nystagmus

Frequent in

Occasional in

Occasional in

8. Eye

Myopia

Frequent in

Occasional in

Blue Sclerae

Frequent in

Occasional in

Microphthalmos

Frequent in

Occasional in

Iris, Unusual Patterning or Coloration

Frequent in

Colobomata of Iris

Frequent in

Occasional in

Glaucoma

Frequent in

Occasional in

Large Cornea

Frequent in

Occasional in

Keratoconus, Microcornea

Frequent in

Occasional in

Corneal Opacity

Frequent in

Occasional in

Cataract, Lenticular Opacities

Frequent in

9. Nose

Low Nasal Bridge

Frequent in

Occasional in

Prominent Nasal Bridge

Frequent in

Occasional in

Broad Nasal Bridge

Frequent in

Broad Nasal Root

Frequent in

Small or Short Nose, With or Without Anteverted Nostrils

Frequent in

Occasional in

Hypoplasia of Nares and/or Alae Nasi

Frequent in

Occasional in

Prominent Nose (Relative)

Frequent in

Occasional in

Choanal Atresia

Frequent in

Occasional in

10. MAXILLA AND MANDIBLE

Malar Hypoplasia

Frequent in

Maxillary Hypoplasia, Often With Narrow or High Arched Palate

Frequent in

Occasional in

Micrognathia

Frequent in

Occasional in

Prognathism

Frequent in

Occasional in

11. ORAL REGION AND MOUTH

Cleft Lip With or Without Cleft Palate

Frequent in

Occasional in

Abnormal Philtrum

Frequent in

Prominent Full Lips

Frequent in

Occasional in

Lower Lip Pits

Frequent in

Occasional in

Downturned Corners of Mouth

Frequent in

Microstomia

Frequent in

Macrostomia

Cleft Palate or Bifid Uvula Without Cleft in Lip

Oral Frenula (Webs)

Frequent in

Occasional in

Cleft or Irregular Tongue

Frequent in

Occasional in

Macroglossia

Frequent in

12. TEETH

Anodontia (Aplasia)

Frequent in

Occasional in

Hypodontia (Including Conical Teeth)

Frequent in

Occasional in

Enamel Hypoplasia

Frequent in

Occasional in

Occasional in

Preauricular Tags or Pits

Frequent in

Occasional in

14. NECK, THORAX, AND VERTEBRAE

Web Neck or Redundant Skin

Frequent in

Hypoplasia of Clavicles

Frequent in

Occasional in

Other Clavicular Anomalies

Frequent in

Occasional in

Pectus Excavatum or Carinatum

Frequent in

Occasional in

Scoliosis

Frequent in

Occasional in

Other Vertebral Defects
(Usually As Part of Generalized
Bone Disorder)

Frequent in

Other Vertebral Defects
(Primarily Segmentation Defects)

Frequent in

Occasional in

Odontoid Hypoplasia/Cervical Spine Instability

Frequent in

Occasional in

15. LIMBS

Arachnodactyly

Frequent in

Occasional in

Fractures

Frequent in

Occasional in

Short Limbs

Frequent in

Occasional in

Limb Reduction, Moderate to Gross

Frequent in

Occasional in

Small Hands and Feet, Including Brachydactyly

Frequent in

Occasional in

Clinodactyly of Fifth Fingers

Frequent in

Occasional in

Thumb Hypoplasia to Aplasia, Triphalangeal Thumb

Frequent in

Occasional in

Radius Hypoplasia to Aplasia

Frequent in

Occasional in

Metacarpal Hypoplasia— All Metacarpals

Frequent in

Occasional in

Metacarpal Hypoplasia—Third, Fourth, and/or Fifth

Frequent in

Occasional in

Metacarpal Hypoplasia—First Metacarpal With Proximal Placement of Thumb

Metatarsal Hypoplasia

Polydactyly

Broad Thumb and/or Toe

Frequent in

Occasional in

Syndactyly, Cutaneous or Osseous

Frequent in

Occasional in

Elbow Dysplasia and Cubitus Valgus

Frequent in

Occasional in

Patella Dysplasia

Frequent in

Occasional in

16. LIMBS: NAILS, CREASES, DERMATOGLYPHICS

Nail Hypoplasia or Dysplasia

Frequent in

Single Crease (Simian), Upper Palm

Frequent in

Occasional in

Distal Palmar Axial Triradius

Frequent in

17. LIMBS: JOINTS

Joint Limitation and/or Contractures; Inability to Fully Extend (Other Than Foot)

Club Foot—Especially
Equinovarus Deformity, Including
Metatarsus Adductus

Frequent in

Clenched Hand: Index Finger Tending to Overlie the Third and the Fifth Finger Tending to Overlie the Fourth

Frequent in

Occasional in

Joint Hypermobility and/or Lax Ligaments

Frequent in

Occasional in

Joint Dislocation

Frequent in

Occasional in

18. SKIN AND HAIR

Loose Redundant Skin

Frequent in

Edema of Hands and Feet

Frequent in

Occasional in

Altered Skin Pigmentation, Melanomata

Frequent in

Occasional in

Thin Skin, Skin Defects

Frequent in

Altered Sweating

Frequent in

Occasional in

19. CARDIAC

Cardiac Malformation

Frequent in

Cardiomyopathy

Occasional in

Abnormal Connective Tissue/Storage

Frequent in

Occasional in

Arrhythmia/Abnormal EKG

Frequent in

Occasional in

20. ABDOMINAL

Inguinal or Umbilical Hernia

Frequent in

Occasional in

Hepatomegaly

Frequent in

Occasional in

Pyloric Stenosis

Frequent in

Incomplete Rotation of Colon (Malrotation)

Frequent in

Occasional in

Duodenal Atresia

Occasional in

Hirschsprung Aganglionosis

Frequent in

Occasional in

Aarskog S. 128
Deletion 13q S. 60
Fryns S. 210
Metaphyseal Dysplasia, McKusick
  Type 384
Nager S. 258
Senter-KID S. 554

Tracheoesophageal-Fistula/ Esophageal Atresia

Frequent in

VATER Association 664

Occasional in

Apert S. 418
CHARGE Association 668
DiGeorge Sequence 616
Down S. 8
Dyskeratosis Congenita S.
  (esophageal stenosis) 538
Fanconi Pancytopenia S. 320
Maternal PKU Fetal Effects 580
Metaphyseal Dysplasia, McKusick
  Type 384
Monozygotic (MZ) Twinning and
  Structural Defects—General 652
Opitz S. 132
Trisomy 18 S. 14
Waardenburg S. 248

Diaphragmatic Hernia

Frequent in

Fryns S. 210

Occasional in

Beckwith-Wiedemann S.
  (eventration) 164
Craniofrontonasal Dysplasia 422
de Lange S. 88
Deletion 9p S. 47
DiGeorge Sequence 616
Ehlers-Danlos 482
Escobar S. 306
Hydrolethalus S. 190
Iniencephaly Sequence 608
Kabuki S. (eventration) 116

Killian/Teschler-Nicola S. 208
Lethal Multiple Pterygium S. 178
Marfan S. 472
Microphthalmia—Linear Skin
  Defects S. 536
Miller S. 256
Simpson-Golabi-Behmel S. 168
Trisomy 9 Mosaic S. 28
Trisomy 13 S. 18
Trisomy 18 S. 14

Single Umbilical Artery

Frequent in

Exstrophy of Cloaca Sequence 628
Monozygotic (MZ) Twinning and
  Structural Defects—General 652
Sirenomelia Sequence 634
Trisomy 18 S. 14
VATER Association 664

Occasional in

Fetal Hydantoin S. 559
Jarcho-Levin S. 598
Meckel-Gruber S. 184
Multiple Lentigines S. 530
Trisomy 13 S. 18
Zellweger S. 212

Short Umbilical Cord

Frequent in

Amnion Rupture Sequence 636
Limb—Body Wall Complex 640
Neu-Laxova S. 180
Pena-Shokeir Phenotype 174
Restrictive Dermopathy 182

Occasional in

Amyoplasia Congenita Disruptive
  Sequence 608
Lethal Multiple Pterygium S. 178

21. RENAL

Kidney Malformation

Frequent in

Aniridia—Wilms Tumor Association 56
Bardet-Biedl S. 590

Renal Insufficiency

Frequent in

Occasional in

Hypertension

Occasional in

22. GENITAL

Ambiguous Genitalia/ Hypospadias/Bifid Scrotum

Frequent in

Occasional in

Micropenis, Hypogenitalism, Other Than Conditions Cited Above

Frequent in

Occasional in

Cryptorchidism

Frequent in

Occasional in

Hypoplasia of Labia Majora

Frequent in

Occasional in

Bicornuate Uterus and/or Double Vagina

Frequent in

Occasional in

Vaginal Atresia

Frequent in

Occasional in

Anal Defects or Anorectal Malformations

Frequent in

Occasional in

Various Calcifications

Frequent in

Albright Hereditary Osteodystrophy
(subcutaneous, basal ganglia) 446
Autosomal Recessive
Chondrodysplasia Punctata 390
Cerebro-Oculo-Facio-Skeletal
(COFS) S. 176
Chondrodysplasia Punctata,
X-Linked Dominant Type 388
Encephalocraniocutaneous
Lipomatosis (cranial) 516
Fetal Warfarin S. (epiphyses) 568
Fibrodysplasia Ossificans
Progressiva S. 492
Gorlin S. (falx cerebri, cerebellum) ... 528
Linear Sebaceous Nevus Sequence
(cerebral) 500
Sturge-Weber Sequence (cerebral) 495
Tuberous Sclerosis S. (subependymal)
.... 506
Von Hippel-Lindau S. 511
Werner S. 142
Zellweger S. 212

Occasional in

Acrodysostosis (epiphyseal) 444
Cerebro-Costo-Mandibular S.
(epiphyseal) 596
CHILD S. (epiphyseal) 308
Cockayne S. (cranial) 144
Dyskeratosis Congenita S. 538
Klippel-Trenaunay-Weber S.
(cranial) 512
Oculo-Auriculo-Vertebral Spectrum
(falx cerebri) 642
Oculodentodigital S. (basal ganglia)
.... 268
Smith-Lemli-Opitz S. (epiphyseal) 112
Trisomy 9 Mosaic S. (developing
cartilage) 28

Lipoatrophy (Loss or Lack of Subcutaneous Fat)

Frequent in

Berardinelli Lipodystrophy S. 600
Cockayne S. 144
Fetal Alcohol S. 555
Lenz-Majewski Hyperostosis S. 404
Leprechaunism S. 599

Progeria S. 138
Werner S. 142

Occasional in

Klippel-Trenaunay-Weber S. 512
Marfan S. 472

Hyperlipemia

Frequent in

Arteriohepatic Dysplasia
(cholesterol) 586
Berardinelli Lipodystrophy S. 600

Hyperthermia

Frequent in

Hypohidrotic Ectodermal
Dysplasia S. 543

Occasional in

Freeman-Sheldon S. (malignant) 214
Noonan S. (malignant) 122
Oromandibular-Limb Hypogenesis
Spectrum 646
Rapp-Hodgkin Ectodermal
Dysplasia S. 543
Schwartz-Jampel S. (malignant) 218

24. IMMUNE DEFICIENCY

Immunoglobulin Deficiency

Frequent in

Ataxia-Telangiectasia S. (IgA, IgE) ... 196
Dyskeratosis Congenita S. 538
Shwachman S. 387

Occasional in

Bloom S. (IgA, IgM) 104
Deletion 18p S. (IgA) 64
Deletion 18q S. (IgA) 66
Kartagener S. (IgA) 604
Mulibrey Nanism S. 100
Radial Aplasia–
Thrombocytopenia S. 322

Cell-Mediated Immune Deficiency

Frequent in

Occasional in

25. HEMATOLOGY-ONCOLOGY

Anemia

Frequent in

Occasional in

Thrombocytopenia

Frequent in

Occasional in

Other Bleeding Tendency

Occasional in

Leukocytosis

Occasional in

Lymphoreticular Malignancy

Occasional in

Other Malignancies

Frequent in

Occasional in

26. UNUSUAL GROWTH PATTERNS

Obesity

Frequent in

Occasional in

Hydrops Fetalis

Frequent in

Occasional in

Early Macrosomia, Overgrowth

Frequent in

Occasional in

Asymmetry

Frequent in

Occasional in

INDEX

Note: Page numbers in *italics* indicate figures; page numbers followed by t indicate tables.

ISBN 0-7216-6115-7

90069

9 780721 661155

FETAL DEVELOPMENT

AGE weeks	LENGTH cm C-R	LENGTH cm Tot.	WT gm	GROSS APPEARANCE	CNS	EYE, EAR	FACE, MOUTH	CARDIO-VASCULAR	LUNG
7½	2.8				Cerebral hemisphere. Infundibulum, Rathke's	Lens nearing final shape	Palatal swellings. Dental lamina, Epithel	Pulmonary vein into left atrium	
8	3.7				Primitive cereb. cortex. Olfactory lobes. Dura and pia mater	Eyelid. Ear canals	Nares plugged. Rathke's pouch detach. Sublingual gland	A-V bundle. Sinus venosus absorbed into right auricle	Pleuroperitoneal canals close. Bronchioles
10	6.0				Spinal cord histology. Cerebellum	Iris. Ciliary body. Eyelids fuse. Lacrimal glands. Spiral gland different	Lips, Nasal cartilage. Palate		Laryngeal cavity reopened
12	8.8				Cord—cervical & lumbar enlarged, Cauda equina	Retina layered. Eye axis forward. Scala tympani	Tonsillar crypts. Cheeks. Dental papilla	Accessory coats, blood vessels	Elastic fibers
16	14				Corpora quadrigemina. Cerebellum prominent. Myelination begins	Scala vestibuli. Cochlear duct	Palate complete. Enamel and dentine	Cardiac muscle condensed	Segmentation of bronchi complete
20						Inner ear ossified	Ossification of nose		Decrease in mesenchyme. Capillaries penetrate linings of tubules
24		32	800		Typical layers in cerebral cortex. Cauda equina at first sacral level		Nares reopen. Calcification of tooth primordia		Change from cuboidal to flattened epithelium. Alveoli
28		38.5	1100		Cerebral fissures and convolutions	Eyelids reopen. Retinal layers complete. Perceive light			Vascular components adequate for respiration
32		43.5	1600	Accumulation of fat		Auricular cartilage	Taste sense		Number of alveoli still incomplete
36		47.5	2600						
38		50	3200		Cauda equina, at L-3. Myelination within brain	Lacrimal duct canalized	Rudimentary frontal maxillary sinuses	Closure of foramen ovale, ductus arteriosus, umbilical vessels, ductus venosus	
First postnatal year +					Continuing organization of axonal networks. Cerebrocortical function, motor coordination. Myelination continues until 2–3 years	Iris pigmented, 5 months. Mastoid air cells. Coordinate vision, 3–5 months. Maximal vision by 5 years	Salivary gland ducts become canalized. Teeth begin to erupt 5–7 months. Relatively rapid growth of mandible and nose	Relative hypertrophy left ventricle	Continue adding new alveoli